MR Spectroscopy of Pediatric Brain Disorders

Stefan Blüml • Ashok Panigrahy
Editors

MR Spectroscopy of Pediatric Brain Disorders

Springer

Editors
Stefan Blüml
Dept. of Radiology, Children's Hospital Los Angeles
Keck School of Medicine,
University of Southern California
Los Angeles, CA, USA

Ashok Panigrahy
Dept. of Pediatric Radiology
Children's Hospital of Pittsburg of UPMC
Pittsburgh, PA, USA

ISBN 978-1-4419-5863-1 ISBN 978-1-4419-5864-8 (eBook)
DOI 10.1007/978-1-4419-5864-8
Springer New York Heidelberg Dordrecht London

Library of Congress Control Number: 2012954293

Printed on acid-free paper

Springer is part of Springer Science+Business Media (www.springer.com)

Foreword

For each generation new vistas appear that were almost inconceivable to that which went before. Nuclear magnetic resonance, a physical technique first described some 60 years ago and best known to physicians since the 1980s as MRI, is now so ubiquitous that few can be unaware of its impact across the entire field of medicine. But most conspicuously MRI has contributed to observing the brain and its dysfunctions. This is because the radiofrequency pulses and magnetic responses which create MRI are safe and effective well beyond the bony skull, which has rendered so many prior technologies either relatively useless or has at the very least confined them to the brains of adults where exposure to ionizing radiation or radioactive isotopes can usually be justified. Pediatric brain imaging with MRI, even of the fetus in utero is feasible, safe, and permissible and here also MRI has been most valuable in neurological applications. Because of this, we are not surprised that myriads of MRI textbooks have appeared describing pediatric brain disorders. Drs. Blüml and Panigrahy offer us not another textbook of pediatric MRI but what must qualify as the first textbook devoted exclusively to magnetic resonance spectroscopy of pediatric brain disorders. And a very compelling topic it is.

Magnetic resonance spectroscopy (MRS), it may surprise readers of this volume to discover, existed long before MRI. Under the term *nuclear magnetic resonance* and as practiced by chemists and biochemists, MRS is preeminently a tool for nondestructive chemical analysis and metabolic profiling. It is this property of NMR that first excited the interest of neonatologists and pediatricians searching for a better way to describe their patients than was provided by indirect assays of arterial or venous blood and lumbar puncture-derived cerebrospinal fluid. As first described in *The Lancet* nearly 3 decades ago, unlocalized phosphorus MRS opened a new chapter by demonstrating directly ATP, phosphocreatine, inorganic phosphate (and hence intracerebral pH), and some other novel phosphorylated membrane constituents of the human brain previously only known to the "invasive" neurochemist. Moreover, MRS confirmed that oxygen deprivation dramatically altered the ambient concentrations of high energy phosphates and brain pH of newborns subjected to perinatal asphyxia, thereby providing prognostic information. Subsequent pioneering studies used proton (hydrogen) MRS to quantify brain lactate concentration, a more powerful predictor of post-ischemic neurological outcome and, perhaps most valuable of all, *N*-acetyl aspartate (NAA), a then barely known amino compound, now recognized as the most reliable neuronal marker available to the neurologist. These discoveries and the rapid resolution of engineering challenges involved in constructing stable MR scanners suited to a hospital environment should have revolutionized the practice not only of pediatric neurology but adult neurology also. In fact, many thousands of children, infants, and newborns have undergone MRS examinations of the brain so that a compendious database exists. The missing element, and one addressed directly by this book, has been any serious attempt to systematize the knowledge so that practicing pediatric neurologists and others can evaluate their need or otherwise for the information provided: does MRS alter clinical management as required of any new technology in medicine if it is to leave the purely research realm and enter practice? In their authoritative new book, Blüml and Panigrahy do an outstanding job on each of these critical elements in turn. First, in selected chapters from a range of expert contributors, they define what MRS can and cannot do, naming peaks and defining the state of knowledge on their individual functions. Second, using their own deep knowledge of the technical challenges which confront all MRS examinations on patients, they systematically provide the tools that investigators working with newborns and older children will need to ensure technical excellence in the clinical environment. Third, they provide visual examples of the key pathologies which MRS has helped to define—with varying degrees of certainty, and in some situations, have not yet reached the clinical "frontier"—a masterful inspection of the theoretic basis of ADHD is one such example. Finally, and for me, the most valuable, is the unstated exploration of the role of MRS in pediatric neurological differential diagnosis and decision making. This is contained in a unique collection termed Case Reports from which the practicing pediatric neurologist or intensivist can devise his or her own diagnostic algorithms. It is to be hoped that this book will reach a wide audience, beyond the conventional practitioners of the MRS art, who tend to be physicists with only indirect impact on patient care—because, as is now abundantly clear, pediatric neurological magnetic resonance spectroscopy is ready for prime time. This book will greatly assist a new generation of practitioners.

Pasadena, CA, USA
Boston, MA, USA

B. D. Ross

Preface

Several books are available that describe principles and methodology as well as applications of Magnetic Resonance Spectroscopy (MRS). However, these are, to the best of our knowledge, focused on adults. MRS in the pediatric population is different from adults for two main reasons. Particularly in the newborn phase, the brain undergoes biochemical maturation with dramatic changes of the "normal" biochemical fingerprint. Secondly, brain diseases in the pediatric population are different from adult disorders. Stroke, dementia, and brain tumors cover most of the abnormalities observed in the adult brain. This is in contrast to pediatrics, where the normal profile changes with age, tumors originate from many different cell types, inborn errors and leukodystrophies are encountered, and generally, injury in the context of ongoing brain development adds complexity to the interpretation of a study.

The basic physics of MRS is purposely kept concise to extent possible. This acknowledges the fact that improved hardware performance and convenient "push-button" setup of MRS on most modern clinical scanners allow any interested person to obtain good quality data. Thus, the target audiences for this book are not MR physicists but clinicians and researchers focusing on pediatric brain disorders. This includes radiologists, neurologists, neurooncologists, neurosurgeons, and more broadly the neuroscience and neurobiology community. The individual chapters selected for this book provide a comprehensive state-of-the-art overview of the findings and potential of MR spectroscopy for various pediatric brain diseases. This book also contains a large number of case studies, important for clinicians who may want to see example spectra for various conditions and want to use MRS as a tool to improve management of individual patients.

Los Angeles, CA, USA

Stefan Blüml

Acknowledgments

SB: This book would not have been possible without the support of mentors, colleagues, and collaborators. B. D. Ross introduced me to MR spectroscopy and influenced profoundly my thinking and approach to this methodology. Starting with my first day at Children's Hospital Los Angeles, M. D. Nelson provided a highly stimulating environment and has supportive all endeavors. I also want to acknowledge collaborators across the different disciplines. Without the support of J. L. Finlay, F. H. Gilles, J. G. McComb, and I. Seri there would have been no MR spectroscopy program at CHLA.

Finally, I like to thank my dear wife Gloria whose gentle encouragements always came at the right time and my delightful daughters Isabel and Sabrina.

AP: I would also like to acknowledge the support of mentors, colleagues, and collaborators. Dr. Stefan Blüml introduced me to MR spectroscopy, enabled me to further development as a clinical researcher, and continues to be a life-long colleague. I would also like also thank H. C. Kinney, M. D. Nelson, F. H. Gilles, J. L. Finlay, I. F. Pollack, R. Jakacki, and M. Painter for the mentorship and support over the last few years.

I would also like to thank my partner Al for all of the advice, support, and encouragement to be the best that I can be.

We also like to recognize Adrian Liou for his help with compiling case reports and Julia Castro for her organizational and administrative skills that made this book possible.

Contents

Contributors

Jeffry R. Alger, Ph.D. Department of Radiological Sciences, UCLA, Los Angeles, CA, USA

Theodoros N. Arvanitis, Ph.D. School of Electronic, Electrical & Computer Engineering, The University of Birmingham, Birmingham, UK

Stephen Ashwal, M.D. Division of Pediatric Neurology, Department of Pediatrics, Loma Linda University School of Medicine, Loma Linda, CA, USA

Brenda Bartnik-Olson, Ph.D. Department of Radiology, Loma Linda University Medical Center, Loma Linda, CA, USA

Stefan Blüml, Ph.D. Department of Radiology, Children's Hospital of Los Angeles, Keck School of Medicine, University of Southern California, Los Angeles, CA, USA

Kim M. Cecil, Ph.D. Department of Radiology, Pediatrics, Neuroscience and Environmental Health, Cincinnati Children's Hospital Medical Center, University of Cincinnati College of Medicine, Cincinnati, OH, USA

Andre D. Furtado, M.D. Division of Pediatric Neuroradiology, Department of Radiology, Children's Hospital of Pittsburgh at UPMC, Pittsburgh, PA, USA

Simrandip K. Gill School of Cancer Sciences, University of Birmingham, Birmingham, UK

Floyd H. Gilles, M.D. Neuropathology Section, Keck School of Medicine of USC, Children's Hospital, Los Angeles, CA, USA

Barbara Holshouser, Ph.D. Department of Radiology, Section of Magnetic Resonance Imaging, Loma Linda University School of Medicine, Loma Linda, CA, USA

Alena Horská, Ph.D. The Russell H. Morgan Department of Radiology and Radiological Science, Johns Hopkins University, Baltimore, MD, USA

Richard Koch, M.D. USC Keck School of Medicine, Los Angeles, CA, USA

Jennifer G. Levitt, M.D. Department of Psychiatry, Semel Institute for Neuroscience and Human Behavior, UCLA, Los Angeles, CA, USA

Catherine Limperopoulos Ph.D. Advanced Pediatric Brain Imaging Research Center, Washington, DC, USA

George Washington University Health Center, Washington, DC, USA

Children's National Medical Center, Washington, DC, USA

Alexander P. Lin, Ph.D. Department of Radiology, Brigham and Women's Hospital, Boston, MA, USA

Diana M. Lindquist, Ph.D. Department of Radiology, Cincinnati Children's Hospital Medical Center, University of Cincinnati College of Medicine, Cincinnati, OH, USA

E. Mark Mahone, Ph.D. Department of Neuropsychology, Kennedy Krieger Institute, Baltimore, MD, USA

Elka Miller, M.D. Department of Diagnostic Imaging, Children's Hospital of Eastern Ontario, Ottawa, ON, Canada

Arabhi Nagasunder, M.S. Children's Hospital Los Angeles, Los Angeles, CA, USA

Rudi Schulte Research Institute, Santa Barbara, CA, USA

Joseph O'Neill, Ph.D. Division of Child and Adolescent Psychiatry, Semel Institute for Neuroscience and Human Behavior, UCLA, Los Angeles, CA, USA

Ashok Panigrahy, M.D. Department of Pediatric Radiology, Children's Hospital of Pittsburgh of UPMC, Pittsburgh, PA, USA

Department of Radiology, University of Pittsburgh School of Medicine, Pittsburgh, PA, USA

Andrew C. Peet, Ph.D., F.R.C.P.C.H. Institute of Child Health, University of Birmingham, Whittall Street, Birmingham, B4 6NH, UK

Niveditha Pinnamaneni, B.A, B.S. Department of Radiology, Children's Hospital of Pittsburgh, University of Pittsburgh Medical Center, Pittsburgh, PA, USA

Vera R. Sperling, M.D. Department of Pediatric Radiology, Children's Hospital of Pittsburgh of UPMC, Pittsburgh, PA, USA

Gayathri Sreedher, M.B.B.S., M.D. Department of Radiology, Children's Hospital of Pittsburgh at the University of Pittsburgh Medical Center, Pittsburgh, PA, USA

Elysa Widjaja, M.B.B.S., M.R.C.P., F.R.C.R., M.D. Department of Medical Imaging, University of Toronto, Toronto, ON, Canada

Department of Diagnostic Imaging, Hospital for Sick Children, Toronto, ON, Canada

Jessica L. Wisnowski, Ph.D. Brain and Creativity Institute and Dornsife Cognitive Neuroscience Imaging Center, University of Southern California, Los Angeles, CA, USA

Giulio Zuccoli, M.D. Department of Radiology, Children Hospital of Pittsburgh at the University of Pittsburgh Medical Center, Pittsburgh, PA, USA

Part I

Introduction

The Developing Human Brain: Differences from Adult Brain

1

Floyd H. Gilles

The purpose of this chapter is to introduce the reader to the great differences between the fetal, neonatal, childhood, adolescent, and adult brain.

Overview

Human brain development is innately beautiful and bewildering in its complexity. To assemble its integrated parts and circuits all neurons must move from their ventricular wall origin to other locations, sometimes over considerable distances, or complicated trajectories. Once appropriately deployed, the neurons usually extend one long process (if they have not done so during migration), sometimes over great lengths, and other shorter processes usually nearby the cell. All of these cellular movements are tightly choreographed genetically, from the timing of origin in ventricular wall to the ultimate destination of their processes [1]. Activation of gene sets in different combinations and sequences of at least one half of our entire human genome of 20–30,000 genes (only a third more than the roundworm *C. elegans*) is devoted to producing this most complex organ that will constitute only 2% of our body weight. The adult human brain probably contains at least one hundred billion neurons, perhaps five to ten times as many neuroglial cells, and trillions of synaptic connections. During intrauterine growth, a great excess of neurons is produced, but these are culled towards the third trimester end and the first few postnatal months. For the 9 months of intrauterine life and for a short but indeterminate postnatal period, brain growth and development is largely genetically determined. However, environmental factors begin taking a role shortly after conception and become increasingly important with advancing development.

These rapidly evolving changes throughout the developing brain lead to humans who are distinguished from other primates by cognitive capacities that have consummated in language, an *advanced* technology, and complex social behavior. The adult brain comprises only a few percent of body mass but expends one-fifth of the body's energy. The developing brain is just the opposite. The newborn brain, representing only one-fifth body mass, expends four-fifths of the baby's energy.

Particular vulnerabilities relate to distinct stages in brain development such as neurogenesis, neural migration, forebrain or hindbrain growth, gray matter or white matter maturation, dendritic sprouting, synaptogenesis, and possibly lifelong neural stem cell production and migration.

Conceptual Limitations

Neither pathologists nor neuroradiologists can see *hypoxia*, *hypoxischemia*, or *ischemia*. These diagnoses are merely interpretations needing confirmation, that is, autopsy verification of imaging findings. Nevertheless, decreasing autopsy rates coupled with a serious decline in neuroanatomy training for neuropathologists and neuroradiologists result in a cascade of confusion in recognizing anatomic location of brain lesions and specific brain functions. The result often is serious misunderstanding of pathologic processes. For instance, a commonly used term *periventricular*, as an anatomic location, is of little value since all brain and spinal cord is periventricular, and the term includes gray as well as white matter. Additionally, not all necrosis is infarct, even though all infarction is necrosis. Furthermore, designations such as *stroke*, *brain attack*, *frontoparietal*, or *prefrontal* have no anatomic or pathologic specificity and their use as outcomes is of little value in epidemiologic, statistical, or functional imaging studies. In neuroimaging, terms are often conflated to mean something else, such as *periventricular*

F.H. Gilles, M.D. (✉)
Neuropathology Section, Keck School of Medicine of USC, Children's Hospital, Los Angeles, CA, USA
e-mail: fgilles@usc.edu

S. Blüml and A. Panigrahy (eds.), *MR Spectroscopy of Pediatric Brain Disorders*,
DOI 10.1007/978-1-4419-5864-8_1,

leucomalacia (multiple focal white matter necroses, as originally defined [2–4]) to mean diffuse white matter astrocytosis, or diffuse neuroimaging changes.

Labels used as antecedents or *causes* need to be specific. For instance, some 34 different pathologic abnormalities, ranging from hemorrhage to necrosis, have been attributed to anoxia, hypoxia, hypoxischemia, and asphyxia without adequate clinical or pathologic definitions of any of these conditions. This suggests the possibility of having overlooked other risk factors which might have been potentially modifiable by the obstetrician or neonatologist [5].

Growth

Growth is generally a continuous process; however, one cannot sample a single growing fetus repeatedly except for some forms of neuroimaging. For pathologists, this limits us to providing best estimates of growth at different times in development from images or autopsied fetuses. The traditional strategy of measuring growth uses the independent variable of estimated gestational age. Unfortunately, the argument of defining *normal* brain weight as a ratio relative to some other body parameter (allometric relationship) continues. If brain weight is defined as a ratio to body weight alone, adverse influences affecting both the brain and body are likely to be missed because both might be influenced similarly.

Brain growth is a dynamic active process varying not only in time and space but also from one neural subdivision to another. Growth consists of a proportional daily (or weekly) gain in mass (weight) and is a very complex process for each organ [6]. During development, an individual's body size, shape, and proportions change due to differential growth of body parts. Growth cannot be discussed without considering its relation to rate. Since most human embryonic and fetal growth processes cannot be measured continuously, mathematical growth models are used. The advantage of such models is that growth curve characteristics such as maximum rate and points of inflection can be estimated. Growth rate is the percentage increase in weight and spatial dimensions per unit of time, which varies over time, particularly for specific brain parts. Inflection points reflect major changes in growth acceleration or deceleration. The models also estimate unobserved values, smooth measurement values, and minimize stochastic errors.

Both neuropores close at the end of the first postovulatory month, and most cranial nerve ganglia are present at this time [7]. The future cerebral hemispheres begin to bulge from the diencephalic ventricle at approximately 32 days. In prosencephalon, the hypothalamic, amygdaloid, hippocampal, and olfactory anlage are discernible. Both ganglionic eminences (medial and lateral) arise at approximately 33 days, and epithalamus, dorsal thalamus, ventral thalamus, and subthalamus are apparent. Spinal axodendritic synapses arise first in cervical region [8, 9]. The neurohypophysis evaginates at approximately 37 days, and 4 days later olfactory bulb and first amygdaloid nuclei become evident and a deep longitudinal interhemispheric fissure is conspicuous. The future corpus striatum, inferior cerebellar peduncle, and dentate nucleus are evident at approximately 44 days. Slightly later, the fourth ventricular choroid plexuses appear followed by lateral ventricular plexuses 3 days later (about 51 days). The cortical plate is visible in cerebral hemispheres at approximately 52 days and 2 days later axons in the internal capsule and olfactory tract appear. The embryonic period ends at approximately 57 days, with the cortical plate extending over most of cerebral surface.

When does the developing brain require particular large amounts of metabolites necessary to support rapid tissue growth? The weight of all brain components during the growing period must be considered, including the entire vascular bed and the intravascular blood necessary to support the brain's remarkable growth and activity [10]. The brain, and its various subdivisions, new cells, axons, dendrites, neural supporting cells, and vasculature all individually contribute to weight gain with each component added during separate developmental times. At term the brain is growing at its greatest rate; during the second year it will triple its birth weight. Myelin deposition in large amounts in the last gestational weeks and over the first few months of life probably accounts for a large proportion of weight gain. This transient and special variety of tissue (myelinating white matter) is potentially vulnerable to a unique array of insults, and estimation of its degree of maturation is of great importance to the neuroradiologist and neuropathologist.

Growth Functions

The Gompertz function is superior to the logistic, and also to several nonsigmoid functions, such as the generalized exponential and the polynomial, even though the latter has been considered important [11]. The first and second Gompertz function derivatives provide prenatal brain instantaneous and maximum growth rate and acceleration. The prenatal brain growth model is

$$Y = 1{,}190e^{-e^{(1.99-0.0437X)}}$$

where Y is brain weight in grams and X is gestational age in weeks (Fig. 1.1a). Maximum growth acceleration occurs at 24.5 weeks and maximum growth rate occurs at or just after term. This model confirmed the Dobbing and Sands original smaller study [12] and was corroborated in a second larger fetal brain population [11]. The inflection point and rates of maximal growth are similar to the original Gompertz model (above), namely second trimester's end and end of term gestation.

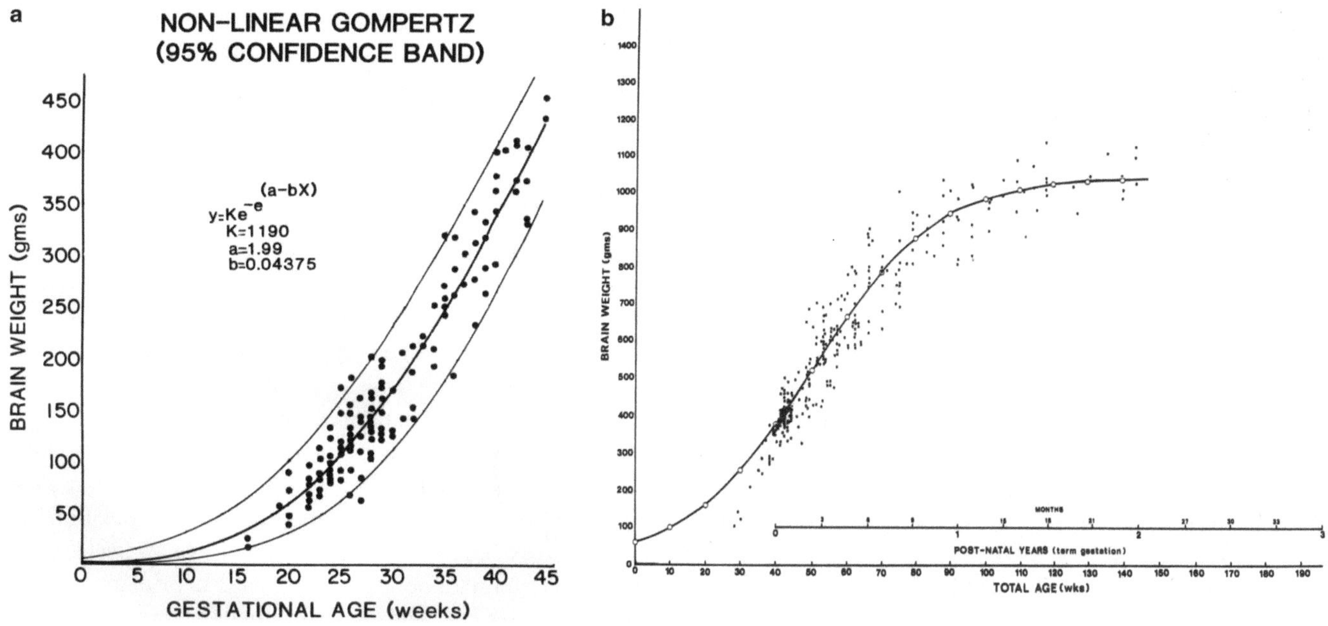

Fig. 1.1 (**a**) Nonlinear Gompertz (**b**) Sigmoid growth curve

In a separate newborn and childhood group, a sigmoid growth curve was generated from birth to 2 postnatal years (Fig. 1.1b) (McLennan and Gilles, 1983, unpublished data). Postnatal brain growth in our model is similar to Dobbing and Sands, although they had only a small number of cases beyond 12 months [12]. Again, there is a wide range in brain weight at each specific week. The significant implication is that most postnatal brain growth is completed within the first 2 postnatal years, similar to other reports [13, 14].

New Tissue Addition

If one assumes a large figure for the ultimate human neuronal number (for instance, estimated at 10^{11}—L. Swanson, personal communication, 2009), then during the first half of gestation, neuronal precursor cells develop in ventricular zone, move to some new location, mature in very large numbers (for example, many hundreds of thousands every second), and make innumerable connections.

Gyri, Cortical Thickness, Neuronal Maxima, and Synapses

Cortical layer thickness increases linearly with age and cortical neuronal density reaches a maximum at 20–28 weeks and then declines by about 70% [15], with additional decreases during adolescence [16]. The human infant's cerebral cortex at term has a gyral pattern similar to the adult cortex, but has only one third the total surface area. The gyral pattern is probably unique for each hemisphere and for each individual. Postnatal cortical expansion varies considerably from lobe to lobe and within lobes: regions of lateral temporal, parietal, and frontal cortex expand nearly twice as much as locations in insular and medial occipital cortex [17]. Within cerebral cortex, homotypical association cortices mature only after heterotypical agranular somatic motor and granular sensory and visual cortices are developed, and phylogenetically older brain areas mature earlier than newer ones [18]. Thus, primary sensory and motor areas generally attain peak cortical thickness before adjacent secondary areas, and before other polymodal association areas. Specifically, in brain behind the central sulcus, the first region to reach peak thickness is granular somatic sensory cortex (8 years), followed by calcarine cortex, containing striate granular primary visual area (7 years on the left and 8 years on the right), and then the remaining homotypical parieto-occipital cortex, with polymodal regions (such as the posterior parietal cortex) reaching peak thickness later (9–10 years). In the frontal cortex, the primary agranular motor cortex attains peak cortical thickness early (9 years), followed by the supplementary motor areas (10 years) and most of the frontal pole (10 years). High-order cortical areas, such as the dorsolateral homotypical frontal cortex and cingulate cortex, reach peak thickness later (10.5 years). The anterior insular transition cortex reaches its maximum thickness at 18 years. In the medial views, the occipital and frontal poles attain peak thickness early, and then a wave sweeps from these areas, with the medial frontal and cingulate cortex attaining peak thickness last. There is also a marked dorsal to ventral progression of development [19].

Studies in nonhuman animals suggest that cortical dimensions during critical periods for the development of cognitive functions reflect experience-dependent molding of the architecture of cortical columns along with dendritic spine and axonal remodeling [20–24]. Such morphological events likely contribute to the childhood phase of increase in cortical thickness, which occurs in regions with either a cubic or quadratic trajectory. The phase of cortical thinning, dominating adolescence, likely reflects the use-dependent selective elimination of synapses that could refine neural circuits, including those supporting cognitive abilities [19, 25–27].

Functionally, the posterior medial orbitofrontal areas have been linked with the limbic system and autonomic nervous system control. These areas are thought to monitor the outcomes associated with behavior, particularly punishment or reward [28, 29], cognitive functions so fundamental that they are unlikely to undergo prolonged development. In contrast, isocortical regions often support more complex psychological functions, which show clear developmental gradients, characterized by rapid development during critical periods. The delineation of critical periods for human skill development is complex, but late childhood is a period of particularly rapid development of executive skills of planning, working memory, and cognitive flexibility, an age period which coincides with an increase in cortical thickness in the lateral frontal cortex [30]. In contrast, the critical period for certain visual functions (such as letter acuity and global motion detection) has been estimated as ending in middle childhood (age 6 or 7) [31]. Likewise, the period of increase in cortical thickness in the visual cortex also ends around this time (approximately ages 7–8).

The fate of all cerebral cortical cells is tied to the cortical vasculature, which supplies oxygen and nutrients, maintains homeostasis, and removes metabolic waste. Considering the increasing surface area of neuronal soma, dendrites, and axons that accompany brain enlargement, it has been estimated that each human neocortical neuron consumes 3.3 times more ATP to fire a single spike than in rats, and 2.6 times more energy to maintain resting potentials [32].

Synaptic Maxima

There is regional dendritic variation in neonatal human isocortex [33]. Synaptogenesis occurs concurrently with dendritic and axonal growth and with subcortical white matter myelination. Postnatal synaptic density rises after birth, reaches a plateau in childhood and then decreases to adult levels by late adolescence. In macaque monkeys, subsets of terminal synapses, as well as a subset of en passant synapses, appear and disappear each week with no net change in overall density, suggesting ongoing processes of synaptogenesis and elimination [34]. Huttenlocher's examination of visual cortex synapse number and density in brain tissue of deceased infants, children, and adults shows an exuberant growth of number and density of synapses between birth and about 8 months of age from a neonatal level at about 30–40% of the adult level to about 80% above the adult level at 6–8 months followed by a gradual decline to the norm, an approximate plateau from adolescent to adult age [25]. Synapse formation in granular auditory cortex and homotypical middle frontal gyrus begins before conceptual age 27 weeks, and reaches a maximum before 1 year of age in primary auditory and visual cortices, and at approximately three and a half years of age in the middle frontal gyrus. Interestingly, whereas in the human auditory cortex synaptic elimination is complete by 12 years of age, pruning continues until mid-adolescence in the middle frontal gyrus. The frontal cortex develops somewhat more slowly and declines somewhat later. Further, in human brains there is a separation in time of a few years between peaks in visual cortex synapse density and metabolic rate [35].

Myelination

Fetal and postnatal myelination is dramatic [36–38]. In autopsy material, tracts in which 50% of cases contained grossly visible myelin at second trimester end included: medial longitudinal fasciculus, fasciculus gracilis, fasciculus cuneatus, trapezoid body, and inferior cerebellar peduncle. In term infants, 50% of cases contained grossly visible myelin in the following tracts: proprius, spinocerebellar, spinothalamic, medial lemniscus, spinal trigeminal, lateral lemniscus, parathalamic posterior limb, parasagittal cerebellum, superior cerebellar peduncle, capsule of red nucleus, optic chiasm, optic tract, ansa lenticularis, inferior olivary nucleus amiculum, and habenulointerpeduncular tract. The additional tracts at 1 year in which 50% of cases were grossly myelinated included: hilus inferior olivary nucleus, auditory radiation, transverse gyrus of Heschl, transpontine, middle cerebellar peduncle, cerebellar hemisphere, dentate hilus, pontine corticospinal, occipital optic radiation, cingulum, corona radiata, distal radiation to precentral gyrus, posterior frontal, occipital pole, calcarine subcortical association fibers, and body, splenium, and rostrum of corpus callosum. Similarly, additional myelinated tracts at 2 years included: inferior colliculus brachium, lateral crus pedunculi; midbrain, cervical, and thoracic corticospinal; lateral olfactory stria; deep white matter in posterior parietal, temporal, and temporal and frontal pole deep white matter; external capsule; subcortical association fibers in frontal, temporal, and occipital poles, parietal, and posterior frontal; and stria medullaris thalami. Late or slowly myelinating tracts (> 2 years) included: central tegmental, solitary, medial crus pedunculi, lumbar corticospinal, putamen, globus pallidus, alveus, fimbria, fornix, extreme capsule, temporal subcortical association fibers, and anterior commissure [39].

Prematurity and Its Long-term Complications

More than half a million babies are born prematurely each year in the United States and the rate of premature birth has been increasing since 1980. Premature babies face an increased risk of lasting disabilities, such as mental retardation, learning and behavioral problems, neurologic deficit, lung problems, and vision and auditory problems. These long-term problems occur in greater proportions of premature births as the gestational age decreases. For instance, babies born at the end of the second trimester have brain weights half of those born at term and are more likely to have developmental delays [40], but even adults who were born at 34–36 weeks gestation are more likely than those born full-term to have mild disabilities and to earn lower long-term wages.

These neurologic and cognitive delays are accompanied by delays in myelination and development of *N*-acetylaspartate [41] that are accompanied by delays in motor skills at 6 years [42]. Structural abnormalities including cerebellar size, persist throughout childhood [43, 44], and small brain volume and corpus callosum persist into adulthood [45, 46].

Neonatal Brain Edema Likely Differs from That in Adults

Clinically important cerebral swelling, without concomitant necrosis or hematoma, is thought to contribute to necrosis. The few pathologic studies of fetal, term, or neonatal brain edema are in conflict, and whether edema occurs without necrosis remains in dispute. This confusion resulted from supposed analogies to adult swelling, poorly defined criteria, and high fetal brain water content relative to myelinated adult brain. Furthermore, the fetal and neonatal brain adds weight during fixation, often attaining a postfixation weight 30% greater than fresh weight [47]. What some call edema in fixed fetal or neonatal brain (cerebral hemisphere enlargement, sulcal and ventricular narrowing) likely reflects initial high brain water content plus fluid accumulated during fixation. Since immature brain differs from mature brain so markedly in its structure and composition as well as in its responses to insult, one cannot directly extrapolate information from the adult to neonatal brain.

Many neonatal brain edema experimental studies used lethal asphyxia or anoxia (for example, [48–50]). Whether or not this adequately measures uncomplicated water accumulation in cerebral tissue is a moot point; it certainly measures tissue swelling associated with functional endothelial and other cellular loss. Following asphyxia in an airtight jar until death, 5-day-old rat pup brain exhibits only a minimal increase in water content, but no brain weight change. Similar results were obtained with nitrogen anoxia and asphyxia with CO_2. As expected with cellular death, shifts in sodium and potassium occur concomitantly with water shift. Whether the fluid and electrolyte changes concomitant with complete cellular function loss are tantamount to uncomplicated edema, as the term is used for the mature brain, is not clear. Other experiments support the conclusion that “neonatal brain does not have a tendency to edema” [51–53].

A prospective study of all neonatal autopsies in a maternity hospital, defining brain swelling as cerebral hemisphere enlargement, gyral flattening, and sulcal narrowing observed that, without intraventricular hemorrhage, swelling was not found under 33 weeks [54, 55]. Yet, at about term, 89% of brains were “pathologically swollen.” They did not attribute the swollen brain proportion to prolonged postmortem interval, but found that flattened gyri were more likely in stillbirths than early neonatal deaths. The most swollen brains contained the least water.

Diseases Differ Between the Child and Adult

Metabolic and Mitochondrial Inborn Errors

Many metabolic diseases affecting the infant or child have milder presentations in later life. Metabolic errors are generally grouped according to defects in their biochemical pathways. Those caused by energy failure can involve citric acid cycle or respiratory chain, such as mitochondrial disorders, or defects in glycogen mobilization, such as glycogen storage disease, or fats, such as fatty acid oxidation defects. Defects in amino acid metabolism include the urea cycle defects, such as citrullinemia, organic acidemias, such as methylmalonic acidemia, or aminoacidopathies, such as phenylketonuria. Finally, there are disorders of carbohydrate metabolism such as galactosemia. The lysosomal storage disorders, characterized by large carbohydrate–lipid complex accumulation, such as Hurler’s disease, constitute the next general group. Peroxisomal biogenesis disorders include Zellweger’s syndrome and adrenoleukodystrophy. Finally, there is a group of white matter disorders such as metachromatic leukodystrophy.

Brain Tumors

Brain tumors in children differ in location and kind from those in adults. Starr pointed out their predominance below the tentorium in the nineteenth century [56]. Schultz and Cushing recognized that the types of neoplasms also differed from those in adults [57, 58]. The clinical courses, symptoms, and signs in children with brain tumors were sufficiently distinct to prompt Bailey, Buchanan, and Bucy to introduce their classic monograph with the statement that "experience … early taught us that in the case of intracranial neoplasms also, one should not reason in the same manner when confronted with a child suffering from such a lesion as when dealing with an adult" [59]. The distributions of brain tumor locations also differ by age within childhood [60].

Kernicterus and Liver Disease

Bilirubin encephalopathy is a newborn syndrome, in which increased plasma levels of unconjugated bilirubin outstrip albumin-binding capacity and gain access to the brain. Jaques Hervieux described brain jaundice in 31 of his 44 autopsied jaundiced babies in 1847. Orth, an assistant to Virchow, in 1875 found intense yellow staining in basal ganglia, third ventricular wall, hippocampus, and deep cerebellar nuclei in a jaundiced term infant. In 1903, Schmorl reported 120 autopsies of jaundiced infants [3]. Schmorl coined the term kernicterus (basal ganglia jaundice) for this staining pattern. Although the following century of scientific study has added an enormous amount of information about the epidemiology and pathophysiology of neonatal jaundice and kernicterus, the contributions of Hervieux, Orth, and Schmorl will likely continue to be seen as historic landmarks in our quest for understanding of these phenomena [61, 62]. Commonly involved are the cerebellar roof nuclei, cranial nerve nuclei, inferior olives, dorsal funicular nuclei, globus pallidus, thalamus, and subthalamus. Hippocampus, putamen, and lateral geniculate are less often involved. Yellow staining of central nervous system nuclei also occurs in some neonatal brains, despite low levels of serum bilirubin [63].

The relative importance of blood–brain barrier, unconjugated bilirubin levels, serum binding, and tissue susceptibility in this process is only partially understood. Even at dangerously high serum levels, bilirubin traverses the intact blood–brain barrier slowly, requiring time for encephalopathy to occur [64]. Unconjugated bilirubin, the end product of heme catabolism in mammals, causes neonatal jaundice when it accumulates in their plasma. Under low unbound conditions it is a potent antioxidant, but when slightly elevated is toxic to astrocytes and neurons, damaging mitochondria (causing impaired energy metabolism and apoptosis) and plasma membranes (causing oxidative damage and disrupting neurotransmitter transport). With higher concentrations, unbound bilirubin accumulates in neurons and glial cells in several specific brain regions resulting in kernicterus. Unconjugated bilirubin accumulation in cerebrospinal fluid and central nervous system is limited by its active export, probably mediated by multidrug resistance-associated protein present in choroid plexus epithelia, capillary endothelia, astrocytes, and neurons [65–67]. The mechanism(s) by which severe hyperbilirubinemia engenders cytotoxic effects in selected brain regions is poorly understood but has been attributed previously to differences in permeability of blood–brain barrier and blood–cerebrospinal fluid barrier, regional blood flow, and bilirubin oxidation rates.

Brain Trauma

Falls or head blows in the adult result in brain contusions – wedge-shaped brain necroses, usually hemorrhagic, with the base of the wedge located at a gyral apex or the apices of several gyri. For the first half or two-thirds of the first postnatal year, falls or head blows result in unmyelinated white matter tears rather than cortically based contusions [68, 69].

Therapeutic Effects Differ in Children

One of the major limiting factors in treatment of childhood brain tumors is the sensitivity of the young brain to the effects of conventional radiation [70, 71]. The complications include defects in cognition, endocrine, and neurologic sequelae. Another major concern is the induction of secondary tumors in long-term survivors [72], Moyamoya disease [73], and arterial disease leading to infarction. Even very low brain irradiation doses in childhood can diminish later adult intellectual function [74].

Chemotherapy is not spared. Methotrexate is associated with a leucoencephalopathy [75–77], as is L-asparaginase [78, 79], ifosfamide [80, 81], and amphotericin B [82].

Conclusions

The great dissimilarities between infant and adult brains include the remarkable facts of fetal and childhood brain development, the long-term structural and functional abnormalities associated with premature birth, and the differences in gyral development, cortical thickness, neuronal maxima and loss, synaptic maxima and loss, functional cortical regional growth, metabolic and mitochondrial diseases, tumors, kernicterus, and differing therapeutic responses of childhood and adult brains.

References

1. Bui K, Wappler I, Peters H, Lindsay S, Clowry G, Bayatti N. Investigating gradients of gene expression in early human cortical development. J Anat. 2010;217(4):300–11.
2. Virchow R. Zur pathologischen anatomie des gehirns: I. Congenitale encephalitis und myelitis. Virch Arch. 1867;38:129–38.
3. Schmorl CG. Zur kenntniss des ikterus neonatorum, inbesondere der dabei auftretenden gehirnveranderungen. Verhandl deutsch Path Gesellsch. 1904;6:109–15.
4. Banker BQ, Larroche JC. Periventricular leukomalacia of infancy. A form of neonatal anoxic encephalopathy. Arch Neurol. 1962;7:386–410.
5. Gilles FH. Lesions attributed to perinatal asphyxia in the human. In: Gluck L, editor. Intrauterine asphyxia and the developing fetal brain. Chicago: Year Book Medical Publishers, Inc; 1977. p. 99–107.
6. Donaldson HH. The growth of the Brain. London and New York: Walter Scott LTD and Charles Scribner's Sons; 1986.
7. O'Rahilly R, Müller F. The embryonic human brain: an atlas of developmental stages. New York: Wiley-Liss; 1994.
8. Humphrey T. The spinal tract of the trigeminal nerve in human embryos between 7.5 and 8.5 weeks of menstrual age and its relation to fetal behavior. J Comp Neurol. 1952;97:143–209.
9. Humphrey T. Pattern formed at upper cervical spinal cord levels by sensory fibers of spinal and cranial nerves. Arch Neurol Psychiatr. 1955;73:36–46.
10. Kehrer M, Krageloh-Mann I, Goelz R, Schoning M. The development of cerebral perfusion in healthy preterm and term neonates. Neuropediatrics. 2003;34(6):281–6.
11. McLennan JE, Gilles FH, Neff R. A model of growth of the human fetal brain. In: Gilles FH, Leviton A, Dooling EC, editors. The developing human brain: growth and epidemiologic neuropathology. Boston: Wright PSG; 1983. p. 43–58.
12. Dobbing J, Sands J. Quantitative growth and development of human brain. Arch Dis Child. 1973;48(10):757–67.
13. Voigt J, Pakkenberg H. Brain weight of Danish children. A forensic material. Acta Anat (Basel). 1983;116(4):290–301.
14. Coppoletta JM, Wolbach SB. Body length and organ weights of infants and children: Study of body lengths and normal weights of more important vital organs of body between birth and 12 years of age. Am J Pathol. 1933;9:55–70.
15. Rabinowicz T, de Courten-Myers GM, Petetot JM, Xi G, de los Reyes E. Human cortex development: estimates of neuronal numbers indicate major loss late during gestation. J Neuropathol Exp Neurol. 1996;55(3):320–8.
16. Rabinowicz T, Petetot JM, Khoury JC, de Courten-Myers GM. Neocortical maturation during adolescence: change in neuronal soma dimension. Brain Cogn. 2009;69(2):328–36.
17. Hill J, Inder T, Neil J, Dierker D, Harwell J, Van Essen D. Similar patterns of cortical expansion during human development and evolution. Proc Natl Acad Sci USA. 2010;107(29):13135–40.
18. Gogtay N, Giedd JN, Lusk L, Hayashi KM, Greenstein D, Vaituzis AC, et al. Dynamic mapping of human cortical development during childhood through early adulthood. Proc Natl Acad Sci USA. 2004;101(21):8174–9.
19. Shaw P, Kabani NJ, Lerch JP, Eckstrand K, Lenroot R, Gogtay N, et al. Neurodevelopmental trajectories of the human cerebral cortex. J Neurosci. 2008;28(14):3586–94.
20. Chklovskii DB. Synaptic connectivity and neuronal morphology: two sides of the same coin. Neuron. 2004;43(5):609–17.
21. Chklovskii DB, Mel BW, Svoboda K. Cortical rewiring and information storage. Nature. 2004;431(7010):782–8.
22. Mataga N, Mizuguchi Y, Hensch TK. Experience-dependent pruning of dendritic spines in visual cortex by tissue plasminogen activator. Neuron. 2004;44(6):1031–41.
23. Hensch TK, Fagiolini M. Excitatory-inhibitory balance and critical period plasticity in developing visual cortex. Prog Brain Res. 2005;147:115–24.
24. Sur M, Rubenstein JL. Patterning and plasticity of the cerebral cortex. Science. 2005;310(5749):805–10.
25. Huttenlocher PR, Dabholkar AS. Regional differences in synaptogenesis in human cerebral cortex. J Comp Neurol. 1997;387(2): 167–78.
26. Fagiolini M, Fritschy JM, Low K, Mohler H, Rudolph U, Hensch TK. Specific GABAA circuits for visual cortical plasticity. Science. 2004;303(5664):1681–3.
27. Hensch TK, Stryker MP. Columnar architecture sculpted by GABA circuits in developing cat visual cortex. Science. 2004;303(5664): 1678–81.
28. Rolls ET. The functions of the orbitofrontal cortex. Brain Cogn. 2004;55(1):11–29.
29. Kennerley SW, Walton ME, Behrens TE, Buckley MJ, Rushworth MF. Optimal decision making and the anterior cingulate cortex. Nat Neurosci. 2006;9(7):940–7.
30. Burton H, Snyder AZ, Diamond JB, Raichle ME. Adaptive changes in early and late blind: a FMRI study of verb generation to heard nouns. J Neurophysiol. 2002;88(6):3359–71.
31. MacKay TL, Jakobson LS, Ellemberg D, Lewis TL, Maurer D, Casiro O. Deficits in the processing of local and global motion in very low birthweight children. Neuropsychologia. 2005;43(12):1738–48.
32. Sherwood CC, Stimpson CD, Raghanti MA, Wildman DE, Uddin M, Grossman LI, et al. Evolution of increased glia-neuron ratios in the human frontal cortex. Proc Natl Acad Sci USA. 2006;103(37): 13606–11.
33. Travis K, Ford K, Jacobs B. Regional dendritic variation in neonatal human cortex: a quantitative Golgi study. Dev Neurosci. 2005; 27(5):277–87.
34. Stettler DD, Yamahachi H, Li W, Denk W, Gilbert CD. Axons and synaptic boutons are highly dynamic in adult visual cortex. Neuron. 2006;49(6):877–87.
35. Chugani HT. A critical period of brain development: studies of cerebral glucose utilization with PET. Prev Med. 1998;27(2): 184–8.
36. Flechsig P. Anatomie des menschlichen Gehirns und Ruchenmarks. Leipzig: Georg Thieme; 1920.
37. Brody BA, Kinney HC, Kloman AS, Gilles FH. Sequence of central nervous system myelination in human infancy, I: an autopsy study of myelination. J Neuropathol Exp Neurol. 1987;46:283–301.
38. Kinney HC, Brody BA, Kloman AS, Gilles FH. Sequence of central nervous system myelination in human infancy, II: patterns of myelination of autopsied infants. J Neuropathol Exp Neurol. 1988;47: 217–34.
39. Gilles FH, Shankle W, Dooling EC. Myelinated Tracts: Growth Patterns. In: Gilles FH, Leviton A, Dooling EC, editors. The developing human brain: growth and epidemiologic neuropathology. Boston: Wright PSG; 1983. p. 117–83.
40. Petrini JR, Dias T, McCormick MC, Massolo ML, Green NS, Escobar GJ. Increased risk of adverse neurological development for late preterm infants. J Pediatr. 2009;154(2):169–76.
41. Huppi PS, Schuknecht B, Boesch C, Bossi E, Felblinger J, Fusch C, et al. Structural and neurobehavioral delay in postnatal brain development of preterm infants. Pediatr Res. 1996;39(5):895–901.
42. Marlow N, Roberts BL, Cooke RW. Motor skills in extremely low birthweight children at the age of 6 years. Arch Dis Child. 1989; 64(6):839–47.
43. Skranes JS, Nilsen G, Smevik O, Vik T, Brubakk AM. Cerebral MRI of very low birth weight children at 6 years of age compared with the findings at 1 year. Pediatr Radiol. 1998;28(6):471–5.
44. Allin M, Matsumoto H, Santhouse AM, Nosarti C, AlAsady MH, Stewart AL, et al. Cognitive and motor function and the size of the cerebellum in adolescents born very pre-term. Brain. 2001;124 (Pt 1):60–6.

45. Fearon P, O'Connell P, Frangou S, Aquino P, Nosarti C, Allin M, et al. Brain volumes in adult survivors of very low birth weight: a sibling-controlled study. Pediatrics. 2004;114(2):367–71.
46. Nosarti C, Rushe TM, Woodruff PW, Stewart AL, Rifkin L, Murray RM. Corpus callosum size and very preterm birth: relationship to neuropsychological outcome. Brain. 2004;127(Pt 9):2080–9.
47. Gilles FH, Leviton A, Dooling EC. Developing human brain: growth and epidemiologic neuropathology. Boston: John Wright-PSG Publishing Co; 1983.
48. Myers RE, Beard R, Adamsons K. Brain swelling in the newborn rhesus monkey following prolonged partial asphyxia. Neurology. 1969;19(10):1012–8.
49. De Souza SW, Dobbing J. Cerebral oedema in developing brain. 3. Brain water and electrolytes in immature asphyxiated rats treated with dexamethasone. Biol Neonate. 1973;22(5):388–97.
50. De Souza SW, Dobbing J. Cerebral edema in developing brain. II. Asphyxia in the five-day-old rat. Exp Neurol. 1973;39(3):414–23.
51. Spector RG. Water content of the immature rat brain following cerebral anoxia and ischemia. Br J Exp Pathol. 1962;43:472–9.
52. Streicher E, Wisniewski H, Klatzo I. Resistance of immature brain to experimental cerebral edema. Neurology. 1965;15:833.
53. Tweed WA, Pash M, Doig G. Cerebrovascular mechanisms in perinatal asphyxia: the role of vasogenic brain edema. Pediatr Res. 1981;15(1):44–6.
54. Pryse-Davies J, Beard RW. A necropsy study of brain swelling in the newborn with special reference to cerebellar herniation. J Pathol. 1973;109(1):51–73.
55. Pryse-Davies J. Brain swelling in the newborn: artifact, development, or pathology. Arch Dis Child. 1973;48(2):161–2.
56. Starr M. Tumors of the brain in childhood. Med News. 1889;54: 29–37.
57. Schultz O, editor. Tumors of infancy and childhood. Philadelphia: Saunders; 1926.
58. Cushing H. The intracranial tumors of preadolescence. Am J Dis Child. 1927;33:551–84.
59. Bailey P, Buchanan DN, Bucy PC. Intracranial tumors of infancy and childhood. Chicago: The University of Chicago Press; 1939.
60. Childhood Brain Tumor Consortium. A study of childhood brain tumors based on surgical biopsies from ten North American institutions: Sample description. J Neuro-Oncol. 1988;6:9–23.
61. Haymaker W, Margoles C, Pentschew A, et al. Pathology of kernicterus and posticterus encephalopathy. A conference, eleventh annual meeting. New Orleans, Louisiana: Charles C. Thomas; 1961. p. 21–228.
62. Hansen TW. Pioneers in the scientific study of neonatal jaundice and kernicterus. Pediatrics. 2000;106(2):E15.
63. Ahdab-Barmada M, Moossy J. The neuropathology of kernicterus in the premature neonate: diagnostic problems. J Neuropathol Exp Neurol. 1984;43(1):45–56.
64. Wennberg RP. The blood–brain barrier and bilirubin encephalopathy. Cell Mol Neurobiol. 2000;20(1):97–109.
65. Jedlitschky G, Leier I, Buchholz U, Hummel-Eisenbeiss J, Burchell B, Keppler D. ATP-dependent transport of bilirubin glucuronides by the multidrug resistance protein MRP1 and its hepatocyte canalicular isoform MRP2. Biochem J. 1997;327(Pt 1):305–10.
66. Ostrow JD, Pascolo L, Brites D, Tiribelli C. Molecular basis of bilirubin-induced neurotoxicity. Trends Mol Med. 2004;10(2): 65–70.
67. Gennuso F, Fernetti C, Tirolo C, Testa N, L'Episcopo F, Caniglia S, et al. Bilirubin protects astrocytes from its own toxicity by inducing up-regulation and translocation of multidrug resistance-associated protein 1 (Mrp1). Proc Natl Acad Sci USA. 2004;101(8):2470–5.
68. Lindenberg R, Freitag E. Morphology of brain lesions from blunt trauma in early infancy. Arch Pathol. 1969;87:298.
69. Ordia IJ, Strand R, Gilles F, Welch K. Computerized tomography of contusional clefts in the white matter in infants. Report of two cases. J Neurosurg. 1981;54(5):696–8.
70. Mostow EN, Byrne J, Connelly RR, Mulvihill JJ. Quality of life in long-term survivors of CNS tumors of childhood and adolescence. J Clin Oncol. 1991;9(4):592–9.
71. Jannoun L, Bloom HJ. Long-term psychological effects in children treated for intracranial tumors. Int J Radiat Oncol Biol Phys. 1990;18(4):747–53.
72. Rimm IJ, Li FC, Tarbell NJ, Winston KR, Sallan SE. Brain tumors after cranial irradiation for childhood acute lymphoblastic leukemia. A 13-year experience from the Dana-Farber Cancer Institute and the Children's Hospital. Cancer. 1987;59(8):1506–8.
73. Ullrich NJ, Robertson R, Kinnamon DD, Scott RM, Kieran MW, Turner CD, et al. Moyamoya following cranial irradiation for primary brain tumors in children. Neurology. 2007;68(12):932–8.
74. Hall P, Adami HO, Trichopoulos D, Pedersen NL, Lagiou P, Ekbom A, et al. Effect of low doses of ionising radiation in infancy on cognitive function in adulthood: Swedish population based cohort study. BMJ. 2004;328(7430):19.
75. Bresnan M, Gilles FH, Lorenzo A, Watters G, Barlow C. Leukoencephalopathy following combined irradiation and intraventricular methotrexate therapy of brain tumors in childhood. Trans Am Neurol Assoc. 1974;97:204–5.
76. Inaba H, Khan RB, Laningham FH, Crews KR, Pui CH, Daw NC. Clinical and radiological characteristics of methotrexate-induced acute encephalopathy in pediatric patients with cancer. Ann Oncol. 2008;19(1):178–84.
77. Dicuonzo F, Salvati A, Palma M, Lefons V, Lasalandra G, De Leonardis F, et al. Posterior reversible encephalopathy syndrome associated with methotrexate neurotoxicity: conventional magnetic resonance and diffusion-weighted imaging findings. J Child Neurol. 2009;24(8):1013–8.
78. Hourani R, Abboud M, Hourani M, Khalifeh H, Muwakkit S. L-asparaginase-induced posterior reversible encephalopathy syndrome during acute lymphoblastic leukemia treatment in children. Neuropediatrics. 2008;39(1):46–50.
79. Kieslich M, Porto L, Lanfermann H, Jacobi G, Schwabe D, Bohles H. Cerebrovascular complications of L-asparaginase in the therapy of acute lymphoblastic leukemia. J Pediatr Hematol Oncol. 2003;25(6):484–7.
80. Gieron MA, Barak LS, Estrada J. Severe encephalopathy associated with ifosfamide administration in two children with metastatic tumors. J Neurooncol. 1988;6(1):29–30.
81. Shuper A, Stein J, Goshen J, Kornreich L, Yaniv I, Cohen IJ. Subacute central nervous system degeneration in a child: an unusual manifestation of ifosfamide intoxication. J Child Neurol. 2000;15(7):481–3.
82. Mott SH, Packer RJ, Vezina LG, Kapur S, Dinndorf PA, Conry JA, et al. Encephalopathy with parkinsonian features in children following bone marrow transplantations and high-dose amphotericin B. Ann Neurol. 1995;37(6):810–4.

Magnetic Resonance Spectroscopy: Basics

2

Stefan Blüml

In this chapter, the basic principles and procedures of proton magnetic resonance spectroscopy (MRS), with emphasis on clinical and experimental work in humans, are illustrated. An in-depth understanding of the laws of physics and chemistry that make MRS (and MRI) possible is outside the scope.

Overview

MR spectroscopy is a modality that is available on most state-of-the-art clinical MR scanners. For the brain in particular, MRS has been a powerful research tool and has also been proven to provide additional clinically relevant information for several disease families such as brain tumors, metabolic disorders, and systemic diseases [1]. The most widely available MRS method, proton (^{1}H; hydrogen) spectroscopy is an FDA-approved procedure in the US that can be ordered by clinicians for their patients if indicated. Other methods, such as phosphorous-31 (^{31}P), carbon-13 (^{13}C), or fluorine-19 (^{19}F) MRS, have been successfully applied in humans. But with the ever-increasing importance of clinical MR imaging, these *exotic* and time-consuming applications have been push to the side and are only available at a few academic centers. In addition, ^{1}H MRS does *not* require any additional hardware beyond what is already being used for MRI. Thus, proton spectroscopy dominates in vivo MRS and is the focus of this book.

S. Blüml, Ph.D. (✉)
Department of Radiology, Children's Hospital Los Angeles, Keck School of Medicine, University of Southern California, Los Angeles, CA, USA
e-mail: SBluml@chla.usc.edu

What Can Be Measured with Magnetic Resonance Spectroscopy?

MR imaging maps the distribution and interaction of water (its hydrogen atoms) with tissue. In contrast, ^{1}H MRS analyzes signal of the hydrogen protons attached to other molecules. Whereas for MRI only a single peak (water) is being mapped, the output of MRS is a collection of peaks at different radiofrequencies (RF) representing proton nuclei in different chemical environments, the spectrum (Fig. 2.1). Because of the low concentrations of MR-detectable chemicals, MRS is restricted to the analysis of individual regions of interest (ROI) much larger than the resolution of MRI. The typical spatial resolution for MRS is 1–10 cm^3, which is a thousand times larger than what is typically achieved for MRI (1–10 mm^3).

Only small, mobile chemicals (see Chap. 3) with concentrations of $>\approx 0.5$ μmol/g tissue can be observed with in vivo MRS. This leaves most neurotransmitters out of reach for this method. Exceptions may be glutamate, γ-amino butyric acid (GABA), and aspartate. In addition, large immobile macromolecules and phospholipids, myelin, proteins, RNA, and DNA are rendered *invisible* to MRS. The network of small molecular weight amino acids, carbohydrates, fatty acids, and lipids that can be measured is tightly controlled in the brain by enzymes and all but a few key molecules (MR *invisible* messengers and neurotransmitters) are kept at remarkably constant concentrations. It is for this reason that reproducible MR spectra of the brain can be obtained when robust methods are applied. In sequentially studied individual healthy controls, the single greatest variable may not be biological or diet imposed variations, but the practical unavoidable inaccuracy of the positioning of the subject, problems with the identification of a previously selected region of the brain, and the imperfect stability of MR hardware. The biochemical fingerprint of tissue will be abnormal when there is structural damage (trauma, tumor, degenerative diseases, gliosis, etc.), altered physiological

S. Blüml and A. Panigrahy (eds.), *MR Spectroscopy of Pediatric Brain Disorders*,
DOI 10.1007/978-1-4419-5864-8_2, © Springer Science+Business Media, LLC 2013

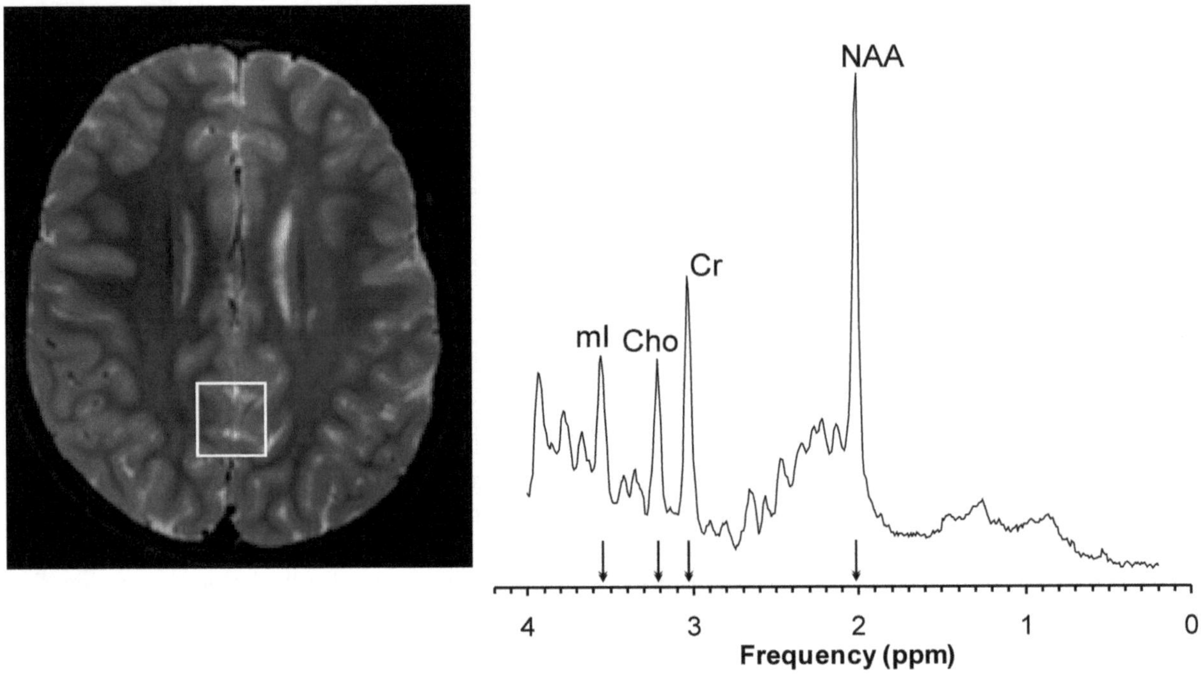

Fig. 2.1 A spectrum is a frequency analysis (=Fourier transform) of the signal that is detected in an MR study. In this case, a *normal* gray matter spectrum, acquired from the region of interest (ROI) indicated by the box on the MR image, acquired with a standard PRESS sequence (TE 35ms) at 1.5T is shown. The height of a peak is equivalent to the strength of the signal. The position on the *x*-axis (or chemical shift axis) measures the chemical shift relative to a reference (tetramethylsilane (TMS) at 0 ppm) and can be used to identify chemicals. The water peak would be at 4.7 ppm. However, the water peak is suppressed in MRS sequences as it would be several orders of magnitude larger than any of the other peaks

conditions (interruption of blood flow, etc.), and biochemical or genetic problems. The metabolic fingerprint also varies with the brain region studied. There are also normal age-dependent changes during brain development, which are discussed in Chap. 3.

Principles of In Vivo Magnetic Resonance Spectroscopy

The main ingredient for both MR imaging and spectroscopy is the strong magnetic field (B_0) created by a superconducting magnet. A net magnetization will develop in any tissue brought into the magnet field. The magnetization can be envisioned as a vector pointing, if undisturbed, along the magnetic field. For any MR sequence, a radiofrequency pulse, which is an additional time-dependent magnetic field, is used to tip the vector out of its equilibrium position. The magnetization vector will then precess around the equilibrium direction with a characteristic frequency (resonance frequency).

Chemical Shift

The resonance frequency of the protons is in a first approximation a function of the main magnetic field strength. However,

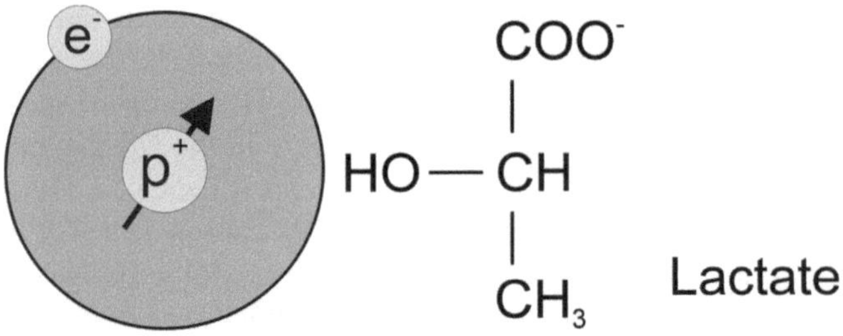

Fig. 2.2 Left: Hydrogen atom with nucleus (proton) and single electron. The electron *modifies* the magnetic field *seen* by the proton. Right: All protons potentially provide an MR detectable signal. The exact frequency of the signal depends on the molecular structure and the position of the proton in the molecule. For example, protons of the CH_3 group of lactate resonate at 1.33 ppm whereas the CH proton resonates at 4.1 ppm

the electronic environments of molecules cause a small modulation of the main magnetic field. If the electrons are close to the proton, there is a *shielding* effect and the proton *sees* a minimally smaller magnetic field (Fig. 2.2). This in turn results in slightly different resonance frequencies for protons in different molecules and even for protons in the same molecule but at different positions. Since the chemical structure of molecules determines the electronic environment this shift in the frequency has been named chemical shift. For in vivo MR spectroscopy, analyzing chemical shifts has been the main method for peak assignment.

J-coupling

In addition to chemical shifts, the spectrum is also modulated by J-coupling (or scalar coupling). J-coupling is the result of an internal indirect interaction of two spins via the intervening electron structure of the molecule. The coupling strength is measured in Hertz (Hz) and is independent of the external B_0 field strength. J-coupling between the same species of spins, e.g., proton and proton is termed *homo-nuclear* J-coupling whereas J-coupling between different species of spins, e.g., proton and phosphorous is referred to as *hetero-nuclear* J-coupling. J-coupling results in a modulation of the signal intensity depending on sequence type and acquisition parameters, particularly the echo time (TE, see below). The most prominent example in proton spectroscopy is lactate where there is a 7 Hz strong coupling between the two MR-detectable proton groups. Other molecules with more complex J-coupling patterns are glutamate and glutamine with three J-coupled proton groups. A spectrum of *N*-acetyl-aspartate (NAA) is shown in Fig. 2.3. NAA has both uncoupled and J-coupled protons.

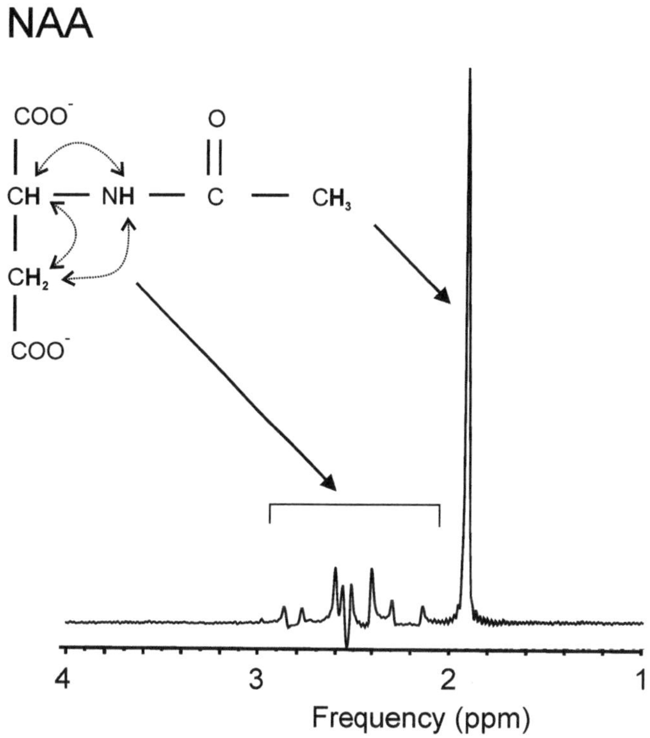

Fig. 2.3 The spectrum of the *N*-acetyl-aspartate (NAA) molecule is shown (standard PRESS, echo time (TE) 35 ms, 1.5 Tesla). The NAA molecule has protons at different positions. The three protons of the $-CH_3$ group are equivalent and their individual signals add-up and give the prominent peak at 2.0 ppm. The other protons attached to carbons of NAA molecule also provide a signal. The protons of the –NH, –CH, and $-CH_2$ are in close proximity in the molecule and do interact via J-coupling (indicated by dashed arrows in above figure). J-couplings split peaks and modulate the phase of a signal. The result is a more complex pattern of multiple peaks, which can be asymmetric or point downwards. The signal from proton next to the nitrogen atom (amide proton) resonates at approx. 8 ppm. Due to rapid exchange with protons from surrounding water molecules, the magnetization disappears quickly and the signal from this proton is very weak

Echo Time and Repetition Time

The main contrast mechanisms in MR imaging are T1-saturation, T2-relaxation, T2*-relaxation, diffusion, and proton density. These properties and the acquisition parameters do affect also the appearance of a spectrum. However, each proton in each molecule has its own set of characteristic MR properties. This and the fact that the spectrum itself provides no reference on how a change of an acquisition parameter may affect the spectrum, complicates this issue considerably (In MRI the anatomy provides a reference. For example, bright ventricles in a T2-weighted MRI help to identify other areas of fluid accumulation by the hyperintense signal, etc.). Metabolite resonances may be prominent with one acquisition sequence whereas the peak amplitude is different when another sequence is used despite spectra being acquired from the same ROI (Fig. 2.4). Therefore, changing sequence parameters or introducing different acquisition sequences should only be done with great caution. Instead, particularly for non-experts, it is important to be consistent and to acquire expertise with one sequence and one set of acquisition parameters.

The most important parameter is the echo time (TE). Indeed, MR spectroscopy can be separated into long TE and short TE methods. As for MR imaging, TE is the time the magnetization is in the transverse plane after an excitation before signal readout. During this time, the signal from each metabolite peak relaxes with its own characteristic T2-relaxation time. In addition, the signal amplitude of protons which are J-coupled is modulated. For example, at a characteristic echo time the signal of a metabolite may be inverted (e.g., lactate at TE = 144 ms, Fig. 2.4). Choosing long echo times simplifies spectra because the number of detectable peaks is reduced and the remaining peaks are more readily identified. Historically, long TE (typically TE > 135 ms) has been easier to use in clinical practice because of a flat baseline and because the three peaks (NAA, creatine (Cr), choline (Cho)) can be unequivocally separated. In addition, long TE MRS has been less sensitive to hardware imperfections (such as eddy currents). More recently, however, significant advances in both hardware and the methods used to analyze spectra have been made. Short TE MRS (TE ≈ 35 ms) allows the detection of an increased number of metabolites and has a signal-to-noise advantage over long TE. Other acquisition parameters that have an impact on the appearance are the repetition time (TR) and the mixing time (TM). TR is the time between each initial excitation of the

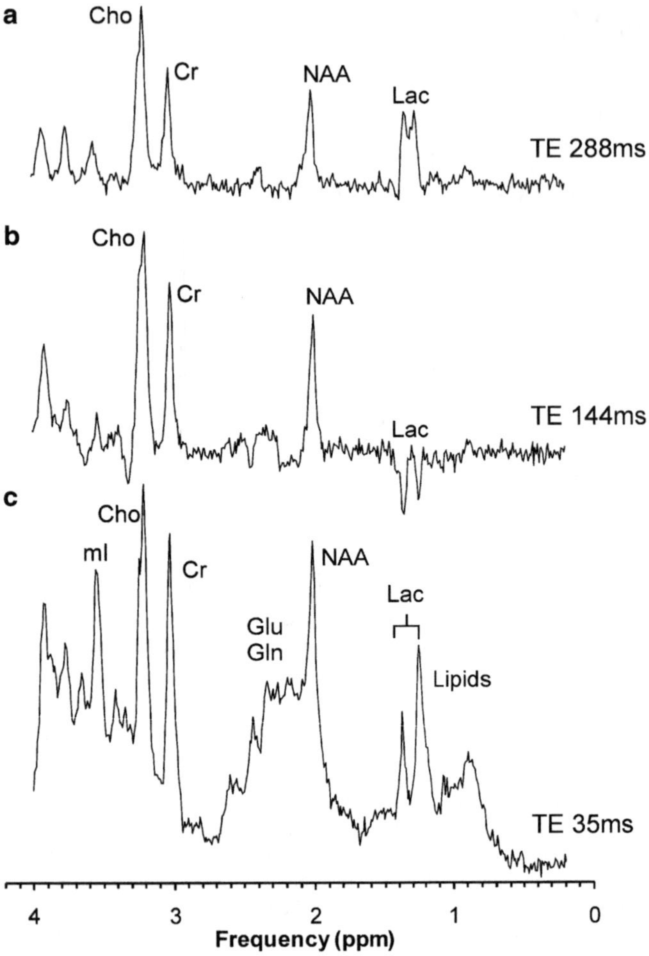

Fig. 2.4 Three single-voxel PRESS spectra of the same ROI acquired with echo times of TE=288 ms (*top*), TE=144 ms (center), and TE=35 ms (*bottom*). The spectrum at short TE (35 ms) is more complex and more challenging to interpret. However, it also contains more information and is the preferred method particularly for single-voxel MRS. For example, lipids are detectable, there is signal from the amino acids glutamate (Glu) and glutamine (Gln), and myo-inositol is detectable. At TE 144 ms the lactate peak is inverted and this echo time is a good choice when the detection of lactate is particularly important. TE 144 ms is frequently selected for chemical shift imaging (see text for details). At TE 288 ms the lactate signal is *in phase* again. However, at this long echo time, spectra are compromised by low signal to noise and a TE of 288 ms is rarely used on modern MR scanners

magnetization. If absolute quantitation is attempted, it is easier to quantify spectra that were obtained with long repetition times. In this case, knowing the individual T1-relaxation times of all peaks is not as crucial. However, spectra that were acquired with repetition times that are substantially longer than the T1-relaxation times (e.g., TR>3× T1) are compromised by lower signal-to-noise ratio. For that reason, repetition times are generally set to approximately 1–1.5 times the T1-relaxation times of metabolites. In contrast to TE, the overall appearance of spectra does change little with the repetition time, which more or less simply causes different scaling of peaks. The mixing time TM is the time delay between the second and the third 90° *RF pulse* in a STEAM sequence. The TE and TM are independent parameters. During TM, the magnetization in a STEAM acquisition points along the magnetic file and there is no signal decay due to T2-relaxation. However, during the mixing period there are still processes possible that have an impact on the final appearance of the spectrum (zero-quantum coherences).

Editing

Editing techniques exploit unique homonuclear (or heteronuclear) J-coupling properties of molecules. Many editing sequences utilize the fact that in an echo sequence the phase of J-coupled spins is modulated during the echo delay. A series of spectra acquired with different echo times each may allow the separation and identification of overlapping signals from different molecules due to their different J-modulation. Metabolite editing confers some specificity on the process of peak identification in high-resolution NMR techniques but has so far contributed little new information to in vivo human brain studies. Practical in vivo sequences have been proposed by Ryner et al. [2] and Hurd et al. [3] and tested in human subjects. While many creative editing sequences from high-resolution NMR are available in the literature, in practice, signal-to-noise limitations preclude their use in vivo. For example, zero-quantum filter for lactate editing is accomplished with a 2:1 signal loss; simple short-echo time sequences without metabolite-specific editing may work just as well. Recent examples of successful in vivo editing include GABA [4, 5] and β-hydroxy butyrate [6].

Data Acquisition

Planning a Magnetic Resonance Spectra

Planning and performing an MRS study is complex and requires extra diligence when compared with the planning of an MRI study. All modern MR scanners allow straightforward planning of MR imaging studies where the operator selects enough slices to cover the whole head and thus all areas of interest. With most acquisition parameters conveniently stored in ready-to-go protocols there is little that can go wrong. In contrast, quality control at the time of data acquisition is essential for MR spectroscopy. For MR spectroscopy, the operator needs to select the *correct* region of interest and may need to adjust scan parameters. Even in case of a focal lesion, such as a tumor, it might be necessary to pick the correct part of the tumor (e.g., avoiding bleeds or calcifications, selecting more cellular parts instead of a necrotic center, staying away from the skull, etc.), adjust the size of the region of interest, and the required scan time. Even with volumetric chemical shift imaging where many spectra from different locations are acquired simultaneously (CSI, discussed in more detail below) it is not possible to cover more than a part of the brain.

Acquisition Methods: Single-Voxel Versus Chemical Shift Imaging

Single-Voxel Magnetic Resonance Spectroscopy

Single-voxel (SV) MRS measures the MR signal of a single selected region of interest whereas signal outside this area is suppressed. For single-voxel MRS, the magnetic field and other parameters are optimized to get the best possible spectrum from a relatively small region of the brain. Manufacturers generally provide PRESS (Point Resolved Spectroscopy) [7, 8], STEAM (Stimulated Echo Acquisition Mode) [9], and ISIS (Image Selected In Vivo Spectroscopy) [10]. These sequences differ in how radiofrequency pulses and so-called gradient pulses are arranged in order to achieve localization. It is beyond the scope of this chapter to discuss details about localization methods and the interested reader is referred to the above-mentioned publications. ISIS is based on a cycle of eight acquisitions, which need to be added and subtracted in the right order to get a single volume. ISIS is considerably more susceptible to motion than STEAM or PRESS and is mostly used in heteronuclear studies, where its advantage of avoiding T2-relaxation is valuable. For ^{1}H MRS, however, ISIS has fallen out of favor.

Both, PRESS and STEAM do not require the addition or subtraction of signals to achieve localization and are thus more robust. PRESS utilizes one 90° and two 180° slice selective pulses along each of the spatial directions and generates signals from the overlap in form of a spin echo. At the same echo time, PRESS has the advantage over STEAM that it recovers the full possible signal and is therefore the method of choice for applications where signal to noise (S/N) is crucial. Since S/N is always crucial in MR, PRESS appears to be the overall winner among the competing localization techniques. STEAM utilizes three 90° slice selective pulses along each of the spatial directions. Signal, in form of a stimulated echo, from the overlap is generated. STEAM allows shorter echo times than PRESS partially compensating for lower S/N. Secondly, the RF bandwidth of 90° pulses is superior to the bandwidth of 180° pulses utilized by PRESS. STEAM is therefore an alternative to PRESS when short echo times, minimal chemical shift artifacts, and robustness are of concern.

2D or 3D Chemical Shift Imaging

With chemical shift imaging (CSI) approaches, multiple spatially arrayed spectra (typically more than 100 spectra per slice) from slices or volumes are acquired simultaneously. Other terms used for CSI are spectroscopic imaging (SI) and MR spectroscopic imaging (MRSI). Slice selection can be achieved with a selective RF pulse as for MR imaging. CSI encodes all spatial information into the phase of the magnetic resonance signal. In contrast to standard 2D MR imaging where one spatial dimension is phase encoded while the second dimension is frequency encoded, data acquisition is performed in the absence of a frequency-encoding gradient so that the chemical shift information can be retained. Due to the phase encoding, many spectra from a slice or from a 3D volume can be acquired simultaneously, and CSI is an excellent technique to obtain metabolic maps (Fig. 2.5). When it is desired to limit the region of interest to a smaller volume, e.g., to avoid bone and fat from the skull, CSI is usually combined with PRESS, STEAM, or ISIS—but with a significantly larger volume selected than for single-voxel MRS. CSI is a very efficient method to acquire information from different parts of the brain. An important feature is that within the examined volume of interest, any ROIs can be selected retrospectively by a process termed voxel-shifting.

When to Use What Method?

Despite evidence for the value of MRS in clinical practice and technical improvements, the application of MR spectroscopy is still hampered by its technically challenging nature. MR spectroscopy is prone to artifacts and processing and interpretation is complex and requires expert knowledge. For MRS to be used in clinical research and practice, standardized acquisition and processing methods need to be employed, easy to follow rules for quality-control applied, and results need to be presented and documented in a timely fashion to have an impact on clinical decision making. Studies should be designed not only to address basic medical or biological questions but also keeping the available resources in mind. Bulky CSI acquisitions with the need to review and interpret hundreds of spectra may require a skilled MR spectroscopist. Therefore, most new investigators will do better in the beginning by employing a single-voxel method. This ensures high quality of individual spectra. Single-voxel MRS performs more robustly when short echo times are selected. Employing a short echo time ensures high S/N of spectra and minimizes the signal loss of fast decaying peaks of metabolites such as myo-inositol, glutamate, and glutamine. Therefore, for single-voxel studies, short echo time PRESS (TE ≤35 ms) or STEAM (TE ≤30 ms) are recommended. However, single-voxel MRS is not a practical

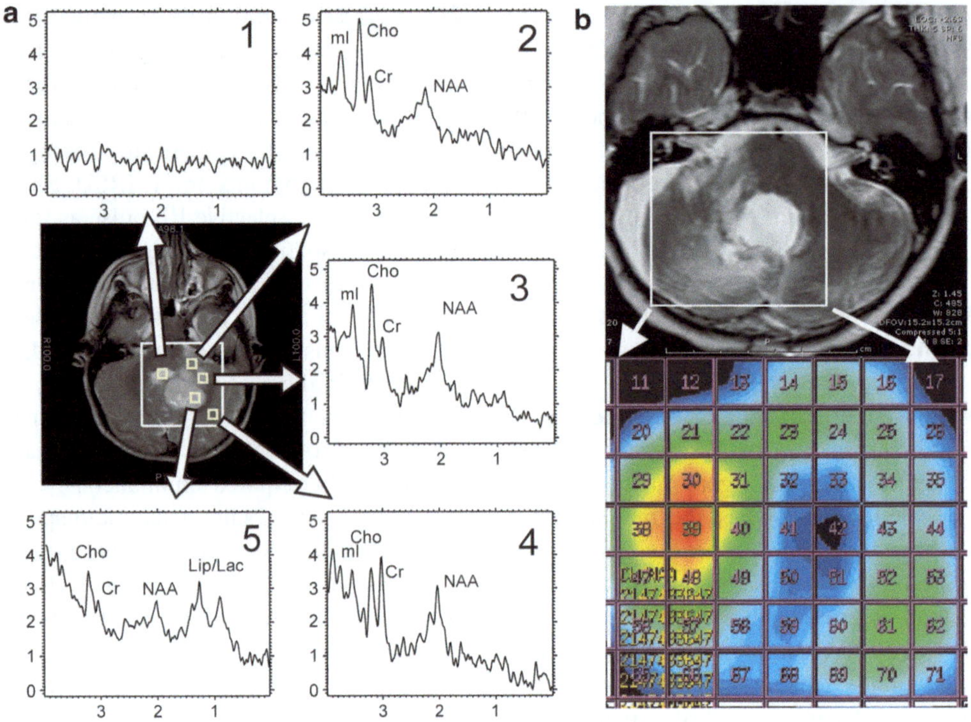

Fig. 2.5 (**a**) 2D CSI of a 3-year-old boy with a posterior fossa astrocytoma. The data were acquired with a PRESS sequence with a repetition time (TR) of 1.0 s, TE = 35ms, field of view = 160 bmm, 20 × 20 phase encoding steps, slice thickness = 8 mm, and two averages resulting in a nominal voxel resolution of 0.5 cc. Acquisition time was 13.3 min. The large *boxes* indicate the excited volume; smaller *boxes* indicate anatomical locations of individual spectra. (**b**) Shown is a 2D CSI of a child with a glioblastoma after radiation therapy. The box on the left image indicates the area from which spectra were acquired. Instead of displaying individual spectra, on the right, the results of the spectroscopy study are displayed as a color map. In this case, areas with increasing prominent choline relative to creatine (tCho/Cr) were colored hot *yellow* to *red* whereas areas with decreasing tCho/Cr are displayed in *green* and *blue*. Acquisition parameters were similar to those used in Fig. 2.5a

approach when maps of the distribution of chemicals within the brain are the goal. The investigator who wants to study many different brain regions or who needs to understand the spatial distribution of metabolites in an efficient matter will need to employ CSI. However, it should be noted that the added information available from CSI acquisitions sampling larger volumes might be compromised by poorer magnetic field homogeneity resulting in less well-defined peaks and nonuniform water suppression.

Signal-to-Noise Ratio

Insufficient signal-to-noise ratio (S/N) is the most significant challenge of in vivo MRS and its main limitation in clinical practice! It is not required for users of MRS to become experts in the discussion of how to best measure absolute S/N. The definition and the measurement of absolute S/N depend on acquisition parameters and steps involved in preprocessing of the data. For our purposes, S/N is the ratio between the amplitude of a resonance and the amplitude of random noise observed elsewhere in the spectrum (Fig. 2.6). In practice, it is more important to know which parameters and how various parameters influence S/N.

Rules (and Qualifiers) for Signal-to-Noise Ratio

1. To improve the S/N by a factor of two, four times the acquisition time is necessary. To have a three-fold signal increase, nine times the acquisition time is necessary.
2. *But:* There are practical limitations to increasing the scan time: If a scan exceeds the time a patient can hold still, nothing will be gained. Patient movements may degrade the quality of a study and the uncertainty of the location and thus the composition of the tissue enclosed in the region of interest compromising the interpretation. Hardware instabilities also take away S/N in scans that take a long time. From our experience, we believe that the acquisition time of a single scan should not exceed 20 min. We acknowledge, however, that under circumstances when a patient is very cooperative scans that last longer can be carried out. More typical and practical acquisition times that are well tolerated are 3–6 min.
3. S/N scales with the volume; half the volume gives half the S/N, doubling the volume doubles the S/N. This is

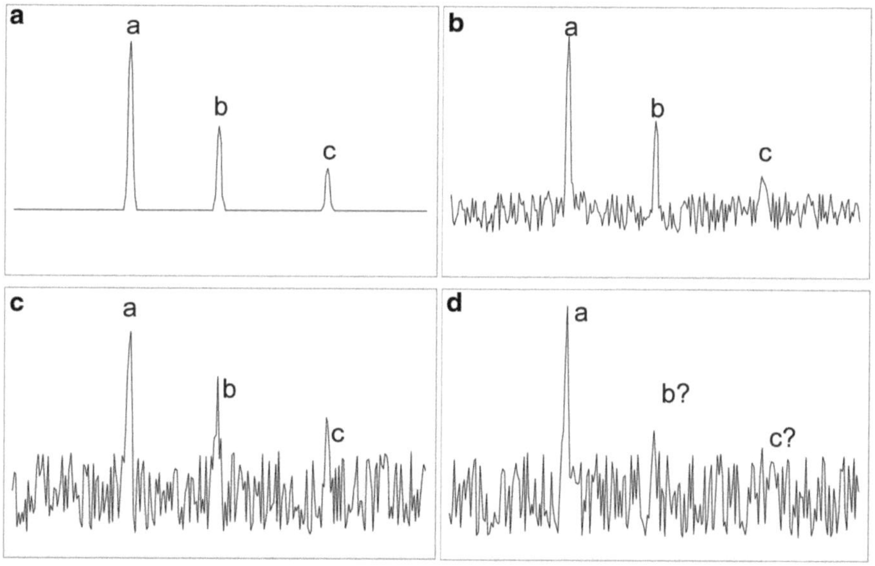

Fig. 2.6 This example illustrates that the S/N of a spectrum needs to be considered before drawing any conclusions. The same simulated spectrum with peaks with amplitude ratios of 4:2:1 is shown in (**a–d**). The hypothetical case of the spectrum with unlimited S/N is shown on the top left (**a**). In the next step random noise at a moderate level was added and peaks with approximate ratios of 4:2:1 are still observed. Spectra (**c**) and (**d**) are two simulations with twice the noise added, respectively. The original amplitude ratios are not reproduced and the spectra can only be interpreted qualitatively. Indeed, peaks b and c have become undetectable in simulation (**d**)

because the signal is proportional to the volume of the selected region. On the other hand, the noise is produced by the entire tissue within the sensitive volume of coil. The noise does not change with selecting different ROIs. (As the noise level in a study is constant, it is possible to compare two spectra that were acquired from different but equally sized ROIs to obtain information about absolute concentrations in both spectra: Scale both spectra such that the noise level is the same in both spectra. Compare the amplitude of the peaks. CAVEAT: This does not work if the linewidths of the peaks of the two spectra are substantially different.)

4. To compensate for a volume reduction by a factor of two the scan time needs to be increased by a factor of four.
5. *But:* A good shim (= process of optimizing the homogeneity of the magnetic field at the region of interest) improves the S/N. The area of a resonance line is constant. Therefore, by improving the shim and narrowing the width and increasing the amplitude of a resonance line the S/N can be improved. Generally, better shims are achieved for smaller ROIs. Thus, increasing the ROI size does not guarantee a linear increase in S/N. Similarly, decreasing the ROI might not result in a linear reduction of S/N.
6. *But:* Another finer point is the shape of a voxel. A cubic voxel can be shimmed better than an odd shaped voxel (very long in one direction and short in another direction). Therefore, ROIs that are closest to a cubic shape have the best S/N among rectangular ROIs with the same volume (spheres would be even better).
7. The S/N decreases with increasing echo times (TE) due to the T2-decay of the signal. Shorter repetition times (TR) cause T1-saturation. This does not necessarily reduce the S/N because more averages can be *packed* into the same acquisition time. T1 and T2 relaxation times vary with metabolites and field strength. In respect to S/N, the shortest possible TE is the best choice (but there are other important considerations). There is no *best* TR. At 1.5T a TR between 1 and 3 s is a good choice; at 3 T a TR between 2 and 5 s is appropriate.
8. If a user wants to acquire several spectra, choosing a large CSI box to cover all regions of interest is more efficient than measuring individual spectra with a single-voxel MRS. On the other hand, spectral quality of CSI is often compromised when single-voxel works fine.
9. With equal TR and TE, a PRESS sequence provides twice the S/N of a STEAM sequence.
10. Increasing the field strength will improve the S/R. Moving from 1.5 to 3 T scanners doubles the magnetization. In practice this does not result in a doubling of the S/R. This is because at 3 T T1-relaxation times are longer (=larger saturation effects), T2-relaxation times are shorter (faster signal decay), and the homogeneity of the magnetic field of 3T magnets does not reach the

homogeneity achieved at 1.5 T. Still, an S/R improvement of at least 50% can probably be achieved with modern 3 T systems.

11. Radiofrequency coils that are optimized (as small as possible without causing inhomogeneous excitation) will provide better S/N when compared with large coils.

Selecting the Region of Interest

On modern MR scanners, MR spectroscopy sequences are fully integrated into protocols and there is little difference between an MRI and an MRS study for patients. For the operator, on the other hand, MRS requires an additional important step. Using an image just obtained, a region of interest (ROI) is selected from which the MR spectrum is obtained. Indeed, selecting an appropriate ROI is probably the most crucial part of an MR spectroscopy study. This is particularly important for diseases with focal lesions. Not only needs the operator decide on the appropriate location, but also other factors such as size (in all three dimensions), number of averages required to obtain a spectrum of sufficient quality, minimizing partial volume with surrounding tissue, avoiding proximity to skull/bone/air transitions (negatively impact quality), avoiding blood and calcifications, and limiting the amount of cerebrospinal fluid (has no metabolites) need to be taken into consideration.

Accuracy in prescribing a region of interest (and proper documentation for longitudinal studies!) is of great importance in particular for single-voxel MRS studies. It is therefore recommended to study brain regions where MRS *works* and where normal MRS data are readily available for comparison. Two very popular choices are parietal white matter and occipital gray matter which have been studied frequently with single-voxel MRS. Frontal white matter and basal ganglia, historically technically more challenging, are also frequently studied brain regions.

How to Acquire *Good* Quality Spectra

Acknowledging that *good* is a relative term, below are a few suggestions on how to ensure that the quality of an MRS study is close to what can be achieved under optimum conditions. In order to acquire good spectra, for MRS the magnetic field within the region of interest is further refined in a process called *shimming*. Whereas in the early days of MRS a skilled spectroscopist would perform this task, today's scanners all have automated procedures that are generally equally good, faster, and more objective. Indeed, shimming as well as other scanner adjustments, such as transmitter and receiver gain setting, water suppression, is now all by default incorporated into the sequence. The user, after selecting the ROI, merely pushes a button and awaits the completion of the study. Good spectra are obtained if the ROI was not selected too small or too large, was not placed over areas of bleeds or calcifications, and away from tissue/bone/air transitions. When the voxel size is too small spectra of inadequate S/N are obtained. It is recommended to use approximately 10 cc at 1.5T for a single-voxel examination with PRESS with 128 averages. Depending on the biological/clinical question, it is possible to have smaller (or larger) ROIs. For example, if the question is whether there is elevated choline in the ROI, but accurate quantitation is not required, a smaller voxel will do. Other applications, for example phenylalanine in phenylketonuria (PKU), require the measurement of metabolites that are at very small concentrations. In this case, the ROI needs to be larger. Bleeds and, to a lesser extent, calcifications distort the magnetic field resulting in broad lines and poor water suppression compromising spectral quality. Similarly, placing the ROI on an area that contains a mixture of tissue, skin, bone, and air will result in poor spectra because the magnetic field cannot be adjusted very well. In summary, careful placement and proper selection of the size of the ROI are the only remaining hurdles for obtaining good quality spectra on modern MR scanners. While experience is useful, this task does certainly not require an MR spectroscopist.

Processing and Quantitation

In the early days of spectroscopy, a file that contains the *raw* result of the spectroscopy study would be stored somewhere on the computer that controls the MR scanner. That file would then be typically copied to an off-line computer for further processing using often custom-designed software. The basic processing steps are:

- Linebroadening: Linebroadening is a filtering process by which the measured signal is multiplied with a function that effectively improves the S/N of a spectrum at the cost of reduced spectral resolution. Alternatively, the filter function improves spectral resolution (negative linebroadening) at the cost of reduced S/N.
- Fourier transform: A Fourier transform is a mathematical operation that decomposes the measured signal in the time domain to its frequencies.
- Phasing: Due to hardware settings and sequence timing following the Fourier transform, a mixture of absorption and dispersion signals is observed in the spectrum. Spectrum analysis and quantitation is performed on the pure absorption signal, which needs to be extracted by a phase correction procedure.

Most modern MR scanners provide semi- or fully automated FDA approved scripts that can be used for processing. When using those, it is highly recommended to be methodological and refrain from *experimenting* with the processing parameters. Phasing and linebroadening do have an impact on the appearance of the spectrum and thus on the interpretation. Users with consistent processing parameters have an advantage particularly when longitudinal studies are being performed.

Recently, sophisticated processing software packages such as LCModel or MRUI [11, 12] have significantly improved automatic assignment and quantitation of metabolites in in vivo MR spectra. Processing of spectra is accomplished by fitting in vivo spectra to linear combinations of typically 15–20 measured or simulated model spectra of metabolites. This list of metabolites includes the major metabolites (e.g., NAA, Cr, Cho, mI) but also less prominent metabolites (e.g., glucose (Glc), or taurine (Tau)). These software packages are particularly appropriate for investigators who work with scanners from different vendors as they ensure equivalent processing and thus comparability. Albeit, these software packages are clearly superior to manufacturer provided solutions, they are not FDA approved and are thus more frequently used in research settings.

Often a neglected step is the proper documentation (preferable on three orthogonal images) of the location of the ROI. If the location of the ROI is not documented the MRS study is not complete. Unfortunately, manufactures do not appreciate the need for good (and automatic!) documentation and the user is settled to use the various, sometimes not intuitive, manual tools available.

Absolute Quantitation

For MR spectroscopy to become an accepted tool for research and clinical application, the information needs to be quantified and condensed in a fashion that allows the nonexpert user to draw adequate conclusions in a timely fashion. The natural parameters appear to be concentrations of metabolites in moles per unit volume, wet weight, or dry weight linking MRS with existing norms of biological chemistry. However, more common are peak ratios by which the signal intensity of one metabolite is expressed as a fraction of another one. Cr has often been used as an internal reference and metabolite ratios relative to Cr are reported. This was based on the assumption that the Cr pool is relatively constant in normal and diseased brain. However, this is not always the case and might be misleading. In particular, tumors may have quite different levels of Cr than normal tissue and ratios may be quite misleading. Even the structurally intact-looking brain might have altered concentrations of creatine—for example, the developing brain or under in *hypo-* and *hyper-*osmolar conditions. Therefore, although in many instances ratios provide important information, absolute quantitation is the preferred method. One commonly employed strategy for absolute quantitation is to acquire the water signal of the brain in the region of interest and measure (or assume) the water content of tissue. This can then be used as an internal concentration reference. For example, the water signal of tissue with a water content of 80% corresponds to a concentration of 55 mol/l × 80% = 44 mol/l. Use of the water signal as an absolute concentration reference eliminates several sources of error, such as differences in voxel size, total gain due to coil loading, receiver gains, hardware changes, etc. However, often the water content, in particular in pathology, is unknown. Therefore, other quantitation methods, using for example an external reference, have been suggested.

Absolute quantitation of CSI data sets is challenging. Whereas for single-voxel MRS sampling the water signal does not add more than a few seconds to the scan time, the situation is different for CSI. To obtain the reference water signal for each region of interest the acquisition of an additional CSI data set with time consuming 2D or 3D phase encoding is necessary. An alternative approach is to skip the extra scan and use the metabolite signal of normal tissue, distant from a focal abnormality, as internal reference. This approach has problems when metabolic changes in apparently normal appearing tissue cannot be ruled out. For a more detailed discussion of quantitation methods, the interested reader is referred to [13, 14].

Miscellaneous

Safety

Three different magnetic fields are applied in MRS:

- Static magnetic field B_0
- Gradient fields for localization purposes
- RF fields to excite the magnetization

These static fields are generally remarkably safe, with no known biological hazards. Fast switching gradients have been considered as associated with risk and nerve stimulation. While there exist *exotic* techniques such as echo planar spectroscopic imaging (EPSI), the vast majority of MRS techniques switches gradients a magnitude slower than routinely applied in MR imaging. Prolonged irradiation of RF is identified as hazardous to the extent that energy is *deposited* in the human head. But, again, MRS, when compared with MRI uses only few RF pulses and excessive RF deposition is not a problem in ^{1}H MRS.

Magnetic Resonance Spectroscopy at 3T

The main benefit of higher field strength for MRS is the increased SNR. MR spectroscopy also benefits from the

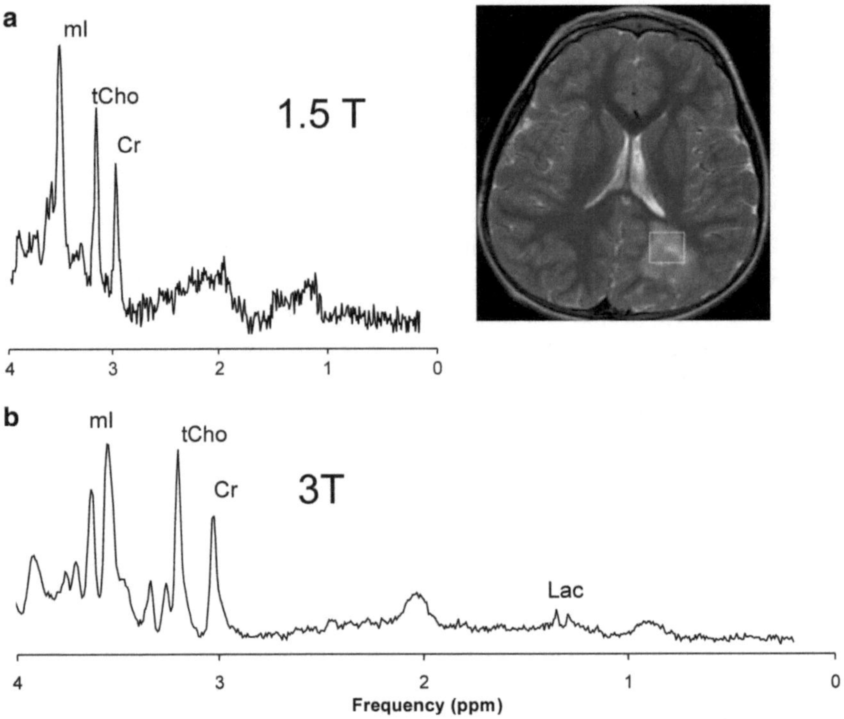

Fig. 2.7 Shown are spectra from the same patient and ROI (*white box* in MRI) acquired at 1.5 T and at 3 T. Both spectra cover the same chemical shift range (0–4 ppm). However, if the *x*-axis would be measured in hertz, the 1.5 T spectrum would cover 260 Hz (4 ppm=4×65 Hz at 1.5 T) whereas the 3 T spectrum would cover 520 Hz (4 ppm=4×130 Hz at 3 T). The acquisition times are comparable. Note, that the 3 T spectrum has considerable better SNR (lower level of random signal outside peaks). In this case the improvement may be exaggerated as the 1.5 T spectrum was acquired on an old system whereas the 3T spectrum was acquired on a state-of-the-art scanner with a smaller head coil. Also, note that while the creatine and choline singlets are rendered unchanged, the appearance of the myo-inositol signal (mI) is different for the two field strength (see also Fig. 2–8)

increased spectral resolution. Essentially, when moving from 1.5 to 3 T, a spectrum is being *stretched* along the chemical shift (*x*-axis) by a factor of two (Fig. 2.7). A disadvantage of the higher field strength is the increased chemical shift artifact. This problem arises from the different frequencies of the resonances associated with various chemical structures. When a gradient is applied to a sample containing chemically shifted species, there will be a displacement of the sensitive volume for each of the different species. The bandwidth of the RF pulse, with respect to the chemical shift range of the chemical structures, sets the percentage of overlap one can expect. Since at 3 T the chemical shift range is two times larger than at 1.5 T there is less (half) overlap (or more chemical shift artifact) at 3 T when the same RF pulse is used for excitation. Increasing the bandwidth of the RF pulse reduces chemical shift artifacts. In addition, whereas the main singlet peaks NAA (2.0 ppm), Cr (3.0 ppm), Cho (3.2 ppm) remain singlets at 3 T, the spectral pattern of other metabolites may change. Unfortunately, for some metabolites, such as taurine, detectability does not improve or may even decrease at higher field (Fig. 2.8).

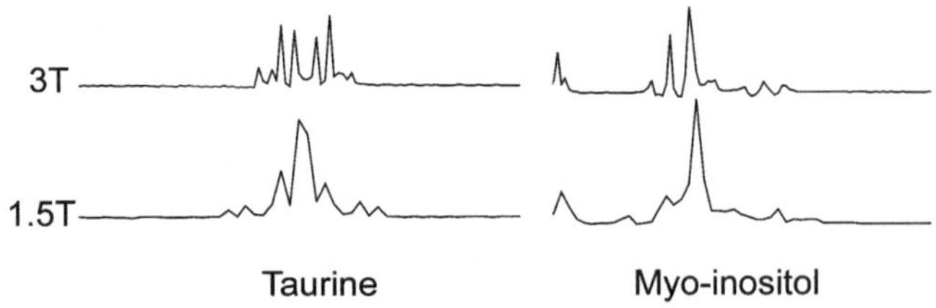

Fig. 2.8 Spectra of chemicals are generally different at different field strength as illustrated here for taurine and myo-inositol. Both spectra were acquired from model solutions with a PRESS TE 35 ms sequence. Changes in patterns need to be taken into consideration when comparing spectra acquired at different field strength

Finally, one has to consider that T1-saturation and T2-relaxation of metabolites are different at 1.5 T and 3 T. To complicate matters, relaxation properties for different metabolites do not change equally. Still, the benefits of improved SNR and spectral resolution at 3 T probably outweigh the disadvantages. Using a 3 T system, when available, is thus recommended.

Basic Questions/Answers

Often questions like "what is the smallest voxel you can measure?, how do I know that the signal-to-noise ratio is sufficient?, how do I know it is an artifact?", etc. are asked. These questions do have in common that there is no definitive answer and, consequently, no definitive answer can be provided in this book. Instead, below, we will try to elucidate a spectroscopist's point of view. Obviously, even within the MRS community there are different opinions and approaches. Thus, it is hereby disclosed that what is written and explained below is biased by the editors' opinions.

What is the smallest voxel that can or should be measured? What is the minimum S/N needed for a study to be conclusive? For global disorders, there is no need to push for the smallest possible voxel. Otherwise, for focal processes, there is—no surprise—no definitive answer to these questions. The approach depends on how much time an investigator is willing to invest and on the importance of the question that is being asked. It also depends on the quality of the shimming and the shape of the voxel. We advise against beginning a study with an acquisition of a spectrum from a very small voxel. Should the result only show random noise it would be unclear whether this is due to insufficient S/N or a feature of the tissue and valuable scan time has been wasted. A better approach might be to acquire a spectrum from a ROI large enough for the investigator to detect the major peaks of a spectrum. In a second step, the investigator can then reduce the voxel size and increase the scan time taking into account the rules given above and judging from the relative peak heights and noise level of the already acquired spectrum. Obviously, for the interpretation, the partial volume of surrounding tissue needs to be considered. To provide a number: We advice to select ROIs smaller than 1 cc only in extreme situations for single-voxel MRS. For CSI we advice against a resolution better than 0.5 cc.

If a spectrum is very noisy, how do I know whether this is due to technical problems or whether presents true biology (e.g., hypocellularity, necrosis, etc.)?
Looking at the noisy spectrum itself may not help to answer this question. Even before an MRS acquisition, MR and CT images (if available) should be inspected for bleeds and for calcifications. These areas should be avoided to the extent possible. Check the size of the ROI. If the volume is less than 1cc and the scan time has not been prolonged substantially, low S/N is the problem. In addition, it should be ruled out that the patient moved considerably during a scan by, for example, comparing MRI studies before and after the MRS study (another reason not to do conduct MRS studies at the very end of an examination). Distortions on MRI may indicate a technical artifact caused by braces (quite common in children) or by other magnetic parts. If this does not explain a *bad* spectrum there is more information that should be reviewed. While metabolites concentrations might be too low to produce peaks in a spectrum there is always enough signal from water. Unfortunately, some manufacturers do not routinely acquire a water spectrum or store it for convenient review. However, all scanners use water for the shimming procedure and the numeric result of the shimming can generally be reviewed. If a spectrum was acquired from a standard-sized voxel and the final shim was within the normal range, the absence of metabolites in the spectrum means that metabolites are low. Good shims are 0.1 ppm or less (6 Hz or less at 1.5 T and 12 Hz or less at 3 T). If shims are 0.15 ppm or worse data should be interpreted very carefully as the absence of certain metabolic features is likely explained by the low quality of the study.

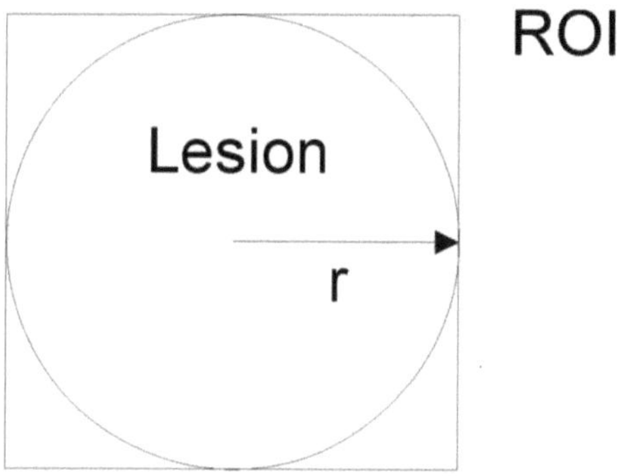

Fig. 2.9 The partial volume of surrounding normal tissue is easily underestimated in MRS. For example, the volume of spherical lesion is $4/3\ r^3\pi$ where r is the radius of the lesion. The volume of a cubic ROI enclosing the lesion is $8\,r^3$. That means that in this case the partial volume is approximately 50%. The resulting spectrum will show a mixed pattern with approximately equal contributions of metabolites from the lesion and from surrounding tissue

How much partial volume do I have?
For the interpretation of an MRS study, a realistic assessment of partial volumes is an absolute prerequisite! For global disorders or any study where standardized regions are examined, partial volumes are a minor problem. Consistency in the methods and accuracy in the placement of a voxel ensure reproducible findings. Partial volume effects are, however, a major challenge for focal processes. A typical scenario is a small focal lesion that is being studied with MRS. As is illustrated in Fig. 2.9, it is easy to underestimate the extent of partial volume.

What is the chemical shift artifact?
The net result of the chemical shift artifact is that the ROIs for the various metabolites in a spectrum do have significant overlap but are not identical. The problem of chemical shift

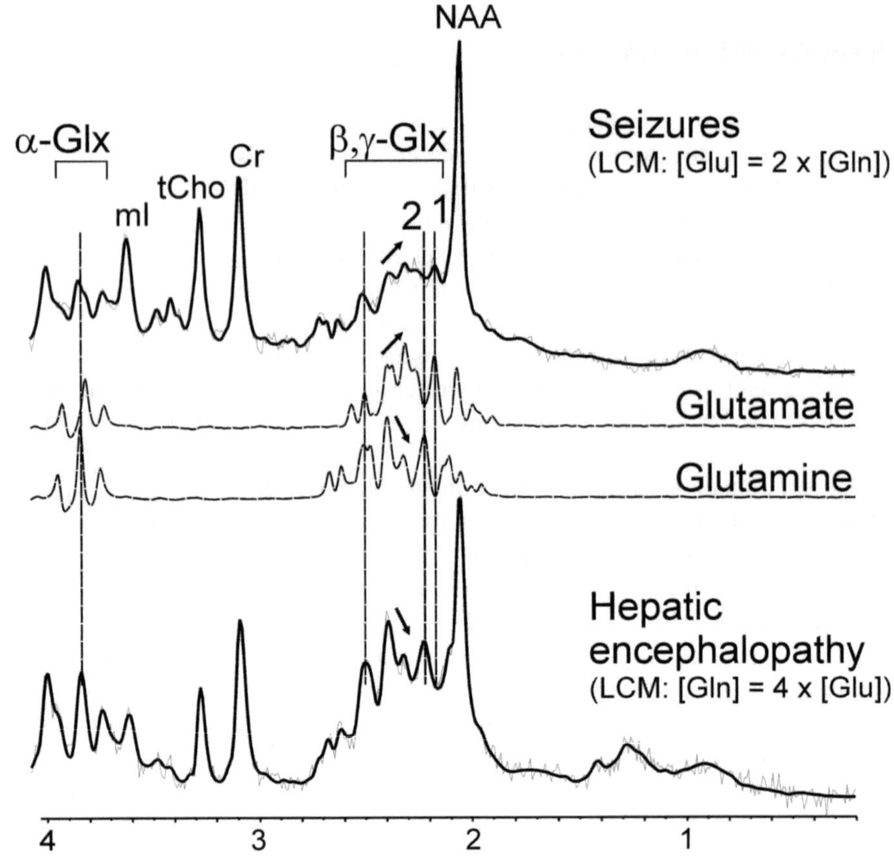

Fig. 2.10 Spectra obtained from a patient with seizures (*top trace*) and a patient with hepatic encephalopathy, a disorder associated with increased glutamine (*bottom trace*). Spectra of model solutions of glutamate and glutamine are shown for comparison (*middle traces*). Note, that in the hepatic encephalopathy spectrum the pattern of the β, γ-Glx region follows the glutamine signal whereas in the seizure case the pattern is more consistent with glutamate. All spectra: Single-voxel PRESS, TE 35 ms, 1.5 T

artifacts arises from the different frequencies of the signal that is observed in MRS. When a gradient for localization is applied there will be a displacement of the sensitive volume for each of the different species. The bandwidth of the RF pulse, with respect to the chemical shift range of the chemical structures, sets the percentage of overlap one can expect. Increasing the bandwidth of the RF pulse reduces chemical shift artifacts. Chemical shift artifacts are a bigger problem at higher field strength. Because most MRS sequences are already optimized, there is not much that can be done to reduce chemical shift artifacts. Chemical shift artifacts can cause problems for MRS of focal lesions. For example, lipids are important markers of tumor malignancy as the lipid signal indicates membrane breakdown and necrosis. The specificity of lipid signal is compromised when the ROI for the spectroscopy is close to skull/bone and lipid signal from the skull can be misinterpreted as signal from the lesion.

I see in the spectrum an unusual peak/signal. Is it real?
Over the years, spectroscopists have been taught by experience what can and what cannot be observed with in vivo MRS in the human brain. Still, occasionally new peaks are *discovered.* The number of unusual peaks observed with in vivo spectroscopy has dropped significantly over time. This is mainly a result if greatly improved hardware and software and thus less artifacts being confused with real signal. If a patient is still on the scanner, a second spectrum should be acquired. If a global disorder is expected, a different brain region should be selected. In case of a focal lesion, a slightly different ROI should be selected. In addition, a spectrum with a different echo time should be acquired if possible.

Scanner stability: Are there Monday morning and Friday afternoon peaks?

Brain metabolism is very well regulated and MRS is remarkable stable. There are no Monday morning or Friday afternoon peaks. Exceptions are glucose, which can increase/decrease with plasma glucose.

Can glutamate and glutamine be separated at 1.5 T?
It depends. Due to their similar chemical structures, glutamate and glutamine form complex and partially overlapping resonances in ^{1}H spectra. However, although the individual spectra of glutamate and glutamine are similar, they are *not* identical (Fig. 2.10). That means, that the quality of a spectrum (linewidth and signal to noise) determines how well the contribution from these two metabolites can be distinguished. Hypothetically, with unlimited signal to noise, perfect separation is possible and a categorical claim that glutamate and glutamine cannot be separated at 1.5 T is wrong. Still, it needs to be acknowledged that only under the best circumstances glutamate and glutamine can be quantified in

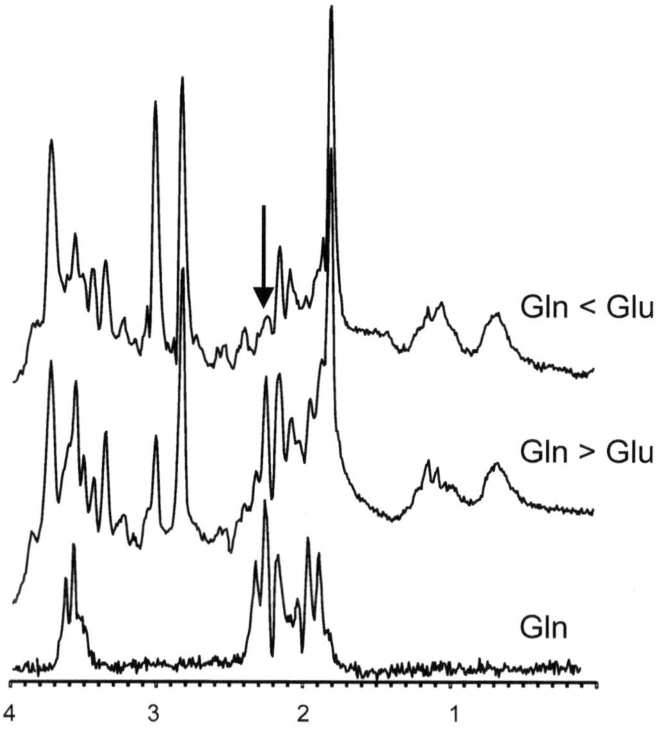

Fig. 2.11 Spectra obtained from a patient with a normal MRI and unremarkable follow-up (*upper trace*) and a patient with acute liver failure (*middle*). A spectrum of a model solution of glutamine is shown for comparison (*bottom*). Note that in the patient with liver failure the signal at around 2.45 pm is consistent with elevated glutamine. Advanced processing with LC Model suggested that glutamine concentration in the liver failure patient is at least three times higher than glutamate. In the control, glutamate concentrations are approximately three times higher than glutamine

individual patients at 1.5 T. Also, it is advised to use sophisticated software, such as LCModel (Provencher 1993) that fits all metabolite resonances simultaneously and provides a measure of the reliability of the analysis (so called Cramer–Rao lower bounds). A prerequisite is to use short TEs to minimize signal decay. Special acquisition methods (*editing*) can be used to improve the separation. However, these methods are not widely available, are compromised by longer acquisition times, and require extra expertise. Separation of glutamate and glutamine improves greatly at 3 T.

Can we distinguish between glutamate and glutamine in spectra acquired at 3 T in individual patients?
Tentatively yes. At 3 T, the glutamate and glutamine signals can be much better distinguished than at 1.5 T. As illustrated (Fig. 2.11), for *PRESS TE 35 ms*, glutamine has, for example, a peak at around 2.45 ppm. Spectra obtained from tissue with high levels of glutamine will show this peak whereas this signal is much less prominent in a situation where glutamate concentration exceeds glutamine. So even without sophisticated software, just by careful inspection of the spectra, it is possible to make a qualitative statement about glutamate and glutamine. But there is an important caveat: Spectra need to be of high quality with the random noise signal below the signal amplitudes of glutamate and/or glutamine.

References

1. Ross BD, Bluml S. Neurospectroscopy. In: Greenberg JO, editor. Neuroimaging second edition; a companion to Adams and Victor's principles of neurology. New York: McGraw Hill; 1999. p. 727–73.
2. Ryner LN, Sorenson JA, Thomas MA. Localized 2D J-resolved 1H MR spectroscopy: strong coupling effects in vitro and in vivo [published erratum appears in Magn Reson Imaging 1995;13(7):1043]. Magn Reson Imaging. 1995;13(6):853–69.
3. Hurd RE, Gurr D, Sailasuta N. Proton spectroscopy without water suppression: the oversampled J- resolved experiment. Magn Reson Med. 1998;40(3):343–7.
4. Rothman DL, Petroff OA, Behar KL, Mattson RH. Localized 1H NMR measurements of gamma-aminobutyric acid in human brain in vivo. Proc Natl Acad Sci USA. 1993;90(12):5662–6.
5. Hetherington HP, Newcomer BR, Pan JW. Measurements of human cerebral GABA at 4.1 T using numerically optimized editing pulses. Magn Reson Med. 1998;39(1):6–10.
6. Shen J, Novotny EJ, Rothman DL. In vivo lactate and beta-hydroxybutyrate editing using a pure-phase refocusing pulse train. Magn Reson Med. 1998;40(5):783–8.
7. Bottomley PA, Inventor. Selective volume method for performing localized NMR spectroscopy. US patent US patent 4 480 2281984.
8. Bottomley PA. Spatial localization in NMR spectroscopy in vivo. Ann N Y Acad Sci. 1987;508:333–48.
9. Frahm J, Merboldt K, Haenicke W. Localized proton spectroscopy using stimulated echos. J Magn Reson. 1987;72:502–8.
10. Ordidge RJ, Connelly A, B. Lohman JA. Image-selected in-vivo spectroscopy (ISIS). A new technique for spatially selective NMR spectroscopy. J Magn Reson. 1986;66:283–94.
11. Provencher SW. Estimation of metabolite concentrations from localized in vivo proton NMR spectra. Magn Reson Med. 1993; 30(6):672–9.
12. Naressi A, Couturier C, Devos JM, et al. Java-based graphical user interface for the MRUI quantitation package. MAGMA. 2001; 12(2–3):141–52.
13. Kreis R. Quantitative localized 1H MR spectroscopy for clinical use. Prog NMR Spectroscopy. 1997;31:155–95.
14. Danielsen ER, Henriksen O. Absolute quantitative proton NMR spectroscopy based on the amplitude of the local water suppression pulse. Quantification of brain water and metabolites. NMR Biomed. 1994;7(7):311–8.

3 Metabolites of Proton Magnetic Resonance Spectroscopy and Normal Age-Dependent Changes

Stefan Blüml

The goal of this chapter is to introduce the main metabolites of proton MRS with emphasis on developmental changes. Understanding how normal metabolite levels may change in the developing brain is important for the interpretation of MR spectra obtained from children.

Because the microscopic composition (density/maturation of cells) of the brain and the activity of the enzymes that regulate its metabolism change during brain development, there are changes of the *normal* metabolic profile with brain maturation. As expected, these changes are most dramatically (illustrated below) at early brain development. Unfortunately, it is also very difficult to obtain normal control data for this age. Albeit completely harmless, magnetic resonance (MR) imaging and MR spectroscopy are expensive and *lengthy* tests that are sensitive to subject motion. Unless there is a clinical justification, MR spectroscopy scans are rarely performed in small children, as they often require sedation to ensure studies with sufficient quality without motion artifacts. This means that there are even fewer studies of normal babies. Consequently, there only few studies describing the normal biochemical maturation are found in the literature [1–7] and the numbers of subjects included in those studies were small and/or the study did cover only a limited age range. At this institution, over a 10-year period, hundreds of spectra were acquired from subjects aged 0 (term) to 18 years (young adults) that were retrospectively considered to be *closest-to-normal* based on the MRI findings (negative) and unremarkable clinical follow-up. These spectra have recently been reviewed and results are provided in this chapter.

Important Limitations

In vivo MR spectroscopy, albeit widely available, is by no means standardized! This includes data acquisition methods, selection of regions of interest (ROI), processing, and quantitation of the spectra. The data provided below were generated with the specific methods (described in detail below) used at Children's Hospital Los Angeles. This means that investigators employing different methods and different strategies for quantitation or measure in different locations may arrive at different numbers. Furthermore, even if identical methods are used and comparable brain regions are examined, but studies are performed on different platforms (e.g., different vendors, different software versions), results may be different. It is beyond the scope of this chapter to explain the underlying causes of these discrepancies. For the interested reader we want to mention that a sequence such as PRESS with an echo time of 35 ms can be implemented in different ways. This includes the timing and amplitude of crusher gradients, type and shape of radiofrequency pulses, and other scanner instructions. These sequence details have an impact on the final spectrum. For example, crusher gradients act equivalent to diffusion gradients in MRI and depending on their strength and timing suppress at varying levels the signal from randomly moving molecules. Thus, as of today, it is not feasible to present universally valid control data rendering this project as "work-in-progress". Despite these limitations, we believe that graphs and tables in this chapter are providing a good first-order approximation of the true metabolic changes occurring in the normal developing brain.

Materials and Methods

Controls/Patients and Brain Regions

The developmental curves for biochemical maturation of the human brain were developed from a database of more than 2,500 subjects undergoing more than 7,000 MR spectroscopy

S. Blüml, Ph.D. (✉)
Department of Radiology, Children's Hospital Los Angeles, Keck School of Medicine, University of Southern California, Los Angeles, CA, USA
e-mail: SBluml@chla.usc.edu

S. Blüml and A. Panigrahy (eds.), *MR Spectroscopy of Pediatric Brain Disorders*,
DOI 10.1007/978-1-4419-5864-8_3, © Springer Science+Business Media, LLC 2013

studies at this institution. Of those, 320 subjects with a gestational age at birth of exactly 40 weeks (term) with no abnormalities on MRI (including no abnormalities on diffusion MRI), as explicitly stated on the MRI report, and unremarkable clinical follow-up (where available) were identified. These subjects were enrolled in various research studies in this institution (a small group of typically siblings of patients) or had clinical indications for MR imaging and spectroscopy. Clinical indications included seizures (retrospectively classified as febrile seizures), suspicions of encephalitis or hypoxic–ischemic episodes, suspected but not confirmed tumor, subdural bleeds, hypotonia, meningitis, and others. All spectra were reviewed for quality and spectra of insufficient quality (large linewidth or insufficient signal to noise) were not included in the analysis. Also eliminated were studies where patients had diseases with persistent clinical symptoms or where spectroscopic abnormalities were reported in the literature despite normal MRI. This included MELAS, gyrate atrophy, and hepatic encephalopathy [8–10].

The MRS studies conducted at this institution routinely included the acquisition of spectra from two standardized brain regions from where spectra of good quality can be obtained. The first location is in the occipital/parietal cortex and contains mostly gray matter (GM). The second region encloses mostly white matter in the parietal/occipital cortex (WM) (Fig. 3.1). Typical MR spectra from these two regions illustrate the main metabolic changes that are detectable by visual inspection are shown in Fig. 3.2.

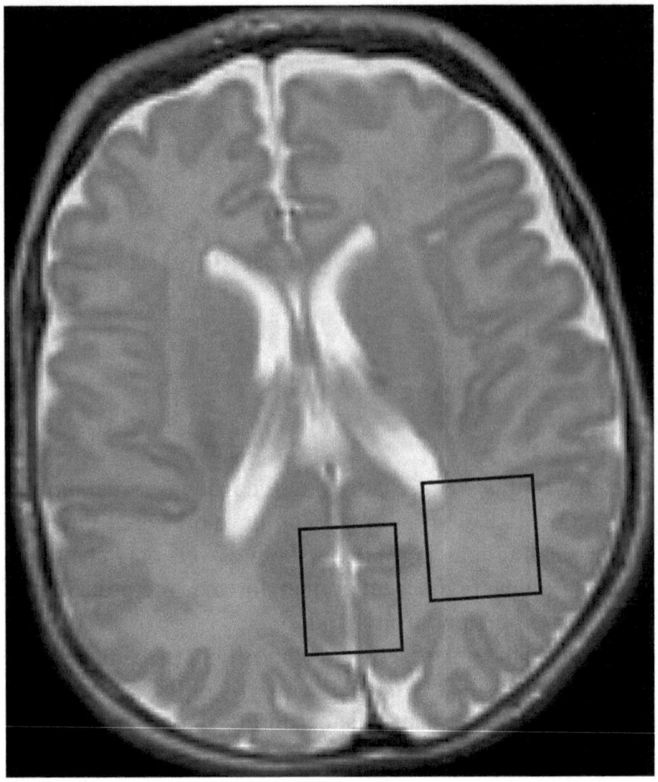

Fig. 3.1 MR image indicating typical parietal white matter (WM) and parietal/occipital gray matter (GM) locations

Presentation of the Data

In MR spectroscopy the signal received is proportional to the number of nuclei present in the region of interest. MRS is thus inherently quantitative, albeit obtaining the correct *scaling* factors to translate signal amplitudes into concentrations is a significant challenge. Indeed, it has been argued that MR spectroscopy cannot be used to quantify chemicals because the same chemical may be either *MR visible*—when capable of moving freely—or *MR invisible* when bound to a membrane or confined in myelin. While this is almost certainly an academic problem that can be overcome in practice by agreeing that the *unbound MR visible* concentrations are being measured, the complexity of MR and the many parameters that can have an impact on the observed signal poses a significant challenge. Consequently, concentrations reported by MRS of the same chemical in the same brain region have varied widely in the past. Due to significant hardware improvements and much iteration to find the best processing and quantitation strategies, the reproducibility of MRS and the consistency of reported concentrations have greatly improved. There might be still systematic differences, depending on how a particular sequence is implemented and which corrections are applied. However, observations such as that choline concentrations are higher and creatine concentrations are lower in parietal white matter than in parietal/occipital gray matter are now universally true (geographically, across vendors, at different field strengths, and irrespectively of the acquisition method used). In this chapter, we report the concentrations as measured with our methods—which we believe are state of the art—to allow the interested reader to make comparisons with data obtained by other measurement techniques. However, we also report concentrations as percentage of concentrations measured in the young adult brain. Reporting relative concentrations is generally more robust as (potential errors in) correction factors have no impact on those numbers. For the interested reader a table is provided (Table 3.1) that summarizes all parameters from which absolute and relative concentrations can readily be calculated for different stages of brain maturation.

Acquisition, Processing, and Quantitation of Magnetic Resonance Spectra

All MR spectroscopy studies were carried out on a 1.5 T MR system (Signa LX, GE Healthcare, Milwaukee, Wis). Patients of age 5 years and below were anesthetized with 100–200 mg/

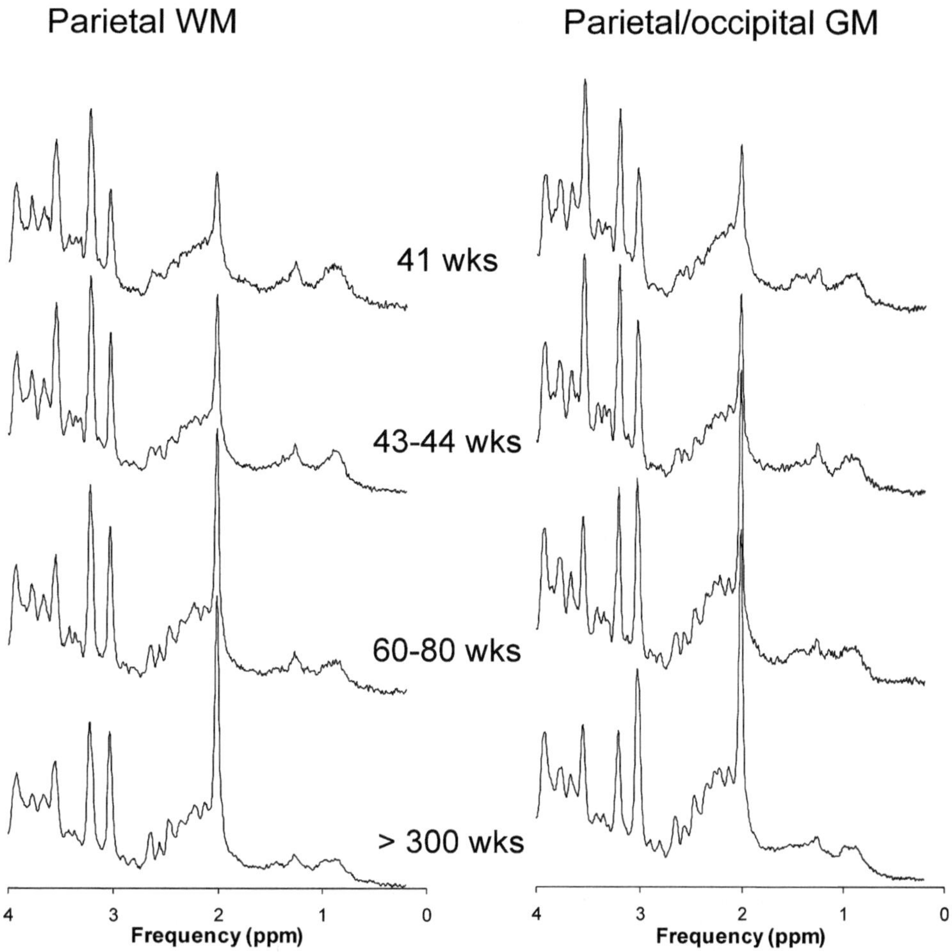

Fig. 3.2 Typical proton MR spectra acquired from parietal WM and parietal/occipital GM in subjects with normal MRI at different stages of brain development

min/kg propofol throughout the MR study. Single-voxel point-resolved spectroscopy (PRESS) with a short echo time of TE = 35 ms, a repetition time of TR = 1.5 s, and 128 signal averages was used for all acquisitions. With these parameters, the total acquisition time, including scanner adjustments was less than 5 min.

Spectra were processed using fully automated LCModel software (Stephen Provencher Inc., Oakville, Ontario, Canada, LCModel Version 6.1–4 F) using the unsuppressed water signal of the brain in the region of interest as an internal concentration reference. For example, the water signal of tissue with a water content of 80% corresponds to a concentration of 55 mol/kg × 80% = 44 mol/kg. Use of the water signal as an absolute concentration reference eliminates several sources of error, such as differences in voxel size, total gain due to coil loading, receiver gains, hardware changes, etc. However, often the water content, as is the case in the developing brain, changes. Data presented in the following paragraphs were thus corrected for the varying water content of the developing human brain by using a look-up table for water content as a function of postconceptional age from published data [11, 12]. Concentrations were also corrected for the varying fractions of cerebrospinal fluid (CSF) in the regions of interest as described earlier [13]. No other corrections were applied.

In a preliminary analysis, data from female and male subjects were analyzed separately. No significant differences were noted and data were thus pooled. Metabolite concentrations measured in each brain region were fitted to empirical functions using the least-squares fit routine provided by MatLab. The functions were minimum χ^2 was determined are reported. Fit functions and fitted parameters (± standard deviation of fit parameters) are summarized in Table 3.1. The standard deviations of the fitted parameters were determined by Monte Carlo simulation as follows. First, typical errors for the quantitation of metabolites (not accounting for systematic errors) were determined by calculating the standard deviations (SD) of metabolites concentrations in subjects older than 10 years when metabolite concentrations were close to constant. For example, gray matter N-acetylaspartate concentrations ([NAA]) in children older than 10 years were 9.89 ± 0.48 mmol/kg. Then random numbers within ± one SD (here ±0.48 mmol/kg) were

Table 3.1 Summary of fitted parameters and fit functions for metabolites with significant changes during brain maturation

		Fit function	A_1 (mmol/kg)	A_2	A_3 (1/years)	A_4 (1/years)	A_5 (years)
NAA	WM	f_1	9.29±0.10	0.27±0.02	0.22±0.03	15.1±1.2	0.812±0.004
	GM		9.87±0.05	0.35±0.03	0.44±0.06	9.1±0.8	0.840±0.005
Cr	WM	f_2	5.13±0.03	–	5.83±0.46	3.7±0.3	0.848±0.006
	GM	f_1	7.01±0.06	0.13±0.02	0.24±0.10	7.2±1.4	0.686±0.018
Cho	WM	f_1	1.64±0.01	−0.30±0.01	0.41±0.05	10.9±1.5	0.544±0.035
	GM		1.24±0.01	−0.50±0.02	1.17±0.09	16.2±1.5	0.667±0.013
mI	WM	f_2	4.85±0.02	−0.65±0.01	3.00±0.10	46.4±2.4	0.737±0.002
	GM		5.89±0.02	−0.62±0.02	3.72±0.12	67.3±8.5	0.748±0.004
Glu	WM	f_2	8.08±0.07	–	5.70±0.51	3.6±0.4	1.005±0.012
	GM	f_3	11.86±0.06	–	9.90±6.19	6.4±4.7	0.805±0.009
Tau	WM	f_4	24.1±0.9	0.015±0.001	2.72±0.04	–	–
	GM		2.36±0.05	0.32±0.04	0.17±0.02	–	–

$$f_1 = \frac{A_1}{A_2 e^{-A_3(\mathrm{PCA}-A_5)} + e^{-A_4(\mathrm{PCA}-A_5)} + 1}, \tag{3.2}$$

$$f_2 = \frac{A_1}{e^{-A_3(\mathrm{PCA}-A_5)} - e^{-A_4(\mathrm{PCA}-A_5)} + 1}, \tag{3.3}$$

$$f_3 = \frac{A_1}{e^{-A_3(\mathrm{PCA}-A_5)} + e^{-A_4(\mathrm{PCA}-A_5)} + 1}, \tag{3.4}$$

$$f_4 = A_1(A_2 + e^{-A_3 \cdot \mathrm{PCA}}), \tag{3.5}$$

where PCA is the postconceptional age in years.

All spectra used to generate these data were acquired on a 1.5 T clinical scanner using a single-voxel PRESS sequence with a TE=35 ms and a TR=1.5 s. Spectra were quantified as described in detail in the text. The standard deviations of the fitted parameters were derived by Monte Carlo simulation as explained in more detail in the text. For functions f_1, f_2, and f_3 the parameter A_1 is equal to the concentration in young adults. For function f_4, $A_1 \times A_2$ is equal to the concentration in young adults. By inserting the postconceptional age (in years) *normal* concentrations for any age can be calculated. To obtain relative concentrations, the obtained concentration needs to be divided by A_1 (f_1, f_2, f_3) or by $A_1 \times A_2$ (f_4). For example, at term (PCA=0.77) NAA in WM is 3.0 mmol/kg which is 32% of concentration observed in young adults. Fit parameters should be only compared for metabolites that were fitted with the same function.

generated and added to all measured data simulating the experimental uncertainty. This synthetic data can be interpreted as a possible result if all subjects were re-examined with MRS taking into account the experimental imperfections. This new data set was then fitted to determine to what extent experimental uncertainty could alter fit parameters. This procedure was typically repeated 2,000 times for each data set and the distribution of the fit parameters was analyzed. Generally, parameters showed a close to Gaussian distribution and the reported uncertainties of the fitted parameters are the standard deviations of the distributions.

Metabolites of ^{1}H Magnetic Resonance Spectroscopy and Their Age-Dependent Changes in *Normal* Brain

N-acetyl-aspartate, *N*-acetyl-aspartyl-glutamate

The most prominent peak of the ^{1}H spectrum of normal tissue is the resonance at 2.02 ppm from the three equivalent protons of the acetyl group of the *N*-acetyl-aspartate (NAA) molecule. The role of NAA, and its regulation in vivo, is not well understood. In the normal brain, NAA is synthesized in neurons, diffuses along axons, and is broken down in oligodendrocytes. NAA is present in high concentrations only in normal neurons and axons [14, 15], and from a MR spectroscopic perspective, it is a marker for adult type *healthy* neurons and axons. Proton spectra of any disease that is associated with neuronal or axonal loss (or replacement, e.g., tumors) will exhibit a reduction of NAA. Although the loss of NAA is not specific for a disease or disease process, the extent of neuronal or axonal loss for an already diagnosed disorder can be quantified. There are several caveats regarding the role of NAA as marker for neuronal/axonal density: NAA is low in normal, developing, newborn brain, despite the presence of neurons. Brain NAA increases rapidly as the brain matures, peaks at ≈10–15 years, and then decreases slightly over time as the number of neurons and axons declines even in the normal brain [16]. Significantly increased NAA is observed only in Canavan disease, where aspartoacylase deficiency, the enzyme that breaks down NAA, results in an accumulation of NAA. Are there other scenarios where NAA could increase or recover? Almost certainly yes! In head trauma, in clinical

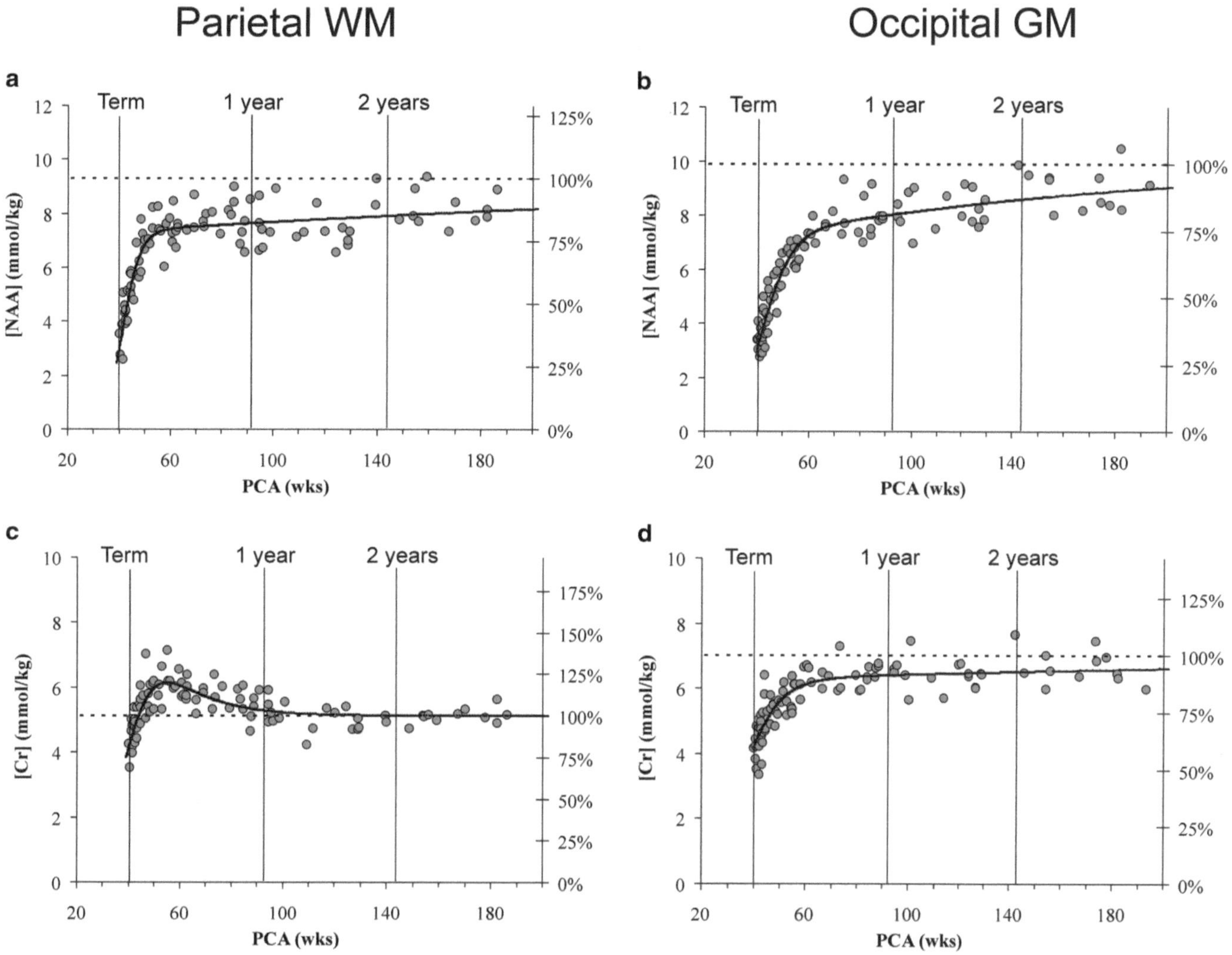

Fig. 3.3 Shown are the measured NAA (**a, b**), Cr (**c, d**), Cho (**e, f**), and mI (**g, h**) concentrations in subjects deemed to be *closest to control* as function of postconceptional age. Only subjects born exactly at term (40 weeks) with normal MRI and unremarkable clinical follow-up are included. Superimposed are curves that were obtained by least-squares fits. Albeit, the curves for white matter and gray matter regions appear to be similar, there were significant differences in the fitted parameters. For example, in contrast to Cr in GM, Cr in WM reaches a transient maximum at early brain development. In addition, the increase of NAA in WM (**a**) preceded the increase in GM (**b**). These concentrations were measured using a single-voxel, TE (35 ms), PRESS sequence on a 1.5 T scanner and LCModel quantitation (see details in text). *NAA N*-acetyl-aspartate, *Cr* creatine, *Cho* choline, *mI* myo-inositol

as well as animal studies, a recovery of NAA in both white and gray matter has been reported at late follow-up [17–19]. Albeit other mechanisms might contribute, one possible explanation is the sprouting of new axons from surviving neurons. Also, for disease or conditions that predominantly affect glial cells but leave neurons and axons intact it might be possible to see an (relative, transient?) increase of NAA. Myelin contains little or no NAA and thus effectively dilutes the MR-detectable NAA. Therefore it is at least conceivable that a selective loss of myelin may result in an *apparent* increase of NAA, as the partial volume of axons may increase.

Very closely linked with NAA is *N*-acetyl-aspartylglutamate (NAAG) found on the shoulder of the NAA peak at approximately 2.04 ppm. Only in spectra of excellent quality can NAAG be separated from NAA. In the past, most investigators have quantified/interpreted the peak at ≈2.0 ppm that comprises both NAA and a smaller amount of NAAG.

NAA in parietal white matter (WM) increased rapidly from approximately 30 to 75% of normal adult levels between 40 weeks (term) and 51 weeks postconceptional age (PCA) (equivalent to a 2.5-month-old baby born at term). Thereafter a more gradual increase to 95% of adult levels by 7–8 years of age was observed. A similar time course was observed for NAA in parietal/occipital gray matter GM, although it appears that the WM increase of NAA precedes the increase in GM slightly (Fig. 3.3a, b). NAA concentrations of the young adult brain are similar for both locations.

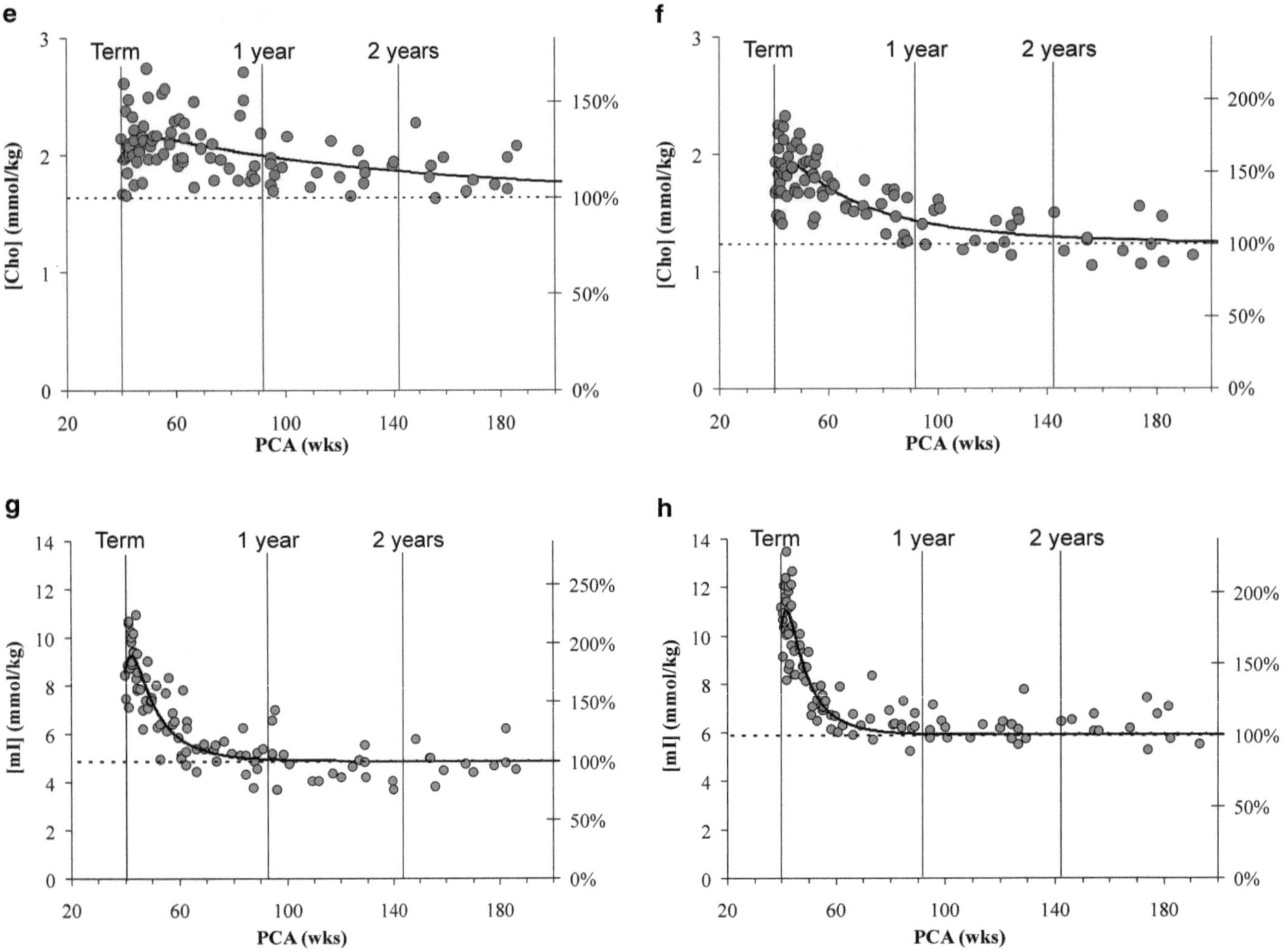

Fig. 3.3 (continued)

Creatine

The next most prominent peak in parietal/occipital gray matter spectra is creatine (Cr) at 3.0 ppm. For normal brain tissue, the creatine peak comprises contributions from free creatine (fCr) and phosphocreatine (PCr) in approximately equal proportions. PCr stores energy. PCr is in rapid chemical exchange with fCr and is used to maintain/replenish adenosine triphosphate (ATP) levels if required by creatine kinase (CK) catalyzed conversion of PCr to fCr:

$$\mathrm{PCr} + \mathrm{ADP} + \mathrm{H+} \rightarrow \mathrm{fCr} + \mathrm{ATP} \tag{3.1}$$

Parietal WM Cr levels at term are approximately 80% of normal adult levels. Creatine rapidly increases thereafter and reaches a transient maximum (≈125% of normal) within the first 6 months of life, then declines gradually, and reaches normal adult levels between 1 and 2 years of age. In a subgroup of this study, MR spectra of right frontal WM were obtained and a similar time course, with a transient maximum concentration within 6 months after birth was observed. In contrast, in parietal/occipital GM, a transient maximum for Cr was not observed. Instead, Cr increased from ≈ 50 to 75% of normal within the first 2–3 months of life and to 95% around 4 years of age (Fig. 3.3c, d). In young adults, the Cr concentration of GM was 7.0 mmol/kg, whereas in WM Cr concentration was lower at 5.1 mmol/kg.

Total Choline

The next prominent peak at 3.2 ppm is commonly referred to as choline (Cho) or trimethylamines (TMA). Choline is a complex peak comprising several choline-containing metabolites and therefore sometimes referred to as total choline. In a previous study using ^{1}H MRS and (phosphorous) ^{31}P MRS in vivo, it was found that the sum of phosphorylated cholines, phosphorylcholine (PCho) and glycerophosphorylcholine (GPC) accounts for most of the choline detected with ^{1}H MRS in normal tissue [20]. Choline-containing compounds are involved in the synthesis and breakdown of phosphatidylcholine (PtdCho = lecithin). PtdCho is the major phospholipid component of eukaryotic cells accounting for approx. 60% of total phospholipids. GPC is also a cerebral osmolyte [21] and a reduction (increase) of GPC in response to hypoosmotic (hyperosmotic) conditions might be reflected by an alteration of total choline. Choline concentrations in white matter are slightly higher than in gray matter and in a normal white matter spectrum Cho is the second most prominent peak after NAA. In tumors, choline levels are generally higher than in normal tissue. Among tumors there appears to be an overall correlation of higher choline concentrations with higher grade tumors. However, it needs to be acknowledged that considerable variations of choline levels within the same tumor type and subtype have been noted [22].

Changes of Cho during early brain development are less dramatic than those observed for NAA and Cr. Choline increased slightly in the first few weeks of life in both parietal WM and parietal/occipital GM and declined gradually thereafter (Fig. 3.3e,f). In parietal WM, initial Cho reached approximately 130% of levels observed in young adults. In GM a maximum of 150% of the Cho levels in young adults was observed. The decline of Cho was more gradual in WM than in GM.

Myo-inositol

Cho, Cr, and NAA can be detected readily and quantified in long *echo time* (TE) MR spectroscopy. Short TE acquisition methods are necessary for reliable quantitation of *myo-inositol* (mI). Myo-inositol is a little-known sugar-like molecule that resonates at 3.6 ppm in the proton spectrum. It has been identified as a marker for astrocytes and is an osmolyte [21, 23]. Myo-inositol is involved in metabolism of phosphatidyl inositol, a membrane phospholipid. Similar to choline, mI is expected to be altered in response to alteration of membrane metabolism or damaged membrane. Myo-inositol is high in the newborn brain but decreases rapidly to normal levels within the first few years of live. Being a marker for astrocytes, mI concentrations are higher in astrocytomas than in normal brain tissue. Myo-inositol is also elevated in gliosis [24] and in some leukodystrophies [25]. An example for reduced mI is hepatic encephalopathy. When interpreting the mI signal in MR spectra, it is important to remember that its signal looks different at different field strengths (cf. Fig. 2.8). Glycine (see below) co-resonates with mI and cannot be distinguished from mI with the method employed in this study. But glycine levels are low and it has previously been reported that it is unlikely that Gly varies significantly during maturation [1].

A small increase of mI to a transient maximum at approximately 200% of normal within the first weeks after term was observed. Myo-inositol concentrations then declined rapidly during further postnatal brain development (Fig. 3.3g, h). Absolute concentrations of mI appear to be slightly higher in GM, particularly at birth, than in WM.

Ratios of NAA, Cho, and mI Relative to Cr

In the literature often ratios relative to Cr have been reported under the assumption that Cr concentrations remain relatively constant. Comparing relative levels of metabolites is also a frequently used strategy for interpreting spectra in clinical practice. Thus, albeit, Cr is clearly not constant in developing brain (or in many diseases), concentration ratios NAA/Cr, Cho/Cr, and mI/Cr are shown in Fig. 3.4. It needs to be emphasized (one more time) that these ratios are specific for the methods used (here: SV-PRESS, TE 35 ms, 1.5 T).

Glutamate and Glutamine

Glutamate (Glu) and *glutamine* (Gln) are important components of the ^{1}H spectrum. Of all metabolites, glutamate is believed to have the highest concentration in normal human brain tissue. Due to their similar chemical structures, glutamate and glutamine form complex and partially overlapping resonances in ^{1}H spectra. Both, glutamate and glutamine have two groups of resonances: The first group (α-Glu and α-Gln) has three peaks between 3.6 ppm and 3.9 ppm whereas the second group (β,γ-Glu and β,γ-Gln) comprises a more complex series of resonances between 2.0 and 2.6 ppm. Accordingly, the quantitation of these chemicals is challenging and often the more robust sum of glutamate + glutamine (Glx) is determined. MR spectra of excellent quality and sophisticated software, such as LCModel [26] that fits all metabolite resonances simultaneously, are essential for reliable independent quantitation of these amino acids. The independent quantitation of Glu and Gln can be considerably improved by moving from 1.5 T to 3 T. Glutamate and glutamine form an important neurotransmitter cycle in the normal brain where glutamate is mainly stored in neurons whereas the glutamine concentration is higher in astrocytes. However, the role of glutamate and glutamine is almost certainly much more complicated. For example, glutamate can be used as a fuel and oxidized to substitute for glucose metabolism in hypoglycemic states [27, 28]. Excessive synaptic glutamate may cause nerve cell damage due to excessive excitation. Glutamine increases under hypoxic stress and under hyperammonemic conditions [29].

Glutamate concentrations increased rapidly from $\approx$25% at term in parietal WM and reached a transient maximum within the first year of life. A transient maximum was not observed for parietal/occipital GM where Glu increased from $\approx$25% to adult levels within the first year of life and remained close to constant thereafter. Glu in GM is approximately 50% higher than in parietal WM (Fig. 3.5a, b). The interpretation of the transient maximum of Glu in WM and an early plateau in GM is unclear. The time courses of Glu concentration suggest that maturation of glutamatergic

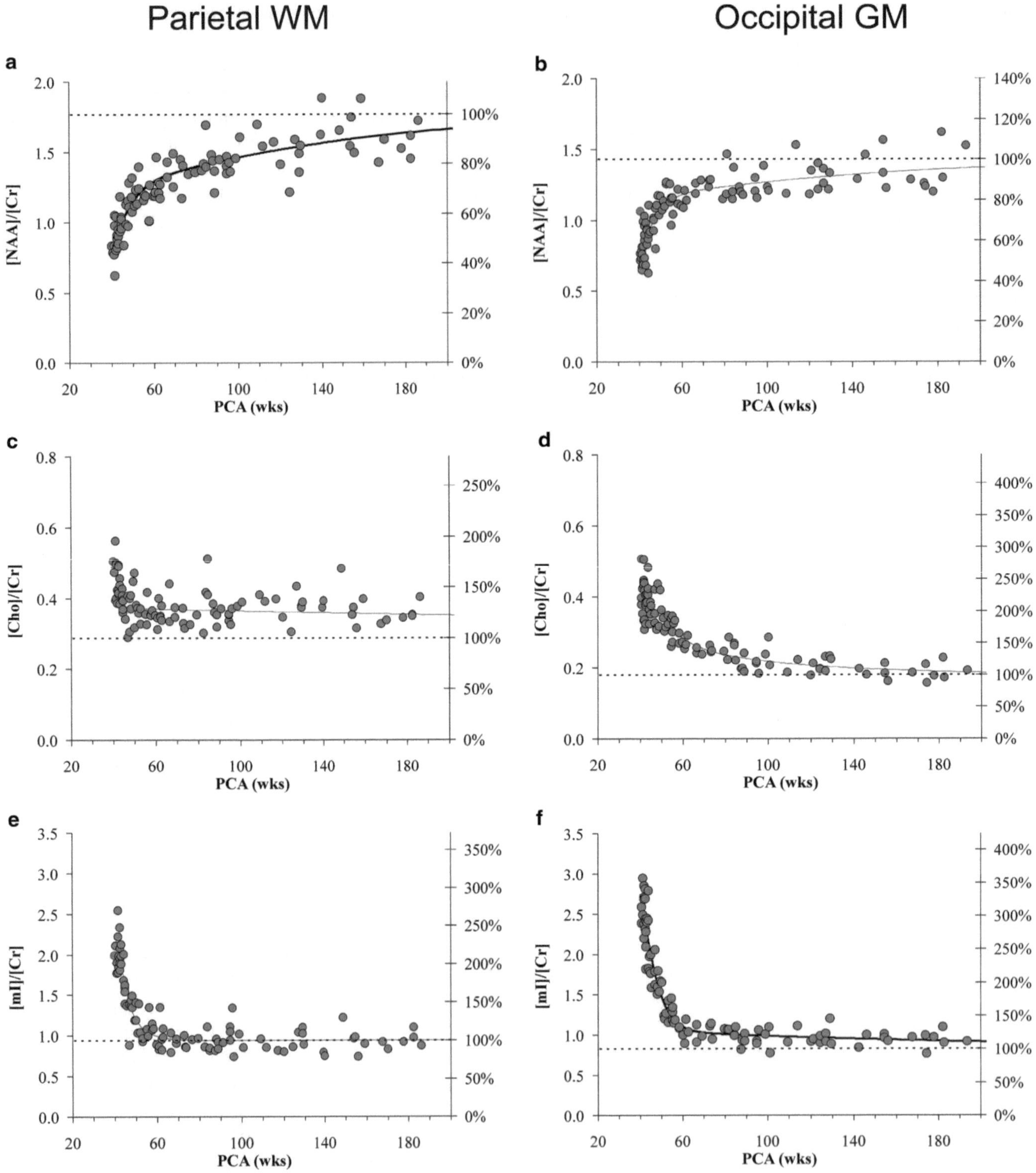

Fig. 3.4 (**a–f**) The concentration ratios of NAA/Cr, Cho/Cr, and mI/Cr are plotted versus postconceptional age. Note these are not intensity ratios! For example, the nine equivalent proton of the choline molecule give three times more signal than the three equivalent protons of creatine (at 3.0 ppm). This means, if visual inspection of a spectrum shows approximately equal Cr and Cho peaks, the concentration ratio [Cho]/[Cr] will be approximately 0.33

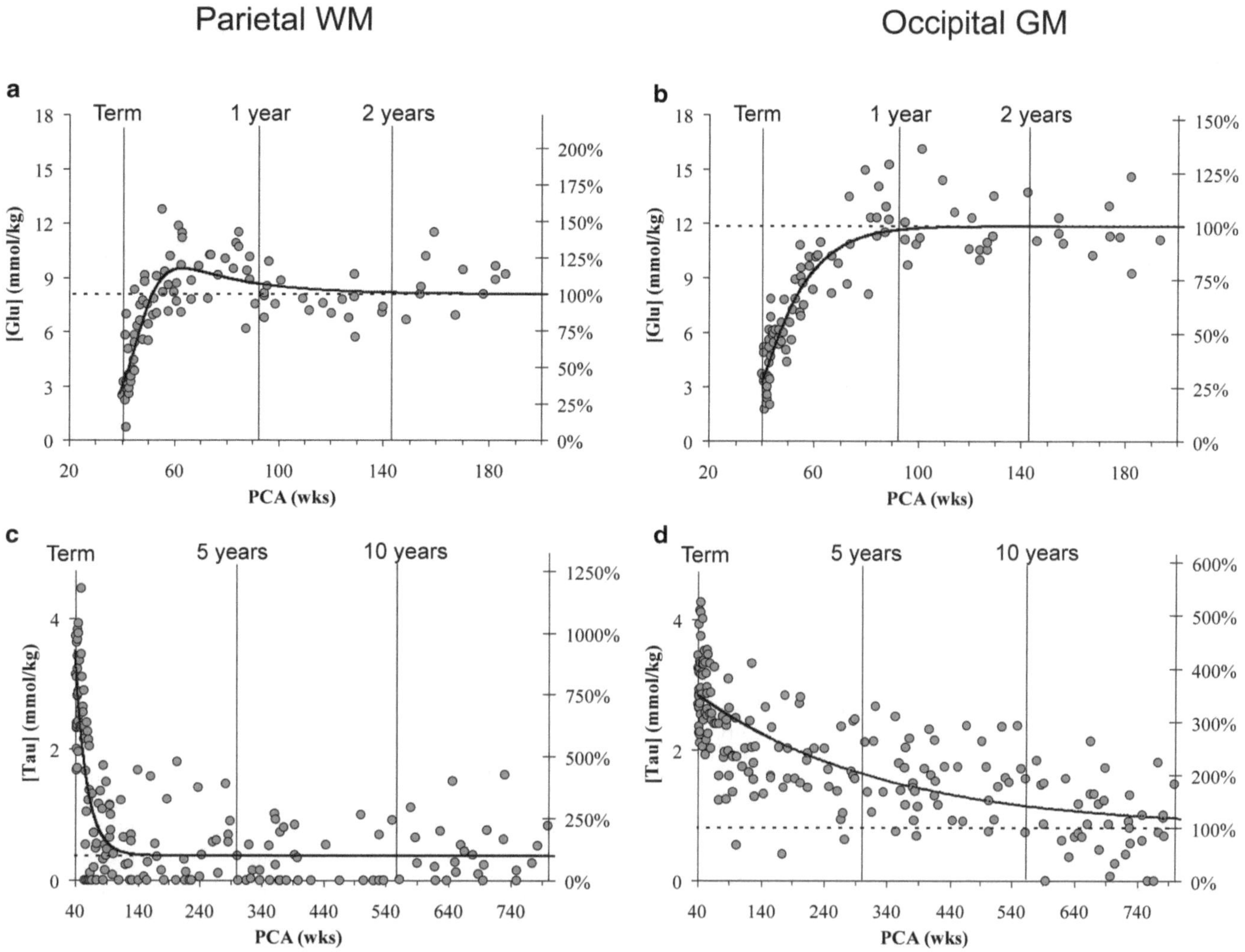

Fig. 3.5 Both in parietal WM (**a**) and parietal/occipital GM (**b**) an initial rapid increase of glutamate is observed. In WM a transient maximum is reached at around 6 months and thereafter glutamates decline gradually to levels observed in young adults. In GM, a significant transient maximum was not observed. Taurine can be detected in white matter at the very early stages of brain development (**c**) but then very quickly declines to concentrations that are at or below the level of detection. In parietal/occipital GM (**d**) a more gradual decline is observed

neurons and the maximum density of their axon/dendrite network, in each location studied are reached within the first year of life. In contrast, NAA, possibly a more general marker for adult-type neurons and axons, has a different developmental curve and does not reach a plateau before 5 years of age for both locations (cf. Fig. 3.3a, b). On the other hand, developmental curves for Cr (cf. Fig. 3.3c,d) are similar to the Glu curves in both locations. A detailed analysis shows, however, that the rise of Cr slightly precedes the increase of Glu in both locations (see fit parameter A_5 in Table 3.1). No significant age-dependent changes were observed for Gln. Consequently, the sum of glutamate + glutamine (Glx) showed a time course similar to that of Glu.

Taurine

Taurine, an aminosulfonic acid, is abundant in developing cerebellum and isocortex [30] and taurine levels are generally high in less differentiated brains of neonates [1]. In adults the detection and quantitation of taurine is difficult due to its low concentration and spectral overlap with scyllo-inositol. Pathologically elevated taurine has been detected in pediatric brain medulloblastoma [31, 32]. Taurine is predominantly obtained from the diet but it can also be synthesized from amino acids in the brain. The taurine signal at ≈ 4 ppm is complex and its pattern changes with the field strength (see Fig. 2.8). Taurine levels decreased in both WM and GM locations. Whereas Tau fell below the limits of detection in WM locations within the first 2–4 years of life, Tau declined more gradually in parietal/occipital GM (Fig. 3.5c, d).

Lactate

Lactate (Lac) is an important metabolite since it indicates anaerobic metabolism. Lactate can be detected at pathologically elevated concentrations, whereas in healthy tissue the lactate concentration is too low for routine detection with currently available methods. Careful positioning of the region of interest is required because the lactate concentration of cerebrospinal fluid (CSF) is approximately 1 mmol/l. Consequently, a spectrum acquired from a voxel with a significant partial volume of CSF might therefore show the typical doublet of lactate at 1.33 ppm even in a healthy control. Lactate is the product of anaerobic glycolysis and increases when subsequent oxidation of lactate in the TCA cycle is impaired (for example by lack of oxygen or mitochondrial disorders). Lactate has great prognostic value for global hypoxic/ischemic injuries. An elevation of lactate even in *normal* appearing tissue would indicate global disruption/impairment of perfusion consistent with hypoxia and eventual poor outcome [33–37].

Consistent with earlier reports [5] we have observed Lac in normal premature babies (Fig. 3.6). At term or shortly thereafter, Lac is hardly detectable with routine MRS methods that are available today (cf. Fig. 3.2).

Glucose

Relative glucose concentration ratios of normal plasma, cerebrospinal fluid, and brain tissue are approximately 3:2:1. Glucose (Glc) has two resonances: one at 3.43 ppm and one at 3.80 ppm, partially overlapping with a-glutamate and a-glutamine (Fig. 3.7). The Glc spectrum is thus quite different from that of Tau and there is little covariance of Glc and Tau. Still, because of low glucose concentrations and low signal intensity, the accuracy of quantitation of glucose in individual spectra is low. Glucose is the principal fuel for cells. It is broken down in a two-step process: glycolysis with the end-product pyruvate, and then complete oxidation in the tricarboxylic acid (TCA) cycle. Elevated and sometimes prominent glucose is obviously observed in diabetes. Glucose may also be above normal in other conditions where energy production from glucose is impaired such as coma or following hypoxic/ischemic injury. Because glucose is taken up from the diet and readily transported into the brain it is unique among the metabolites that are routinely detectable because its tissue concentration can change. No significant age-dependent changes were observed in our control subjects.

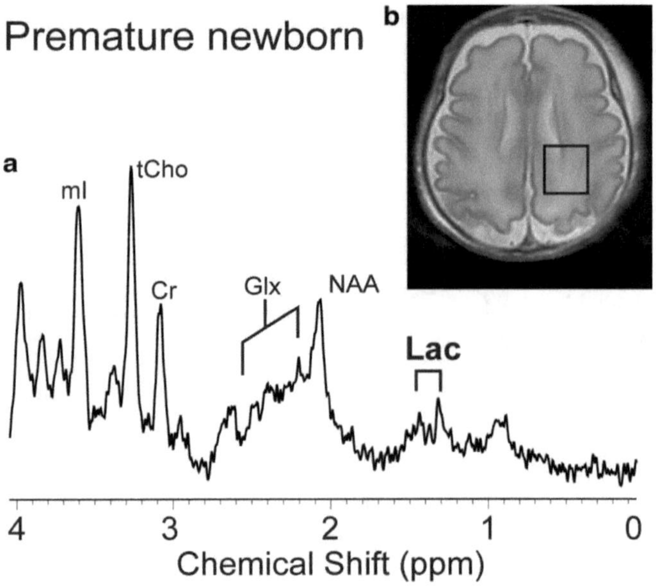

Fig. 3.6 (**a**) Lactate forms a typical doublet at 1.3 ppm and can readily be detected (unless obscured by a huge lipid peak in pathology) if present (cf. Fig 3.7). At 1.5 T lactate is basically undetectable in normal brain. (**b**) However, lactate can be observed in premature babies with normal MRI

Lipids and Macromolecules

The protons of the methyl groups ($-CH_3$) of lipid molecules resonate at 0.9 ppm whereas protons of the methylene groups ($-CH_2-$) resonate at 1.3 ppm in the ^{1}H spectrum. Both resonances are broad and may also comprise contributions from other macromolecules. Thus in the literature, any signal in this part of the spectrum is labeled as "lipids," "MM" (for macromolecules) or "lipids + MM". In normal tissue, the concentration of free lipids is small and there should be very little signal in this part of the spectrum. Lipid signals increase when there is breakdown of cell membrane and release of fatty acids. Lipids (and macromolecules) have short T2-relaxation times. This means that the contribution of lipids to spectra is greatly suppressed when a long echo time is selected (e.g., TE = 144 ms). Visual inspection of spectra in Fig. 3.2 shows that there are little changes of the MR-detectable lipid content during brain maturation.

Citrate, Alanine, Scyllo-Inositol, Glycine

Citrate (Cit) is an intermediate product of the tricarboxylic acid cycle (TCA cycle) and forms a multiplet at around 2.6 ppm. The concentrations of this metabolite are found to be low in the human brain with possible causes of accumulation being metabolic, pathological, or both. Citrate has been observed in pediatric brain tumors with the highest concentrations in diffuse intrinsic brain stem gliomas [38, 39].

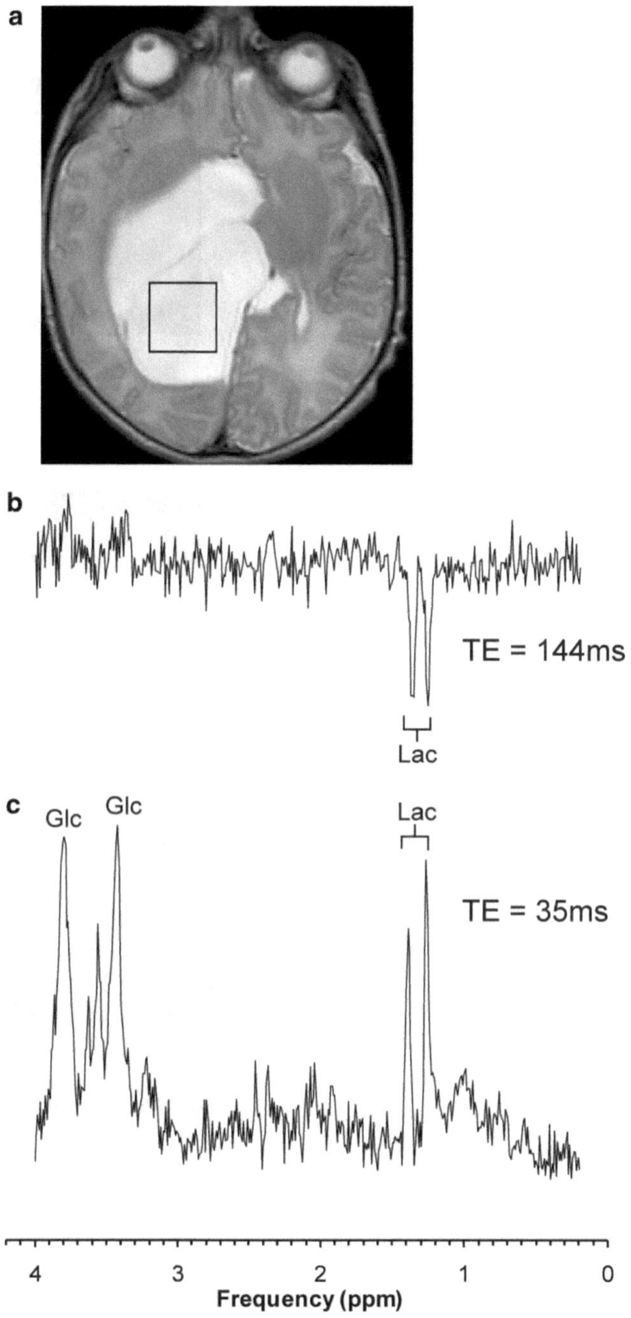

Fig. 3.7 (**a–c**) Glucose is generally too low for reliable detection. However, prominent glucose was observed in this cystic lesion with short TE PRESS (**c**) whereas it is not readily observable with longer echo times (**b**). Both spectra show also the typical doublet for lactate

In controls, there was little or no evidence for citrate in subjects older than 6 months. However, citrate was observed in newborns [38].

Similar to lactate, alanine (Ala) can be observed with current methods only at pathologically elevated concentrations. Alanine forms a characteristic doublet similar to that of lactate at 1.48 ppm and has been detected previously in multiple sclerosis and in tumors [22, 40, 41].

The scyllo-inositol (sI) peak at 3.36 ppm is partially overlapping with taurine. In contrast to taurine, which has a complex pattern, sI is a singlet arising from six equivalent protons of this molecule. The sI peak is usually very weak and can thus not be quantified reliably in individual spectra. Occasionally, prominent sI is observed in tumors and other conditions. The causes and significance of elevated sI are not understood.

Glycine (Gly) is an amino acid with a resonance as a singlet peak around 3.55 ppm and is better observed at 1.5 T with long TE MRS as it overlaps with myo-inositol. It is the smallest amino acid located within the brain and CNS, with a concentration in human adult brain at approximately 1 mM. The roles of glycine include acting as an inhibitory neurotransmitter and antioxidant. The synthesis of the metabolite is from glucose via serine and it is readily converted to creatine [42, 43]. Glycine has been found to be increased in brain tumors, particularly found to be increased with WHO grading. Levels of glycine have been found to be high in medulloblastomas and glioblastomas [43–46].

Other Metabolites Detectable with ^{1}H Magnetic Resonance Spectroscopy

Several other metabolites can be detected with ^{1}H MRS in certain diseases or under certain conditions. This includes leucine, isoleucine, and valine (0.9 ppm), acetate (1.92), and succinate (2.4 ppm) in abscesses from infections (details in Chap. 13, Infection and Encephalitis). MR spectra obtained in patients with metabolic disorders (Chap. 11, Metabolic Disorders) may also show unusual peaks. For example, the branched chain amino acids leucine, isoleucine, and valine are also detectable in Maple Syrup Urine Disease (MSUP). Other additional peaks are observed after the ingestion of alcohol, in unusual diets (ketone bodies such as acetone after ketogenic diet) [47] or following the administration of large amounts of medication such as mannitol or propylene glycol (solvent for drugs).

Regional Variations

Frontal White Matter, Basal Ganglia, Pons, and Cerebellum

Parietal white matter and parietal/occipital gray matter have been popular regions for in vivo MRS because good quality spectra from these brain regions have been obtained early on when MRS was less robust. With the advancers in technology, other brain regions are now being studied more frequently. In this paragraph, we show a few examples for spectra obtained from other brain regions that might be of interest for investigators.

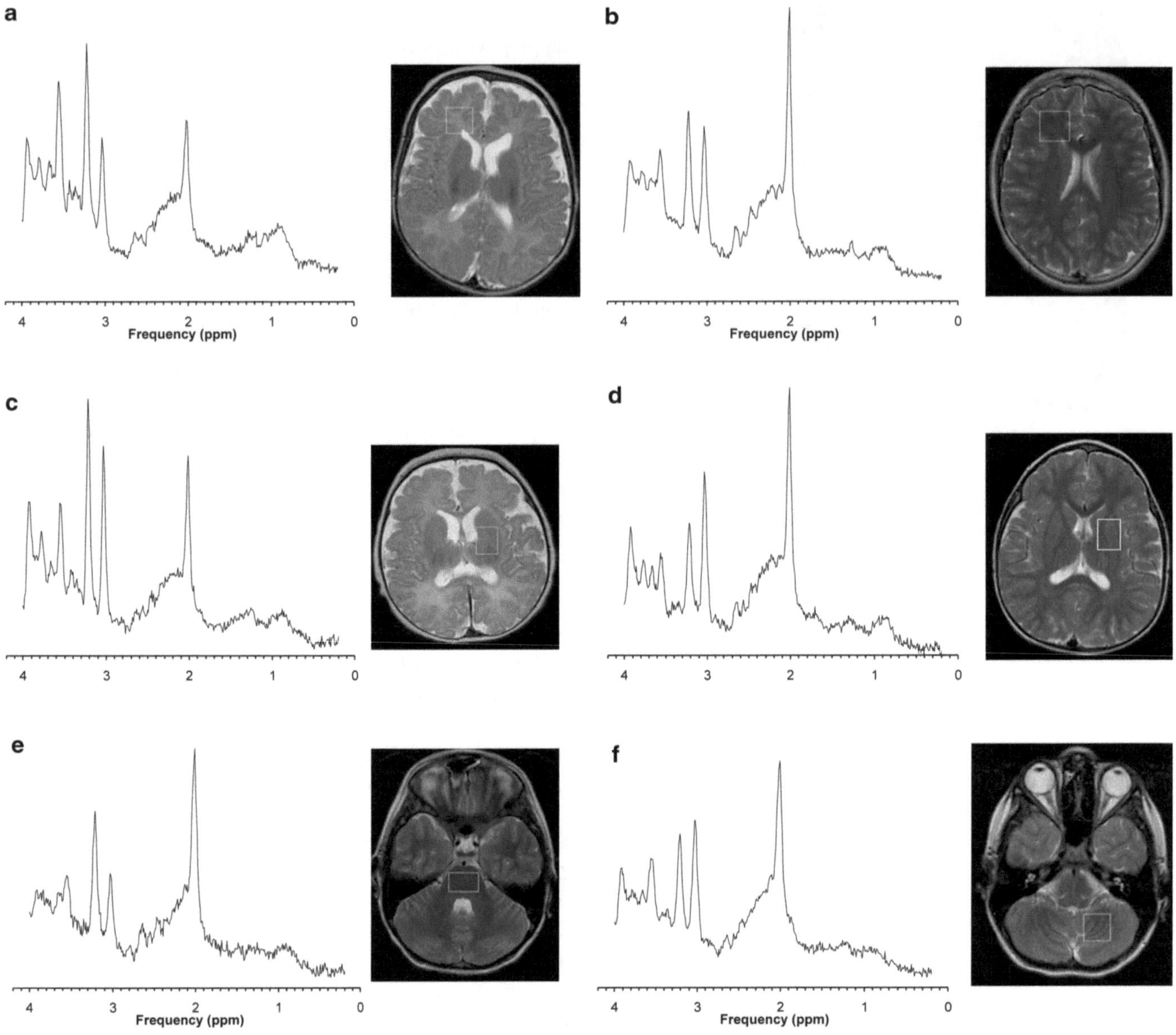

Fig. 3.8 (**a–f**) Shown are typical single-voxel PRESS, TE 35 ms, spectra acquired from various brain regions to demonstrate regional variations

A representative spectrum of frontal WM shortly after birth (average of four studies in patients with normal MRI and unremarkable follow-up) is shown in Fig. 3.8a. In contrast, a typical frontal WM spectrum for children around 10 years of age is shown in Fig. 3.8b. The spectra show a metabolic profile that is comparable with parietal WM spectra (cf. Fig. 3.2). Basal ganglia (BG) spectra of a 4-week-old baby (Fig. 3.8c) and of an 11-year-old child (Fig. 3.8d) show a pattern similar to gray matter spectra (cf. Fig. 3.2). Minor differences between parietal/occipital GM and BG are a slightly lower NAA and myo-inositol in BG. In contrast, a brainstem spectrum acquired at the level of the pons in a 10-year-old child (Fig. 3.8e) shows comparably prominent Cho and low Cr. The complex signal of glutamate and glutamine also appears to be less prominent in the spectrum acquired from the pons. NAA in the cerebellum in healthy controls appears to be lower than in other brain regions (Fig. 3.8f).

References

1. Kreis R, Hofmann L, Kuhlmann B, Boesch C, Bossi E, Huppi PS. Brain metabolite composition during early human brain development as measured by quantitative in vivo ^{1}H magnetic resonance spectroscopy. Magn Reson Med. 2002;48(6):949–58.
2. van der Knaap MS, van der Grond J, van Rijen PC, Faber JA, Valk J, Willemse K. Age-dependent changes in localized proton and phosphorus MR spectroscopy of the brain. Radiology. 1990;176(2):509–15.

3. Huppi PS, Posse S, Lazeyras F, Burri R, Bossi E, Herschkowitz N. Magnetic resonance in preterm and term newborns: [1]H-spectroscopy in developing human brain. Pediatr Res. 1991;30(6):574–8.
4. Toft PB, Leth H, Lou HC, Pryds O, Henriksen O. Metabolite concentrations in the developing brain estimated with proton MR spectroscopy. J Magn Reson Imaging. 1994;4(5):674–80.
5. Cady EB, Penrice J, Amess PN, et al. Lactate, N-acetylaspartate, choline and creatine concentrations, and spin-spin relaxation in thalamic and occipito-parietal regions of developing human brain. Magn Reson Med. 1996;36(6):878–86.
6. Kreis R, Ernst T, Ross BD. Development of the human brain: in vivo quantification of metabolite and water content with proton magnetic resonance spectroscopy. Magn Reson Med. 1993;30(4):424–37.
7. Pouwels PJ, Brockmann K, Kruse B, et al. Regional age dependence of human brain metabolites from infancy to adulthood as detected by quantitative localized proton MRS. Pediatr Res. 1999;46(4):474–85.
8. Castillo M, Kwock L, Green C. MELAS syndrome: imaging and proton MR spectroscopic findings. AJNR Am J Neuroradiol. 1995;16(2):233–9.
9. Nanto-Salonen K, Komu M, Lundbom N, et al. Reduced brain creatine in gyrate atrophy of the choroid and retina with hyperornithinemia. Neurology. 1999;53(2):303–7.
10. Ross BD, Danielsen ER, Bluml S. Proton magnetic resonance spectroscopy: the new gold standard for diagnosis of clinical and subclinical hepatic encephalopathy? Dig Dis. 1996;14 Suppl 1:30–9.
11. Smart JL, Dobbing J, Adlard BP, Lynch A, Sands J. Vulnerability of developing brain: relative effects of growth restriction during the fetal and suckling periods on behavior and brain composition of adult rats. J Nutr. 1973;103(9):1327–38.
12. Lentner C. Geigy scientific tables. In: Ciba G, editor. Units of measurement body fluids nutrition, vol. 1. Ciba-Geigy: Basel, Switzerland; 1981. p. 220. 222, 223.
13. Ernst T, Kreis R, Ross BD. Absolute quantitation of water and metabolites in the human brain. I. Compartments and water. J Magn Reson. 1993;102:1–8.
14. Tallan HH. Studies on the distribution of N-acetyl-L-aspartic acid in brain. J Biol Chem. 1957;224(1):41–5.
15. Baslow MH. Functions of N-acetyl-L-aspartate and N-acetyl-L-aspartylglutamate in the vertebrate brain: role in glial cell-specific signaling. J Neurochem. 2000;75(2):453–9.
16. Kreis R, Ernst T, Ross BD. Absolute quantitation of water and metabolites in the human brain. II. Metabolite concentrations. J Magn Reson. 1993;102:9–19.
17. Brooks WM, Stidley CA, Petropoulos H, et al. Metabolic and cognitive response to human traumatic brain injury: a quantitative proton magnetic resonance study. J Neurotrauma. 2000;17(8):629–40.
18. Gasparovic C, Arfai N, Smid N, Feeney DM. Decrease and recovery of N-acetylaspartate/creatine in rat brain remote from focal injury. J Neurotrauma. 2001;18(3):241–6.
19. Schuhmann MU, Stiller D, Skardelly M, Thomas S, Samii M, Brinker T. Long-time in-vivo metabolic monitoring following experimental brain contusion using proton magnetic resonance spectroscopy. Acta Neurochir Suppl. 2002;81:209–12.
20. Bluml S, Seymour KJ, Ross BD. Developmental changes in choline- and ethanolamine-containing compounds measured with proton-decoupled (31)P MRS in in vivo human brain. Magn Reson Med. 1999;42(4):643–54.
21. Lien YH, Shapiro JI, Chan L. Effects of hypernatremia on organic brain osmoles. J Clin Invest. 1990;85(5):1427–35.
22. Panigrahy A, Krieger MD, Gonzalez-Gomez I, et al. Quantitative short echo time [1]H-MR spectroscopy of untreated pediatric brain tumors: preoperative diagnosis and characterization. AJNR Am J Neuroradiol. 2006;27(3):560–72.
23. Videen JS. Human cerebral osmolytes during chronic hyponatremia. A proton magnetic resonance spectroscopy study. [see comments.]. J Clin Investig. 1995;95(2):788–93.
24. Bitsch A, Bruhn H, Vougioukas V, et al. Inflammatory CNS demyelination: histopathologic correlation with in vivo quantitative proton MR spectroscopy. AJNR: Am J Neuroradiol. 1999;20(9):1619–27.
25. Kruse B, Hanefeld F, Christen HJ, et al. Alterations of brain metabolites in metachromatic leukodystrophy as detected by localized proton magnetic resonance spectroscopy in vivo. J Neurol. 1993;241(2):68–74.
26. Provencher SW. Estimation of metabolite concentrations from localized in vivo proton NMR spectra. Magn Reson Med. 1993;30(6):672–9.
27. Daikhin Y, Yudkoff M. Compartmentation of brain glutamate metabolism in neurons and glia. J Nutr. 2000;130(4S Suppl):1026S–31S.
28. Erecinska M, Silver IA. Metabolism and role of glutamate in mammalian brain. Prog Neurobiol. 1990;35(4):245–96.
29. Kreis R. Metabolic disorders of the brain in chronic hepatic encephalopathy detected with H-1 MR spectroscopy. [see comments.]. Radiology. 1992;182(1):19–27.
30. Flint AC, Liu X, Kriegstein AR. Nonsynaptic glycine receptor activation during early neocortical development. Neuron. 1998;20(1):43–53.
31. Kovanlikaya A, Panigrahy A, Krieger M, et al. Untreated pediatric primitive neuroectodermal tumor in vivo: quantitation of taurine with MR spectroscopy. Radiology. 2005;236(3):1020–5.
32. Moreno-Torres A, Martinez-Perez I, Baquero M, et al. Taurine detection by proton magnetic resonance spectroscopy in medulloblastoma: Contribution to noninvasive differential diagnosis with cerebellar astrocytomas. Neurosurgery. 2004;55:824–9.
33. Ross BD, Ernst T, Kreis R, et al. ^{1}H MRS in acute traumatic brain injury. J Magn Reson Imaging. 1998;8(4):829–40.
34. Holshouser BA, Ashwal S, Luh GY, et al. Proton MR spectroscopy after acute central nervous system injury: outcome prediction in neonates, infants, and children. Radiology. 1997;202(2):487–96.
35. Holshouser BA, Ashwal S, Shu S, Hinshaw Jr DB. Proton MR spectroscopy in children with acute brain injury: comparison of short and long echo time acquisitions. J Magn Reson Imaging. 2000;11(1):9–19.
36. Haseler LJ, Arcinue E, Danielsen ER, Bluml S, Ross BD. Evidence from proton magnetic resonance spectroscopy for a metabolic cascade of neuronal damage in shaken baby syndrome. Pediatrics. 1997;99(1):4–14.
37. Condon B, Oluoch-Olunya D, Hadley D, Teasdale G, Wagstaff A. Early ^{1}H magnetic resonance spectroscopy of acute head injury: four cases. J Neurotrauma. 1998;15(8):563–71.
38. Seymour ZA, Panigrahy A, Finlay JL, Nelson Jr MD, Bluml S. Citrate in pediatric CNS tumors? AJNR Am J Neuroradiol. 2008;29(5):1006–11.
39. Costello LC, Franklin RB, Narayan P. Citrate in the diagnosis of prostate cancer. Prostate. 1999;38(3):237–45.
40. Gill SS, Thomas DG, Van Bruggen N, et al. Proton MR spectroscopy of intracranial tumours: in vivo and in vitro studies. J Comput Assist Tomogr. 1990;14(4):497–504.
41. Howe FA, Barton SJ, Cudlip SA, et al. Metabolic profiles of human brain tumors using quantitative in vivo ^{1}H magnetic resonance spectroscopy. Magn Reson Med. 2003;49(2):223–32.
42. Govindaraju V, Young K, Maudsley AA. Proton NMR chemical shifts and coupling constants for brain metabolites. NMR Biomed. 2000;13(3):129–53.
43. Davies NP, Wilson M, Natarajan K, et al. Non-invasive detection of glycine as a biomarker of malignancy in childhood brain tumours using in-vivo ^{1}H MRS at 1.5 tesla confirmed by ex-vivo high-resolution magic-angle spinning NMR. NMR Biomed. 2010;23(1):80–7.

44. Carapella CM, Carpinelli G, Knijn A, Raus L, Caroli F, Podo F. Potential role of in vitro ^{1}H magnetic resonance spectroscopy in the definition of malignancy grading of human neuroepithelial brain tumours. Acta Neurochir Suppl. 1997;68:127–32.
45. Lehnhardt FG, Röhn G, Ernestus RI, Grüne M, Hoehn M. [1]H- and (31)P-MR spectroscopy of primary and recurrent human brain tumors in vitro: malignancy-characteristic profiles of water soluble and lipophilic spectral components. NMR Biomed. 2001;14(5):307–17.
46. Lehnhardt FG, Bock C, Röhn G, Ernestus RI, Hoehn M. Metabolic differences between primary and recurrent human brain tumors: a ^{1}H NMR spectroscopic investigation. NMR Biomed. 2005;18(6):371–82.
47. Seymour KJ, Bluml S, Sutherling J, Sutherling W, Ross BD. Identification of cerebral acetone by ^{1}H-MRS in patients with epilepsy controlled by ketogenic diet. Magma. 1999;8(1):33–42.

4 Challenges in Pediatric Magnetic Resonance Imaging

Jessica L. Wisnowski, Vera R. Sperling, and Ashok Panigrahy

Recent advances in magnetic resonance imaging (MRI) have vastly improved the delineation of Central Nervous System (CNS) anatomy and the diagnosis and extent of pediatric CNS pathology. MRI is noninvasive and does not utilize ionizing radiation. Relative to other available imaging modalities, MRI provides higher spatial resolution and better contrast between healthy tissue types (i.e., gray and white matter) and between pathology and *normal* tissue. Additionally, physiology, function, and metabolism can now be evaluated and assessed by MRI. Advanced imaging sequences such as diffusion-weighted imaging (DWI) and diffusion tensor imaging (DTI), MR spectroscopy (MRS), perfusion imaging (e.g., Arterial Spin Labeling/ASL or dynamic contrast enhanced/DCE), functional MRI (fMRI), and CSF flow studies all provide complementary information to that obtained from anatomic imaging and provide further characterization of disease pathophysiology, response to therapy, and/or disease progression.

However, numerous challenges exist in pediatric MR imaging, which, generally speaking, stem from two interacting factors: the subject population and the MR environment. To begin, neonatal and pediatric patients are not more compacted versions of adults. Rather, relative to adults, they demonstrate marked differences in both the structure and function of their central nervous systems. Structurally, there is much higher water content and much lower lipid content in the brains of infants and children. This stems from both the composition of the extracellular matrix and the extent of myelination, which begins along specific tracts in the third trimester of fetal gestation and extends well into the postnatal years [1]. Importantly, these differences cause a lengthening of the T2-relaxation time with decreasing age necessitating longer echo times for younger patients. Similarly, the T1-relaxation is longer for infants and young children and varies with the magnetic field strength. In general, this results in the need for longer inversion times (TI) for acquisition of T1-weighted scans in infants. Finally, the higher water content and lower anisotropy necessitates a lower b-value for infants in order to obtain sufficient signal to noise in diffusion-weighted imaging.

In addition to modifying the sequences to allow for differences in the T1-relaxation and T2-relaxation constants, in pediatric MR, sequences are often modified to accommodate a smaller field of view (FOV). However, the smaller FOV is associated with less signal to noise, thereby often necessitating longer scan times in order to obtain adequate signal to noise.

Functionally, or more specifically, psychologically, infants and children respond differently to the MR environment and to the constraints necessary for obtaining adequate MR data. For example, children, particularly when not introduced to the MR environment in an age-appropriate manner, may become afraid of the scanner or the loud sounds that it makes. Additionally, they often find it challenging to hold still during the MR sequences, which may lead to images that are complicated by motion artifact. Infants, though not necessarily afraid, may be startled by the noise associated with MR sequences and lack the capacity to volitionally lie still during the MRI. As a result, for clinically necessitated scans, infants and children are frequently sedated (using conscious sedation or general anesthesia). Alternatives to sedation include

J.L. Wisnowski, Ph.D. (✉)
Brain and Creativity Institute and Dornsife Cognitive Neuroscience Imaging Center, University of Southern California, Los Angeles, CA, USA

V.R. Sperling, M.D.
Department of Pediatric Radiology, Children's Hospital of Pittsburgh of UPMC, 4401 Penn Ave, Pittsburgh, PA 15224, USA
e-mail: sperlingvr@upmc.edu

A. Panigrahy, Ph.D.
Department of Pediatric Radiology, Children's Hospital of Pittsburgh of UPMC, 4401 Penn Ave, Pittsburgh, PA 15224, USA

Department of Radiology, University of Pittsburgh School of Medicine, 4401 Penn Avenue, Suite Floor 2, Pittsburgh, PA 15224, USA
e-mail: Ashok.Panigrahy@chp.edu

S. Blüml and A. Panigrahy (eds.), *MR Spectroscopy of Pediatric Brain Disorders*,
DOI 10.1007/978-1-4419-5864-8_4, © Springer Science+Business Media, LLC 2013

obtaining the MRI scan during natural sleep (e.g., using *feed and bundle* procedures in young infants) or the use of distraction techniques (e.g., watching movies using MR compatible video goggles). Additionally, children often benefit from the opportunity to experience the MR environment and even *practice* before their MRI scans, which may be provided through the use of mock scanners.

In addition to the challenges associated with obtaining scans in pediatric patients, pediatric diseases are rare and accurate diagnosis is complicated by the need to obtain normative data from adequate numbers of diagnosed patients and healthy, typically developing children across the age span (preterm to late adolescent). This is often most challenging for disorders that present between late infancy and early school age, when, in most circumstances, research scans must be obtained without the use of sedation. As alternatives to community samples of healthy children, researchers and clinicians often rely on children who undergo clinically indicated MRIs but are found to have no intracranial pathology (the *nearly normal*) as sources of normative comparison patients in this age range.

Technological Advancements That Aid Pediatric Magnetic Resonance Imaging

In the last 10–15 years, a number of technological advancements have been made, which not only improve the quality of pediatric MR imaging, but also enhance the experience of the child while providing unprecedented information regarding normal development, disease pathophysiology, and treatment response. To begin, in the last decade, high field MR systems (e.g., 3 T) have become almost commonplace in pediatric settings, alongside 1.5 T MR systems. These higher field systems often allow for faster acquisitions at higher spatial resolution due to the inherent increase in signal at 3.0 T relative to 1.5 T. Additionally, multichannel radiofrequency coils and parallel imaging have further accelerated MR acquisition. At the time this chapter was prepared, 96-channel coils were being commercially introduced, allowing for relatively artifact-free image reconstructions based on acquisitions with an acceleration factor of six [2] and potentially eliminating the need for sedation in certain pediatric cases. However, the parallel imaging afforded by multichannel systems provides a paradox for pediatric imaging: the potential for faster imaging, better spatial resolution, and higher signal to noise (SNR), but only in the regions closest to the head coil. In contrast, in adults, SNR in the center of the brain and in the brainstem is no higher in the 96-channel coil than in the 32-channel coil and may result in even lower SNR in the center of the brain when combined with higher acceleration factors during parallel imaging [3]. This latter point is vital, because, in general, pediatric heads are smaller than adult heads and depending on whether the child is positioned so that their brain is truly centered in the coil or positioned toward the back of the coil, there may be too little SNR or marked SNR difference across the child's brain—beyond which is generally corrected for in standard B1 inhomogeneity corrections. The reason for the relatively lower SNR in the center of the brain compared to the periphery (i.e., cortex) stems from the necessity of building smaller and smaller coil elements in order to fit a larger number of coils across the same surface area. As the receive-only coil elements become smaller in size, they become less sensitive at a given distance compared to larger coil elements. Given that the center of the head coil is furthest from all coil elements, any added signal to noise due to the additional elements is counterbalanced by the decreased sensitivity of each of the individual elements, resulting in approximately the same SNR at the center (absent parallel imaging) from these ultramultichannel coils, compared to earlier 32-channel coils. Notably, multichannel pediatric coils are now becoming commercially available, which provide the advantages expected from parallel imaging without the detrimental impact on SNR associated with the adult coils [3].

Aside from multichannel coils and parallel imaging, other ways of improving image quality and decreasing motion artifact in pediatric MR imaging include the use of motion-corrected or *single-shot* sequences. Motion-corrected sequences, such as *periodically rotated overlapping parallel lines with enhanced reconstruction* (PROPELLER) essentially oversample k-space while rotating the phase-encoding lines. The result after reconstruction is an image acquisition that is more robust to patient movement (though not all patient movements) (Fig. 4.1). Another option is a *single-shot* MRI (ssMRI) sequence where the entire raw dataset is acquired within a single excitation pulse and each of the subsequent echoes is given a different phase encoding. ssMRI sequences are useful when large movements are expected such as during fetal MR.

Finally, during the last 2 decades pediatric MR imaging has been aided by the development of technologies and environments specifically designed for the pediatric population. This includes specifically designed pediatric and neonatal head coils (Fig. 4.2) and devices such as MR-compatible incubators that not only allow for the imaging of even the most fragile preterm infants in an environment that mimics the incubators in the neonatal intensive care, but also provides greater ease in transport and minimal manipulation of these infants in the MR suite, as the infants may be placed into the incubators and stabilized while still in the NICU, and then transported directly into the MR scanner without

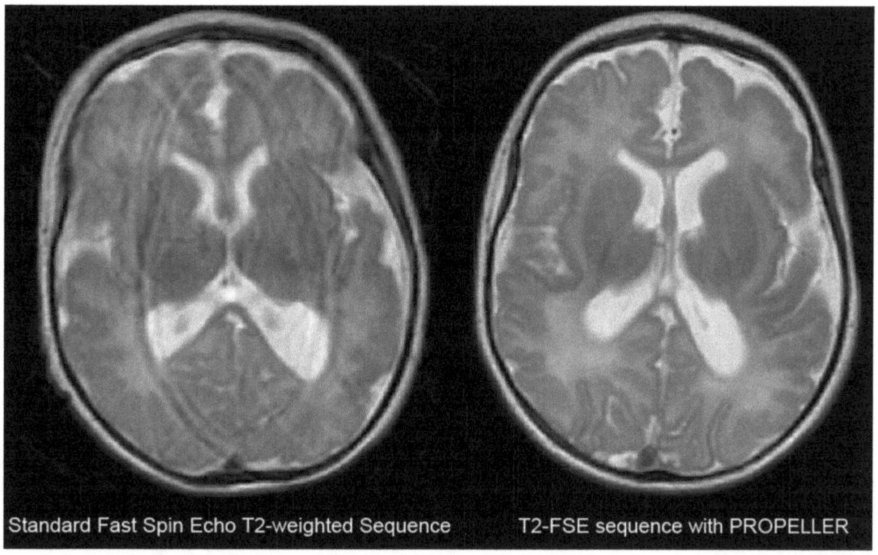

Fig. 4.1 Term infant imaged using a standard T2-weighted Fast Spin Echo (FSE) sequence (*left*) and T2-FSE sequence with PROPELLER (*right*) using a neonatal transmit-receive head coil. Note the polymicrogyria in the bilateral regions apparent on the image obtained with the PROPELLER sequence

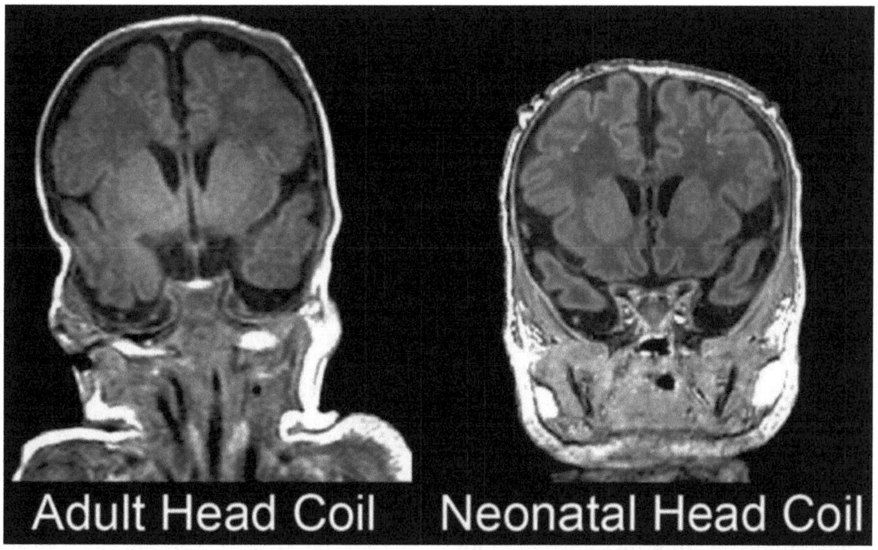

Fig. 4.2 Late preterm infant imaged with a SPGR sequence on the same day using a standard transmit-receive (bird cage) adult head coil and a commercially available transmit-receive neonatal coil. Note that the enhanced contrast between the cortex and the underlying white matter as well as the hyperintense lesions apparent in the SPGR sequence obtained with the neonatal head coil

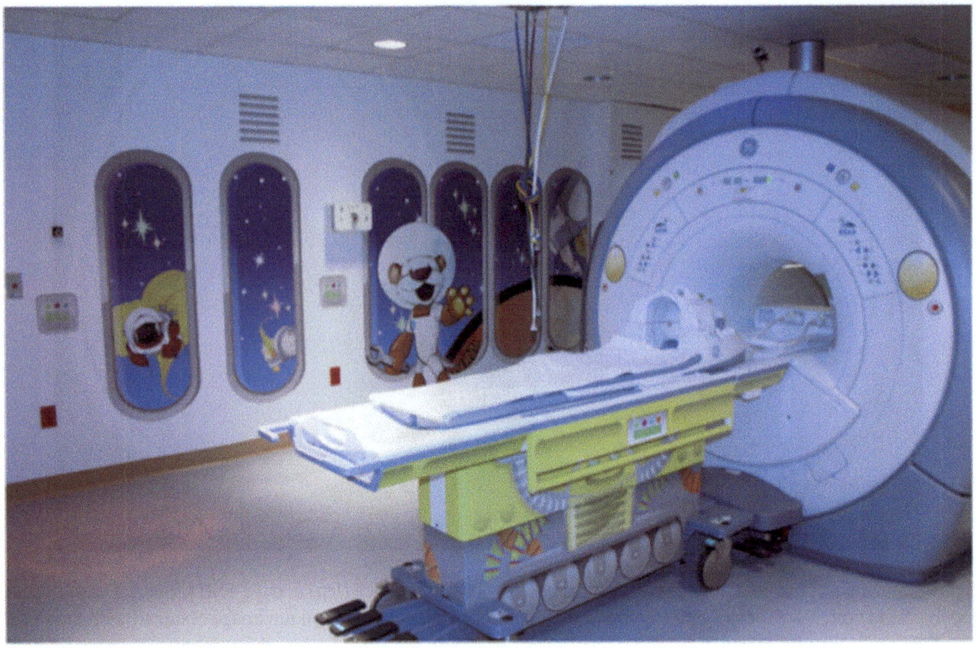

Fig. 4.3 Space-adventure themed MR suite used at Children's Hospital Pittsburgh of UPMC to reduce anxiety in children undergoing clinical and research MRI studies

intervention by MR technologists or staff. In the near future, dedicated modified neonatal MRI scanners, which can be housed in the NICU, will be commercially available. For children, colorful themes and effort toward providing a pediatric-friendly environment (Fig. 4.3), as well as the availability of mock scanners and psychologists or child-life professionals with expertise in reducing the child's anxiety over medical procedures all help overcome the challenges of working with pediatric patients.

Summary

MR imaging of pediatric patients and typically developing children has provided unparalleled insight into normal brain development and pediatric diseases. However, certain modifications of the MR environment are necessary in order to ensure both adequate data acquisition and a positive experience for the child.

References

1. Kinney HC, Brody BA, Kloman AS, Gilles FH. Sequence of central nervous system myelination in human infancy. II. Patterns of myelination in autopsied infants. J Neuropathol Exp Neurol. 1988;47:217–34.
2. Wiggins GC, Polimeni JR, Potthast A, Schmitt M, Alagappan V, Wald LL. 96-Channel receive-only head coil for 3 Tesla: design optimization and evaluation. Magn Reson Med. 2009;62:754–62.
3. Keil B, Alagappan V, Mareyam A, Mcnab JA, Fujimoto K, Tountcheva V, Triantafyllou C, Dilks DD, Kanwisher N, Lin W, Grant PE, Wald LL. Size-optimized 32-channel brain arrays for 3 T pediatric imaging. Magn Reson Med. 2011;66:1777–87.

Part II

Pathologies

5 Magnetic Resonance Spectroscopy of Pediatric Brain Tumors

Simrandip K. Gill, Ashok Panigrahy, Theodoros N. Arvanitis, and Andrew C. Peet

Overview

Pediatric Brain Tumors

Childhood brain tumors are the second most frequent malignancy of childhood, exceeded only by leukemia, and the most common form of solid tumor. There are approximately 2,500 new diagnoses per year in the USA and the incidence of brain tumors has increased slightly over the decades—possibly a result of improved diagnostic imaging. Brain tumors comprise 20–25% of all malignancies occurring among children under 15 years of age and 10% of tumors occurring among 15–19-year-olds. Brain tumors are the leading cause of death from cancer in pediatric oncology. In addition, due to either the effects of the tumor or the treatment required to control it, survivors of childhood brain tumors often have severe neurological, neurocognitive, and psychosocial sequelae. Among brain tumor subjects, approximately 35% of all patients are younger than 5 years and 75% are younger than 10 years. The type of tumors, the overall incidence of brain tumors, and the risks for poor outcome change with the age. Young children are at the highest risk, since tumors tend to be more malignant in their behavior in this age group. Childhood brain tumors display a high pathologic heterogeneity. Whereas most brain tumors in adults are World Health Organization (WHO) grade II astrocytoma, anaplastic astrocytoma, or glioblastoma, a significant portion of pediatric brain tumors are primitive neuroectodermal tumors, such as medulloblastoma, pilocytic astrocytomas, ependymomas, and others (Table 5.1). In addition, the behavior of pediatric brain tumors ranges from relatively indolent growth to rapid growth and tendency to disseminate. Genetic risk factors for brain tumors include neurofibromatosis types 1 and 2 (pilocytic astrocytoma, low-grade gliomas, ependymomas), Turcot syndrome (medulloblastoma and high-grade gliomas), Li–Fraumeni syndrome, Gorlin syndrome, and von Hippel–Lindau syndrome (hemangioblastoma) but account for only a small proportion of tumors. The only confirmed environmental risk factor is previous exposure to ionizing radiation.

Prognoses

Outcome and long-term survival depends on the availability of effective treatment. Diffuse intrinsic brainstem gliomas (also termed diffuse pontine gliomas), often low-grade lesions at presentation [1–6], are inoperable because of their location and are highly resistant to radiation or chemotherapy. They have the worst prognosis of all tumors in pediatric neuro-oncology with a median survival of 9 months and 90% dying by 2 years. There has been no improvement in survival for several decades for these tumors. On the other hand, fast growing and quickly fatal—if untreated—germinomas can be successfully treated by radiation therapy alone. Indeed, for these particular tumors, long-term survival is so high that the long-term side effects of radiation therapy are increasingly becoming a concern—considering that ionizing radiation is the only established environmental risk factor for gliomas in

S.K. Gill
School of Cancer Sciences, University of Birmingham, Birmingham, UK

A. Panigrahy, M.D.
Department of Pediatric Radiology, Children's Hospital of Pittsburgh of UPMC, 4401 Penn Ave, Pittsburgh, PA 15224, USA

Department of Radiology, University of Pittsburgh School of Medicine, 4401 Penn Avenue, Suite Floor 2, Pittsburgh, PA 15224, USA
e-mail: Ashok.Panigrahy@chp.edu

T.N. Arvanitis, Ph.D.
School of Electronic, Electrical & Computer Engineering, The University of Birmingham, Birmingham, UK

A.C. Peet, Ph.D., F.R.C.P.C.H. (✉)
Institute of Child Health, University of Birmingham, Whittall Street, Birmingham, B4 6NH, UK
e-mail: a.peet@bham.ac.uk

S. Blüml and A. Panigrahy (eds.), *MR Spectroscopy of Pediatric Brain Disorders*,
DOI 10.1007/978-1-4419-5864-8_5, © Springer Science+Business Media, LLC 2013

Table 5.1 WHO grade and approximate relative incidence of the most common pediatric brain tumors

Diagnosis	WHO grade	Location	Relative frequency
Medulloblastoma	IV	Posterior fossa	≈20%
Pilocytic astrocytoma	I	Posterior fossa, hypothalamic/third ventricular region, optic nerve, and chiasmal region	≈20%
Astrocytoma		Anywhere in the brain	≈20–25%
low-grade astrocytoma	II		
Anaplastic astrocytoma	III		
Glioblastoma	IV		
Ependymal tumors		Mostly posterior fossa	≈10–15%
Ependymoma	II		
Anaplastic ependymoma	III		
Choroid plexus tumors		Mostly intraventricular, growing out from choroid plexus tissue	≈3%
Papilloma	I		
Carcinoma	III		
Germ cell tumors		Pineal and suprasellar regions, also basal ganglia.	≈3%
Pure germinomas			
Mixed germ cell tumors			
Craniopharyngioma	I	Sellar region, not a primary brain tumor	≈5%
Other			≈5–10%
Neuronal and mixed neuronal-glial tumors, etc.			

Among the more than 100 subtypes of pediatric brain tumors, medulloblastoma, pilocytic astrocytomas, astrocytomas, and ependymomas constitute more than 80%. Note that the incidence of individual tumors changes with age

Data from The 2007 World Health Organization Classification of Tumors of the Central Nervous System

adults [7, 8]. In addition, highly aggressive cerebellar grade IV medulloblastomas have now 5-year survival rates exceeding 60% overall and around 80% for localized tumors. This can be attributed to refined surgical techniques and improved adjuvant treatment with radiotherapy and chemotherapy. Improved ability to assess initial and residual disease with clinical imaging, both together resulting in a higher incidence of complete tumor resection, is an important factor in localized medulloblastoma but particularly in ependymomas, where complete macroscopic resection is a key prognostic factor. Early detection and aggressive treatment of recurrent disease is also an important factor in improving outcomes. A major goal of current clinical trials is to improve outcomes and quality of life for the young high-risk group of patients, where tumors tend to be more aggressive and disease dissemination is particularly challenging to treat. In this age group, chemotherapy regimens aim to avoid or minimize the use of radiation therapy which can have devastating effects [9–13].

The Potential Benefits of Magnetic Resonance Spectroscopy

The emergence of high resolution imaging, firstly computed tomography (CT) and then magnetic resonance imaging (MRI), has been crucial to the improvement of clinical management for children with brain tumors. MRI scans are now performed on these children at multiple points in their clinical management: At presentation to confirm the presence of a mass and aid diagnosis; for some patients, before surgery for staging and surgical planning; just after surgery to assess extent of resection; approximately 3 months during adjuvant treatment to monitor effectiveness; and at similar intervals after the end of treatment to detect recurrence. Although the use of conventional MR imaging has become extensive, there are a number of significant limitations of the information provided. For that reason, MRI is increasingly being supplemented by methods, which might give valuable additional information on the properties of the tumor, such as magnetic resonance spectroscopy (MRS).

When interpreted alongside conventional MRI, MR spectroscopy can add new information to many clinical situations. Noninvasive diagnosis has been the focus of many research studies, but is only the prelude to the improved characterization of tumors. One of the most important strategies in the management of childhood cancer is the identification of prognostic factors, which have improved tumor characterization and allow stratification of treatment according to risk. A number of prognostic MRS biomarkers have been discovered and await formal evaluation in a clinical trial setting. The noninvasive nature of MRS is of particular importance in the monitoring of treatment since scans can be performed on multiple occasions throughout treatment to assess its effectiveness. Early markers of treatment response are particularly attractive and there is increasing evidence that MRS can provide these in some situations. Determining whether posttreatment residual masses on MRI represent active tumor is challenging using conventional MRI and may be aided by MRS. Similarly, distinguishing radiotherapy related changes from recurrent tumor cannot always be achieved by conventional MRI and MRS could provide extra valuable information.

While there are studies that show encouraging results for MRS in most of these clinical scenarios, the technique is still not used routinely in clinical practice in centers without specific interest and expertise. In part, this is due to the difficulty of interpreting MRS data, which is both complex and often presented in a form that is not familiar to radiologists. Alternatively, the introduction of pattern recognition methods has become very popular with research groups for the classification of brain tumors using MRS. They often give excellent accuracy rates for tumor diagnosis but are not currently available for use in a routine clinical setting. The pattern recognition methods used are based on multivariate statistics and can be performed on either the whole MR spectrum or a list of parameters which has been extracted from it, for example metabolite concentrations. The most commonly used multivariate techniques include principal component analysis (PCA) and linear discriminant analysis (LDA) [14]. More complex methods, such as artificial neural networks and support vector machines, have also been used and also shown to have high accuracy [15]. The classifier is strengthened by the use of MRS in combination with imaging, clinical, and other information [16]. Classification using these methods is most effective when a small number of potential diagnoses are being considered and the effect of combining tumor groups in order to give smaller numbers of larger classes [17].

In this chapter, we present the MRS characteristics of common and important tumor types, giving mean spectra or example spectra. Metabolic features, which have been shown to be significantly different from noninvolved brain and other tumor types, are then given. This information provides a resource for the interpretation of MRS data for noninvasive diagnosis. Among other chemicals detectable by MRS, choline, lactate, and lipids have been of particular interest in tumor spectroscopy. Choline-containing compounds are involved in cell membrane synthesis and breakdown and are abnormal in all forms of cancer [18, 19]. Lactate is an indicator for abnormal glycolytic function but can also accumulate in necrotic tissue [20, 21], whereas lipids are believed to be elevated in aggressive, fast growing tumors outgrowing their blood supply and causing necrosis in insufficiently perfused tumor tissue [22].

Acquiring and Processing Magnetic Resonance Spectroscopy Data from Children with Brain Tumors

Single Voxel Spectroscopy Versus Chemical Shift Imaging

In a clinical setting, MRS is performed using either single voxel spectroscopy (SVS), if the tumor is focal and homogenous, or Chemical Shift Imaging (CSI), if the tumor is large and heterogeneous. During SVS, a single voxel is positioned on the region of interest and the spectrum is obtained from the tissue inside the voxel with a high degree of localization. CSI, also sometimes referred to as MRS imaging (MRSI), produces multiple spectra from various locations simultaneously, usually including the region of interest and its surrounding areas. However, the signal from an individual voxel in the CSI grid has potential contributions from signals in adjacent voxels (*voxel bleeding*).

In general, SVS has become the method of choice for most pediatric brain tumor investigations. The acquisition times are comparatively short, with good quality data being acquired from a 2 cm sided cube (8 cc) in 4–6 min. It is comparatively robust and, with a high level of automation, means it is easy to implement into clinical practice [23]. The signal of unsuppressed water can be acquired in a few seconds without any additional set up and used as a reference for the data to allow estimation of concentrations—a technique sometimes called absolute quantitation [24]. A considerable number of publications using SVS are available, thereby aiding interpretation.

Large heterogeneous tumors present a challenge for MRS and, if SVS is to be used, a single region of the tumor needs to be selected or data needs to be acquired from several voxels, each of which has the same acquisition time. The variation in MRS, across such tumors, can be studied more efficiently by using CSI. This technique also has the advantage that data can be collected from surrounding regions, giving information on the presence of infiltrating tumor. Information from CSI can be useful for identifying the best biopsy site or identifying regions of active tumor after treatment. CSI is also useful for investigating lesions identified on conventional MRI following radiotherapy. Such lesions can be multiple and complex and discriminating between the regions of radiation necrosis and tumor recurrence is a major clinical challenge [25]. CSI data interpretation for each voxel is essentially the same as for SVS; however, the sheer amount of data available for the whole CSI grid makes visualization and interpretation challenging. Data is often summarized using color maps created from the matrix of spectra of main metabolite peaks, for example choline (Cho) and *N*-acetyl aspartate (NAA) [26]. Features identified on color maps should always be verified by inspecting the spectra in the voxels involved, since poor quality data can lead to spurious features being present on the color maps.

The appearance of MR spectra is determined by acquisition parameters. Metabolite resonances may be prominent with one acquisition sequence whereas the peak amplitude is different when another sequence is used despite spectra being acquired from the same region of interest (ROI). To allow easy comparison, all spectra presented in this review article were, unless explicitly stated otherwise, acquired using the same acquisition method (point-resolved single-voxel spectroscopy (PRESS), echo time (TE) = 35 ms, repetition time (TR) = 1,500 m) on a 1.5 T clinical scanner. The echo time is the parameter that tends to affect the visual appearance of the spectrum the most. Small variations, in the range of 30 ms to 40 ms, will lead to minor alterations only. For fully automated quantification of metabolite concentrations (e.g., using LCModel [27], TARQUIN [28], or jMRUI [29]) spectra of model solutions of each metabolite measured with the same acquisition parameters are needed. Whereas in the early days of MRS model spectra were obtained for each MR system, simulated spectra are now as accurate as experimentally acquired ones [30]. This greatly simplifies the implementation of fully automated absolute quantitation of MR spectra.

Metabolic Profiles of Pediatric Tumors at Presentation

Posterior Fossa Lesions

Approximately 50% of all pediatric tumors arise from the posterior fossa. In most cases, these tumors are grade IV medulloblastoma, grade I pilocytic astrocytoma, or (less frequently) grade II or III ependymomas. Although medulloblastoma tend to have low signal intensity on T_2w images, indicating a *hyper*cellular tumor, there are instances in which ependymoma may present with similar features. It is common that ependymoma involve the fourth ventricular floor and extend into the foramen of Luschka. However, large medulloblastoma may have a similar growth pattern. Occasionally, a cystic/necrotic medulloblastoma may have imaging characteristics, which overlap with posterior fossa pilocytic astrocytoma (Fig. 5.1). Proton spectroscopy and diffusion imaging appear to be particularly useful for diagnoses. Taurine (Tau) has been consistently observed by several groups in medulloblastoma [31–34] and is an important differentiator of medulloblastoma from other tumors of the posterior fossa. Among the various subtypes of medulloblastoma (Fig. 5.2), desmoplastic medulloblastoma typically have lower taurine levels than classic medulloblastoma albeit there is considerable overlap [35]. The desmoplastic subtype may also have lower choline (Cho) levels. Metabolic features of other subtypes, such as large cell, anaplastic, or medulloblastoma with extensive nodularity, have not been studied sufficiently due to their low incidence. Medulloblastoma have higher levels of choline than other posterior fossa tumors [21, 36]. The hallmark of pilocytic astrocytomas is very low creatine concentrations, low myo-inositol (ml), and low choline concentrations consistent with their low cellularity. Lipids are also low in pilocytic astrocytoma but mean lactate levels are higher than in other tumors. Ependymomas have higher myo-inositol than medulloblastoma or pilocytic astrocytoma and their choline levels are variable but fall generally between medulloblastoma and pilocytic astrocytoma.

Davies et al. [17] found that only myo-inositol was significantly different for all three pair-wise comparisons with highest mean values in ependymomas and lowest in cerebellar pilocytic astrocytomas (higher mI is sometimes observed in pilocytic astrocytoma outside the posterior fossa such as optic pathway gliomas—see below). Analysis of variance (ANOVA) tests revealed that creatine (Cr) concentrations were significantly lower and NAA significantly higher in pilocytic astrocytomas when compared to the respective metabolite concentrations in medulloblastomas and ependymomas. In this study, taurine, choline, and glutamate (Glu) were significantly higher whereas glutamine (Gln) was significantly lower in medulloblastomas when compared to pilocytic astrocytomas.

Tumors Outside the Posterior Fossa

Lesions outside the posterior fossa account for approximately 50% of all pediatric brain tumors. For these tumors, MRS may also potentially improve initial diagnoses. However, this is not well documented in the literature as there are many different tumor types rendering clinical studies with sufficient numbers of subjects and follow-up difficulty. Posterior fossa medulloblastoma tumors belong to the group of *embryonal tumors*. It is likely that the equivalent tumor type outside the posterior fossa (central nervous system primitive neuroectodermal tumors—PNET) does have metabolic profiles comparable with that observed in medulloblastoma (Fig. 5.3), albeit this has not been formally investigated. There is also no established metabolic profile for teratoid/rhabdoid tumors (AT/RT), another type of embryonal tumor, more frequent in young children with particular poor prognosis, albeit it appears that Tau concentrations are low in this type of tumor (Fig. 5.3).

Pilocytic astrocytoma outside the posterior fossa may show a slightly more prominent *myo-inositol* (mI) signal [37] but the metabolic pattern is otherwise quite comparable with that of cerebellar pilocytic lesions (Fig. 5.4). While pilocytic astrocytomas are the most common brain tumors in children (25%), their incidence in adults is very rare, at only 2% of all brain tumors. It is noted that the metabolic profiles of pilocytic astrocytoma and grade

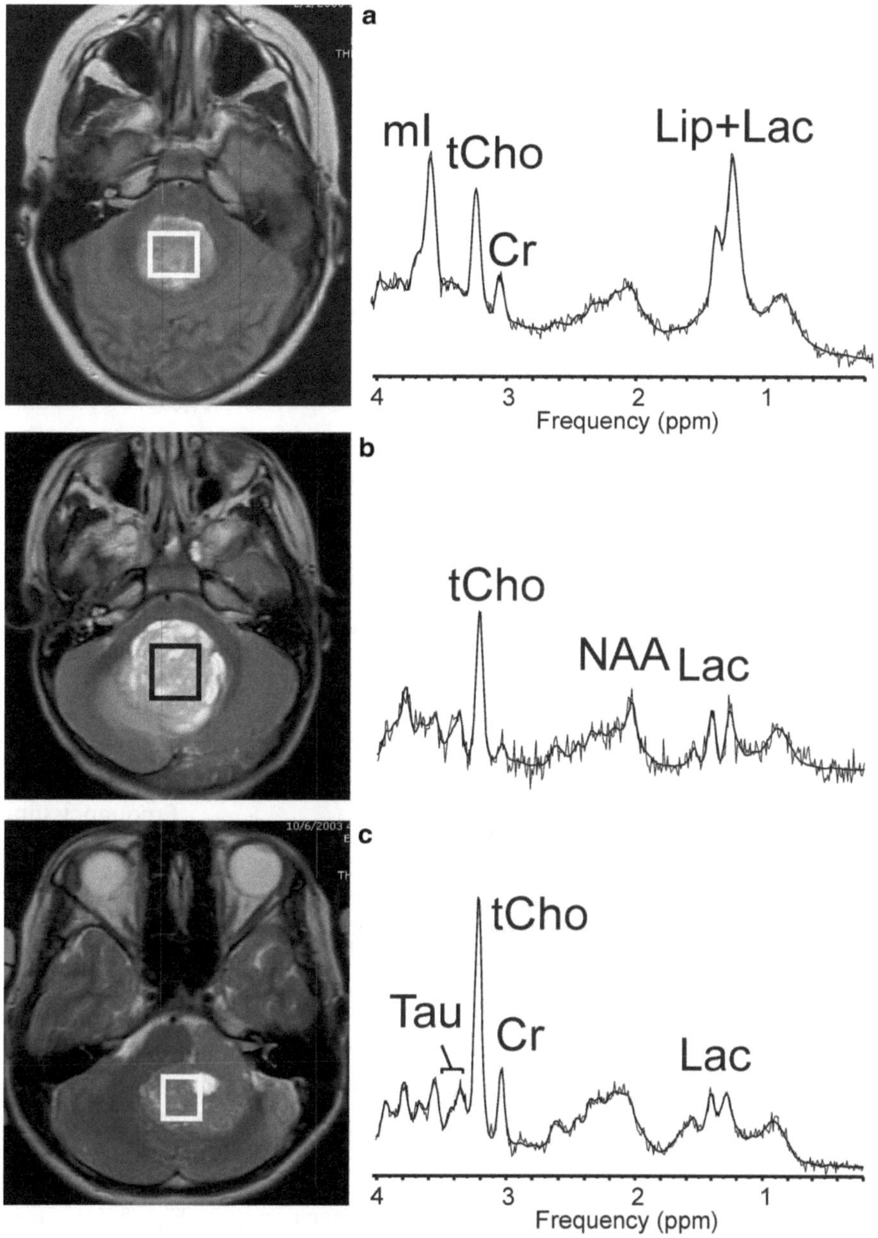

Fig. 5.1 T2-weighted MR images and MR spectra of posterior fossa tumors. (**a**) Ependymoma (grade II). (**b**) Pilocytic astrocytoma. (**c**) Classic medulloblastoma. All spectra were acquired from lesions with no partial volume of surrounding tissue using a single-voxel PRESS sequence with a short echo time of 35 ms. Shown are the original unfiltered spectra (*thin line*) and the LCModel (Stephen Provencher Inc., version 6.1-G4) fits to the data (*thick line*). In all three cases, the MRI report missed the final diagnosis or did not mention the final diagnosis as the most likely tumor

II–IV astrocytoma are quite different. For example, the Cho/Cr ratios increase in astrocytomas II-IV with grade. However, grade I pilocytic astrocytoma, due to the low Cr concentration, have an even more prominent Cho/Cr ratio than grade IV glioblastomas (Fig. 5.5). On the other hand, pilocytic astrocytomas share some of the metabolic features of neurocytoma, ganglioglioma, and diffuse leptomeningeal glioneuronal tumors (see discussion below on rarely encountered tumors) such as a peak at around 2.0 ppm, which is usually assigned to NAA.

Astrocytomas display a wide range of metabolic characteristics, even within the same grade. Mean choline concentrations increase with grade and lipids are more frequently detected in higher grade lesions. However, accurate diagnosis based on MRS alone is unreliable (Fig. 5.5). Diffuse intrinsic pontine gliomas (DIPG) are not biopsied and are usually diagnosed based on clinical symptoms at presenta-

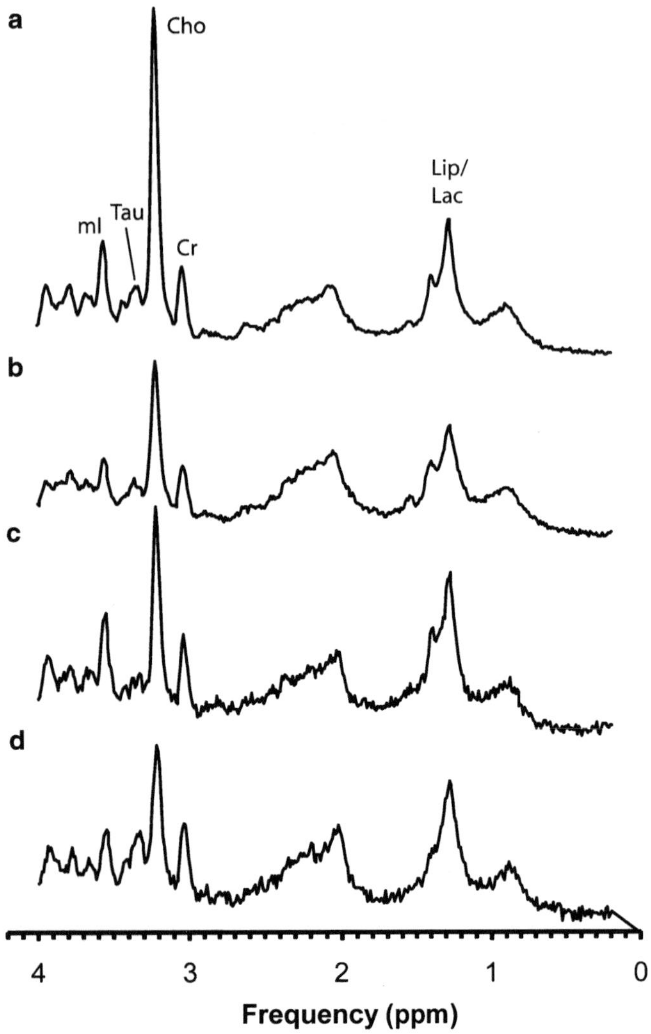

Fig. 5.2 Representative (average of individual spectra) MR spectra of classic (**a**), desmoplastic (**b**), anaplastic (**c**), and large cell (**d**) medulloblastoma

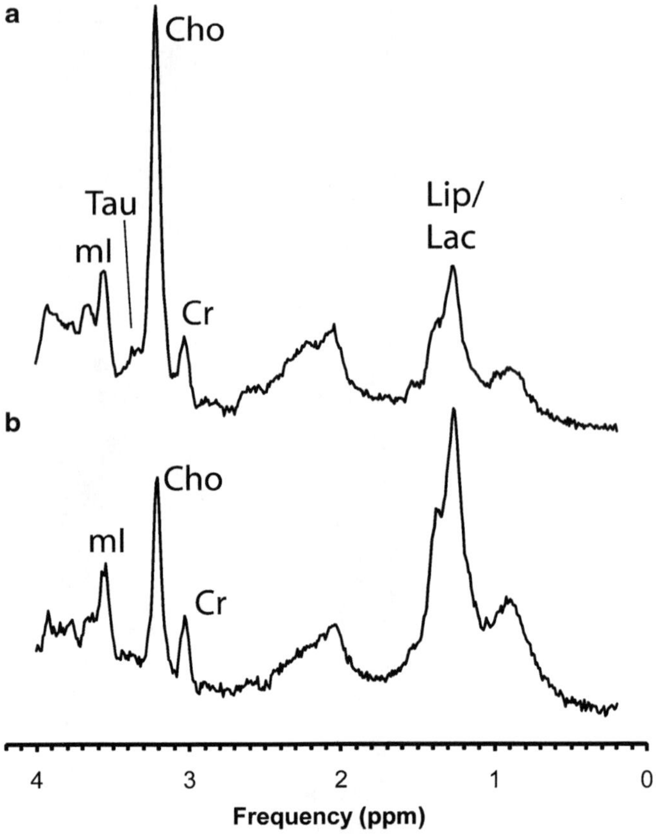

Fig. 5.3 Representative spectra of CNS primitive neuroectodermal tumors (PNET) (**a**) and atypical teratoid/rhabdoid (AT/RT) (**b**). Whereas taurine is detectable in PNET there is no clear evidence for taurine in AT/RT

tion and MR imaging [4, 38–40]. Spectra of DIPG often resemble spectra of low-grade (WHO II) astrocytoma with prominent citrate at presentation [41, 42] (Fig. 5.6). In the vast majority of the cases, conventional MRI and clinical symptoms are sufficient for diagnosis. There may be an incidence of an unusual presentation of an exophytic brainstem tumor, often a pilocytic lesion with much better prognosis, which resembles the MRI features of a diffuse tumor. In these occasions, an MRS study may be useful as the MRS profiles of pilocytic astrocytoma and pontine gliomas are readily distinguishable.

Choroid plexus papilloma (WHO I) do have a highly characteristic metabolic profile (striking myo-inositol) which distinguishes them readily from all other tumors, but also from choroid plexus carcinoma (WHO III) which are cellular and highly perfused tumors with very prominent choline and unremarkable myo-inositol (Fig. 5.7a, b) [21]. Atypical choroid plexus papillomas have a very low incidence and their metabolic profile has not been described in the literature. The spectrum obtained from a single patient at Children's Hospital Los Angeles appears to fall between papilloma and carcinoma spectra (Fig. 5.7c). Secreting germ cell tumors can usually be diagnosed by their midline location, age of the subjects (typically older postpuberty children), and by raised serum tumor markers alpha-fetoprotein (AFP) and β-human chorionic gonadotropin (β-HCP). Nonsecreting germ cell tumors, such as germinomas, are usually diagnosed by biopsy and this is often challenging due their common location in the pineal gland. Noninvasive diagnosis would be an important advance in the management of these tumors, which are usually cured without surgery. Taurine was consistently observed in germinoma spectra as well as prominent lipids features that could be useful for distinguishing these tumors from other tumor types (Fig. 5.8) [21, 43]. Craniopharyngioma (not a primary brain tumor) are found relatively frequently in pediatrics and usually diagnosed by rim calcifications which are well visualized on CT images. However, since surgery is

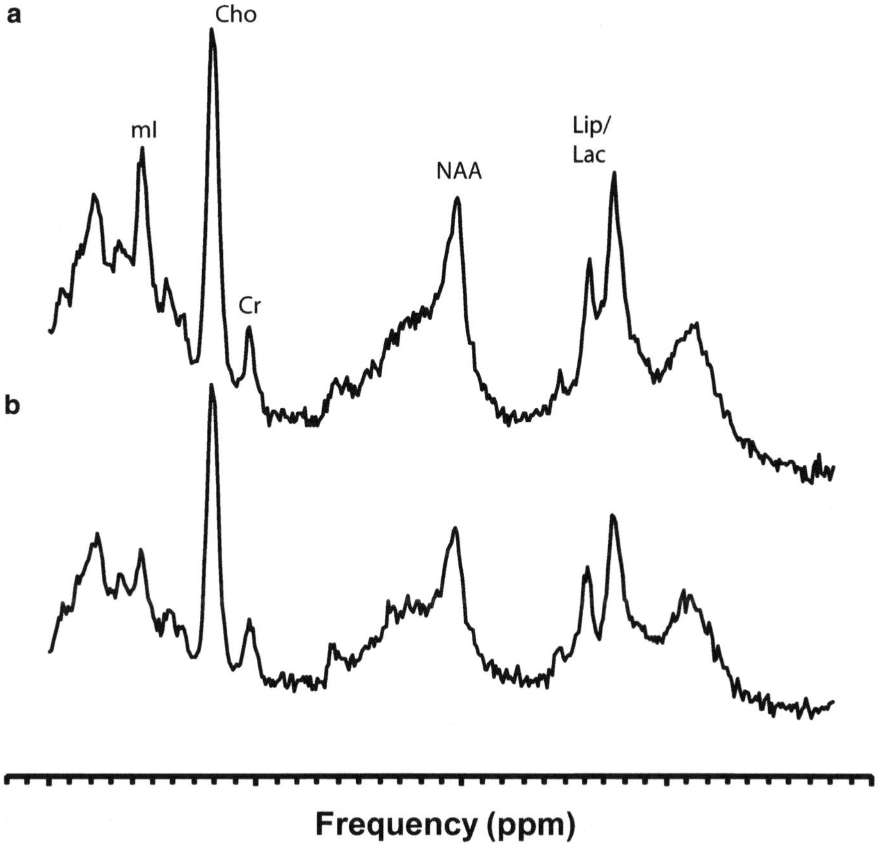

Fig. 5.4 Typical MR spectra of supratentorial (**a**) and infratentorial (**b**) juvenile pilocytic astrocytoma. Myo-inositol (mI) appears to be slightly more prominent in the supratentorial pilocytic astrocytomas

the most important aspect of their treatment, a histopathological diagnosis is usually available. Typical spectra of cystic and solid (rarely encountered) craniopharyngioma are shown in Fig. 5.9.

Apart from tumors discussed above there are more than 100 other less frequently encountered pediatric brain tumors subtypes which have until now not been studied in detail. This includes oligodendrogliomas, oligoastrocytic tumors, neuronal and mixed neuronal-glial tumors, and others. Examples of spectra obtained from some of these rarely encountered tumors are shown in Fig. 5.10.

Prognosis and Risk Stratification

A second probably more important and challenging task, with major implications on treatment strategies and outcome, is *risk assessment.* Patients at high risk for progressive disease need to undergo therapy that is more aggressive, whereas standard risk patients may be treated less aggressively to avoid the often-devastating side effects of therapy in children. Obvious risk factors are the type and grade of the tumor, location of the tumor, age of the subject, disease spread at diagnosis, and completeness of resection if attempted. There are also histological features that allow further subclassification of tumors [44, 45] and researchers are trying to identify genetic risk factors, as well as genetic variations of tumors that could guide therapy in individual subjects. Still, physiological MR methods such as MRS can contribute to better patient stratification, as it is well known that the microenvironment plays a significant role in how diseases progress. For example, *hypoxic* tumors have altered physiologic processes, which include increased angiogenesis and local invasion, switch to more malignant phenotypes, as well as increased formation of distant central nervous system metastases [46–50]. Standard MR imaging, on the other hand, provides limited information about tissue environment at the microscopic/cellular level, such as its metabolic state, hemodynamic properties, and cellularity.

Risk Assessment in Tumors That Are Resectable

It needs to be acknowledged that for those tumors where complete macroscopic resection can be achieved, the major role for MRI is in aiding the surgeon to attain a complete

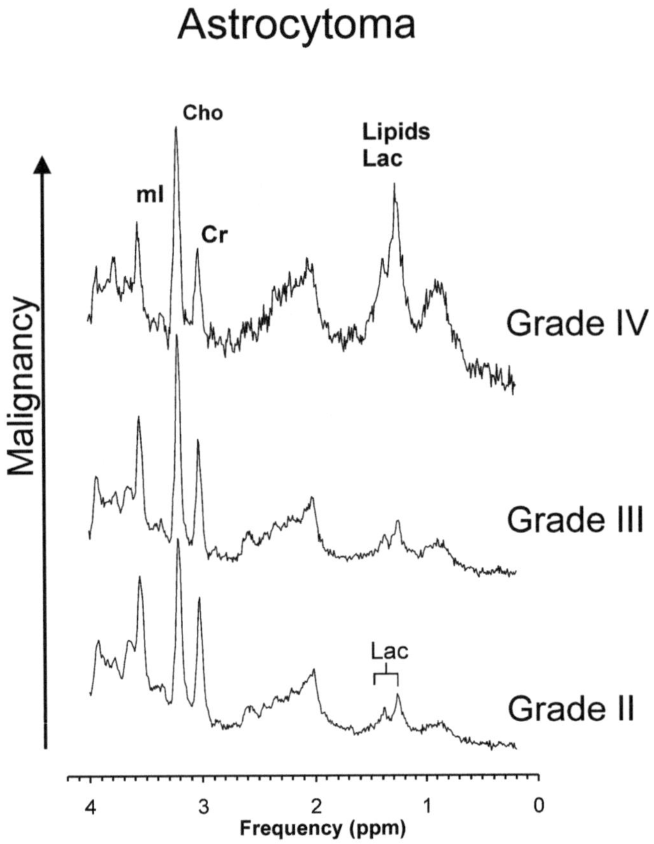

Fig. 5.5 Representative spectra of grade II astrocytoma, anaplastic astrocytoma, and grade IV glioblastoma in pediatric tumors. Spectra shown for grade II astrocytoma and anaplastic astrocytoma were acquired from untreated lesions. Glioblastoma spectra were acquired mostly from recurrent tumors

resection and identifying residual disease, either postoperatively but increasingly intra-operatively. Comparably crude MR markers compete with the highly sophisticated tests that are available in today's biology such as RNA and DNA analyses. It is thus not a surprise that genetic/molecular features are the focus of the neuro-oncology community. Still, identifying *metabolic* risk factors early on is important as it could guide initial surgery, the most important component of treatment for resectable tumors. Risk assessment goes beyond merely identifying the correct tumor type but to predict which tumor within the same group of tumors is more likely to recur or spread. Particularly among the relatively large group of posterior fossa tumors, there is a considerable overlap of traditional clinical risk factors for patients with widely different outcome. A potentially important recently reported finding is that, in medulloblastoma metastatic disease was more frequently encountered in lesions that had high levels of total choline and low lipids [51], albeit this observation needs to be confirmed in a prospective study. Still, overall, very few studies have been carried out to determine the significance of MRS in predicting overall and progression free survival. One of the reasons might be that MR physicists (for a variety of reasons) do often not appreciate the necessity for consistent data acquisition and record keeping over many years required for clinical research. Typical *short-term* clinical measures for outcome in clinical trials are 5-year survival times. The problems are compounded by the presence of multiple confounding factors such as diagnosis, grade, extent of resection, and adjuvant treatment, all of which affect outcome themselves and need to be accounted for if clinically robust conclusions are to be drawn.

Risk Assessment in Inoperable or Only Partially Resectable Tumors

Inoperable or only partially resectable lesions include mostly glial tumors such as diffuse intrinsic pontine glioma, bithalamic astrocytoma, optic chiasm/hypothalamic gliomas, and gliomatosis cerebri. According to Broniscer et al. approximately 8% of low-grade (grade II) gliomas progress to high-grade lesions. There are currently no biomarkers that would predict which low-grade gliomas are likely to progress. The same is true for the small fraction of grade I pilocytic astrocytoma that metastasize. For these tumors, noninvasive *metabolic* risk factors potentially play a more important role [52].

In adults, gliomas at high risk for poor outcome are typically cellular and highly perfused lesions (not discussed in detail here) with prominent choline, low NAA, low myo-inositol, and high lipids [36, 53–61]. How do these observations compare with findings in gliomas in children? MRS studies of biopsy confirmed pediatric astrocytoma grade II-IV demonstrate metabolic patterns that are consistent with what has been established in adults, albeit variations in lesions of the same grade are considerable. Chang et al. performed a small multimodal MR study patients with glioblastoma, of which three had SVS MRS. Analysis of spectra demonstrated a reduction in the amplitude of NAA and elevation of Cho. Low NAA/Cho ratio calculated was found to be a valuable aid for precise targeting of stereotactic biopsies. However, small patient numbers, histological heterogeneity, as well as the clinical heterogeneity (data from untreated, treated, and recurrent lesions) prevent the formation of a clear picture from these studies [62].

Pediatric Astrocytoma

In a recent study, medical records and metabolite concentrations of 29 pediatric astrocytomas were reviewed. When grade II astrocytomas were subdivided in patients with stable disease for more than 2 years and a group of patient with disease progression within 2 years, it was noted that citrate (Cit) concentrations were significantly higher in patients with poor outcome [63]. Prominent citrate may be used for

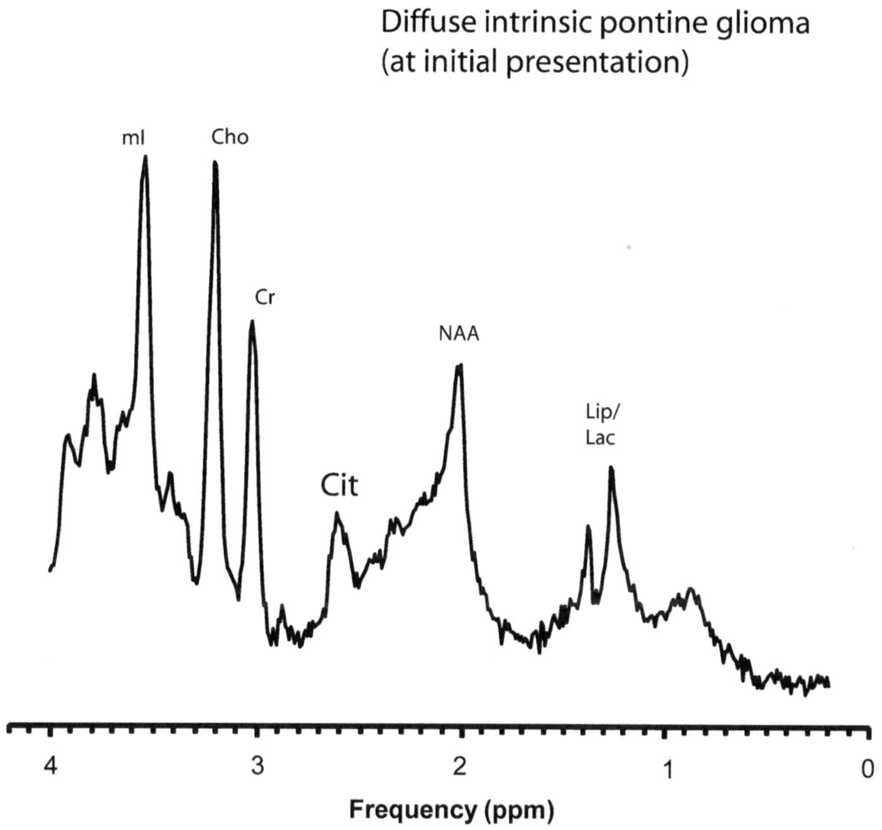

Fig. 5.6 A representative spectrum of diffuse intrinsic pontine glioma at initial presentation

identifying pediatric grade II astrocytomas destined for aggressive behavior (Fig. 5.11). On the other hand, there was no consistent pattern for citrate in anaplastic astrocytoma and glioblastoma with citrate prominent in some lesions, whereas undetectable in others. Furthermore, moderate or even low levels of choline were *not* a predictor for stable disease. Citrate was not specific for poor outcome as it was not detectable in all high-grade astrocytomas, despite poor outcome in all cases. Among high-grade astrocytoma, tumors with prominent citrate may constitute a metabolic subclass. It needs to be noted that the detection of prominent citrate, in low-grade astrocytomas with malignant progression, is consistent with the observation of high citrate in pontine gliomas [41]. Pontine gliomas are tumors with apparently inevitable aggressive behavior, despite presenting frequently with histopathological features typical for grade II diffuse astrocytomas [1–6, 64].

Pilocytic Astrocytoma

Recently, the metabolic profiles of stable and progressive pilocytic astrocytomas, at baseline and follow-up, were compared [37]. It was noted that optic pathway or thalamic pilocytic tumors that progressed had a significantly lower myo-inositol at initial MRS than those with stable disease. Furthermore, myo-inositol levels decreased significantly in progressing lesions between the initial and subsequent MRS. These changes in myo-inositol occurred before clinical and radiological progression and low and decreasing myo-inositol may thus be a noninvasive indicator for high risk for progression.

Although pilocytic astrocytoma (PA) in both children and adults are classified as WHO grade I, these tumors in adults are slightly more aggressive in nature. The reason for this difference is unclear. Porto et al. [65] investigated the differences in MRS between PAs in adults and children. A trend towards higher Cho levels in adults was found, although not significant. Similarly, albeit mean Cr was not significantly different in the two groups, some pediatric PAs had higher values than those seen in adults.

High-Grade Versus Low-Grade Tumors

Recent observations have also demonstrated robust biomarkers of tumor grade. The presence of glycine has been found to be increased in brain tumors, particularly increasing with WHO grading. Davies et al. retrospectively compared two cohorts of brain tumors that were confirmed to have high

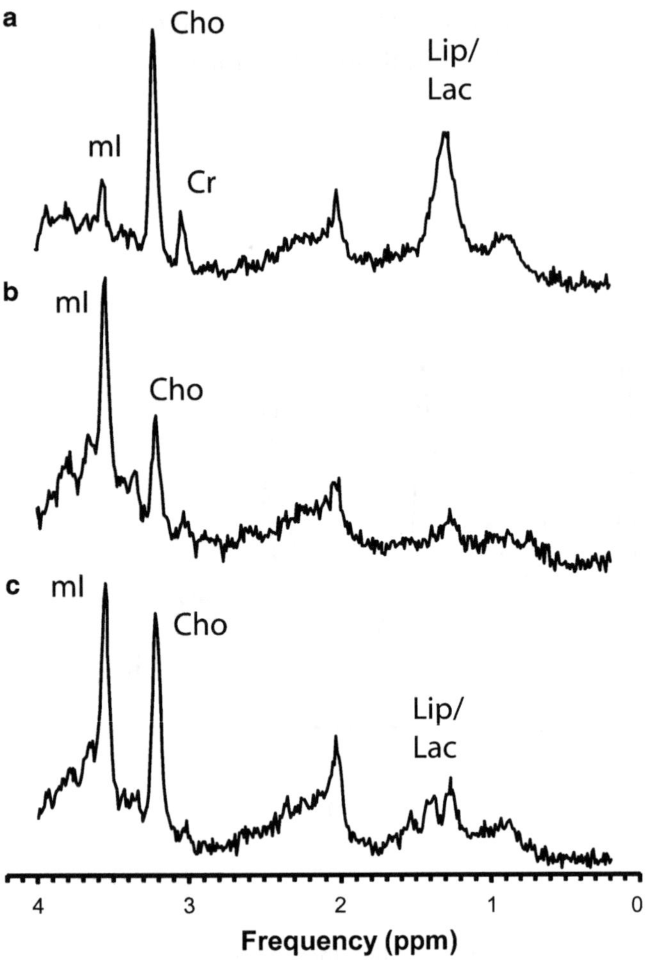

Fig. 5.7 Representative MR spectra of choroid plexus carcinoma (**a**) and choroid plexus papilloma (**b**). These tumors are readily distinguishable as myo-inositol (mI) is prominent in choroid plexus papilloma whereas Cho is the most prominent peak in choroid plexus carcinoma. A spectrum acquired from a single patient with an atypical choroid plexus papilloma appears to fall between carcinoma and papilloma spectra (**c**)

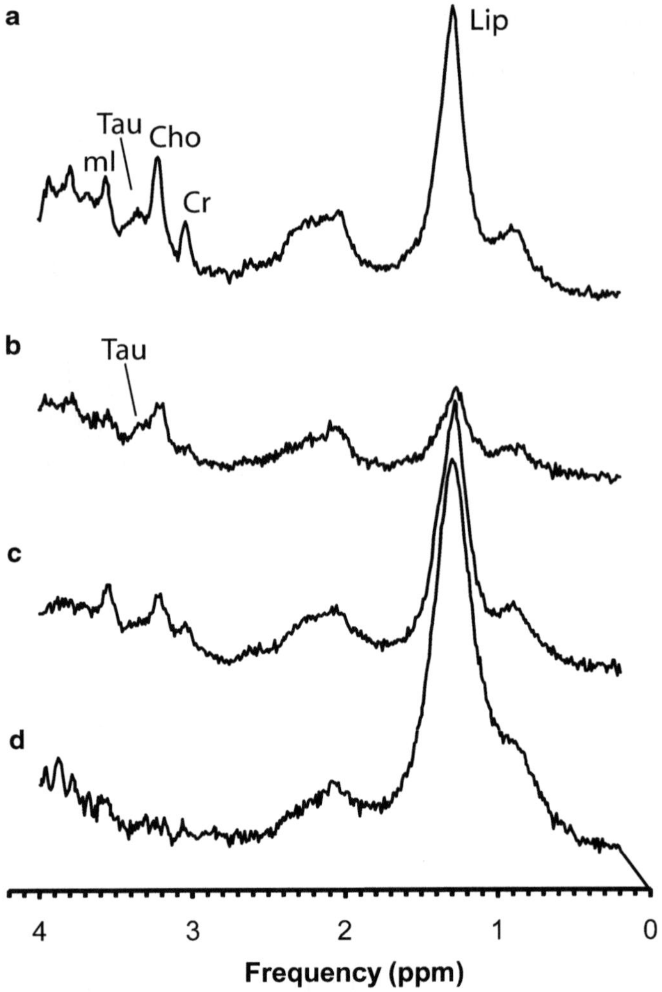

Fig. 5.8 Representative spectra for pure pineal germinoma (**a**), pineal mixed malignant germ cell tumors (**b**), for nonpineal pure germinomas (**c**), and mixed malignant nonpineal germ cell tumors (**d**). Taurine is detectable in pure germinomas and possibly also in mixed germ cell tumors. MR spectra of germ cell tumor are sometimes of low quality. Note, that no metabolites might be detectable in subgroups of these tumors

grade (III or IV) and low grade (I or II) using WHO grading for the presence of glycine. Analysis revealed that high- and low-grade tumors had highly significant differences in the levels of glycine (Gly) in particular higher normalized Gly concentration in the high-grade tumors. The differences in glycine concentration between high-grade tumors demonstrated a prominent singlet peak at 3.55 ppm from glycine clearly distinguishable from the multiplet peak of myo-inositol which could not be seen in low-grade tumors (very small number of low-grade tumors quantified to have low levels of glycine) [66].

A study by Astrakas et al. performed using CSI also compared high- and low-grade tumors determined by histopathology. Using an intermediate echo time of 65 ms to minimize the contribution of the lactate signal, it was found that Cho and lipids + lactate were significantly elevated in the high-grade tumors. Logistical regression revealed that both biomarkers were significant independent predictors of the grade of tumors. While grade is strongly associated with prognosis, tumors with the same grade can behave very differently. Studies of event free survival and overall survival are required to establish the accuracy of putative prognostic biomarkers [67]. A follow-up study performed largely on the same cohort showed that high Cho and lipids + lactate were associated with poor overall survival. However, a number of important tumor groups were excluded from the study and many metabolites of interest were not quantified due to the relatively long echo time used. Overall, systematic studies are required which incorporate MRS into multicenter clinical trials where specific patient groups are treated in a uniform manner with robust follow-up data [68].

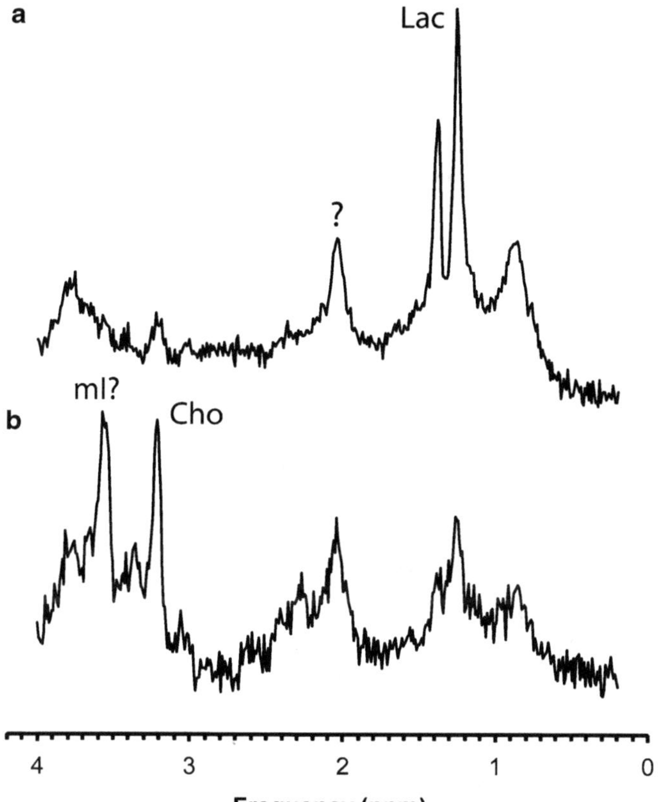

Fig. 5.9 Representative spectra for cystic (**a**) and solid (**b**) craniopharyngioma

Assessment of Effectiveness of Therapy

What Does Successful Therapy Do to the Spectrum?

Conventional imaging does not reliably distinguish between recurrent/residual disease and postoperative changes or necrosis after radiation. Postradiation changes do sometimes occur many months after therapy and the correct diagnosis is a major challenge for the optimum management of pediatric patients. It is well known that spectroscopy is an important tool to assess response to therapy in pediatric and adult brain tumors [69–75]. Most metabolites are intracellular. Effective therapy causing cell death will thus result in generally reduced metabolite concentrations (including Cho) and increased lipids due to the release of fatty acids from cell membranes. On the other hand, increasing levels of Cho (or Cho/NAA) are indicators for failed therapy and high risk for progressing disease.

A study by Weybright et al. used 2D MRSI to evaluate new areas of contrast enhanced lesions in previously treated brain tumors. MRS was performed on both a contrast enhancing lesion and normal appearing white matter in 28 patients aged between 4 and 54 years with range of tumor diagnoses. Results demonstrated that lesions in the recurrence or residual tumor group had significantly higher Cho/Cr than those with radiation injury and in turn the radiation injury group had significantly higher Cho/Cr ratios than normal appearing white matter. The lesions in the tumor group also had significantly higher Cho/NAA ratios than those in the radiation injury group and significantly higher Cho/NAA ratios than normal appearing white matter. NAA/Cr ratios were significantly lower in the lesion group compared to those in the radiation injury group. Using Cho/Cr or Cho/NAA ratios with a cut-off for the cohort, 27 out of 28 patients were correctly classified with either recurrent tumor or radiation injury assuming radiation injury was diagnosed accurately [76, 77]. These studies have demonstrated the potential for MRS to be an effective tool in discriminating between tumor recurrence and radiation changes.

While the concept of assessing response to therapy with MRS is straightforward (for any tumor for adults and pediatrics), there are significant limitations that need to be acknowledged. Absolute quantitation, requiring data processing beyond the tools provided by the manufacturers, is required to measure metabolite concentrations accurately and reliably. Chemical shift imaging, technically more demanding and time consuming, might be necessary to study large and inhomogeneous lesions. Still, the extent and shape of a lesion (or multiple lesions) may make MRS impractical. MRS may not work in lesions close to the skull or lesions with bleeds and calcifications. In addition, MRS, being a methodology of low sensitivity, can assess the bulk response of tissue but does not provide certainty that every single tumor cell has been successfully treated.

Pontine Gliomas

Diffuse intrinsic pontine gliomas are unique in pediatric neuro-oncology as they are inoperable and rarely being biopsied. They are a relatively *clean* tumor group to be studied with MR spectroscopy because lesions are always in the same region, generally large and homogeneous, and MR studies are technically not compromised by biopsies or surgery. These tumors are well suited for longitudinal studies to evaluate metabolic changes over the disease course. Please see Chap. 6 for details about MRS findings in these tumors.

Current Challenges

Major obstacles for management and clinical research are the biological and physiological diversity of tumors, the small number of patients in each category due to the relatively low incidence of these tumors (≈ 9 per 100,000 in the US) [78], as well as the general difficulties of conducting

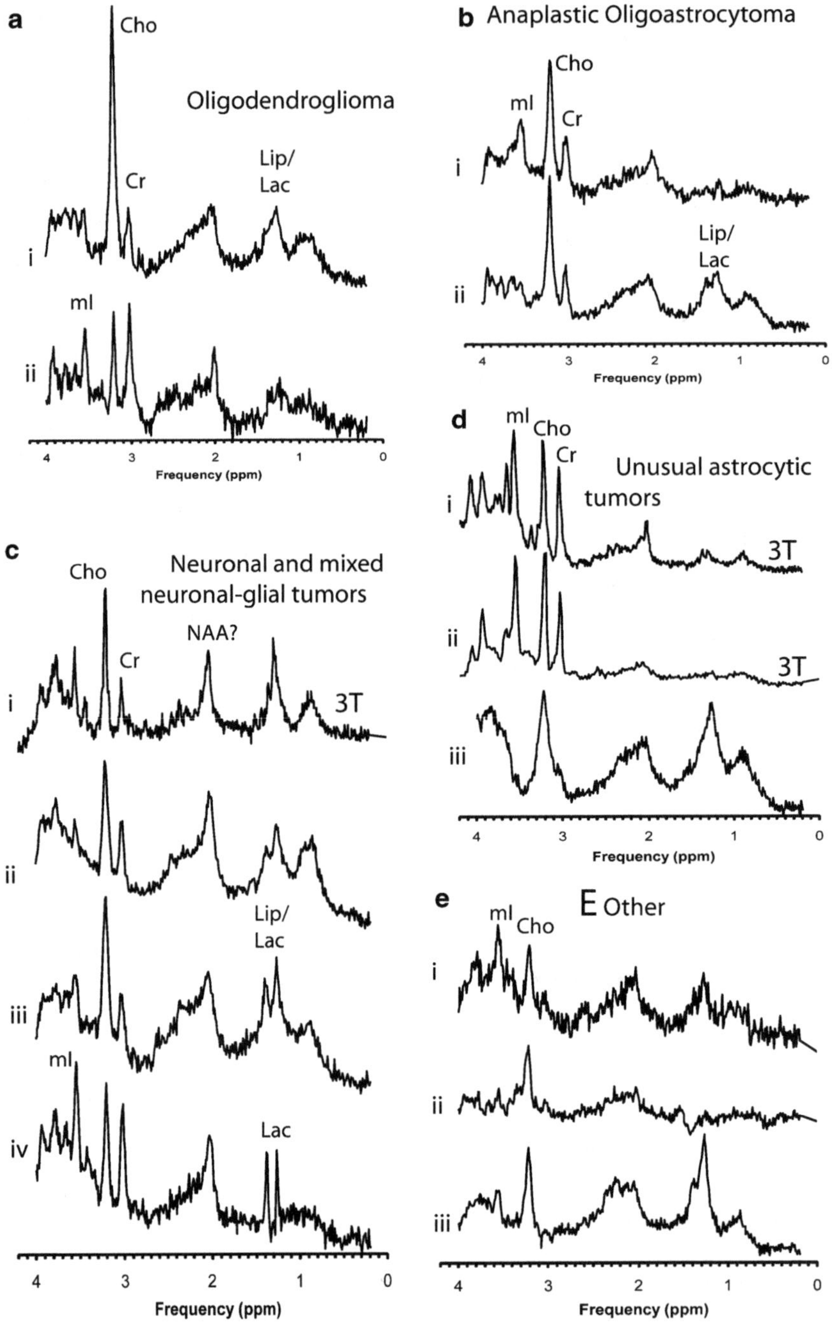

Fig. 5.10 Examples for MR spectra obtained from less frequently encountered pediatric brain tumors. All spectra were obtained enclosing only tumor tissue in the region of interest. The spectral patterns should not be generalized as they have been obtained from individual patients and significant variations of the metabolic profiles within tumor types or subtypes cannot be ruled out. (**a**) Recurrent oligodendroglioma (i) and oligodendroglioma at initial diagnosis. (**b**) Anaplastic oligoastrocytoma with progressive disease (i) and anaplastic oligoastrocytoma with stable disease >5 years (ii). (**c**) Neurocytoma (i – note spectrum acquired at 3T), diffuse leptomeningeal glioneuronal tumor (ii), ganglioglioma (iii), dysembryoplastic neuroepithelial tumor (iv). (**d**) Gemistocytic astrocytoma (i – note spectrum acquired at 3T), angiocentric astrocytoma (ii – note spectrum acquired at 3T), pleomorphic xanthoastrocytoma (iii). (**e**) Schwannoma (i), mesenchymal inflammatory myofibroblastic tumor (ii), fibrous histocytoma (iii)

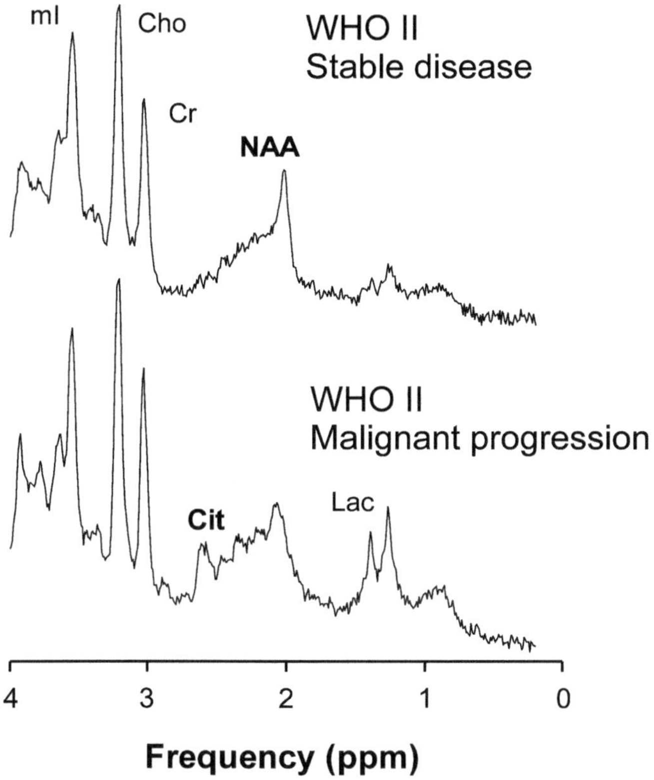

Fig. 5.11 Shown are averaged spectra computed from grade II astrocytoma with stable disease and with malignant progression. Citrate (Cit) at ≈ 2.6 ppm was significantly more prominent in aggressive astrocytoma. Other chemicals that can be quantified with in vivo MR spectroscopy include N-acetyl-aspartate (NAA), creatine (Cr), lactate (Lac), choline (Cho), and myo-inositol (mI). Note that NAA in aggressive astrocytoma was significantly lower than in stable astrocytoma but to a much lesser extent than citrate. Despite the more prominent appearance of lactate in grade II astrocytomas with malignant significance was not reached due to considerable scatter of measured concentrations. All spectra are scaled to the measured concentrations to allow direct comparison

clinical research in children. Current basic research focuses on identifying specific molecular targets critical for cellular changes, which result in uncontrolled growth and spread—moving away from the traditional approach of administering cytotoxic agents at maximum tolerated dose. Another current strategy is to utilize agents that influence the environment of tumors such as antiangiogenic drugs, which are likely to be effective in tumors with increased angiogenesis. However, taking advantage of the numerous new potential targets remains challenging due to small patient populations, questions about the dosage and which targets to choose, how to get agents across the blood–brain barrier (BBB), and how to monitor/measure response [79]. The main challenge for the MR community is to demonstrate that conventional and advanced MR is a pivotal tool for overcoming these bottlenecks in pediatric neuro-oncology and to contribute actively to improved patient management. MRS offers a unique noninvasive approach to assess features of tumors at microscopic levels by quantifying cellular metabolites. Thus, MRS is an essential noninvasive tool that should be included in the portfolio of imaging methods that aim to characterize and monitor disease status in clinical trials. Of the various MR modalities, MRS is among the more demanding techniques, as it is technically challenging and requires extra training and expertise for proper interpretation of results. However, due to recent technical advances as well as fully automated processing software, MRS has become increasingly robust and good quality spectra can now be obtained from nonexperts on clinical scanners in less than 5 min. MRS is thus well positioned to contribute significantly in the field of pediatric (and adult) brain tumors in the future.

Summary

MR spectroscopy can provide noninvasive metabolite profiles of childhood brain tumors and these are highly characteristic for tumor type. This information is increasingly being used to provide a noninvasive diagnostic aid but since tumor pathologies differ in children to adults, child-specific classifiers are required. Despite the strong dependence of the MRS metabolite profile on tumor type, some metabolites are also biomarkers of prognosis both within and across tumor groups. Some evidence is also emerging that MRS can also provide biomarkers of treatment response where prior to changes on conventional MRI. Further translation into routine clinical practice requires these biomarkers of prognosis and treatment response to be evaluated in robust clinical trials of specific tumor groups.

Acknowledgments CRUK and EPSRC Cancer Imaging Programme at the Children's Cancer and Leukaemia Group (CCLG) in association with the MRC and Department of Health (England) (C7809/A10342).

References

1. Farmer JP, Montes JL, Freeman CR, Meagher-Villemure K, Bond MC, O'Gorman AM. Brainstem Gliomas. A 10-year institutional review. Pediatr Neurosurg. 2001;34(4):206–14.
2. Freeman CR, Farmer JP. Pediatric brain stem gliomas: a review. Int J Radiat Oncol Biol Phys. 1998;40(2):265–71.
3. Mandell LR, Kadota R, Freeman C, Douglass EC, Fontanesi J, Cohen ME, Kovnar E, Burger P, Sanford RA, Kepner J, Friedman H, Kun LE. There is no role for hyperfractionated radiotherapy in the management of children with newly diagnosed diffuse intrinsic brainstem tumors: results of a Pediatric Oncology Group phase III trial comparing conventional vs. hyperfractionated radiotherapy. Int J Radiat Oncol Biol Phys. 1999;43(5):959–64.
4. Pan E, Prados M. Brainstem Gliomas. In: Gupta N, Haas-Kogen D, Banerjee A, editors. Pediatric CNS tumors, vol. 3. Berlin: Springer; 2004. p. 49–61.
5. Nelson Jr MD, Soni D, Baram TZ. Necrosis in pontine gliomas: radiation induced or natural history? Radiology. 1994;191(1):279–82.

6. Yoshimura J, Onda K, Tanaka R, Takahashi H. Clinicopathological study of diffuse type brainstem gliomas: analysis of 40 autopsy cases. Neurol Med Chir (Tokyo). 2003;43(8):375–82. discussion 382.
7. Wen PY, Kesari S. Malignant gliomas in adults. N Engl J Med. 2008;359(5):492–507.
8. Fisher JL, Schwartzbaum JA, Wrensch M, Wiemels JL. Epidemiology of brain tumors. Neurol Clin. 2007;25(4):867–90. vii.
9. Sands SA, van Gorp WG, Finlay JL. Pilot neuropsychological findings from a treatment regimen consisting of intensive chemotherapy and bone marrow rescue for young children with newly diagnosed malignant brain tumors. Childs Nerv Syst. 1998;14(10):587–9.
10. Dhall G, Grodman H, Ji L, Sands S, Gardner S, Dunkel IJ, McCowage GB, Diez B, Allen JC, Gopalan A, Cornelius AS, Termuhlen A, Abromowitch M, Sposto R, Finlay JL. Outcome of children less than three years old at diagnosis with non-metastatic medulloblastoma treated with chemotherapy on the "Head Start" I and II protocols. Pediatr Blood Cancer. 2008;50(6):1169–75.
11. Gardner SL, Asgharzadeh S, Green A, Horn B, McCowage G, Finlay J. Intensive induction chemotherapy followed by high dose chemotherapy with autologous hematopoietic progenitor cell rescue in young children newly diagnosed with central nervous system atypical teratoid rhabdoid tumors. Pediatr Blood Cancer. 2008;51(2):235–40.
12. Fangusaro J, Finlay J, Sposto R, Ji L, Saly M, Zacharoulis S, Asgharzadeh S, Abromowitch M, Olshefski R, Halpern S, Dubowy R, Comito M, Diez B, Kellie S, Hukin J, Rosenblum M, Dunkel I, Miller DC, Allen J, Gardner S. Intensive chemotherapy followed by consolidative myeloablative chemotherapy with autologous hematopoietic cell rescue (AuHCR) in young children with newly diagnosed supratentorial primitive neuroectodermal tumors (sPNETs): report of the Head Start I and II experience. Pediatr Blood Cancer. 2008;50(2):312–8.
13. Zacharoulis S, Levy A, Chi SN, Gardner S, Rosenblum M, Miller DC, Dunkel I, Diez B, Sposto R, Ji L, Asgharzadeh S, Hukin J, Belasco J, Dubowy R, Kellie S, Termuhlen A, Finlay J. Outcome for young children newly diagnosed with ependymoma, treated with intensive induction chemotherapy followed by myeloablative chemotherapy and autologous stem cell rescue. Pediatr Blood Cancer. 2007;49(1):34–40.
14. Opstad KS, Ladroue C, Bell BA, Griffiths JR, Howe FA. Linear discriminant analysis of brain tumour (1)H MR spectra: a comparison of classification using whole spectra versus metabolite quantification. NMR Biomed. 2007;20(8):763–70.
15. Huang Y, Lisboa PJG, El-Deredy W. Tumour grading from magnetic resonance spectroscopy: a comparison of feature extraction with variable selection. Stat Med. 2003;22(1):147–64.
16. Reynolds GM, Peet AC, Arvanitis TN. Generating prior probabilities for classifiers of brain tumours using belief networks. BMC Med Inform Decis Mak. 2007;7:27.
17. Davies NP, Wilson M, Harris LM, Natarajan K, Lateef S, Macpherson L, Sgouros S, Grundy RG, Arvanitis TN, Peet AC. Identification and characterisation of childhood cerebellar tumours by in vivo proton MRS. NMR Biomed. 2008;21(8):908–18.
18. Ackerstaff E, Glunde K, Bhujwalla ZM. Choline phospholipid metabolism: a target in cancer cells? J Cell Biochem. 2003;90(3):525–33.
19. Podo F. Tumour phospholipid metabolism. NMR Biomed. 1999;12(7):413–39.
20. Hwang JH, Egnaczyk GF, Ballard E, Dunn RS, Holland SK, Ball Jr WS. Proton MR spectroscopic characteristics of pediatric pilocytic astrocytomas. AJNR Am J Neuroradiol. 1998;19(3):535–40.
21. Panigrahy A, Krieger MD, Gonzalez-Gomez I, Liu X, McComb JG, Finlay JL, Nelson Jr MD, Gilles FH, Bluml S. Quantitative short echo time 1H-MR spectroscopy of untreated pediatric brain tumors: preoperative diagnosis and characterization. AJNR Am J Neuroradiol. 2006;27(3):560–72.
22. Negendank W, Sauter R. Intratumoral lipids in 1H MRS in vivo in brain tumors: experience of the Siemens cooperative clinical trial. Anticancer Res. 1996;16(3B):1533–8.
23. Barker PB. Fundamentals of MR spectroscopy. In: Gillard JH, Waldman AD, Barker PB, editors. Clinical MR neuroimaging—diffusion, perfusion and spectroscopy. Cambridge: Cambridge University Press; 2005. p. 15–20.
24. Panigrahy A, Nelson MJ, Blüml S. Magnetic resonance spectroscopy in pediatric neuroradiology: clinical and research applications. Pediatr Radiol. 2010;40(1):3–30.
25. Martínez-Bisbal MC, Celda B. Proton magnetic resonance spectroscopy imaging in the study of human brain cancer. Q J Nucl Med Mol Imaging. 2009;53(6):618–30.
26. McRobbie DW. It's not just squiggles: in vivo spectroscopy. In: McRobbie DW, Moore EA, Graves MJ, Prince MR, editors. MRI From Picture to Proton; 2008. p 306–324.
27. Provencher SW. Estimation of metabolite concentrations from localized in vivo proton NMR spectra. Magn Reson Med. 1993;30(6):672–9.
28. Wilson M, Reynolds G, Kauppinen RA, Arvanitis TN, Peet AC. A constrained least-squares approach to the automated quantitation of in vivo ^{1}H magnetic resonance spectroscopy data. Magn Reson Med. 2011;65(1):1–12.
29. Naressi A, Couturier C, Devos JM, Janssen M, Mangeat C, de Beer R, Graveron-Demilly D. Java-based graphical user interface for the MRUI quantitation package. MAGMA. 2001;12(2–3):141–52.
30. Wilson M, Davies NP, Sun Y, Natarajan K, Arvanitis TN, Kauppinen RA, Peet AC. A comparison between simulated and experimental basis sets for assessing short-TE in vivo ^{1}H MRS data at 1.5 T. NMR Biomed. 2010;23(10):1117–26.
31. Moreno-Torres A, Martinez-Perez I, Baquero M, Campistol J, Capdevila A, Arus C, Pujol J. Taurine detection by proton magnetic resonance spectroscopy in medulloblastoma: Contribution to non-invasive differential diagnosis with cerebellar astrocytomas. Neurosurgery. 2004;55:824–9.
32. Wilke M, Eidenschink A, Muller-Weihrich S, Auer DP. MR diffusion imaging and 1H spectroscopy in a child with medulloblastoma. A case report. Acta Radiol. 2001;42(1):39–42.
33. Tong Z, Yamaki T, Harada K, Houkin K. In vivo quantification of the metabolites in normal brain and brain tumors by proton MR spectroscopy using water as an internal standard. Magn Reson Imaging. 2004;22(5):735–42.
34. Kovanlikaya A, Panigrahy A, Krieger M, Gonzalez-Gomez I, Ghugre N, McComb J, Gilles F, Nelson M, Blüml S. Untreated pediatric primitive neuroectodermal tumor in vivo: quantitation of taurine with MR spectroscopy. Radiology. 2005;236(3):1020–5.
35. Ashok P, Finlay JL, Nelson MD, Gilles FH, Gonzalez-Gomez I, Krieger MD, Bluml S. In vivo MR spectroscopy and diffusion MR imaging of the desmoplastic subtype of medulloblastoma. Dallas, Texas, US: Society of Neuro-Oncology; 2007.
36. Wang Z, Sutton LN, Cnaan A, Haselgrove JC, Rorke LB, Zhao H, Bilaniuk LT, Zimmerman RA. Proton MR spectroscopy of pediatric cerebellar tumors. AJNR Am J Neuroradiol. 1995;16(9):1821–33.
37. Harris LM, Davies NP, Macpherson L, Lateef S, Natarajan K, Brundler MA, Sgouros S, English MW, Arvanitis TN, Grundy RG, Peet AC. Magnetic resonance spectroscopy in the assessment of pilocytic astrocytomas. Eur J Cancer. 2008;44(17):2640–7.
38. Albright AL, Packer RJ, Zimmerman R, Rorke LB, Boyett J, Hammond GD. Magnetic resonance scans should replace biopsies for the diagnosis of diffuse brain stem gliomas: a report from the Children's Cancer Group. Neurosurgery. 1993;33(6):1026–9. discussion 1029–1030.
39. Jallo GI, Biser-Rohrbaugh A, Freed D. Brainstem gliomas. Childs Nerv Syst. 2004;20(3):143–53.
40. Barkovich AJ, Krischer J, Kun LE, Packer R, Zimmerman RA, Freeman CR, Wara WM, Albright L, Allen JC, Hoffman HJ. Brain

stem gliomas: a classification system based on magnetic resonance imaging. Pediatr Neurosurg. 1990;16(2):73–83.
41. Seymour ZA, Panigrahy A, Finlay JL, Nelson Jr MD, Bluml S. Citrate in pediatric CNS tumors? AJNR Am J Neuroradiol. 2008;29(5):1006–11.
42. Panigrahy A, Nelson Jr MD, Finlay JL, Sposto R, Krieger MD, Gilles FH, Bluml S. Metabolism of diffuse intrinsic brainstem gliomas in children. Neuro Oncol. 2008;10(1):32–44.
43. Harris LM, Davies N, MacPherson L, Wilson S, English M, Brundler M-A, Arvanitis TN, Grundy R, Peet AC. Short echo time single voxel 1H Magnetic Resonance Spectroscopy in the diagnosis and characterisation of pineal region tumours. Pediatric Blood Cancer. 2011;57(6):972–7.
44. Brown WD, Gilles FH, Tavare CJ, Rorke LB, Davis RL, Adelman L, Hedley-Whyte ET, Leviton A. Prognostic limitations of the Daumas-Duport grading scheme in childhood supratentorial astroglial tumors. J Neuropathol Exp Neurol. 1998;57(11):1035–40.
45. Gilles FH, Leviton A, Tavare CJ, Adelman L, Rorke LB, Sobel EL, Hedley-Whyte ET, Davis RL. Definitive classes of childhood supratentorial neuroglial tumors. The childhood brain tumor consortium. Pediatr Dev Pathol. 2000;3(2):126–39.
46. Hockel M, Schlenger K, Mitze M, Schaffer U, Vaupel P. Hypoxia and radiation response in human tumors. Semin Radiat Oncol. 1996;6(1):3–9.
47. Hockel M, Schlenger K, Aral B, Mitze M, Schaffer U, Vaupel P. Association between tumor hypoxia and malignant progression in advanced cancer of the uterine cervix. Cancer Res. 1996;56(19):4509–15.
48. Sutherland RM, Ausserer WA, Murphy BJ, Laderoute KR. Tumor hypoxia and heterogeneity: challenges and opportunities for the future. Semin Radiat Oncol. 1996;6(1):59–70.
49. Jain RK, di Tomaso E, Duda DG, Loeffler JS, Sorensen AG, Batchelor TT. Angiogenesis in brain tumours. Nat Rev Neurosci. 2007;8(8):610–22.
50. Winkler F, Kozin SV, Tong RT, Chae SS, Booth MF, Garkavtsev I, Xu L, Hicklin DJ, Fukumura D, di Tomaso E, Munn LL, Jain RK. Kinetics of vascular normalization by VEGFR2 blockade governs brain tumor response to radiation: role of oxygenation, angiopoietin-1, and matrix metalloproteinases. Cancer Cell. 2004;6(6):553–63.
51. Peet AC, Davies NP, Ridley L, Brundler MA, Kombogiorgas D, Lateef S, Natarajan K, Sgouros S, Macpherson L, Grundy RG. Magnetic resonance spectroscopy suggests key differences in the metastatic behaviour of medulloblastoma. Eur J Cancer. 2007;43(6):1037–44.
52. Broniscer A, Baker SJ, West AN, Fraser MM, Proko E, Kocak M, Dalton J, Zambetti GP, Ellison DW, Kun LE, Gajjar A, Gilbertson RJ, Fuller CE. Clinical and molecular characteristics of malignant transformation of low-grade glioma in children. J Clin Oncol. 2007;25(6):682–9.
53. Castillo M, Smith JK, Kwock L. Correlation of myo-inositol levels and grading of cerebral astrocytomas. AJNR Am J Neuroradiol. 2000;21(9):1645–9.
54. Tzika AA, Vigneron DB, Dunn RS, Nelson SJ, Ball Jr WS. Intracranial tumors in children: small single-voxel proton MR spectroscopy using short- and long-echo sequences. Neuroradiology. 1996;38(3):254–63.
55. Negendank WG. Studies of human tumors by MRS: a review. NMR Biomed. 1992;5:303–24.
56. Negendank WG, Sauter R, Brown TR, Evelhoch JL, Falini A, Gotsis ED, Heerschap A, Kamada K, Lee BC, Mengeot MM, Moser E, Padavic-Shaller KA, Sanders JA, Spraggins TA, Stillman AE, Terwey B, Vogl TJ, Wicklow K, Zimmerman RA. Proton magnetic resonance spectroscopy in patients with glial tumors: a multicenter study. J Neurosurg. 1996;84(3):449–58.
57. Nelson SJ, Vigneron DB, Dillon WP. Serial evaluation of patients with brain tumors using volume MRI and 3D 1H MRSI. NMR Biomed. 1999;12:123–38.
58. Sijens PE, Knopp MV, Brunetti A, Wicklow K, Alfano B, Bachert P, Sanders JA, Stillman AE, Kett H, Sauter R, et al. 1H MR spectroscopy in patients with metastatic brain tumors: a multicenter study. Magn Reson Med. 1995;33(6):818–26.
59. Taylor JS, Ogg RJ, Langston JW. Proton MR spectroscopy of pediatric brain tumors. Neuroimaging Clin N Am. 1998;8(4):753–79.
60. Taylor JS, Langston JW, Reddick WE, Kingsley PB, Ogg RJ, Pui MH, Kun LE, Jenkins JJ, Chen G, Ochs JJ, Sanford RA, Heideman RL. Clinical value of proton magnetic resonance spectroscopy for differentiating recurrent or residual brain tumor from delayed cerebral necrosis. Int J Radiat Oncol Biol Phys. 1996;36(5):1251–61.
61. Shimizu H, Kumabe T, Tominaga T, Kayama T, Hara K, Ono Y, Sato K, Arai N, Fujiwara S, Yoshimoto T. Noninvasive evaluation of malignancy of brain tumors with proton MR spectroscopy. AJNR Am J Neuroradiol. 1996;17:737–47.
62. Chang YW, Yoon HK, Shin HJ, Roh HG, Cho JM. MR imaging of glioblastoma in children: usefulness of diffusion/perfusion-weighted MRI and MR spectroscopy. Pediatr Radiol. 2003;33(12):836–42.
63. Blüml S, Panigrahy A, Laskov M, Dhall G, Krieger MD, Nelson Jr MD, Finlay JL, Gilles FH. Elevated citrate in pediatric astrocytomas with malignant progression. Neuro-Oncol. 2011;12(10):1107–17.
64. Hargrave D, Bartels U, Bouffet E. Diffuse brainstem glioma in children: critical review of clinical trials. Lancet Oncol. 2006;7(3):241–8.
65. Porto L, Kieslich M, Franz K, Lehrbecher T, Vlaho S, Pilatus U, Hattingen E. Spectroscopy of untreated pilocytic astrocytomas: do children and adults share some metabolic features in addition to their morphologic similarities? Childs Nerv Syst. 2010;26(6):801–6.
66. Davies NP, Wilson M, Natarajan K, Sun Y, Macpherson L, Brundler MA, Arvanitis TN, Grundy RG, Peet AC. Non-invasive detection of glycine as a biomarker of malignancy in childhood brain tumours using in-vivo (1)H MRS at 1.5 Tesla confirmed by ex-vivo high-resolution magic-angle spinning NMR. NMR Biomed. 2009;23(1):80–7.
67. Astrakas LG, Zurakowski D, Tzika AA, Zarifi MK, Anthony DC, De Girolami U, Tarbell NJ, Black PM. Noninvasive magnetic resonance spectroscopic imaging biomarkers to predict the clinical grade of pediatric brain tumors. Clin Cancer Res. 2004;10(24):8220–8.
68. Marcus KJ, Astrakas LG, Zurakowski D, Zarifi MK, Mintzopoulos D, Poussaint TY, Anthony DC, De Girolami U, Black PM, Tarbell NJ, Tzika AA. Predicting survival of children with CNS tumors using proton magnetic resonance spectroscopic imaging biomarkers. Int J Oncol. 2007;30(3):651–7.
69. Lazareff JA, Gupta RK, Alger J. Variation of post-treatment H-MRSI choline intensity in pediatric gliomas. J Neurooncol. 1999;41(3):291–8.
70. Warren KE, Frank JA, Black JL, Hill RS, Duyn JH, Aikin AA, Lewis BK, Adamson PC, Balis FM. Proton magnetic resonance spectroscopic imaging in children with recurrent primary brain tumors. J Clin Oncol. 2000;18(5):1020–6.
71. Tzika AA, Astrakas LG, Zarifi MK, Zurakowski D, Poussaint TY, Goumnerova L, Tarbell NJ, Black PM. Spectroscopic and perfusion magnetic resonance imaging predictors of progression in pediatric brain tumors. Cancer. 2004;100(6):1246–56.
72. Wald LL, Nelson SJ, Day MR, Noworolski SE, Henry RG, Huhn SL, Chang S, Prados MD, Sneed PK, Larson DA, Wara WM, McDermott M, Dillon WP, Gutin PH, Vigneron DB. Serial proton magnetic resonance spectroscopy imaging of glioblastoma multiforme after brachytherapy. J Neurosurg. 1997;87(4):525–34.
73. Preul MC, Leblanc R, Caramanos Z, Kasrai R, Narayanan S, Arnold DL. Magnetic resonance spectroscopy guided brain tumor resection: differentiation between recurrent glioma and radiation change in two diagnostically difficult cases. Can J Neurol Sci. 1998;25(1):13–22.
74. Isobe T, Matsumura A, Anno I, Nagatomo Y, Yoshizawa T, Itai Y, Nose T. Changes in 1H-MRS in glioma patients before and after irradiation: the significance of quantitative analysis of choline-containing compounds. No Shinkei Geka. 2003;31(2):167–72.

75. Schlemmer HP, Bachert P, Herfarth KK, Zuna I, Debus J, van Kaick G. Proton MR spectroscopic evaluation of suspicious brain lesions after stereotactic radiotherapy. AJNR Am J Neuroradiol. 2001;22(7):1316–24.
76. Weybright P, Sundgren PC, Maly P, Hassan DG, Nan B, Rohrer S, Junck L. Differentiation between brain tumor recurrence and radiation injury using MR spectroscopy. Am J Roentgenol. 2005;185(6):1471–6.
77. Smith EA, Carlos RC, Junck LR, Tsien CI, Elias A, Sundgren PC. Developing a clinical decision model: MR spectroscopy to differentiate between recurrent tumor and radiation change in patients with new contrast-enhancing lesions. Am J Roentgenol. 2009;192(2):W45–52.
78. Central Brain Tumor Registry of the United States. Statistical report: primary brain tumors in the United States, 1997–2001. 2004.
79. Warren K. Molecularly targeted therapy for pediatric brain tumors. J Neurooncol. 2005;75(3):335–43.

6 Diffuse Intrinsic Pontine Gliomas

Stefan Blüml

Diffuse intrinsic pontine gliomas (DIPG) are unique in pediatric neuro-oncology as they are inoperable and rarely being biopsied. They are a relatively *clean* tumor group to be studied with magnetic resonance (MR) spectroscopy because lesions are always in the same region, generally large and homogeneous, and MR studies are technically not compromised by biopsies or surgery. These tumors are well suited for longitudinal studies to evaluate metabolic changes over the disease course. The absence of tissue samples, unfortunately, also means that definitive correlation between physiological features and tissue biology and histology is not possible. In this chapter, an overview of the MR spectroscopic features of DIPG at baseline and at follow-up is given.

Pontine Gliomas

The majority of childhood brainstem gliomas (approximately 80%) are diffuse intrinsic tumors that involve the pons, often with contiguous involvement of other brainstem sites [1–4]. It is believed that at diagnosis most DIPG present as low- or high-grade astrocytoma but the frequency of each is unclear because biopsies are usually not obtained. At autopsy most lesions have progressed to glioblastoma, with extensive brainstem involvement [5–7]. On T1-weighted MR images, these lesions are hypointense with indistinct margins, reflecting the infiltrative nature of this tumor. Contrast enhancement is variable and has no prognostic implication [8]. On T2-weighted MRI, these lesions are indiscrete hyperintense (Fig. 6.1). Among pediatric brain tumors, DIPG carry the worst prognosis and outcomes have not improved for decades. The brainstem is responsible for basic vital life functions such as breathing, heartbeat, and blood pressure. Therefore, intrinsic brainstem tumors are considered inoperable due to the unavoidable damage to essential structures. In addition, brainstem gliomas are highly resistant to chemo- and radiation therapy. Thus, without effective and lasting treatment options, the majority of the patients die within 6–18 months after diagnoses. Reports of several years of survival after diagnosis are rare and there is only anecdotal evidence for complete and lasting disease remission. Consequently, current management aims to preserve the quality of life for patients and to reduce the burden on the families. Since biopsies for diagnostic purposes and to monitor disease progression are risky and have failed to show any benefits for patients, noninvasive MR imaging is considered the gold standard for diagnosing these types of tumors. Still, magnetic resonance imaging (MRI) and other currently available imaging modalities are often of limited value to assess disease progression or response to therapy. This lack of appropriate monitoring tools compromises clinical research considerably. Despite the inevitably fatal outcome of these tumors, there are still important treatment decisions that have to be made which have a significant impact on the quality of life of a patient. Whether advanced MR methods such as MR spectroscopy can be used for early substratification of brainstem gliomas is still unclear.

Other Brainstem Gliomas

Other tumors of the brainstem have a more favorable prognosis. These include:

(a) Focal cystic or solid tumors with demarcated lesions on MRI in the midbrain, pons, and medulla. Enhancement after administration of contrast of these tumors is variable. These tumors are less infiltrative and are histologically mostly benign (e.g., pilocytic astrocytoma). However, primitive neuroectodermal tumors (PNET) and anaplastic ganglioglioma have been also reported [9].
(b) Dorsally exophytic brainstem gliomas arise from subependymal glial tissue and have features on MRI similar

S. Blüml, Ph.D. (✉)
Department of Radiology, Children's Hospital Los Angeles, Keck School of Medicine, University of Southern California, Los Angeles, CA, USA
e-mail: SBluml@chla.usc.edu

S. Blüml and A. Panigrahy (eds.), *MR Spectroscopy of Pediatric Brain Disorders*,
DOI 10.1007/978-1-4419-5864-8_6, © Springer Science+Business Media, LLC 2013

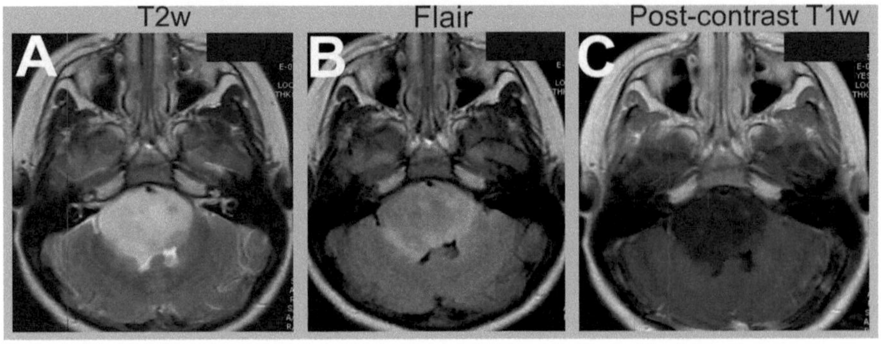

Fig. 6.1 T2-weighted, FLAIR, and postcontrast T1-weighted MR images of a pontine glioma at diagnosis. These lesions are generally hyperintense on T2w MRI and hypointense on T1w MRI

to that of focal brainstem tumors. As focal brainstem tumors, they are mostly low-grade lesions.

(c) Cervicomedullary brainstem gliomas center either in the medulla or cervical spinal cord. These tumors are mostly low-grade astrocytomas with almost no infiltrative capacity [10]. Brainstem tumors associated with neuro fibromatosis I (NF-1) also carry a more favorable diagnosis. These lesions often have an indolent course similar to that of the low-grade astrocytoma in the hypothalamic/optic chiasm region.

Magnetic Resonance Spectroscopy of Diffuse Intrinsic Pontine Gliomas

Only few groups have attempted to study pediatric brainstem tumors by MR spectroscopy and only few patients were examined longitudinally. Laprie et al. [11] performed long echo time (TE = 144 ms) 2D and 3D CSI. Four DIPG patients were studied before radiation therapy, upon completion of treatment, and at the time of recurrence (determined by clinical status). In their study, only ratios of choline to NAA (Cho/NAA) and Cho to Cr (Cho/Cr) were determined and the presence/absence of lipid or lactate peaks was reported. They found that the Cho/NAA ratio decreased from studies at diagnosis to the time of response to radiation therapy but then again increased at the time of relapse. Curless et al. [12] studied five patients with long TE = 135 ms single voxel MRS and determined NAA/Cr and Cho/Cr ratios. They concluded that MRS provided additional information, which might be useful for determination of the malignant potential of the brainstem lesions. In particular, it was reported that more aggressive tumors have larger values of Cho/Cr. Recently, 40 MRS studies acquired with short TE = 35 ms PRESS at baseline and at various times of follow-up of a larger cohort of 16 patients were reviewed [13]. At baseline, creatine and choline were significantly lower in DIPG than in astrocytoma elsewhere in the central nervous system. Serial MRS in individual subjects revealed increasing levels of Cho and lipids and reduced ratios of NAA, creatine, and myo-inositol relative to Cho (Fig. 6.2). Similar to the earlier studies by [11, 14], it was also noted that metabolic progression, defined by increased Cho concentration in serial MRS, preceded clinical deterioration. It appears that, as seen by MR spectroscopy, DIPG at baseline have typically metabolic profiles consistent with low-proliferative tumors. This is consistent with earlier reports of histopathological features often typical for grade II diffuse astrocytomas [4–7, 15–17]. However, clearly, these tumors do have the capability to transform to tumors that are more malignant within a short period, which is then also reflected by an altered metabolic profile more typical for higher grade gliomas.

Monitoring Treatment Response

It needs to be emphasized that the metabolic progression observed in most DIBSG patients is consistent with the fact that radiation therapies and other treatments applied for this disease are essentially ineffective. However, patients treated with radiation therapy have a longer median survival than what would have been attained in the absence of radiation therapy, albeit they are not cured. Although, the outcomes are generally poor, there are significant differences of survival times in individual patients. One may wonder whether the metabolic profile at diagnosis and/or the metabolic progression of patients with significant different survival periods is different. Indeed, preliminary data suggest that *metabolic* degeneration appears to be less apparent in patients with longer survival [18] (Figs. 6.2 and 6.3).

Distinguishing Diffuse Intrinsic Pontine Gliomas from Other Brainstem Tumors

Due to their typical appearance (and the accompanying clinical symptoms), DIPG are generally readily diagnosed by anatomical MRI alone. However, occasionally, in individual patients the appearance of an exophytic brainstem tumor

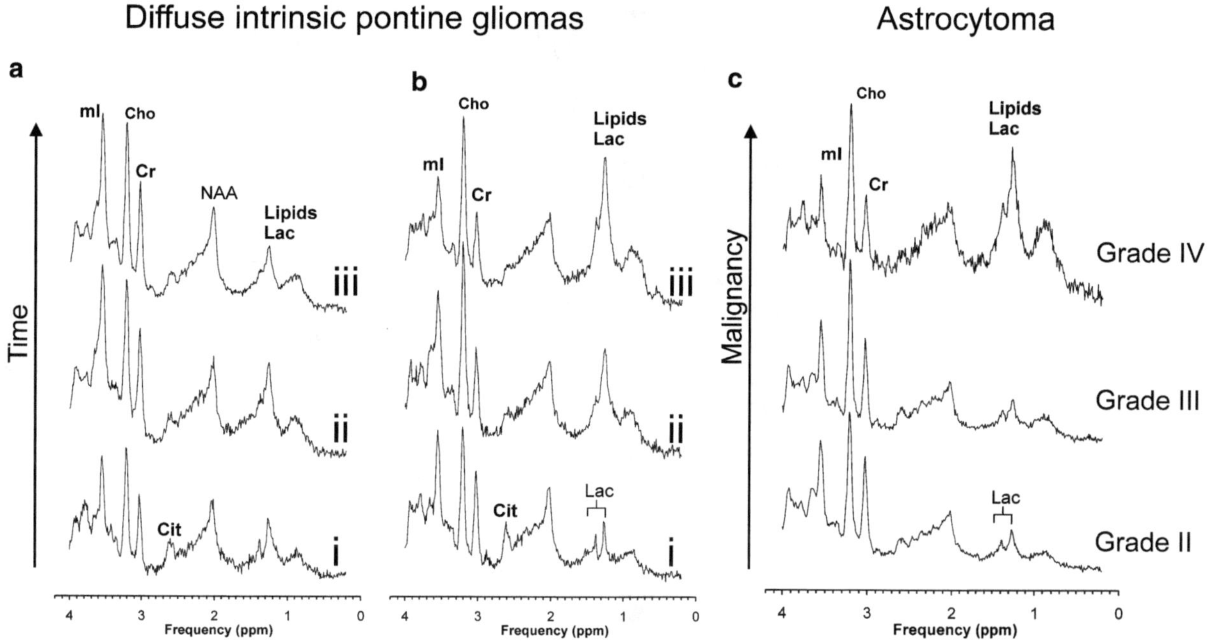

Fig. 6.2 Shown in this figure are typical metabolic profiles of diffuse intrinsic pontine gliomas (**a**, **b**) and of biopsy-confirmed grade II-IV astrocytomas (**c**). Spectra from DIPG were obtained from 12 patients that were studied repeatedly at diagnosis and thereafter. The DIPG patients were subdivided in two groups (each six patients) based on their overall survival time. Mean survival time for group A (14±3 months) was significantly longer than for group B (9±2 months). Only minor alterations were noticed for group A. Group B showed changes consistent with malignant transformation (compare with MR pattern of confirmed grade II–IV astrocytoma (C)). Note, that moderate Cho and Cho/Cr and the absence of lipids in the baseline spectrum is more typical for low-grade tumors. Cho and Cho/Cr as well as lipids and lactate subsequently increase. The time of MRS examinations was at baseline (i), postradiation therapy up to 6 months after initial diagnosis (ii), and thereafter (iii). Overall, for both groups, serial MRS is consistent with unavailability of any effective therapy and the poor clinical course of DIPG. Citrate is detectable at approximately 2.6 ppm

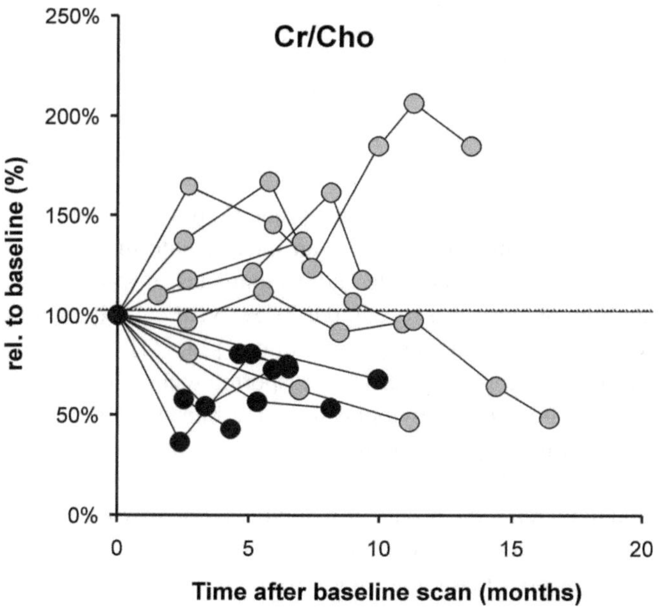

Fig. 6.3 Shown is the time course of the creatine to choline ratio (Cr/Cho) relative to the value measured at diagnosis (baseline). Generally, there is a significant scatter. However, measured Cr/Cho was more often above baseline in patients who did clinically better (*gray circles*) than in patients with shorter overall survival times (*black circles*). The data shown here are from the same 12 patients illustrated in Fig. 6.2

may mimic the features of a DIPG. Considering that many of the non-DIPG tumors are pilocytic astrocytomas, which are readily distinguishable from regular astrocytoma by their unique metabolic profile [19], MRS can be very useful for reaffirming diagnoses (Figs. 6.4 and 6.5) [20].

Transformation to higher grade gliomas is exceedingly rare in children in the setting of neurofibromatosis 1 (NF1) [21]. Although the diagnosis of neurofibromatosis has generally already been made, one may wonder whether the metabolic profile of tumors of the brainstem (or elsewhere in the brain) in NF1 patients is substantially different. It appears that spectra of lesions in the pons of NF1 patient have a pattern comparable with that of low-grade gliomas. However, lactate levels appeared to be lower and there was no evidence for citrate in a small number of patients studied at Children's Hospital Los Angeles (Fig. 6.6).

Citrate

The presence of *citrate* (Cit) in in vivo spectra of pediatric brain tumors was recently reported [22]. Citrate levels were reported to be particularly high in DIPG [22], tumors with

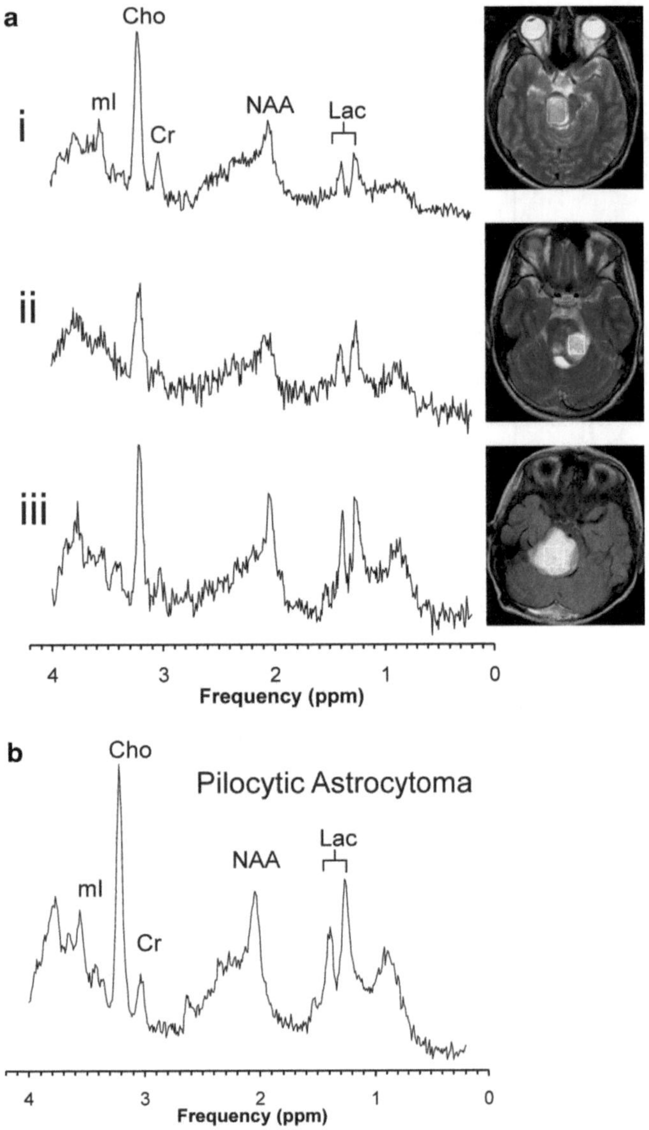

Fig. 6.4 MR spectra and MR images indicating the ROIs of three exophytic brainstem tumors are shown (**a**). Note, that the MRS pattern in each case does not resemble the profile observed for DIPG. Particularly, creatine concentrations are very low in these tumors. In addition, myo-inositol is below normal tissue concentrations and there is a residual NAA peak of the same intensity as creatine. This pattern is more suggestive for pilocytic astrocytoma. A typical spectrum of infratentorial pilocytic astrocytoma is shown for comparison (**b**). All three patients (i–iii) are still alive as of today more than 6 years after their initial diagnoses

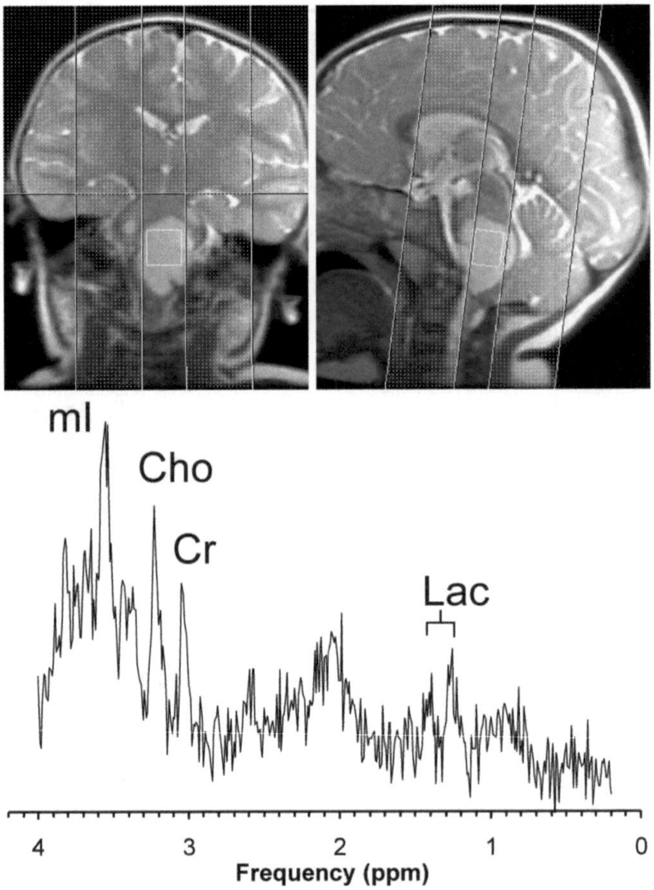

Fig. 6.5 MR images and MR spectrum of a brainstem glioma. The location and appearance on MRI was slightly unusual and it was felt that this tumor might be an exophytic possibly pilocytic astrocytoma. MRS was, however, not consistent with pilocytic astrocytoma. This was subsequently confirmed by biopsy which was suggestive for a grade II or III astrocytoma (Case courtesy of Dr. Giulio Zuccoli, Pittsburgh Children's Hospital.)

apparently inevitable aggressive behavior despite presenting frequently with histopathological features typical for grade II diffuse astrocytomas [4–7, 15–17] (Fig. 6.2a). Citrate was also detected in biopsy-proven grade II,III astrocytoma outside the brainstem. Citrate is an intermediate in the tricarboxylic acid (TCA) cycle and accumulates in tissue where the glycolytic rate exceeds the TCA cycle activity, a long known feature of malignant tumors [23, 24]. Excessive citrate can be used by cells to transport mitochondrial acetyl-CoA carbons to the cytoplasm for the biosynthesis of fatty acids ultimately needed for the de novo synthesis of cell membranes. This is an essential step to support cell divisions and to increase the production of biomass of growing tumors [25]. Of potential importance is the observation that citrate levels at presentation are not only high in DIPG (generally

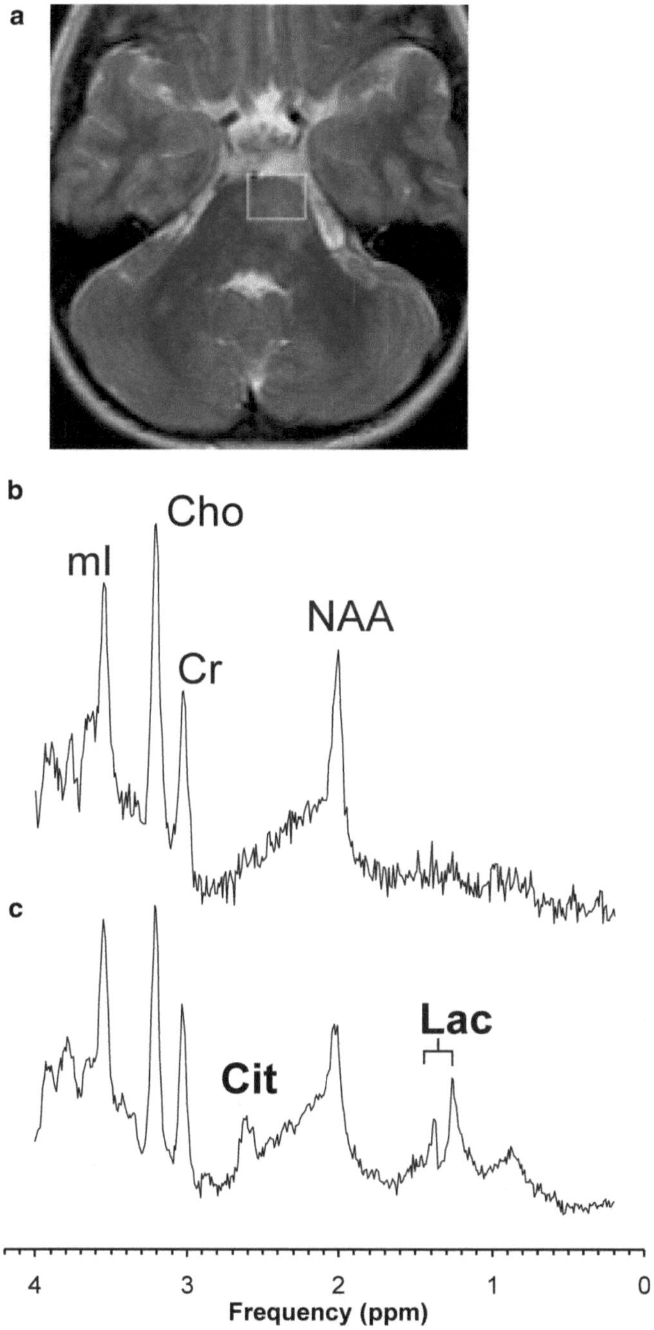

Fig. 6.6 Shown is an MRI (**a**) of a patient with neurofibromatosis I (NF1) and a lesion in the brainstem. Lesions in NF1 of often benign and progression to higher grade lesion is exceedingly rare including lesions of the brainstem. A typical MRS from NF1 brainstem lesion (**b**) is comparable with spectra from DIPG at baseline (**c**). However, there is no evidence for citrate in NF1 and lactate is unremarkable

assumed to progress) but also remarkably prominent in cases of low-grade (grade II) astrocytoma outside the brainstem with sometimes unexpected rapid disease progression (Fig. 6.7) [26]. In repeatedly studied DIPG patients, citrate concentrations declined significantly as the disease progressed (Fig. 6.8).

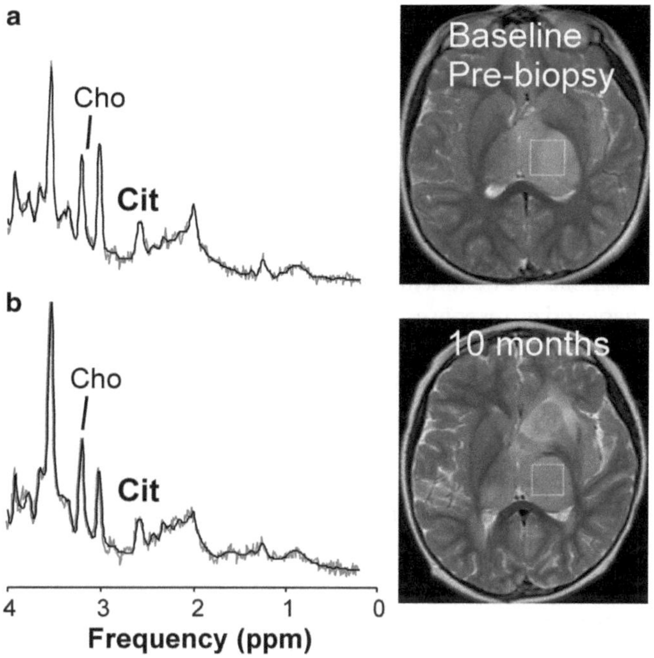

Fig. 6.7 MR spectra and T2-weighted MRI indicating the region of interest from which spectra were obtained of a grade II bithalamic astrocytoma with aggressive behavior. A spectrum acquired from a nonenhancing diffuse astrocytoma at initial presentation (**a**) shows no evidence of elevated lipids or lactate (Lac) and choline (Cho) levels are moderate. On the other hand, citrate (Cit) is readily detectable at baseline. Progressive disease was apparent on MRI within one year after initial diagnosis (**b**) and the patient died within 2 years after diagnosis. Note that choline, lactate, and lipid (Lip) levels increased as the disease progressed whereas citrate did not increase but may have decreased slightly in this patient (cf. Fig. 6.8)

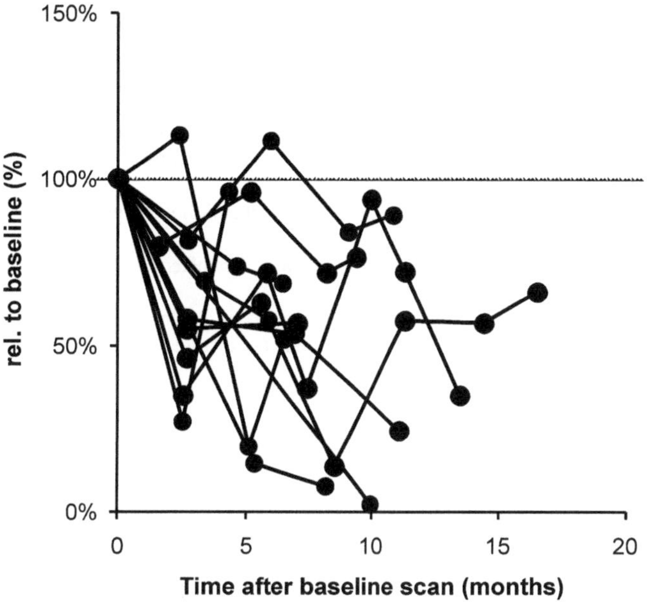

Fig. 6.8 Citrate concentrations decrease significantly over time in DIPG

Conclusions

The majority of DIPG have metabolic fingerprints at initial presentation consistent with tumors with low proliferative rates. The metabolic changes thereafter are consistent with a malignant transformation. This is observed despite transient clinical improvement and is consistent with ineffectiveness of all current treatments. MRS may be an important tool to characterize response to therapy and tumor progression in small groups of patients. This may compensate for the relatively small number of patients available for studies, and allow a faster completion of clinical trials, thus enhancing development of effective therapy for this disease. DIPG can readily be distinguished from other brainstem such as exophytic pilocytic astrocytoma.

References

1. Cohen ME, Duffner PK, Heffner RR, Lacey DJ, Brecher M. Prognostic factors in brainstem gliomas. Neurology. 1986;36(5):602–5.
2. Albright AL, Guthkelch AN, Packer RJ, Price RA, Rourke LB. Prognostic factors in pediatric brain-stem gliomas. J Neurosurg. 1986;65(6):751–5.
3. Halperin EC, Wehn SM, Scott JW, Djang W, Oakes WJ, Friedman HS. Selection of a management strategy for pediatric brainstem tumors. Med Pediatr Oncol. 1989;17(2):117–26.
4. Freeman CR, Farmer JP. Pediatric brain stem gliomas: a review. Int J Radiat Oncol Biol Phys. 1998;40(2):265–71.
5. Farmer JP, Montes JL, Freeman CR, Meagher-Villemure K, Bond MC, O'Gorman AM. Brainstem gliomas. A 10-year institutional review. Pediatr Neurosurg. 2001;34(4):206–14.
6. Nelson Jr MD, Soni D, Baram TZ. Necrosis in pontine gliomas: radiation induced or natural history? Radiology. 1994;191(1):279–82.
7. Yoshimura J, Onda K, Tanaka R, Takahashi H. Clinicopathological study of diffuse type brainstem gliomas: analysis of 40 autopsy cases. Neurol Med Chir (Tokyo). 2003;43(8):375–82. discussion 382.
8. Fischbein NJ, Prados MD, Wara W, Russo C, Edwards MS, Barkovich AJ. Radiologic classification of brain stem tumors: correlation of magnetic resonance imaging appearance with clinical outcome. Pediatr Neurosurg. 1996;24(1):9–23.
9. Matson D. Neurosurgery of infancy and childhood. Springfield, Il: CC. Thomas; 1969. p. 469–77.
10. Jallo GI, Biser-Rohrbaugh A, Freed D. Brainstem gliomas. Childs Nerv Syst. 2004;20(3):143–53.
11. Laprie A, Pirzkall A, Haas-Kogan DA, et al. Longitudinal multivoxel MR spectroscopy study of pediatric diffuse brainstem gliomas treated with radiotherapy. Int J Radiat Oncol Biol Phys. 2005; 62(1):20–31.
12. Curless RG, Bowen BC, Pattany PM, Gonik R, Kramer DL. Magnetic resonance spectroscopy in childhood brainstem tumors. Pediatr Neurol. 2002;26(5):374–8.
13. Panigrahy A, Nelson Jr MD, Finlay JL, et al. Metabolism of diffuse intrinsic brainstem gliomas in children. Neuro Oncol. 2008;10(1):32–44.
14. Thakur SB, Karimi S, Dunkel IJ, Koutcher JA, Huang W. Longitudinal MR spectroscopic imaging of pediatric diffuse pontine tumors to assess tumor aggression and progression. AJNR Am J Neuroradiol. 2006;27(4):806–9.
15. Mandell LR, Kadota R, Freeman C, et al. There is no role for hyperfractionated radiotherapy in the management of children with newly diagnosed diffuse intrinsic brainstem tumors: results of a Pediatric Oncology Group phase III trial comparing conventional vs. hyperfractionated radiotherapy. Int J Radiat Oncol Biol Phys. 1999;43(5):959–64.
16. Pan E, Prados M. Brainstem gliomas. In: Gupta N, Haas-Kogen D, Banerjee A, editors. Pediatric CNS tumors, vol. 3. Berlin, Heidelberg, New York: Springer; 2004. p. 49–61.
17. Hargrave D, Bartels U, Bouffet E. Diffuse brainstem glioma in children: critical review of clinical trials. Lancet Oncol. 2006;7(3):241–8.
18. Panigrahy A, Finlay J, Dhall G, Krieger M, Nelson M, Bluml S. Post-therapeutic metabolic changes in diffuse intrinsic brain stem glioma: initial experience. Neuro-Oncology, Abstracts from the Thirteenth International Symposium on Pediatric Neuro-Oncology (ISPNO). 2008:393.
19. Panigrahy A, Krieger MD, Gonzalez-Gomez I, et al. Quantitative short echo time 1 H-MR spectroscopy of untreated pediatric brain tumors: preoperative diagnosis and characterization. AJNR Am J Neuroradiol. 2006;27(3):560–72.
20. Jackson HA, Panigrahy A, Lui X, Nelson M, D, Blüml S. Quantitative short echo time1H magnetic resonance spectroscopy of pediatric pontine gliomas: diagnosis and characterization. Paper presented at: Western Neuroradiological Society2005; Carlsbad, CA.
21. Dirks PB, Jay V, Becker LE, et al. Development of anaplastic changes in low-grade astrocytomas of childhood. Neurosurgery. 1994;34(1):68–78.
22. Seymour ZA, Panigrahy A, Finlay JL, Nelson Jr MD, Bluml S. Citrate in pediatric CNS tumors? AJNR Am J Neuroradiol. 2008;29(5):1006–11.
23. Warburg O. On the origin of cancer cells. Science. 1956; 123(3191):309–14.
24. Busch H, Davis JR, Olle EW. Citrate accumulation in slices of transplantable tumors of the rat. Cancer Res. 1957;17(7):711–6.
25. Vander Heiden M, Cantley L, Thompson C. Understanding the Warburg effect: the metabolic requirements of cell proliferation. Science. 2009;324(5930):1029–33.
26. Nagasunder AC, Joseph A, Panigrahy A, et al. Prominent citrate predicts malignant progression of low-grade astrocytomas in children. International Society of Magnetic Resonance in Medicine (ISMRM)2010; Stockholm, Sweden.

Traumatic Brain Injury and Concussion

7

Alexander P. Lin and Stefan Blüml

Traumatic brain injury (TBI) results when forces acting upon the head interrupt normal brain function. This type of injury is especially prevalent in children, resulting in over 475,000 emergency department visits each year [1]. In its most severe form, head trauma accounts for 80% of the traumas that lead to death in children, including falls, motor vehicle accidents, and abuse, making it one of the leading causes of death. In addition, "mild" traumatic brain injury (mTBI), otherwise known as concussions, are also a great concern, especially in children ages 0–4 years where the rates of head injury are highest compared to all ages, including adults. Sports-related head injuries are also becoming of increasing concern, especially in older children where 18% of head injuries were sports-related and where the long term effects are unknown.

Magnetic resonance spectroscopy (MRS) offers a unique tool for ascertaining the physiological changes that occur after a traumatic brain injury. What is the metabolic profile of the brain after traumatic injury? Studying head trauma with MRS, as with any tool, is inherently challenging. The type and severity of injury and the time after injury when an MRS study is performed will vary unavoidably. It is therefore expected that the pattern of MR spectroscopy of head trauma is heterogeneous reflecting the different location, degree, and stage of injury and different physiologic and pathologic response of the brain to injury in individuals. There is no single characteristic "finger print" for trauma. As studies emerge, it appears that the brain biochemistry is reflective of this spectrum of traumatic brain injury. As such, this chapter will focus on the metabolic changes observed in the acute and chronic stages of *severe* traumatic brain injury as well as the acute and chronic stages of *mild* traumatic brain injury.

A.P. Lin, Ph.D. (✉)
Department of Radiology, Brigham and Women's Hospital, Boston, MA, USA

S. Blüml, Ph.D.
Department of Radiology, Children's Hospital Los Angeles, Keck School of Medicine, University of Southern California, Los Angeles, CA, USA

Severe Traumatic Brain Injury

Traumatic Brain Injury Is (Almost) Always Associated with a Decrease of NAA in White Matter and Gray Matter

Reduced NAA (or NAA/Cr ratio) after traumatic injury due to diffuse axonal injury and neuronal loss has been consistently reported [2]. The qualifier, "almost", should not be interpreted as an indicator that there is traumatic head injury without any neuronal/axonal loss. Slightly varying normal levels of NAA in individual subjects, inaccuracies of the MR method, and the absence of a pre-injury baseline scans make it difficult to detect small decreases of NAA in less severe injury [3]. Also, if MRS is carried out soon (within 24 h) after initial injury, a loss of NAA may not yet be established [4].

Is recovery of NAA a marker for healthy neurons and axons? If yes, what is the interpretation? Clinical as well as animal studies are indeed strongly suggestive for a recovery of NAA in both white and gray matter [5–7]. In patients with moderate to severe traumatic brain injury, a continuing decrease of NAA consistent with continuing neuronal loss (or metabolic dysfunction) was observed for gray and white matter at 1.5 and 3 months after injury in longitudinal studies. However, in both brain regions an increase of NAA, albeit to levels that were still less than normal, was observed at the 6-months follow-up study [5].

Assuming that there is no neurogenesis this observation is likely due to one or a combination of the following mechanisms:

(a) Surviving neurons can sprout healthy fibers into the spaces once occupied by damaged axons. This increases the partial volume of healthy axons and will thus increase the measured NAA concentration. This mechanism would predict a more substantial recovery in fibrous white matter than in gray.
(b) Neurons that reestablish their connections start to increase communication with each other. A tight coupling between cerebral glucose metabolism and (glutamate) neurotransmitter flux in humans has been proposed

S. Blüml and A. Panigrahy (eds.), *MR Spectroscopy of Pediatric Brain Disorders*, DOI 10.1007/978-1-4419-5864-8_7, © Springer Science+Business Media, LLC 2013

by Magistretti [8]. Although this theory is not universally accepted, it would explain a higher rate of glycolysis and TCA-cycle activity as neurons resume their communication with neighboring neurons. Since NAA reduction has been associated with mitochondrial dysfunction in experimental head trauma [9], it can at least be speculated that mitochondrial NAA synthesis may increase with a normalization of neuronal activity.

(c) After injury, consolidation of remaining intact tissue and atrophy is well documented by neuropathological studies and by cortical atrophy on MR images. Thus the relative number of healthy neurons and axons per tissue volume will actually increase and a more prominent NAA peak will be observed.

(d) NAA can increase or decrease in response to hyper-osmolar or hypo-osmolar states.

Total Choline Is Elevated

Most of the choline in human brain is stored in large, water insoluble molecules and rendered MR *invisible* under normal circumstances. Elevated total choline would be expected in head trauma because of at least three mechanisms:

(a) In acute injury, choline-containing metabolites may be released to the MR-visible pool as a result of shear injury and damage to cell membranes and myelin. It is known that free choline accumulates rapidly in necrotic tissue [10, 11]. This mechanism therefore offers an explanation for elevated choline in acute and sub-acute injury. In the spectrum of acute and severe injury (Fig. 7.1), tCho was 35% above normal. Free choline can be taken up by the cells and recycled to form phosphatidylcholine (PtdCho).

(b) Increased synthesis of cell membranes during repair might result in higher levels of total choline. For example, both the newborn (fast growing) brain and many tumors with a high rate of cell duplication have elevated total choline indicating up-regulation of membrane precursor production. Of the choline containing compounds, it is now phosphocholine (PC) which is expected to be above normal. Unfortunately the MR signal of free choline and PC cannot be separated with proton MRS in vivo. Proton-decoupled phosphorous MRS would be required for this task, which is available only at very few sites.

(c) In patients with more chronic injury, an alternative explanation could be diffuse glial proliferation which is known to be associated with increased tCho but also with elevated mI and Cr [12–14]. Indeed, Ross et al. [15] observed in some subjects elevated mI, tCho, and Cr persistently in white matter even 18 months after injury. In that study mI, tCho, and Cr were essentially normal in gray matter. This would be consistent with glial proliferation predominantly in the white matter. The authors of that study also offered as an alternative explanation for the generally elevated metabolite concentration: the possibility that the white matter is in a *hyper-osmolar* state.

Indeed, elevated tCho or tCho/Cr ratios were reported by a number of investigators [5, 15–19]. In longitudinal patient studies, tCho was significantly increased at 1.5 months for both gray and white matter and remained elevated 3 and 6 months after injury, with a trend (not significant) to lower tCho concentrations [5].

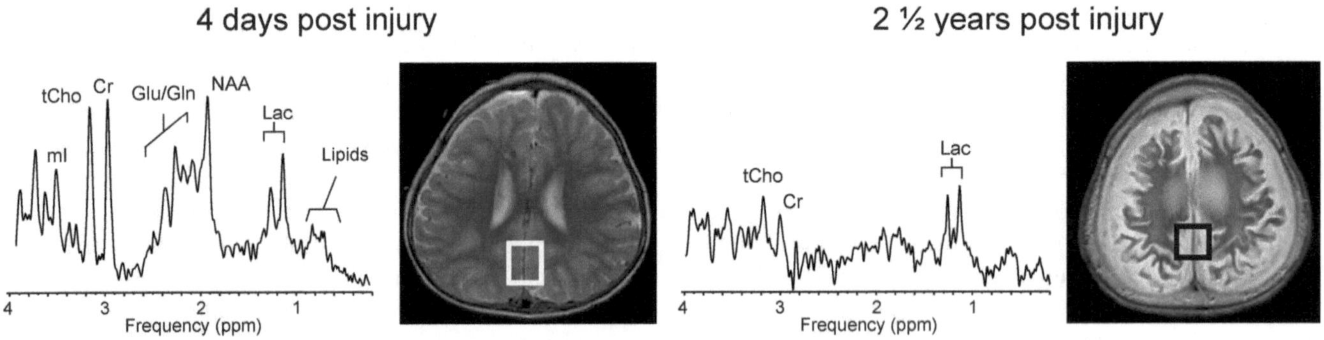

Fig. 7.1 The MRS and T2-weighted MRI of a child (17 months old at time of event) 4 days after traumatic brain injury (*left*) and 2½ years after injury (*right*). The MRI report at baseline mentions an increase of signal intensity in the parietal lobes at the vertex bilaterally. The sulci were effaced in that region as well. MRS changes were dramatic. NAA was reduced to 35% of normal and lactate, not detectable in normal brain, was strikingly prominent. Cr and mI were also reduced to 75% of normal whereas tCho was elevated (135% of normal). Glutamine was threefold higher than normal. There is only a small increase in the lipid signal at this early stage after injury. MRS is consistent with severe hypoxic injury subsequent to low/disrupted perfusion and poor outcome was predicted in the MRS report. Follow-up MRI shows general volume loss. The ROI selected for MRS is similar to the anatomy chosen for the initial study. Due to the massive atrophy little brain tissue is included and the spectrum shows lactate (possible from CSF) and only traces of creatine and choline. No trace of NAA is detected indicating that any tissue within the ROI does not contain viable neurons or axons. Clinical outcome was poor (nonverbal, seizures, dystonia, spasticity, profound cognitive loss). Spectra were acquired using a PRESS sequence with TE=35 ms. at Children's Hospital Los Angeles

Magnetic Resonance Spectroscopy of Acute Severe Brain Injury with Disruption or Significantly Impaired Perfusion Resembles That of Hypoxic Brain Injury and Lactate Is a Predictor for Poor Outcome

In acute and severe injury, increased lactate and lipids also accompanies the reduction of NAA in gray and white matter ROI's are markers of neuronal/axonal loss and cell death. Lactate is the product of anaerobic glycolysis and increases when subsequent oxidation of lactate in the TCA-cycle is impaired (for example by lack of oxygen or mitochondrial disorders). As a result, the MRS pattern of lactate resembles that of hypoxic injury due to global anoxia (Fig. 7.1). Several groups found that lactate found in acute injury may be useful to predict outcome [15, 17, 20–22].

Lipid signals increase when there is breakdown of cell membrane and release of fatty acids. Lipids are therefore important markers for severe brain injury. Lipids appear to be more prominent in children. Particularly prominent lipid peaks were reported by Haseler et al. [21] in "shaken babies" with poor outcome.

Concentrations of Cerebral Metabolites Are Reduced in Patients with Clinically Diagnosed Syndrome of Inappropriate Antidiuretic Hormone Secretion and Low Serum Sodium

Syndrome of Inappropriate Antidiuretic Hormone Secretion (SIADH) is a frequently observed feature of head injury. Because the metabolites of the ^{1}H spectrum can also function (to variable degrees) as osmolytes, systemic changes can be observed. Absolute quantitation of metabolite concentrations is necessary to depict this condition because a reduction of all metabolites is not apparent when peak ratios are analyzed. The reduction persisted weeks after Na+returned to normal [15].

MRS Can Detect Widespread Injury: In Radiologically Normal Appearing Tissue!

MRS confirms that traumatic brain injury is associated with damage at the microscopic level throughout the brain. This has been—unintentionally—confirmed by all those single-voxel MRS studies of normal appearing tissue where investigators selected different regions of interest (although most investigators pick well established parietal white matter and occipital gray matter locations). Spectral abnormalities were reported in all those studies. Obviously, it is more elegant to employ CSI where widespread metabolic abnormalities apparently affecting radiologically normal appearing tissue is readily detectable in individual subjects (Fig. 7.2).

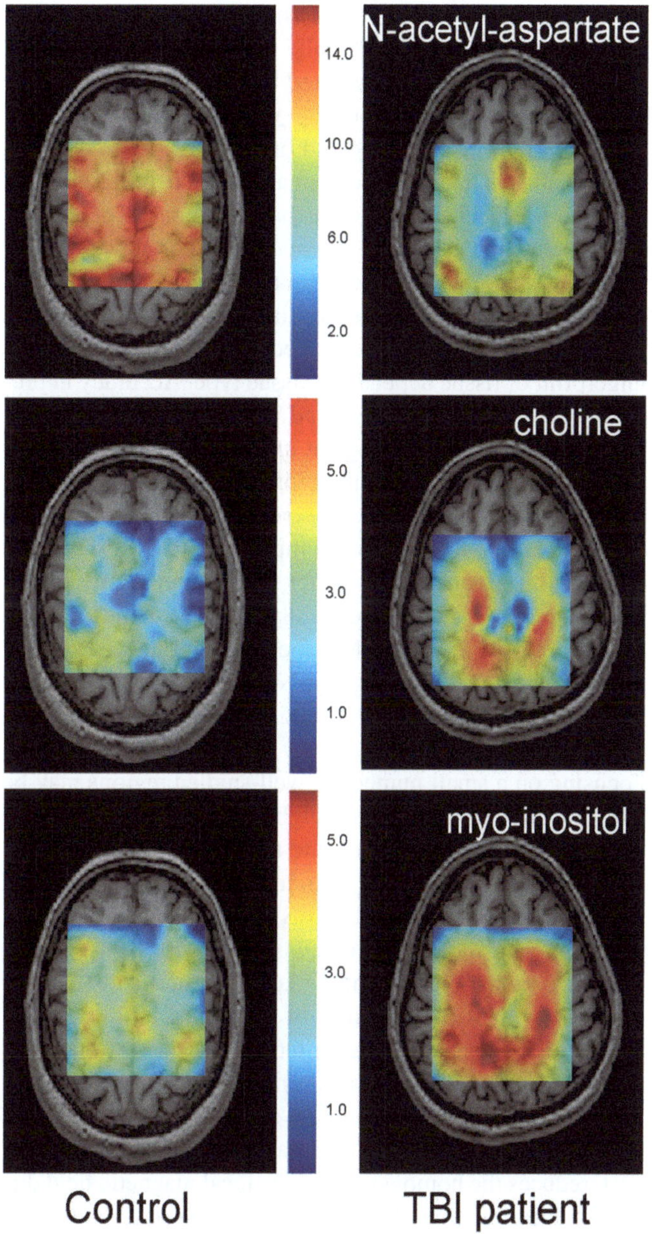

Fig. 7.2 Three Tesla magnetic resonance spectroscopic imaging data (STEAM, TE=20 ms) in traumatic brain injury. The data in the right panels were acquired from a 20-year-old male patient who had suffered a motor-cycle accident (Glasgow Coma Scale=3) 84 days previously. Although the primary site of injury was frontal, the metabolite images show widespread decreased *N*-acetyl-aspartate and elevated choline and myo-inositol throughout this radiologically normal-appearing brain slice. Comparison metabolite data from an uninjured 27-year-old male are shown in the *left panels*. The color map corresponds to metabolite concentrations expressed in institutional units (unpublished data, Hoglund Imaging Center, University of Kansas Medical Center)

Widespread injury is consistent with the fact that recovery of patients is not well explained by purely focal injury. Rather, it is more likely that the overall behavioral recovery is related to the severity and location of the injury averaged over the whole brain.

Returning to the question of where to measure, the added value of measuring the metabolic profile of apparently normal tissue has been demonstrated by Holshouser et al. [23]. They used susceptibility (T2*) weighted MRI to depict regions of non-hemorrhagic and of hemorrhagic tissue after injury. CSI was then utilized to analyze biochemical changes in hemorrhagic and non-hemorrhagic regions. They found that biochemical changes in *apparently* normal appearing tissue predict outcome better than alterations in lesions.

The selection of an appropriate region of interest is another problem. As mentioned above, the metabolic fingerprint of tissue depends on tissue type. Accuracy in prescribing a region of interest (and proper documentation for longitudinal studies!) is of great importance in particular for single voxel studies. It is therefore recommended to study brain regions where MRS *works* and where normal MRS data are readily available for comparison. Two very popular choices are parietal white matter and occipital gray matter which have been studied frequently in head trauma with single voxel MRS [5, 15, 21]. MR spectra of normal gray matter and white matter differ slightly. NAA is present in approximately equal concentration. Creatine is ≈20% higher in gray matter whereas tCho is slightly higher in white matter. Focusing on a small number of well-studied regions may be less of a limitation than one might think. As shown below, alterations of the metabolic state throughout the brain have been observed in traumatic brain injury. When studying head trauma (with single-voxel MRS) one should also avoid acquiring MR spectra from ROIs with obvious focal injury for two reasons: (1) It is most likely, and unsurprising, that metabolism will be abnormal in visibly injured areas and hence MRS does not add very much to MRI. (2) A prerequisite for good quality spectra is a highly homogeneous magnetic field within the region of interest. The presence of blood or blood products, often associated with lesions in TBI, reduces the homogeneity of the local magnetic field due to iron accumulation. Accurate prescription of the region of interest is less a problem for CSI where spectra from a whole slice are being obtained and the position of individual voxels can be adjusted retrospectively via voxel shifting. However, currently CSI is less reproducible than single voxel methods, particularly at the short echo times necessary to evaluate glutamate levels.

Magnetic Resonance Spectroscopy, a Predictor of Outcome?

Considering that the extent of the decrease of NAA can be seen as a quantitative marker for neuronal loss, questions arise whether MRS can be used to predict outcome and if so, at what (earliest) time after injury can prognostic information be obtained. Significant reduction of NAA, the presence of lipids and elevated lactate are markers of severe (hypoxic) brain injury and MRS as early as 2–5 days after injury (Fig. 7.1) might be a useful tool for triage of patients who remain unconscious several days after injury [15, 17, 20–22]. In less devastating injury, Friedman et al. [18] found that NAA concentrations in occipital gray matter measured 1½ months after injury predicted overall neuropsychological performance measured at 6 months after injury (Fig. 7.3) and correlated with the Glasgow Outcome Score (GOS).

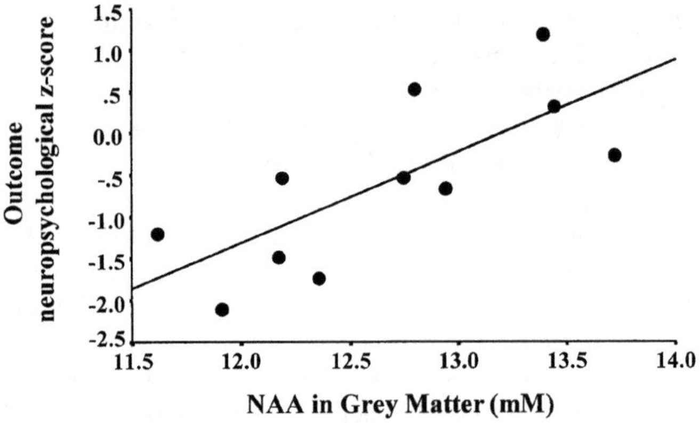

Fig. 7.3 NAA concentrations at 1.5 months after injury versus the composite neuropsychological z-score. A significant correlation was found. Patients with lower NAA concentration have significantly poorer overall cognitive function. (Figure provided by Seth Friedman Ph.D. and reproduced with permission from S.D. Friedman, W.M. Brooks, R.E. Jung, et al. Quantitative proton MRS predicts outcome after traumatic brain injury Neurology 1999;52(7):1384–1391, with permission.)

Other measures of metabolites were not predictive in this study. The prognostic value of MRS in occipital gray matter alone is quite remarkable, considering that other important parts of the brain sensitive to shearing injury were not evaluated in this study. For example, marked decreases of NAA have been reported for sites such as the corpus callosum [24] and frontal lobe [16, 19, 25]. Still, in this cross-sectional study considerable differences of NAA were observed in patients with comparable neuropsychological scores. This cannot be seen as evidence that NAA is an imperfect marker for neuronal loss. As mentioned above, variations of baseline NAA levels (and baseline neurological function) are obviously not accounted for. Therefore the *loss* of NAA, which is supposedly proportional to the loss of neurons, can only be determined relative to mean NAA in a control group. One wonders whether subjects with high risk for head injury should be studied with prospective MRS to obtain baseline values for NAA.

Another study by Shutter et al. [26] has demonstrated that other metabolites such as glutamate and glutamine and choline have shown predictive value, particularly when incorporating different metabolites from different areas of the brain. For example, GOS at 1 month was best predicted from ratios of NAA/Cr and Glx/Cr from the posterior white matter with

Table 7.1 Meta-analysis of current MRS studies in mild traumatic brain injury

Reference	MRS Method	Post injury	Location	Findings
Cecil et al. 1998 [52]	1.5 T; STEAM SV, TE=31 ms	9 days—several years	Splenium (WM)	↓NAA/Cr
Garnett et al. 2000 [53]	1.5 T; STEAM SV, TE=30 ms	3–35 days	Centrum semiovale (WM)	↓NAA/Cr, ↑Cho/Cr, ↓NAA/Cho
Govindaraju et al. 2004 [54]	1.5 T; volumetric CSI, TE=70 ms	2–30 days	WM regions	↓NAA/Cr, ↑Cho/Cr, ↓NAA/Cho
Kirov et al. 2007 [55]	3 T, PRESS CSI, TE=135 ms	6 days–8 years	Thalamus	↓[NAA], ↓[Cr], ↓[Cho]
Cohen et al. 2007 [56]	1.5 T, Whole brain NAA, TE=0 ms	1 day–8 years	Whole brain	↓[NAA]
Nakabayashi et al. 2007 [57]	1.5 T, STEAM SV, TE=144 ms	1week, 1 month	Frontal and temporal WM	↓NAA/Cr early ↑Cho/Cr late
Vagnozzi et al. 2008 [37]	3 T, PRESS SV, TE=144 ms	3, 15, and 30 days	Frontal WM	↓NAA/Cr
Gasparovic et al. 2009 [58]	3 T, PRESS SV and CSI, TE=40 ms	4–19 days	GM, WM, Splenium	↑Cr in WM, Spl ↓Glx in GM

Abbreviations: *STEAM* stimulated echo acquisition method, *PRESS* point-resolved spectroscopy, *SV* single voxel, *CSI* chemical shift imaging, *TE* echo time, *ms* milliseconds, *WM* white matter, *GM* gray matter, *NAA*: *n*-acetyl aspartate, *Cr* creatine, *Cho* choline; *Glx* glutamate/glutamine, *Spl* splenium

an accuracy of 78% in comparison with motor GCS, which had an accuracy of 62%. However, GOS at 6 months was best predicted with NAA/Cho and Cho/Cr from the posterior white matter combined with Glx/Cr from the occipital gray matter, increasing the accuracy up to 94% compared with motor GCS which remained low at 67% at 6 months. It is also important to note, however, that MRS is not a replacement for clinical evaluation as this same study found that the combination of MRS ratios and motor GCS provided the most accurate prediction of outcome (97%) when utilized together. This demonstrates that MRS is highly complementary to existing TBI measures and used in conjunction may provide the greatest diagnostic value to TBI victims.

Mild Traumatic Brain Injury

Mild traumatic brain injury (mTBI) is defined by the Mild Traumatic Brain Injury Committee of the Head Injury Interdisciplinary Special Interest Group of the American Congress of Rehabilitation Medicine as a TBI where the severity of the injury does not exceed the following [27]:

- Posttraumatic amnesia not greater than 24 h
- After 30 min, an initial Glasgow Coma Scale (GCS) of 13–15
- Loss of consciousness of approximately 30 min or less

In addition, persons that have undergone mild TBI will suffer at least one of the following conditions: any period of loss of consciousness; any loss of memory for events immediately before or after the accident; any alteration in mental state at the time of the accident (e.g., feeling dazed, disoriented, or confused); and focal neurological deficit(s) that may or may not be transient.

Mild traumatic brain injury is the most prevalent form of TBI, accounting for approximately 70% of the TBI that occur. Furthermore, 15–30% of mild TBI are so-called *malingering* TBI where symptoms persist beyond 1 year or more. Even though this type of TBI is called "mild", the effect on the family and the injured person can be significant, resulting in symptoms such as headache, difficulty thinking, memory problems, attention deficits, mood swings, and frustration.

While a majority of the MR spectroscopy studies have focused on severe traumatic brain injury, recent literature has increasingly focused on this more mild form of brain injury, showing long-term effect sometimes decades after the initial injury. Table 7.1 summarizes some of the major studies of mild TBI.

In summary, these mTBI studies find that NAA, a putative neuronal/axonal marker, is decreased in white matter (WM) regions such as the splenium, centrum semiovale, and frontal white matter. Decreases in NAA have been found in other diseases as well [28] and although there is some debate, it is generally accepted in the literature as an indicator of neuronal/axonal health. These studies show that in mTBI, there is definitive axonal/neuronal loss particularly in the WM where fiber tracts are found which correlates well with diffusion tensor imaging studies that have found similar results [29]. Secondary findings such as changes in choline, a marker for cellular proliferation or tissue damage, are inconsistent throughout the studies. It is important to note that some studies have shown changes in creatine, an energy marker but more importantly a commonly used internal reference used for metabolite ratios (i.e., NAA/Cr, Cho/Cr). The assumption is that Cr is generally unchanged in normal brain tissue however if it is affected by mTBI, metabolite ratio measurements would not be accurate as it would be difficult to assess if changes in ratios is due to the metabolite of interest or Cr itself.

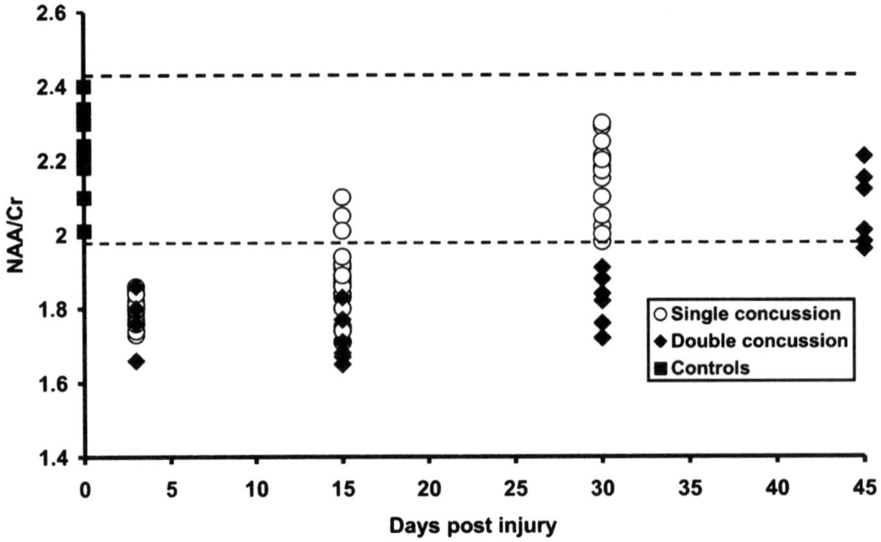

Fig. 7.4 Scatterplot demonstrating the different time course of NAA recovery in athletes having single or double concussive injury, as expressed by the NAA-to-Cr ratio determined by 1 H-MR spectroscopy. The second concussion (occurring between the 10th and the 13th d after the first insult) either provoked a further slight NAA decrease or significantly delayed the process of NAA restoration, which was completed at 45 days instead of at 30 days post-injury. (From Vagnozzi R, Signoretti S, Tavazzi B, et al. Temporal Window of Metabolic Brain Vulnerability to Concussion: A Pilot 1 H-Magnetic Resonance Spectroscopic Study in Concussed Athletes-Part III. *Neurosurgery.* 2008;62(6):1286–1296, with permission.)

Acute Sports-Related Concussion

An estimated 1.8–3.8 million sports-related concussions occur each year in the United States [30]. There is increasing recognition of immediate and long-term neurological problems from these injuries, including headaches, dizziness, behavioral changes, and problems with memory and attention [31]. Some evidence is being accumulated on neurochemical effects of head trauma in general and concussion in particular, including a number of changes in key neurochemical levels in the brain (see below).

Sports-related concussions are a major problem in pediatrics [32]; according to the Center for Disease Control, 10–15 year olds have the highest rate of SRC compared to other age groups [33], and studies have shown that younger athletes require longer recovery times [34]. Despite the magnitude of the clinical problem, there is no information on the neurochemical effects of concussion in this age group, which may be pronounced due to their earlier developmental stage.

Sports-related TBI are generally milder head injuries. To date, there are only three studies that have focused specifically on sports-related TBI: Cimatti et al. [35] found that NAA decreased in two of six adult athletes after head trauma. Henry et al. [36] showed a significant decrease in Glx and NAA in the primary motor cortex and NAA in the prefrontal cortex in 14 concussed compared with non-concussed athletes (ages 20–25 years). Vagnozzi et al. [37] showed in 13 concussed athletes (ages 22–25) a decrease of 18.5% in NAA, with modest recovery at 15 days and full recovery at 30 days. Most importantly, this study also showed that in those with second concussive injuries that took up to 45 days to fully recover, NAA levels did not seem to return to the same level as in those with a single head injury (Fig. 7.4). This has significant implications for the hypothesized cumulative effects of head injury. Unfortunately there are no studies that have been conducted in children and therefore it is unclear whether the same mechanisms are invoked after head injury.

Chronic Sports-Related Head Injury

It is believed that the cumulative head trauma experienced by these athletes is responsible for neurodegenerative changes, which, over time, result in a progressive decline of memory and executive functioning [38]; mood and behavioral disturbances that include depression, apathy, impulsivity, anger, irritability, suicidal behavior [39], and aggressiveness [40, 41]; gait changes that resemble Parkinsonism [40]; and, eventually, progression to dementia [40]. Previously referred to as dementia pugilistica due to its strong association with boxing [42, 43], the chronic effects of head injury has been identified as chronic traumatic encephalopathy (CTE). Autopsy studies by the Boston University Center for the Study of Traumatic Encephalopathy (BUCSTE) and others also reveal a distinct pattern of neuropathological changes in CTE, including: extensive tau-immunoreactive inclusions scattered throughout the cerebral cortex in a patchy, superficial distribution, with focal epicenters at the depths of sulci and around the cerebral vasculature; extensive tau-immunoreactive inclusions in limbic and paralimbic regions as well as brainstem nuclei; gener-

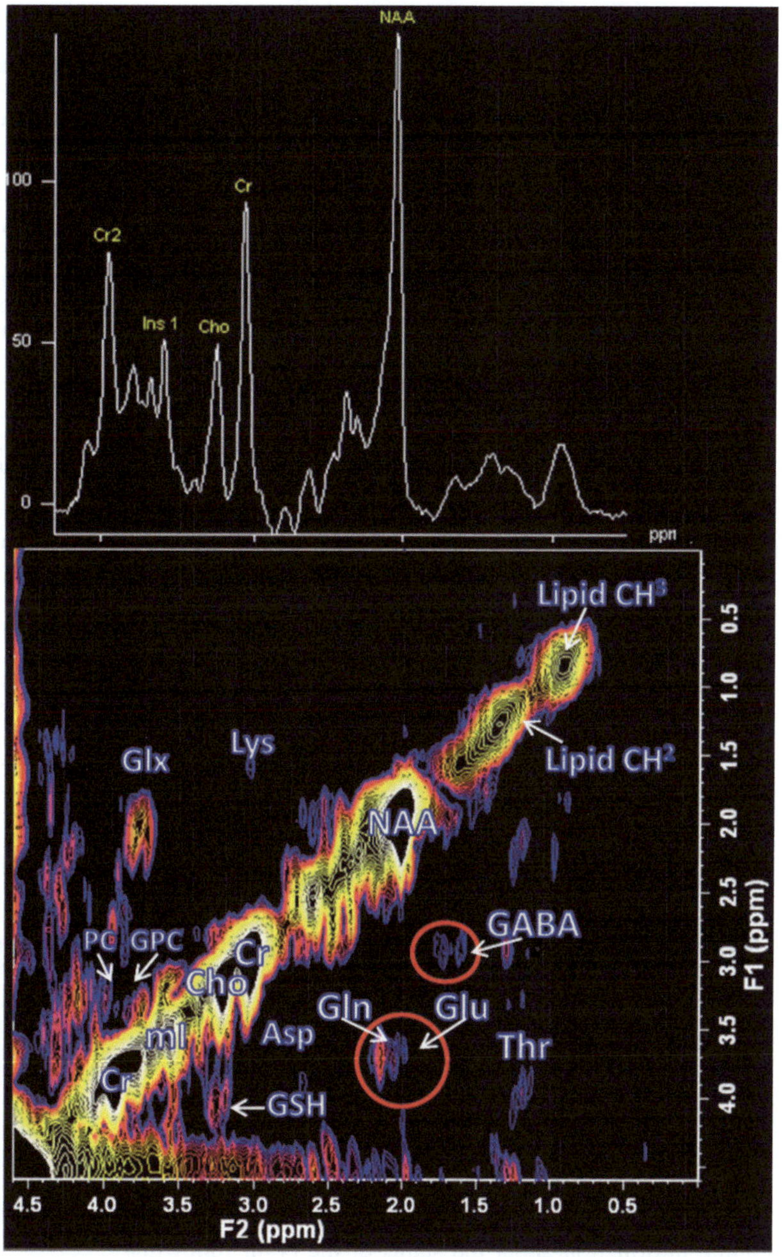

Fig. 7.5 Representative spectrum of conventional 1D MRS (top) and 2D COSY MRS (bottom) of a 34-year-old male professional motorcross racer with a long history of repetitive head injury starting at age 9 and through high school and college. Symptoms of CTE include memory loss, anger issues, and confusion. Data acquired at Brigham and Women's Hospital

alized atrophy and enlarged ventricles; specific atrophy of the frontal and medial temporal lobes; degenerations of white matter fiber bundles; cavum septum pellucidum, often with fenestrations; thinning of the hypothalamic floor and shrinkage of the mammillary bodies; and a relative absence of beta-amyloid (Aβ) deposits. [40] The BUCSTE has examined over 24 brains of deceased athletes. Neuropathological evidence of CTE has been found in 12 of 12 football players examined to date, three of whom only played in high school and college. CTE was also found in a deceased former professional hockey player, and we have found the initial evidence of the disease in an 18-year-old boy who died after having had multiple sports-related concussions. These initial findings suggest that CTE may be more common than previously known, and may develop without involvement in professional sports. Given the millions of youth, high school, and collegiate athletes participating in contact sports involving head trauma, CTE may represent an important and previously under-recognized public health issue.

Recently MRS was used to study neurochemical levels in five professional athletes, ages 31–54 years, with histories of concussions and subconcussive trauma. The higher Cho and Glx are statistically significant. In 1D MRS many of the resonances are composite or overlap. Two dimensional (2D) MRS, COrrelated SpectroscopY (COSY), can be employed to separate them in a second frequency [44, 45] (Fig. 7.5).

While it is possible to use spectral editing techniques to identify metabolites that overlap in 1D MRS, the advantage of the 2D COSY method is that the second frequency reveals all chemical species within a single scan [46].

In addition to the Cho and Glx changes, the following neurochemicals have been shown to be involved in severe traumatic brain injury, and can be measured with 2D COSY:

- Aspartate (Asp): An excitatory amino acid released into extracellular space after head injury [47].
- Possibly threonine (Thr): A structural amino acid that appears to be released when tissue is damaged [48].
- Lipids (Lip) and macromolecules (mac): Acute brain injury initiates a metabolic cascade that includes activation of phospholipase resulting in the accumulation of lipid and macromolecules [49].
- Possibly gamma-aminobutyric acid (GABA) and histidine (His): Both are inhibitory neurotransmitters. GABA is initially increased in the brain after head injury and thought to play a neuroprotective role [50]. Histidine has been shown to be excreted for an extended period of time after head injury [46, 51].

It is thought that blows to the skull cause an immediate disruption of neuronal membranes resulting in a massive efflux of potassium into extracellular space that triggers the calcium-dependent release of excitatory amino acids, further stimulating potassium efflux and resulting in a cascade of neurochemical effects on both the acute and long-term level [32]. The ability to measure these metabolites in vivo and noninvasively will provide an important window into the molecular pathophysiology of pediatric sports concussion.

Conclusions

MRS is a unique non-invasive method to study metabolism of tissue in vivo. Proton spectroscopy and in particular the quantitation of NAA, lactate, total choline, and lipids provide unique information about the status of the brain following acute and chronic head trauma.

References

1. Langlois JA, Rutland-Brown W, Thomas KE. The incidence of traumatic brain injury among children in the United States: differences by race. J Head Trauma Rehabil. 2005;20(3):229–38.
2. Brooks WM, Friedman SD, Gasparovic C. Magnetic resonance spectroscopy in traumatic brain injury. J Head Trauma Rehabil. 2001;16(2):149–64.
3. Govindaraju V, Gauger GE, Manley GT, Ebel A, Meeker M, Maudsley AA. Volumetric proton spectroscopic imaging of mild traumatic brain injury. AJNR Am J Neuroradiol. 2004;25(5):730–7.
4. Macmillan CS, Wild JM, Wardlaw JM, Andrews PJ, Marshall I, Easton VJ. Traumatic brain injury and subarachnoid hemorrhage: in vivo occult pathology demonstrated by magnetic resonance spectroscopy may not be "ischaemic". A primary study and review of the literature. Acta Neurochir (Wien). 2002;144(9):853–62. discussion 862.
5. Brooks WM, Stidley CA, Petropoulos H, et al. Metabolic and cognitive response to human traumatic brain injury: a quantitative proton magnetic resonance study. J Neurotrauma. 2000;17(8):629–40.
6. Gasparovic C, Arfai N, Smid N, Feeney DM. Decrease and recovery of N-acetylaspartate/creatine in rat brain remote from focal injury. J Neurotrauma. 2001;18(3):241–6.
7. Schuhmann MU, Stiller D, Skardelly M, Thomas S, Samii M, Brinker T. Long-time in-vivo metabolic monitoring following experimental brain contusion using proton magnetic resonance spectroscopy. Acta Neurochir Suppl. 2002;81:209–12.
8. Magistretti PJ, Pellerin L, Rothman DL, Shulman RG. Energy on demand. Science. 1999;283(5401):496–7.
9. Signoretti S, Marmarou A, Tavazzi B, Lazzarino G, Beaumont A, Vagnozzi R. N-Acetylaspartate reduction as a measure of injury severity and mitochondrial dysfunction following diffuse traumatic brain injury. J Neurotrauma. 2001;18(10):977–91.
10. Miller BL. A review of chemical issues in 1 H NMR spectroscopy: N-acetyl-L-aspartate, creatine and choline. NMR Biomed. 1991;4(2):47–52.
11. Jope RS, Jenden DJ. Choline and phospholipid metabolism and the synthesis of acetylcholine in rat brain. J Neurosci Res. 1979;4(1):69–82.
12. Brand A, Richter-Landsberg C, Leibfritz D. Multinuclear NMR studies on the energy metabolism of glial and neuronal cells. Dev Neurosci. 1993;15(3–5):289–98.
13. Badar-Goffer RS, Ben-Yoseph O, Bachelard HS, Morris PG. Neuronal-glial metabolism under depolarizing conditions. A 13C-n.m.r. study. Biochem J. 1992;282(Pt 1):225–30.
14. Pfefferbaum A, Adalsteinsson E, Spielman D, Sullivan EV, Lim KO. In vivo spectroscopic quantification of the N-acetyl moiety, creatine, and choline from large volumes of brain gray and white matter: effects of normal aging. Magn Reson Med. 1999; 41(2): 276–84.
15. Ross BD, Ernst T, Kreis R, et al. 1 H MRS in acute traumatic brain injury. J Magn Reson Imaging. 1998;8(4):829–40.
16. Garnett MR, Blamire AM, Corkill RG, Cadoux-Hudson TA, Rajagopalan B, Styles P. Early proton magnetic resonance spectroscopy in normal-appearing brain correlates with outcome in patients following traumatic brain injury. Brain. 2000;123(Pt 10):2046–54.
17. Holshouser BA, Ashwal S, Shu S, Hinshaw Jr DB. Proton MR spectroscopy in children with acute brain injury: comparison of short and long echo time acquisitions. J Magn Reson Imaging. 2000;11(1):9–19.
18. Friedman SD, Brooks WM, Jung RE, et al. Quantitative proton MRS predicts outcome after traumatic brain injury. Neurology. 1999;52(7):1384–91.
19. Ricci R, Barbarella G, Musi P, Boldrini P, Trevisan C, Basaglia N. Localised proton MR spectroscopy of brain metabolism changes in vegetative patients. Neuroradiology. 1997;39(5):313–9.
20. Holshouser BA, Ashwal S, Luh GY, et al. Proton MR spectroscopy after acute central nervous system injury: outcome prediction in neonates, infants, and children. Radiology. 1997;202(2):487–96.
21. Haseler LJ, Arcinue E, Danielsen ER, Bluml S, Ross BD. Evidence from proton magnetic resonance spectroscopy for a metabolic cascade of neuronal damage in shaken baby syndrome. Pediatrics. 1997;99(1):4–14.
22. Condon B, Oluoch-Olunya D, Hadley D, Teasdale G, Wagstaff A. Early 1 H magnetic resonance spectroscopy of acute head injury: four cases. J Neurotrauma. 1998;15(8):563–71.
23. Holshouser BA, Tong KA, Ashwal S. Proton MR spectroscopic imaging depicts diffuse axonal injury in children with traumatic brain injury. AJNR Am J Neuroradiol. 2005;26(5):1276–85.
24. Cecil KM, Hills EC, Sandel ME, et al. Proton magnetic resonance spectroscopy for detection of axonal injury in the splenium of the

corpus callosum of brain-injured patients. J Neurosurg. 1998;88(5): 795–801.
25. Choe BY, Suh TS, Choi KH, Shinn KS, Park CK, Kang JK. Neuronal dysfunction in patients with closed head injury evaluated by in vivo 1 H magnetic resonance spectroscopy. Invest Radiol. 1995;30(8):502–6.
26. Shutter L, Tong KA, Holshouser BA. Proton MRS in acute traumatic brain injury: role for glutamate/glutamine and choline for outcome prediction. J Neurotrauma. 2004;21(12):1693–705.
27. Kay T, Harrington DE, et al. Definition of mild traumatic brain injury. J Head Trauma Rehabilitat. 1993;8(3):86–7.
28. Lin A, Ross BD, Harris K, Wong W. Efficacy of proton magnetic resonance spectroscopy in neurological diagnosis and neurotherapeutic decision making. NeuroRx. 2005;2(2):197–214.
29. Kraus MF, Susmaras T, Caughlin BP, Walker CJ, Sweeney JA, Little DM. White matter integrity and cognition in chronic traumatic brain injury: a diffusion tensor imaging study. Brain. 2007; 130(10):2508–19.
30. Langlois JA, Rutland-Brown W, Wald MM. The epidemiology and impact of traumatic brain injury: a brief overview. J Head Trauma Rehabil. 2006;21(5):375–8.
31. Iverson GL, Gaetz M, Lovell MR, Collins MW. Cumulative effects of concussion in amateur athletes. Brain Inj. 2004;18(5):433–43.
32. Meehan 3rd WP, Bachur RG. Sport-related concussion. Pediatrics. 2009;123(1):114–23.
33. CDC. Nonfatal traumatic brain injuries from sports and recreation activities–United States, 2001–2005. MMWR. 2007;56(29):733–7.
34. Field M, Collins MW, Lovell MR, Maroon J. Does age play a role in recovery from sports-related concussion? A comparison of high school and collegiate athletes. J Pediatr. 2003;142(5):546–53.
35. Cimatti M. Assessment of metabolic cerebral damage using proton magnetic resonance spectroscopy in mild traumatic brain injury. J Neurosurg Sci. 2006;50(4):83–8.
36. Henry LC, Tremblay SB, Boulanger Y, Ellemberg D, Lassonde M. Neurometabolic changes in the acute phase following sports concussions correlate with symptom severity. J Neurotrauma. 2009;27:65–76.
37. Vagnozzi R, Signoretti S, Tavazzi B, et al. Temporal window of metabolic brain vulnerability to concussion: A pilot 1 H-magnetic resonance spectroscopic study in concussed athletes-Part III. Neurosurgery. 2008;62(6):1286–96.
38. Belanger HG, Spiegel E, Vanderploeg RD. Neuropsychological performance following a history of multiple self-reported concussions: A meta-analysis. J Int Neuropsychol Soc. 2009;11:1–6.
39. Omalu BI, Bailes J, Hammers JL, Fitzsimmons RP. Chronic traumatic encephalopathy, suicides and parasuicides in professional American athletes: The role of the forensic pathologist. Am J Forensic Med Pathol. 2010;31:130–2.
40. McKee A, Cantu R, Nowinski C, et al. Chronic traumatic encephalopathy in athletes. J Neuropath and Exp Neurol. 2009;68:709–35.
41. Guskiewicz KM, Marshall SW, Bailes J, et al. Recurrent concussion and risk of depression in retired professional football players. Med Sci Sports Exerc. 2007;39(6):903–9.
42. Martland HS. PUNCH DRUNK. J Am Med Assoc. 1928;91(15): 1103–7.
43. Millspaugh J. Dementia Pugilistica. US Naval Medical Bulletin. 1937;35(3):297–303.
44. Ramadan S, Mountford CE. Two-dimensional magnetic resonance spectroscopy on biopsy and in vivo. In: Webb GA, editor. Annual reports on NMR spectroscopy, vol. 65. Burlington: Academic; 2009. p. 161–99.
45. Thomas MA, Hattori N, Umeda M, Sawada T, Naruse S. Evaluation of two-dimensional L-COSY and JPRESS using a 3 T MRI scanner: from phantoms to human brain in vivo. NMR Biomed. 2003;16(5):245–51.
46. Lin A, Ramadan S, Stanwell P, et al. In vivo L-COSY MR distinguishes glutamate from glutamine and shows neuropathic pain to cause a buildup of glutamine in the brain. Proc Int Soc Magn Reson Med. 2010;18:381.
47. Gopinath SP, Valadka AB, Goodman JC, Robertson CS. Extracellular glutamate and aspartate in head injured patients. Acta Neurochir. 2000;76:437–8.
48. Bullock R, Zauner A, Woodward JJ, et al. Factors affecting excitatory amino acid release following severe human head injury. J Neurosurg. 1998;89(4):507–18.
49. Shohami E, Shapira Y, Yadid G, Reisfeld N, Yedgar S. Brain phospholipase A2 is activated after experimental closed head injury in the rat. J Neurochem. 1989;53(5):1541–6.
50. Nilsson P, Hillered L, Ponten U, Ungerstedt U. Changes in cortical extracellular levels of energy-related metabolites and amino acids following concussive brain injury in rats. J Cereb Blood Flow Metab. 1990;10(5):631–7.
51. Deutschman CS, Konstantinides FN, Raup S, Thienprasit P, Cerra FB. Physiological and metabolic response to isolated closed-head injury. Part 1: Basal metabolic state: correlations of metabolic and physiological parameters with fasting and stressed controls. J Neurosurg. 1986;64(1):89–98.
52. Cecil KM, Hills EC, Sandel ME, et al. Proton magnetic resonance spectroscopy for detection of axonal injury in the splenium of the corpus callosum of brain-injured patients. J Neurosurg. 1998;88(5): 795–801.
53. Garnett MR, Blamire AM, Rajagopalan B, Styles P, Cadoux-Hudson TAD. Evidence for cellular damage in normal-appearing white matter correlates with injury severity in patients following traumatic brain injury: a magnetic resonance spectroscopy study. Brain. 2000;123(7):1403–9.
54. Govindaraju V, Gauger GE, Manley GT, Ebel A, Meeker M, Maudsley AA. Volumetric proton spectroscopic imaging of mild traumatic brain injury. Am J Neuroradiol. 2004;25(5):730–7.
55. Kirov I, Fleysher L, Babb JS, Silver JM, Grossman RI, Gonen O. Characterizing 'mild' in traumatic brain injury with proton MR spectroscopy in the thalamus: Initial findings. Vol 21: Informa Healthcare; 2007:1147–1154.
56. Cohen BA, Inglese M, Rusinek H, Babb JS, Grossman RI, Gonen O. Proton MR spectroscopy and MRI-volumetry in mild traumatic brain injury. Am J Neuroradiol. 2007;28(5):907–13.
57. Nakabayashi M, Suzaki S, Tomita H. Neural injury and recovery near cortical contusions: a clinical magnetic resonance spectroscopy study. J Neurosurg. 2007;106(3):370–7.
58. Gasparovic C, Yeo R, Mannell M, et al. Neurometabolite concentrations in gray and white matter in mild traumatic brain injury: a 1H Magnetic resonance spectroscopy study. J Neurotrauma. 2009; 26:1635–43.

8 Proton Magnetic Resonance Spectroscopy: Applications in Neonatal Medicine

Stephen Ashwal, Brenda Bartnik-Olson, and Barbara Holshouser

The perinatal period remains one of the highest risk periods for a child to suffer an acute brain injury whether it be related to an intrapartum (e.g., placenta previa, nuchal cord), neonatal (aspiration with cardiorespiratory arrest) or postnatal (cerebral hypoxemia associated with congenital heart disease) insult. In addition to hypoxic-ischemic brain injury (HII), metabolic disorders (e.g., hypoglycemia, inborn errors of metabolism) and hyperbilirubinemia may cause brain injury. Other neonates may suffer intracranial hemorrhage or hydrocephalus leading to progressive deterioration and long-term neurological deficits. With the advent initially of phosphorus and then proton MRS, several of these conditions have been studied intensively over the past two decades in an attempt to characterize the severity of injury and to better understand its evolution.

Several excellent reviews on the role of magnetic resonance imaging (MRI) and fetal and neonatal brain maturation [1–4] as well as its usefulness in assessing brain injury [1, 5–10] have recently been published. Likewise, recent reviews have also examined technical and clinical aspects of the role of magnetic resonance spectroscopy (MRS) in the newborn [11–13]. In the following sections, we review some of the more common and devastating disorders affecting the neonate and the role of MRS in their evaluation.

S. Ashwal, M.D. (✉)
Division of Pediatric Neurology, Department of Pediatrics, Loma Linda University School of Medicine, Loma Linda, CA, USA
e-mail: sashwal@llu.edu

B. Bartnik-Olson, Ph.D.
Department of Radiology, Loma Linda University School of Medicine, Loma Linda, CA, USA
e-mail: bbartnik@llu.edu

B. Holshouser, Ph.D.
Department of Radiology, Section of Magnetic Resonance Imaging, Loma Linda University School of Medicine, Loma Linda, CA, USA
e-mail: bholshouser@llu.edu

Hypoxic Ischemic Injury and Arterial Ischemic Stroke

Neonatal hypoxic ischemic injury (HII) remains a frequent and devastating condition with serious long-term sequelae of cerebral palsy, epilepsy, and mental retardation. The two primary forms of neonatal HII are neonatal hypoxic ischemic encephalopathy (HIE, 2–4 cases per 1,000 births) and arterial ischemic stroke (AIS; 1 in 4,000 births). This remains an important clinical problem as up to 80% of infants surviving severe HII develop serious neurological complications and 10–20% remain moderately impaired. Even those infants with moderately severe HIE are at risk; about 30–50% have serious and 10–20% have minor long-term complications [14]. In AIS, follow-up studies of known full-term neonatal stroke patients beyond 3 years of age indicate that most develop neurologic deficits [15]. One report found delayed mental and motor development (88%), epilepsy (50%), spastic hemiparesis (88%), and major cognitive deficits (88%) [16]. Impaired visual function (28%) is also a common complication [17].

Overview of Pathophysiology

A detailed review of the pathophysiology of neonatal HII and AIS is beyond the scope of this chapter; however, several reviews have recently been published [18–20]. The initiating events involve acute reductions in cerebral blood flow as well as subsequent alterations in cerebral autoregulatory responses that result in acute cell energy failure and loss of ion homeostasis, particularly causing intracellular calcium release which activates numerous pathways associated with cell necrosis and apoptosis. Activation of these distinct pathways lead to cellular injury by way of (1) excitotoxic injury cascades involving the NMDA and AMPA receptors, (2) oxidative and nitro-oxidative pathways that increase free radical injury, (3) arachidonic acid pathways that also increase free radical injury, (4) caspase dependent and independent mechanisms

S. Blüml and A. Panigrahy (eds.), *MR Spectroscopy of Pediatric Brain Disorders*,
DOI 10.1007/978-1-4419-5864-8_8, © Springer Science+Business Media, LLC 2013

that accelerate apoptotic injury, and (5) activation of glial and other cellular inflammatory pathways that can cause delayed secondary injury. Depending on innumerable factors including local differences in regional cerebral blood flow and metabolism, varying patterns and gradients of injury severity can be seen after HII. Similar pathophysiological cascades can also occur in newborns with AIS depending on the severity and the anatomical location and size of the cerebral arteries that are occluded (e.g., main vs. distal branch).

Magnetic Resonance Imaging for Outcome Prediction after Neonatal Hypoxic Ischemic Injury and Arterial Ischemic Stroke

A variety of clinical biomarkers have been used to assess the severity of neonatal HIE but because of their well-recognized limitation [21], attention is now focused on using neuroimaging to assess the evolution, pathogenesis and severity of injury. MRI has allowed the identification of various patterns of brain injury; however investigators recognize that a better understanding of the regional evolution of injury and the optimal timing of when scans should be acquired will improve the sensitivity/specificity of these techniques.

A normal neonatal MRI scan after HIE has been associated with a normal neonatal EEG [22] as well as normal development and normal serial MRI studies at age 4 months and 4 years [23]. MRI abnormalities associated with poor long-term outcomes include cortical highlighting, diffuse loss of gray/white differentiation, loss of signal in the posterior limb of the internal capsule, severe diffuse injury, and injury to the thalamus and basal ganglia [24–26]. Involvement of deep subcortical nuclei particularly the basal ganglia has been regarded as a strong indicator of poor outcome [23, 27]. Even in children who appear normal at age two years, the presence of mild/moderate basal ganglia or moderate/marked white matter lesions has been associated with long-term minor neurological dysfunction and/or perceptual-motor difficulties at school age [25]. The MRI scoring system developed by Barkovich and colleagues at UCSF is often used, and has been shown to discriminate between good and poor neuromotor and cognitive outcome at 3 and 12 months [28]. However, even in this study, as in all studies evaluating the role of neonatal MRI after HIE, MRI was acquired postnatally over a wide time interval (e.g., 1–17 days; mean, 7 days). Others have suggested that the pattern of brain injury is best seen between 1 and 4 weeks after birth [22, 29].

Predictors of outcome after neonatal stroke are not well established. In one study, no correlation was found between site and laterality of the vascular distribution of the lesion on neonatal CT [15]. Several studies have suggested a direct correlation between the extent of infarction seen on MRI [30] especially if cortical involvement is present [31]. Another MRI study found that diffusion abnormalities in the posterior limb of the internal capsule in newborns after AIS correlated with subsequent development of hemiplegia [32]. Involvement of the main branch of the MCA [33] and bilateral infarction also have been shown to correlate with a lower probability of walking [34]. Other factors that correlate with outcome after neonatal AIS include the occurrence of seizures [15], presence of an abnormal EEG [30], presence of neonatal encephalopathy [35], and possibly the presence of a prothrombotic disorder [36].

Proton Magnetic Resonance Spectroscopy in Hypoxic Ischemic Injury

MRS has proved to be a sensitive tool for early evaluation of brain injury in neonates after an acute HI insult. Although no standard protocol has been established, it is useful to study metabolite changes in regions of the brain with high metabolic demands that are vulnerable to injury following hypoxia [27] such as the basal ganglia (BG) and thalami (Thal). Some investigators have sampled the entire BG/Thal region using a single voxel spectroscopy (SVS) technique while others have used a 2D CSI technique through the level of the BG in order to sample the areas separately with smaller voxel sizes. The increased resolution of smaller voxel sizes, however, comes at the expense of lower signal to noise. SVS has also been used to sample occipital and parietal gray and white matter regions also known to be vulnerable after HIE. Some studies have used an echo delay time (TE) that is considered short (TE $<$ 30 ms) so that metabolites with short T2 relaxation times such as myo-Inositol (Ins), glutamate (Glu), glutamine (Gln), lipids and macromolecules can be detected. Otherwise, typical long echo times of 135/144 or 270 ms have been commonly used. A more complete discussion of MRS techniques and parameters can be reviewed in Chap. 2 of this book.

Early studies reported that neonates with HIE demonstrate alterations in metabolites measured with MRS such as N-acetylaspartate (NAA), a neuronal marker; total creatine (Cr, creatine and phosphocreatine), bioenergetic markers; choline-containing compounds (Cho), intermediates in phospholipid metabolism; lactate (Lac), a terminal metabolite in glycolysis, Ins a glial marker and osmolyte; and Glx (glutamate and glutamine), neurotransmitters [37–41]. Neonates studied early after injury (mean of 7 days or less) consistently showed that increased lactate and decreased NAA in the BG or Thal correlated with poor outcome [40–45]. Accurate detection of lactate after HII is important for prognostication. Although increased lactate levels generally correlate with poorer outcomes, small lactate peaks have been reported in spectra from healthy pre-term newborns [46] and in one case of an asphyxiated neonate [41] with good outcome. Two studies comparing MRS techniques concluded that using longer

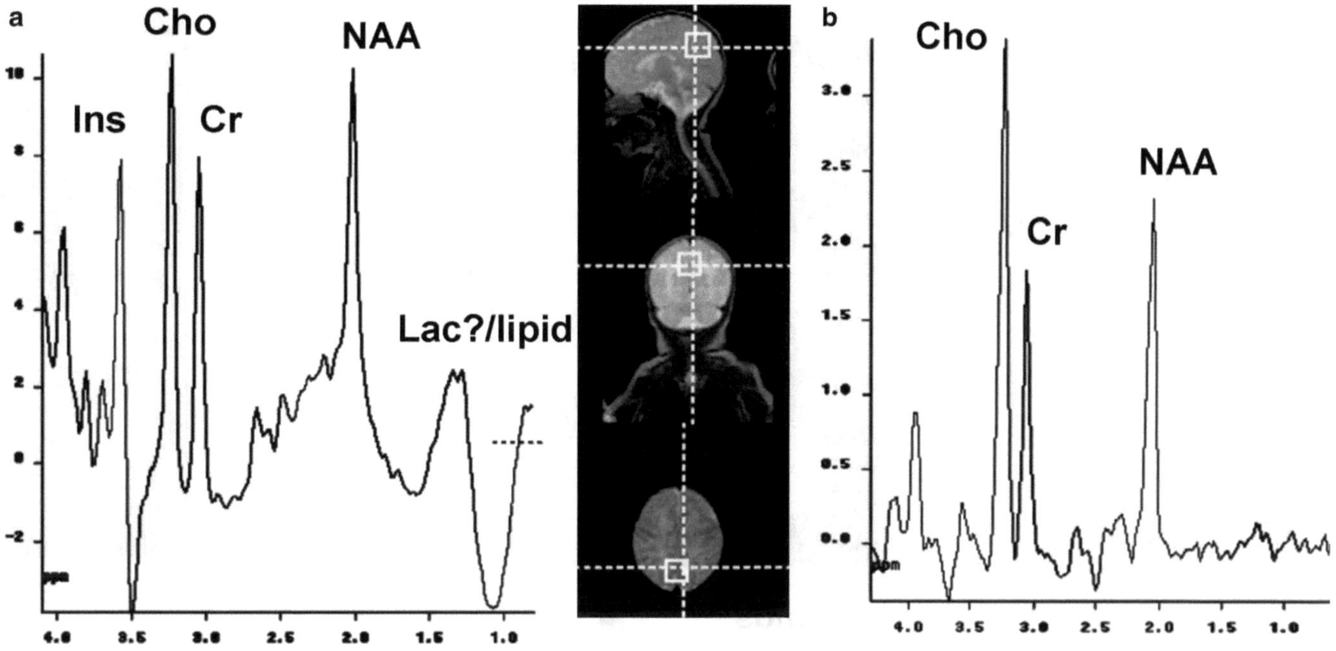

Fig. 8.1 (**a**) Short echo time SVS (STEAM; TR/TE/TM = 3,000/20/13 ms) spectrum in mid-occipital gray matter from a 16 day old neonate shows a large artifact between 1.0 and 1.5 ppm representing lipid contamination from subcutaneous fat around the skull. It is not possible to determine if lactate is present. (**b**) Long echo time SVS (PRESS; TR/TE = 3,000/144 ms) in the same location without interference from skull lipids shows no evidence of lactate. Metabolite levels and ratios were within two standard deviations of normal for a term neonate. A neurologic evaluation at 8 months was normal

echo times to acquire MRS data in neonates provided superior prognostic capabilities because although long echo time acquisitions generally have lower signal to noise than short echo acquisitions, lactate is more easily detected without interference from lipid and macromolecule signals [46, 47]. Figure 8.1 compares spectra from the occipital cortex in a 16 day old neonate evaluated for HIE. The short echo time spectrum (Fig. 8.1a) displays a large artifact from skull lipid contamination in the area of the lactate resonance whereas the long echo time spectrum (Fig. 8.1b) is free from lipid contamination and confirms that lactate is not present.

Conversely, short echo time MRS allows the study of Ins and Glx after hypoxic injury. Robertson et al. found that increased Ins/Cr ratios in the BG of neonates with HIE correlated with poor one-year outcome [48], while other investigators have shown that increased Glx ratios in the BG correlated with severe HIE [49–51]. A recent study demonstrated a strong correlation between HIE and the degree of increase in the Glx-α peak detected at 3.75 ppm. In particular, the Glx-α/Cr ratio in basal ganglia had a significant negative correlation with outcome [52]. The cerebral cortex which is undergoing active myelination at term may also be at increased risk for injury [27]. As shown in Fig. 8.2, MRS taken in the parieto-occipital gray matter of newborns with HIE showed that decreased NAA/Cho and increased Cho/Cr correlated with poor outcome as did the presence of Lac [39, 53].

Relative Importance of Different Metabolites

Numerous previous studies have suggested that changes in lactate may be an extremely early and persistent sensitive biomarker of injury that correlates with outcome. Overall most studies have shown that the Lac/Cr, Lac/NAA, and NAA/Cr correlated best with long-term developmental outcome severity [38, 40, 42, 49, 54–60]. Recently, Thayyil and colleagues [61] have reported on an extensive meta-analysis on MRI and MRS in neonatal encephalopathy. They found that the most sensitive MRS indicators of injury (in 10 of 16 studies that had such data) were the deep gray matter (i.e., Thal or BG) Lac/NAA ratio (days 1–30) which had 82% overall pooled sensitivity (95% CI: 74–89%) and 95% specificity (95% CI: 88–99%). Six of 16 studies reported Thal or BG Lac/Cr and had a pooled sensitivity of 77% (95% CI: 64– 86%) and 94% specificity (95% CI: 85– 98%). They also compared MRI and MRS and found that Lac/NAA had a significantly higher specificity than conventional MRI (98% [95% CI: 87–100%] vs. 76% [95% CI: 61–88%]) and that Lac/NAA sensitivity (86% [95% CI: 72–95%]) was comparable to that for conventional MRI (80% [95% CI: 65–90%]). Their overall impression was that deep gray matter Lac/NAA and Lac/Cr ratios were the most accurate quantitative prognostic indicator during the neonatal period (days 1–30). They also stated that Lac/NAA had better diagnostic accuracy than conventional MRI performed at any

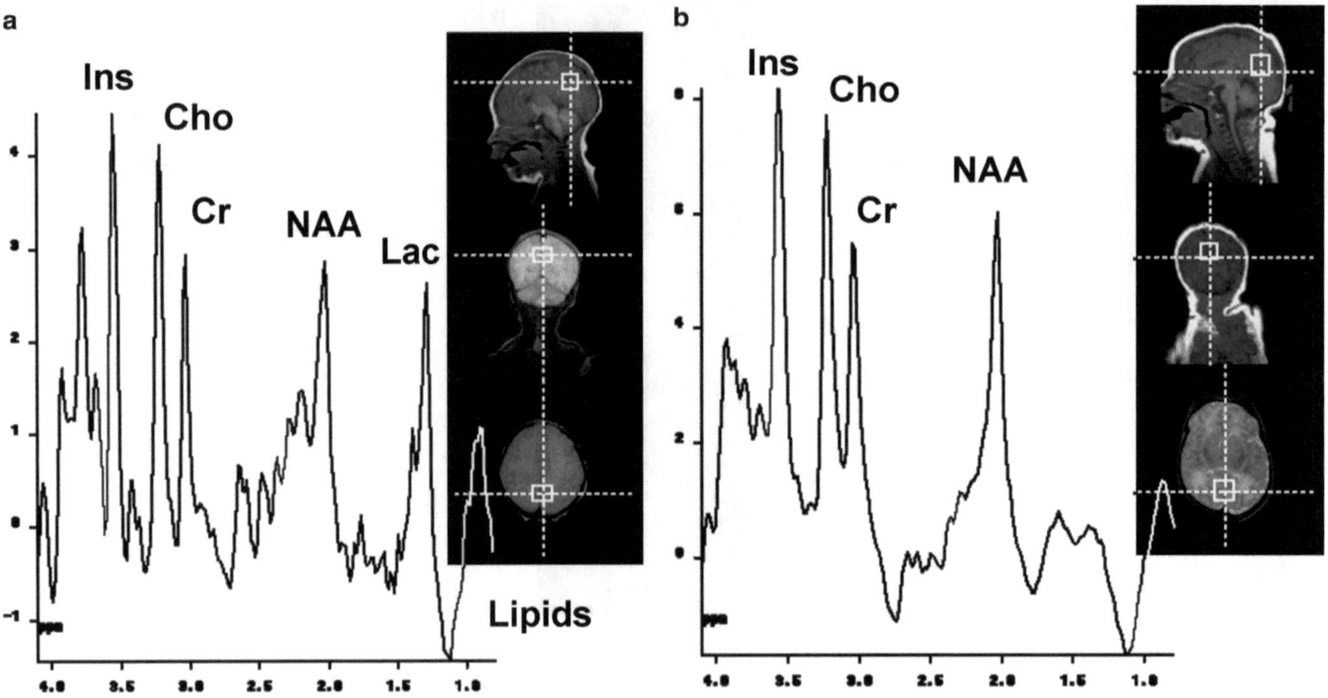

Fig. 8.2 SVS (STEAM; TR/TE/TM = 3,000/20/13 ms) acquisitions in the occipital gray matter of two neonates being evaluated for HIE. (**a**) A spectrum from a 4 day old neonate with a poor long-term outcome shows decreased NAA below normal levels for a neonate, a large lactate peak and lipid/macromolecules (0.9 ppm) indicating cellular breakdown. (**b**) A spectrum from an 8 day old neonate with a normal long-term outcome shows normal metabolite levels and ratios for a term neonate

time during the neonatal period. A recent critique of using MRI and MRS as biomarkers outlined the limitations of such studies to predict prognosis noting that many studies had small sample size, selection bias, vague and overly inclusive outcome assessment and potential self-fulfilling prophecies [62]. It is possible that as 3D MRSI becomes increasingly used [63] and that as the ability to use computational algorithms to more rapidly analyze data becomes available, such methods that integrate spectroscopic data across many critical brain regions may improve the sensitivity and specificity of these methods. Other factors that need to be taken into account that might affect metabolite levels are the coexistence of seizures in neonates with HII [64, 65] and possibly adverse socioeconomic factors [45].

Timing of Magnetic Resonance Spectroscopy

Timing of MRS after injury may be critical following HII as serial studies have shown that increased Lac may be seen as early as 18 h after injury and peaks approximately 4–5 days after injury [42, 66]. Related studies have shown that persistence of lactate 1 month after neonatal HII is also associated with a very poor neurological outcome [67]. Increased brain lactate likely reflects increased anaerobic glycolysis associated with disruption of the mitochondrial electron transport chain and oxidative phosphorylation; but macrophage infiltration or an altered redox state may also contribute [55]. Therefore many studies in neonates have concentrated on early acquisition of MRS [56]. Although early MRS is sensitive for detection of Lac, changes in NAA evolve more slowly and may not diminish significantly until beyond 48 h [40]. As lactate changes may resolve over the first week after injury, many investigators prefer using NAA derived metabolite ratios as a more accurate indicator of neuronal loss and hence a better spectroscopic indicator of acute neuronal loss that would correlate with long-term outcome [39, 68].

Magnetic Resonance Spectroscopy in Combination with Other Magnetic Resonance Imaging Biomarkers

Originally, most investigators examined the role of MRS as an independent indicator of injury or in combination with various clinical variables that reflected the acute clinical status of the newborn. For example, in our own early studies we examined the importance of various clinical variables (admission serum glucose level, Sarnat score, 5-min Apgar score, and electroencephalographic results) and found that these data alone predicted outcome in 78% of neonates and that adding MRS data improved the ability to predict outcome to 83% [68]. In a later study of 37 neonates, 18 of whom had HII, we found that the MRS metabolite ratio data, added to either the Sarnat or EEG scores, enhanced the correlation between these prognostic factors and 6–12 month outcomes [39].

In a third study of 33 neonates, all with HII, we found that combining spectroscopy ratios with the Sarnat and EEG scores to predict 24 month outcome significantly improved the sensitivity but not the specificity in term neonates [53]. In contrast another study did not find any correlation between MRS variables and EEG polygraphic studies [69]. Other investigators have reported on a strong correlation between the 1- and 5-min Apgar scores and BG NAA/Cho ratios but outcome data were not included in this study [70].

Other investigators have examined MRI abnormalities in conjunction with MRS data. In one study of 9 neonates with severe HII, multiple MRI parameters were acquired (T1, T2, DWI, ADC) of the BG and parietal white matter in conjunction with BG MRS [71]. Seven of the nine infants with poor outcomes had various combinations of MRI and MRS abnormalities. Other investigators have developed MRI scoring systems and correlated their results with MRS (i.e., increased lactate and or reduced NAA) and clinical outcome results (i.e., poor outcomes) [72]. In contrast, another group of investigators did not find a correlation between ADC values and outcome although metabolite data (e.g., lactate ratios) did correlate with outcome [73].

Magnetic Resonance Spectroscopy as a Biomarker of Treatment

It is clear that MRS data contribute to the objective assessment of the extent and severity of brain injury in newborns and a logical extension of this is to determine if MRS data can also serve as a surrogate early biomarker of response to treatment. In such instances, resolution of elevated lactate peaks and normalization of NAA, Cr, Glx, and Ins might be used to quantify an early therapeutic response. The value of such an approach is to determine if such data could allow early treatment modifications if no improvement of a neonate's metabolite status is observed or as an early indicator of improved long-term neurological and neuropsychological outcomes. This approach could have an enormous advantage in clinical trials as it could shorten the length of time needed to demonstrate improved functional outcomes.

This possibility is suggested in one of our recent studies [74]. We examined the neuroprotective effects of opioids in a group of 28 neonates (8 opioid-treated, 20 non-opioid treated) with HII who had also undergone painful tissue-damaging procedures (TDPs) such as endotracheal intubation and suctioning, arterial line placement and intramuscular injections, commonly performed in the neonatal intensive care unit (NICU) and known to result in cardiovascular stress [75, 76]. Compared to neonates who received opioids, we found that asphyxiated neonates not treated with opioids showed significantly lower mean NAA/Cr due to lower NAA measured quantitatively at short TE and had Lac in occipital gray matter (OGM) (40% vs 0) suggesting that opioids may provide a neuroprotective effect. Using long echo MRSI (TE = 144 ms) in the BG and Thal in the same cohort of patients, trends of decreased NAA/Cr and NAA/Cho ratios (neuronal loss or dysfunction), increased Cho/Cr (membrane disruption) and increased Glx/Cr ratios were noted but were not significant except between non-treated and control neonates. The number of exposures to TDPs in the first 4 days of life was correlated with brain metabolite data to examine the hypothesis that exposure to pain and stress alters brain biochemistry. We found that a higher TDP incidence was associated with decreased Cr in the OGM suggesting altered energy metabolism and decreased NAA/Cho in the BG. These findings suggest that TDPs may increase the amount of neonatal pain and stress augmenting neonatal brain injury associated with hypoxia-ischemia. Spectra acquired within 7 days from the BG of neonates with HIE show the decrease of NAA and Cr seen with increased severity of injury and outcome (Fig. 8.3).

Hypothermia is now the only accepted treatment for neonatal HII, however, as recently reviewed there is a clear cut need to do such studies to optimize hypothermia treatment [77]. We recently had the opportunity to study 40 neonates with HII of whom 21 underwent total body cooling and 19 did not and compared these metabolite data to a group of neonatal controls ($n=9$) using both short-echo SVS in the OGM and 2D MRSI of the BG and Thal within 2–14 days (mean 6.9 ± 3.1 days) after birth and 1–6 days (mean 2.7 ± 1.6 days) after hypothermia [78]. We found no significant difference in BG NAA/Cr ($p=0.98$) or NAA/Cho ($p=0.59$) between the non-treated HII and hypothermia-treated HII, with both groups showing significantly lower ratios compared to the neonatal controls. However, in the Thal and OGM, hypothermia-treated HII neonates had higher levels of NAA/Cr compared to non-treated neonates with HII which were not significantly different from neonatal controls (Thal, $p=0.39$; OGM, $p=0.15$). These findings suggest that hypothermia treatment may preserve neuronal energy metabolism in the gray matter of HII neonates. Studies are currently underway to determine the sensitivity and specificity of MRS data to predict long-term outcome in these hypothermia-treated HII neonates. Figure 8.4 shows spectra from the BG and Thal that illustrate the spectral findings discussed above in hypothermia-treated neonates compared to non-treated neonates and controls.

Proton Magnetic Resonance Spectroscopy and Arterial Ischemic Stroke

Few studies have examined MRS findings in neonates with AIS. In one study of 4 neonates (3 term, 1 preterm), MRS (SVS) was done 7–49 days postnatally and the distribution of injury involved either the middle cerebral artery ($n=3$) or the posterior cerebral artery [79]. As would be expected

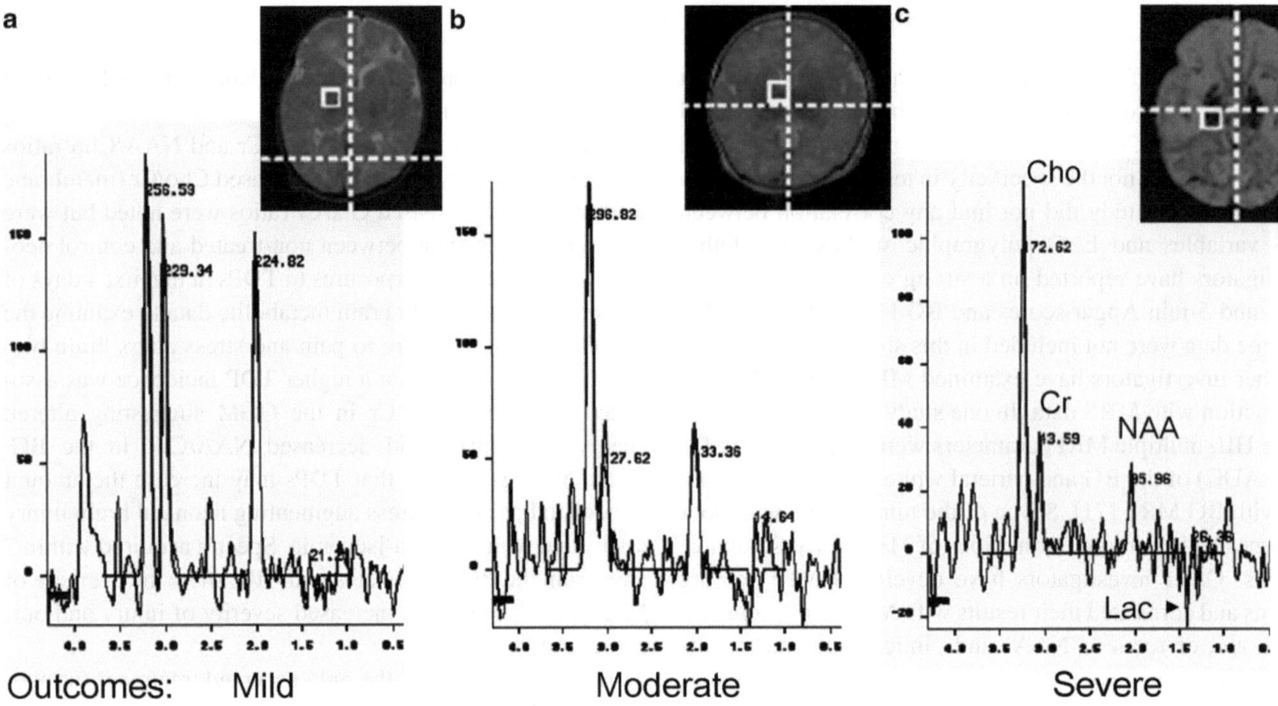

Fig. 8.3 MRSI (PRESS; TR/TE=3,000/144 ms) spectra from the basal ganglia from three neonates with HIE showing (**a**) normal metabolite ratios at 9 days in a neonate with a mild disability long-term outcome, (**b**) markedly reduced NAA and Cr at 4 days in a neonate with moderate disabilities at follow-up, and (**c**) markedly reduced NAA and Cr and presence of Lac at 17 days in a neonate with severe long-term disabilities

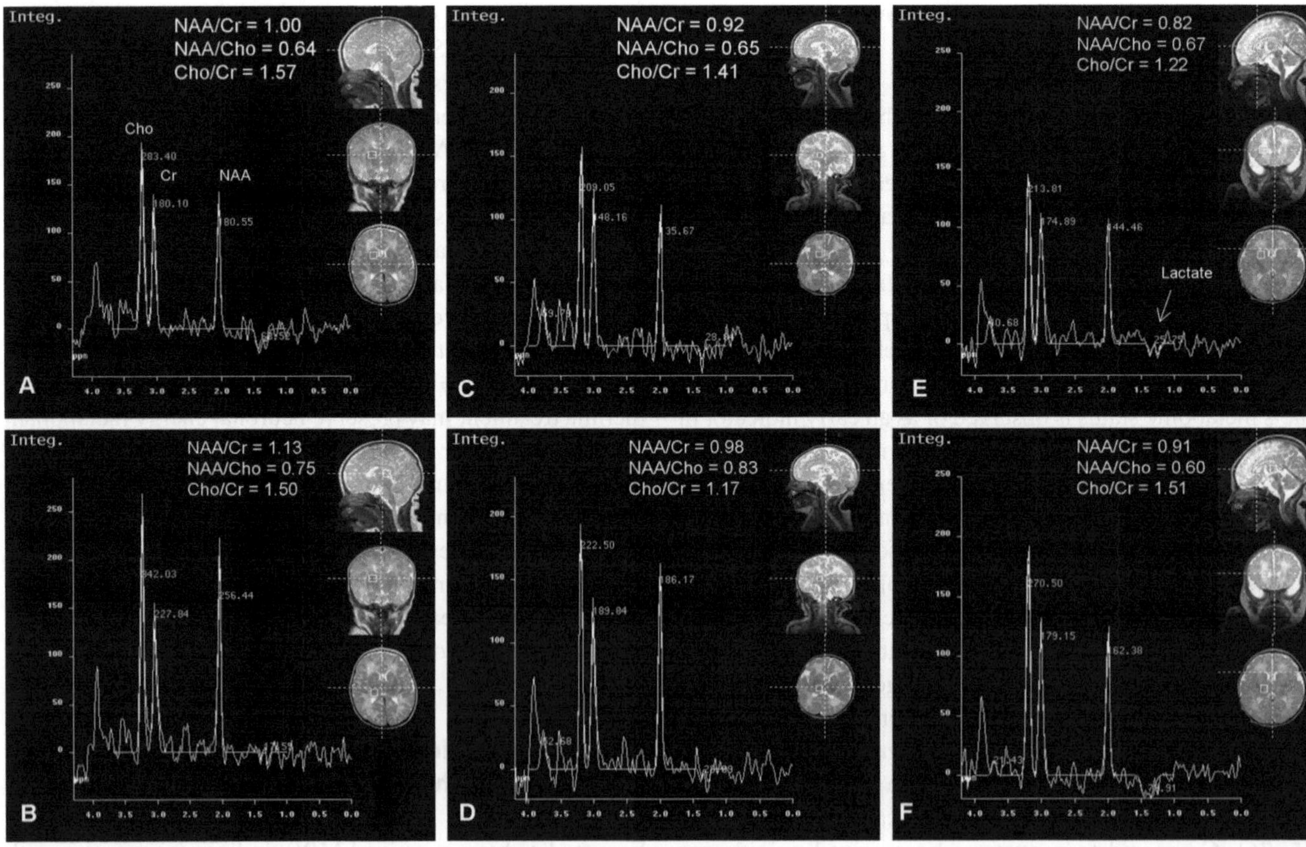

Fig. 8.4 MRSI (PRESS; TR/TE=3,000/144 ms) spectra from the basal ganglia and thalami of (**a**, **b**) a healthy neonate, (**c**, **d**) a neonate with HIE treated with 72 h of whole body hypothermia, and (**e**, **f**) a neonate with HIE and no hypothermia therapy. NAA/Cr is decreased in the basal ganglia of the hypothermia-treated neonate (**c**) and in the basal ganglia and thalamus of the neonate with HIE and no hypothermia (**e**, **f**), compared to the healthy neonate. Lactate is present in the basal ganglia and thalamus of the neonate with HIE and no hypothermia (**e**, **f**). Note: The number beside each peak is the integral (Integ.) measurement of the peak after baseline fitting and represents a relative measure of metabolite concentration

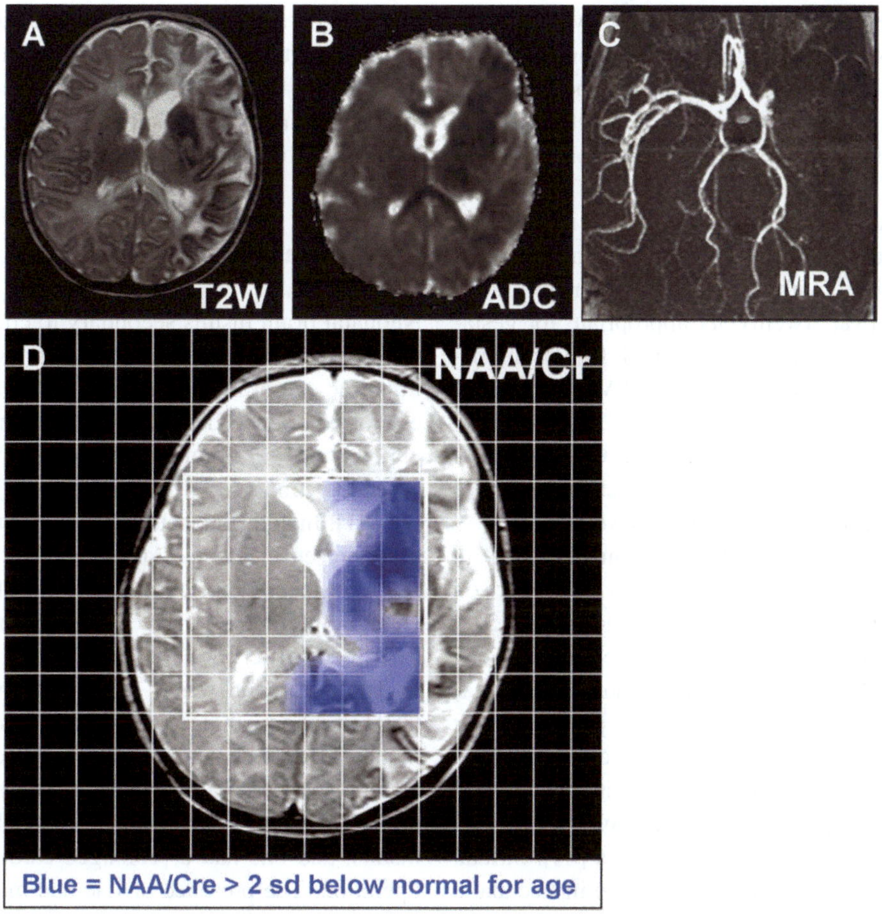

Fig. 8.5 (**a**) T2 weighted (T2W) image, (**b**) apparent diffusion coefficient (ADC) map, and (**c**) maximum intensity projection of a magnetic resonance angiography (MRA) study in a 7 week old infant with a left middle cerebral artery stroke. (**d**) A metabolite image created from a 2D MRSI (PRESS; TR/TE=144 ms; 1.5 T) in which only voxels that have abnormally low NAA/Cr ratios (below 2 standard deviations of normal for age) are colored in blue. Voxels with no coloring have normal NAA/Cr ratios. Note: Metabolite images produced with manufacturers' software will display the metabolite integrals or ratios for each voxel with no comparison to control data. The metabolite image shown here was created with custom software written in our laboratory and compared to age-matched control data acquired at our institution

based on studies of neonatal HII, increased lactate and reduced NAA/Cho were found. In a case study of a suspected intrauterine stroke, no lactate was found on MRS [70]. Another report of 11 term neonates with stroke reviewed the clinical and imaging findings and indicated that the MRI (e.g., DWI data) was more helpful than spectroscopy in defining the extent of injury [80]. The discrepancies between outcome and MRS data after stroke may be a result of the anatomic location sampled after stroke. Spectra taken within the stroke volume would be expected to show decreased NAA (neuronal loss or dysfunction) and increased Lac, the degree of which depends on the severity of the injury and the timing of the MRS, whereas spectra outside the involved region may show normal metabolite levels and ratios. Long-term outcomes of neonates with stroke depend not only on the volume injured but also the volume of brain spared. MR spectroscopic imaging which has the advantage of sampling large areas of brain may better show the extent of injury compared to single voxel MRS. Figure 8.5 is an example of an MRSI study of a 7 week old infant in which only voxels with abnormally low NAA/Cr ratios are colored demonstrating the extent of brain area affected after a left MCA stroke.

Preterm Infants

The majority of MRS studies have involved term neonates with HII but several have examined the role of MRS in preterm neonates. The few studies in preterm neonates is due in large part to the increased technical difficulties in transporting these neonates to the MRI scanner, the fact that they are medically more unstable than their term counterparts, and the lack of control normative data.

In one study of 18 preterm neonates, studies were done at two postnatal weeks of age (i.e., 32.5 weeks) and again at term (40 weeks) [81]. Changes in MRS metabolites were noted in the preterm infants at term compared with full-term infants suggesting a structural as well as a functional delay in brain development.

Another study examined the hypothesis that intrauterine growth retardation caused by placental insufficiency affected MRS and was associated with adverse two-year neurodevelopmental outcomes [82]. Twenty-six appropriate for gestational neonates were compared with 14 small for gestational neonates and had long and short echo time SVS (BG and in the periventricular white matter) acquired at 32 and 41 weeks postgestational age. NAA/Cho, Lac/Cho, mI/Cho, and Glx/Cho ratios were not significantly different between the two groups nor were there differences in neurodevelopment.

Other investigators have examined white matter injury in the preterm neonate using MRS. In the study by Robertson and colleagues, 30 preterm neonates (gestational age 27.9 weeks) were studied at postnatal age of 9.8 weeks [83]. Peak area ratios of Lac/Cr, NAA/Cr, Ins/Cr, and Cho/Cr were measured with short echo time SVS in the posterior periventricular white matter (WM). In the 12 infants with white matter injury, Lac/Cr and Ins/Cr were higher than in those infants without injury. The occurrence of germinal matrix hemorrhage (GMH) can also affect brain MRS in preterm neonates [84]. Striatal MRS in 12 preterm neonates found an increase in Lac and a reduction in NAA which were more pronounced on the side with the larger hemorrhage than contralaterally when the neonates were first studied at 32 weeks gestation. Repeat studies at 54.1 weeks showed that fewer neonates had lactate and that the degree of NAA reduction was less evident. The authors concluded that GMH is initially followed by Lac accumulation and possibly a delay in maturation as indicated by the transiently low Cr and NAA indices. Moreover, the presence of increased Cho at the corrected age of 3 months indicates a more persistent metabolic change after small GMH.

One caveat that should be noted is the observation that preterm neonates who undergo sedation with pentobarbital have lower BG Lac/Cho and Lac/NAA ratios [85]. This is an important consideration when trying to interpret metabolite data in preterm neonates by comparison to term control or other treatment groups. Whether pentobarbital sedation has an effect in neonates treated with hypothermia has not yet been reported.

Two other clinical reports address the long-term effects of prematurity on the developing nervous system as measured with MRS. In one study of 36 very low birth weight preterm neonates (gestational age $\leq$32 weeks), long echo time MRSI through the level of the BG was acquired at 35–43 weeks. Metabolite ratios from the BG and Thal showed no correlation with Bayley scores at 18–24 months adjusted age [86]. A second study of 21 adolescents who were all born prematurely found evidence of hippocampal atrophy and significantly lower NAA and Cr levels in the medial temporal lobe with short echo time SVS compared to a control group [87]. Presumably, complications associated with prematurity affected or injured the brain during the perinatal period and resulted in long-term measurable sequelae.

Congenital Heart Disease

Neonatal brain insults secondary to congenital heart disease (CHD) can occur by a variety of mechanisms related to impaired cerebral blood flow causing reduced oxygen delivery to the brain either preoperatively, intraoperatively (associated with profound hypothermia/circulatory arrest or extended times of low-flow bypass) or postoperatively [88–91]. In addition, some forms of congenital heart disease may present with central nervous system malformations. MRS has been reported in several small series of patients in an attempt to define the extent of injury similar to that described earlier for neonatal HII.

The first report was of nine infants with various forms of CHD in whom single voxel occipital gray and parietal white matter MRS was acquired 9 days after surgery [92]. Four patients had cerebral insults before operation, one had both a preoperative and a perioperative insult, three had perioperative insults, and one had a prolonged cardiac arrest 2 days after operation. The presence of Lac and markedly reduced NAA ratios were predictive of severe outcomes at 6–12 month follow-up whereas the absence of lactate and mild or no changes in metabolite ratios suggested recovery to a mild disability.

A second study examined 24 term infants with CHD in whom all had MRI and 19 had MRS [93]. Preoperative MRI showed periventricular leukomalacia (PVL, $n=4$) and stroke ($n=2$). Preoperative MRS revealed elevated Lac in 53%. Early postoperative MRI ($n=21$) identified new PVL in 48%, new infarct in 19%, and new parenchymal hemorrhage in 33%. New lesions or worsening of preoperative lesions occurred in 67% of subjects. No patient or procedure-related factors for the development of early postoperative lesions were identified. A late postoperative MRI ($n=17$) demonstrated resolution of early lesions in 8 and mild cerebral atrophy in 2.

In a third study, MRS was used to determine whether low [10] versus high [20] perfusate hematocrits during bypass resulted in changes in brain metabolites and whether this correlated with neurologic injury [94]. Long and short echo time single voxel MRS was acquired in the OGM preoperatively and 2 and 5 days postoperatively. No significant differences in metabolite ratios between the low versus high hematocrit groups and the lower vs. higher flow rate groups were noted. In all 11 children, MRS detected a significant decrease in quantitatively measured brain NAA and increases in Ins and Glx after surgery that returned to near baseline levels at 5 days. Furthermore, in infants in which a low flow rate was maintained for more than 3 min, the NAA/Cho ratio was significantly decreased ($p=0.02$) on day 2 and returned to baseline on day 5.

In a fourth study, MRS was acquired preoperatively and postoperatively in ten newborns with transposition of the great arteries (TGA) at a median of 5 days and 19 days of age [95]. Lac/Cho was higher in the TGA neonates compared to controls and decreased postoperatively but remained elevated. Those with preoperative brain injury on MRI had lower NAA/Cho than those with normal MRIs and five newborns had a decline in NAA/Cho postoperatively. A larger study from the same group of investigators involving 41 term neonates with CHD (29 with transposition of the great arteries; 12 with single-ventricle physiology) acquired MRS and diffusion tensor imaging (DTI) preoperatively [96]. As compared with control newborns, those with CHD had a 10% decrease in NAA/Cho, a 28% increase in Lac/Cho, a 4% increase in mean diffusivity and a 12% decrease in white matter fractional anisotropy. Preoperative brain injury, as seen on MRI, was not associated with MRS or DTI findings. The implication of this study was that term neonates with CHD have widespread brain abnormalities before they undergo cardiac surgery. Similar findings have been reported by a separate group of investigators who studied 16 term neonates with TGA examining NAA/Cr, Cho/Cr, and Ins/Cr from parietal white matter and occipital gray matter and correlating these findings with delayed neurodevelopmental outcomes at one year [97].

Related indirectly to CHD is the use of extracorporeal membrane oxygenation (ECMO) as a temporary procedure to maintain neonatal oxygenation until the underlying pulmonary or cardiac disease sufficiently improves. With this procedure the right carotid artery is ligated and concerns about preferential brain injury to that hemisphere despite an intact circle of Willis have always been raised. Previous studies have reported abnormal neuroimaging findings (e.g., right hemispheric ischemic or hemorrhagic injury) in 28% to 52% of neonates undergoing ECMO [98]. There is only one MRS study that examined post-ECMO metabolite data. In this study of nine neonates, no difference in BG metabolite ratios between the two hemispheres were observed and no long-term neurodevelopmental abnormalities were reported [41]. These are hopeful findings but additional investigations using MRS in a larger cohort of patients are necessary to confirm these findings. In addition, using MRS with other MRI methods (e.g., DWI, DTI) would be helpful to reexamine this issue.

Phosphorus Spectroscopy and Hypoxic Ischemic Injury

The use of phosphorus-31 (^{31}P) MRS in HII neonates preceded that of ^{1}H, with the first published reports appearing in the early 1980s. ^{31}P MRS can be used to measure the relative concentrations of phosphorus containing metabolites associated with brain energy metabolism, such as ATP, phosphocreatine (PCr), and inorganic phosphate (P_i). PCr contains a high-energy phosphate bond that exists in steady state exchange with ATP and in situations of increased energy demand, PCr will transfer its phosphate to ADP to maintain cellular ATP levels. P_i is produced by a number of phosphodiesterases and its metabolic function is to participate as a substrate for mitochondrial ATPase in the synthesis of ATP and in substrate level phosphorylation by glyceraldehyde-3-phosphate dehydrogenase [99]. Importantly, the intracellular pH (pH_i) also can be estimated as the resonance of P_i is pH dependent [100]. ^{31}P MRS of the brain also reveals peaks corresponding to the phosphomonoesters (PME), phosphorylethanolamine and phosphorylcholine and the phosphodiesters (PDE), glycerol 3-phosphorylethanolamine and glycerol 3-phosphorylcholine. PME are considered to be phospholipid precursors whereas PDE metabolites include phospholipids themselves and their decomposition products [101, 102]. While the advantage of ^{31}P MRS in the measurement of changes in oxidative phosphorylation following injury remains important, the use of ^{31}P in clinical practice has lessened due to the need for a double resonant volume or surface coil that operates at both hydrogen and phosphorous frequencies, which is not standard on clinical MR scanners. In addition ^{1}H MRS has a higher sensitivity than ^{31}P MRS, thus smaller regions can be studied using shorter acquisition times. Most important, the changes in brain metabolism following HII that are detected by both ^{1}H and ^{31}P MRS occur along a similar time course [44] and provide complimentary information in the diagnosis and prognosis of outcome in these neonates.

In a study by Buchli and colleagues [103], developmental changes of phosphorus metabolite concentrations were measured in the neonate (mean post-conceptional age 42 weeks; $n=16$), infant (mean age 11 months; $n=17$), and adult (mean age 32 years; $n=28$) human brain. Compared to adults, neonates and infants had higher concentrations (mmol/L) of PME and lower concentrations of PDE which corresponds to the development and maturation of the brain. The individual metabolite concentrations of P_i, PCr, ATP, and total phosphorous as well as the resultant PCr/ATP, PCr/P_i, and PDE/PME ratios also increased from birth to adulthood.

Early reports of ^{31}P MRS in neonates with HII identified significant reductions in PCr/P_i (ranging from 0.2–0.7), PCr/total P, and ATP/total P ratios with increased pH in the neonatal brain indicative of abnormal oxidative phosphorylation following birth asphyxia [104, 105]. Of note, these findings were not seen on the first day of life but only became apparent within the subsequent days following injury. This suggested that ^{31}P MRS observable changes in oxidative phosphorylation were related to secondary energy failure due to biochemical and electrophysiology mechanisms including free radical activation, calcium influx, and excitatory neurotransmitter toxicity.

Studies using ^{31}P to determine the prognostic significance of alterations in oxidative phosphorylation on survival and 12 month neurodevelopmental outcomes have been performed [106, 107]. In a study of 61 newborns with suspected HII [106], those neonates with PCr/P_i ratios within the 95% CI of normal had good neurodevelopmental outcomes with neonates with PCr/P_i ratios outside the 95% CI showing multiple major impairments or death [106]. In a later study of 23 asphyxiated neonates, the absolute concentration of PCr and ATP showed a highly significant ($p<0.001$) relationship to the severity of the HIE, with Spearman correlation coefficients of $r=0.85$ and 0.89, respectively [108]. Moreover, the accuracy of outcome prediction was significantly increased when the results from the ^{31}P MRS were added to the neurological assessments.

Neonatal Metabolic Disorders

Common Metabolic Disorders

This section will review MRS studies in three common metabolic disorders that affect the neonate including hyperbilirubinemia, hypoglycemia, and hypothyroidism. In contrast to studies of neonatal HII or AIS, there are few clinical/MRS studies of these conditions.

Hyperbilirubinemia

Although less commonly seen, hyperbilirubinemia remains a serious disorder in the preterm and term infant as it can be hard to detect particularly as newborns spend less time in the hospital after birth. In addition, coexistent conditions (e.g., acidosis, hypoxia, hemorrhage, hypoglycemia) increase the risk of developing kernicterus [109–111].

Several small case series have examined the effects of elevated bilirubin levels on MRS. In one report of five neonates with severe hyperbilirubinemia, the one neonate who had MRI abnormalities and subsequently developed cerebral palsy had decreased NAA/Cho and elevated Lac/NAA [112]. A second study, in six neonates, aged 3 days to 3 weeks, with hyperbilirubinemia and symptoms of kernicterus had MRS acquired from the BG [113]. Ratios of taurine/Cr, Glx/Cr, and Ins/Cr were increased and the Cho/Cr ratio was decreased. These findings were interpreted by the investigators as characteristic for kernicterus. A third and more recent study examined 24 neonates with bilirubin encephalopathy [85]. Nineteen of the 24 patients had abnormal T1 hyperintensity in the globus pallidus that appeared normal on T2. BG NAA/Cho and NAA/Cr were significantly decreased compared to controls however no long-term correlation with outcomes was reported.

Hypoglycemia

Hypoglycemia remains common in seriously ill newborns and is frequently due to an inborn error of metabolism (IEM). Brain injury secondary to hypoglycemia depends on many intrinsic factors related to the overall health of the newborn, coexistent medical problems, gestational age, associated metabolic disturbances (e.g., acidosis), etc. [114–116]. Hypoglycemia in the newborn has traditionally been categorized into four subgroups: (1) poor adaptation to extrauterine life; (2) hyperinsulinism; (3) increased glucose consumption due to illness; and (4) inborn errors of metabolism. The clinical signs and symptoms of neonatal hypoglycemia are protean and variable. Treatment regimens and the need for careful monitoring are well established although still somewhat controversial [117].

Considering how frequent and serious a problem hypoglycemia is, it is surprising that relatively few MRS studies have been reported. In part this is due to the fact that many neonates with hypoglycemia also have other coexistent conditions or an inborn error of metabolism or hyperinsulinemia. In one report of two neonates with a "hypoglycemic encephalopathy," MRI, DWI, and MRS revealed a predominance of abnormalities in the parieto-occipital lobes and underlying white matter including the splenium of the corpus callosum [118]. MRS abnormalities included an increase in the lactate-lipid peak and decreased NAA. Similar findings were reported in a case report of one neonate [119].

Hypothyroidism

Hypothyroidism is increasingly rare in countries that have implemented newborn screening programs but remains a serious issue in developing countries [120]. In some situations, coexistent medical conditions in the newborn can adversely affect thyroid hormone synthesis and this may have long-term consequences [121]. Only one study has used long echo time SVS in neonates with congenital hypothyroidism. This study examined eight neonates that were born to mothers living in iodine-deficient areas [122]. Parietal white matter and thalamic NAA/Cr and NAA/Cho levels were lower in the neonates with hypothyroidism compared to control but no differences were observed in the Cho/Cr ratios. Treatment with thyroxine for 8 weeks was associated with normalization of the initial spectral abnormalities.

Inborn Errors of Metabolism

Many IEMs have been studied using MRS and a detailed discussion of these conditions and their spectral signatures are beyond the scope of this chapter. Over the past two decades, several reviews have been published that catalogue these entities and provide algorithmic approaches to using MRS to help establish a diagnosis and to monitor disease evolution or the response to treatment [123–131]. Table 8.1

Table 8.1 MRS findings in neonates and infants with inborn errors of metabolism[a]

Inborn error of metabolism	Findings
Argininosuccinate lyase deficiency [149]	MRS showed elevated cerebral guanidinoacetate signals indicating that increased levels of this compound in brain are not limited to creatine deficiencies
Canavan disease [150]	Comprehensive report of 28 patients with aspartoacylase deficiency leading to increased NAA on MRS that provides data on the natural history of brain metabolite changes as well as MRI parameters (DWI, DTI)
Cobalamin deficiency [151]	3 of 7 patients showed increased lactate in the basal ganglia or periventricular white matter
Creatine transporter deficiency [152]	9-day-old neonate had reduced creatine on MRS and is a carrier of the R514X nonsense mutation
Galactosemia [153, 154]	MRS detected presence of 8 mmol galactitol per kilogram of brain tissue, an amount potentially relevant to the pathogenesis of brain edema
	12 patients (4 neonates, 8 patients on galactose-restricted diets, age 1.7–47 years). Results demonstrated that a markedly elevated brain galactitol level may be present only in neonates who exhibit massive urinary galactitol excretion
Glutaric acidemia type II [155, 156]	Neonate with hypoketotic hypoglycemia, metabolic acidosis, profound hypotonia, and progressive cardiomyopathy. MRI revealed underdeveloped frontal and temporal lobes with delayed myelination and hypoplasia of the corpus callosum. MRS showed elevated lactate and high Cho/Cr suggestive of dysmyelination
	Report of 4th case of combined D-and L-2-hydroxyglutaric aciduria presenting with neonatal encephalopathy, subependymal cysts, and abnormal MRS
Isovaleric acidemia [157]	Initial abnormal MRS studies resolved with treatment and patient made a good recovery
Maple syrup urine disease [158]	6 patients with MSUD had an abnormal branched-chain amino acid and branched-chain alpha-keto acids peak at 0.9 ppm on MRS and elevated lactate was seen in 4 patients
Methylenetetrahydrofolate reductase deficiency [159]	Presented in neonatal period with lethargy, poor feeding, and hypomethioninemia. Treated with methionine and MRS at 5 months showed normal metabolites
Mitochondrial respiratory chain deficiency [160, 161]	49 children (newborn to 15 years old) divided into three groups (definite, 24; probable, 14; possible,11) who had 81 MRI and 67 MRS studies. Significant differences in the frequency of MRS abnormalities seen among three groups (81%; 31%; 0%)
	11 patients of varying ages with cerebellar ataxia in whom MRS found a cerebellar lactate peak in 9/11 cases, whereas no lactate was seen in the putamen in 8/11
Nonketotic hyperglycinemia [162–167]	MRS showed a markedly increased peak intensity at 3.55 ppm (glycine) and serial studies indicated that glycine/Cho and glycine/Cr ratios correlated with the clinical course
	MRS showed a glycine peak at 10 month and a repeat study at 13 month showed an increase in this peak and a prominent Glx peak
	Reported quantitative MRS absolute glycine concentrations in different brain regions
	Neonate with encephalopathy who had intraventricular hemorrhage making cerebrospinal fluid diagnosis improbably. MRS detected elevated glycine in brain parenchymal confirming diagnosis
	Case report of neonate studied at 15 days and 6 months. MRI revealed progressive atrophy, callosal thinning, and delayed myelination. Glycine peaks were shown by MRS at 3.56 ppm
	Case report of two neonates with MRI and DWI. MRS showed characteristic glycine peaks. MRI and MRS data felt to be helpful for management
Propionic acidemia [168, 169]	Neonate who presented with feeding difficulties, hypotonia, and respiratory insufficiency. MRI showed delayed myelination and atrophy. Basal ganglia MRS showed decreased NAA and Ins and increased Glx
	Five newborns and children in whom lactate was detected by MRS
Pyruvate dehydrogenase deficiency [170]	Neonate demonstrated elevated pyruvate (at 2.37 ppm) on MRS
Smith-Lemli-Opitz syndrome [171]	Disorder of cholesterol biosynthesis (7-dehydrocholesterol reductase deficiency). 16/18 patients had MRS. Cho/NAA, lipid/NAA and lipid/Cho ratios correlated with disease severity and progression
Sulfite oxidase deficiency [172, 173]	Elevated lactate, decreased NAA/Cho and NAA/Cr and increased Cho/Cr preceded development of severe cystic encephalomalacia
Sulfite oxidase deficiency	MRS done in two neonates and one 5 month old infant and demonstrated reduced NAA and Cr
Urea cycle disorders [174]	Two infants (citrullinemia and ornithine transcarbamylase deficiency) showed a prominent increase of Glx and lipid/lactate complex. NAA, Cr, and Ins were decreased in the infant with citrullinemia

[a]This list is likely not a complete list of MRS of all inborn errors of metabolism but catalogues the major reported entities that occur in the neonate. Additional information can be obtained from online resources such as PUBMED (http://www.ncbi.nlm.nih.gov/pubmed/), GeneTests (http://www.ncbi.nlm.nih.gov/sites/GeneTests/?db=GeneTests), and subsequent chapters in this text

Table 8.2 ^{1}H NMR spectroscopy findings in urine of neonates with inborn errors of metabolism[a]

Inborn error of metabolism	Findings
Aminoacylase 1 deficiency [175]	Eight patients in which urine accumulation of N-acetylated amino acids was observed
Propionic acidemia [176]	*^{1}H NMR spectroscopy* of urine used to study metabolic changes before and during administration of oral and intravenous L-carnitine
Multiple acyl-CoA dehydrogenase deficiency [177]	The detection of dimethylglycine and sarcosine, intermediates in the oxidative degradation of choline, should discriminate between multiple acyl-CoA dehydrogenase deficiency and related disorders involving fatty acid oxidation

[a]This list is not a complete list of urinary MRS for all inborn errors of metabolism but catalogues the major ones occurring in the neonatal period. Additional information can be obtained from online resources such as PUBMED (http://www.ncbi.nlm.nih.gov/pubmed/), GeneTests (http://www.ncbi.nlm.nih.gov/sites/GeneTests/?db=GeneTests), and other chapters in this text

details MRS findings from some of the IEMs that have been reported in the newborn which are present with neurological symptoms that often mimic a neonatal encephalopathy associated with HII. A full discussion of these can be found in subsequent chapters of this text.

^{1}H NMR Spectroscopy of Urine

Over the past two decades there has been increasing interest in the use of high field ^{1}H NMR spectroscopy to study urine for the purposes of detecting metabolites specific to IEMs [132, 133] and in studying various acquired nervous system insults to determine if there are biomarkers of injury present in the urine [134–136].

Inborn Errors of Metabolism

Table 8.2 lists a number of studies of IEMs that have reported the presence of metabolites specific to the disorder in urine. In these case reports, representative spectra from the urine are depicted.

Acquired Brain Injury

As reviewed by Brown and colleagues, high field ^{1}H NMR spectroscopy has been applied to study urine from premature and sick newborn babies with a variety of clinical disorders. These included severe birth asphyxia, necrotizing enterocolitis, ketosis, and drug treatment [134]. Abnormal levels of metabolites such as lactate, ketone bodies, betaine, dicarboxylic acids, and 4-hydroxyphenolic acids have been detected.

The field of metabonomics (the rapid identification of metabolic profiles of biological fluids through the use of high-throughput analytical techniques combined with statistical pattern recognition tools) has been applied to acquired neonatal brain diseases. Coen and colleagues used this approach in a group of patients with suspected CNS infections and their results demonstrated that such spectroscopic profiling from cerebrospinal or ventricular fluid (from patients with ventriculitis) could distinguish patients with bacterial or fungal meningitis from patients with viral meningitis and control subjects as well as those with postsurgical ventriculitis from postsurgical control subjects [137].

Other investigators have examined the association between urine Lac/Cr ratios in neonates with HII and neurodevelopmental outcome and also determined whether hypothermia affected this ratio [138]. Lac/Cr was higher in neonates who died or had moderate/severe neurodevelopmental disability. Lac/Cr decreased between 6–24 h and 48–72 h of age for all infants and was not affected by hypothermia

Structural Disorders and Other Neonatal Conditions

Hydrocephalus and Other Structural Disorders

Two studies have examined MRS findings in neonates with hydrocephalus. The first study in 24 children and adults with progressive, arrested, or normal pressure hydrocephalus found that the metabolite ratios of patients were within the 95% confidence interval of controls and that a small Lac resonance was detected in 20% of controls and patients with hydrocephalus [139]. The authors concluded that MRS could not detect cerebral metabolic abnormalities in patients with hydrocephalus. The second study only examined preterm and term neonates with hydrocephalus ($n = 13$) and found elevated Lac, Glx, and alanine compared with age-matched controls [140] and the authors concluded that MRS was of limited value in predicting outcome in these infants but that MRS might be useful in identifying subsets of hydrocephalic neonates that have severe neurologic disease and poor prognosis.

Few studies have been done on other structural disorders and all consist of case reports [141]. These include neonates with subcortical heterotopias, megalencephaly [142], the growth-restricted human fetus [143], incontinentia pigmenti [144], brain tumors [145], Turner syndrome [146], and rhizomelic chondrodysplasia punctata [147, 148]. It is likely that other case reports are in the literature, particularly in those neonates and infants who have epilepsy or other specific neurological conditions.

References

1. Panigrahy A, Nelson Jr MD, Bluml S. Magnetic resonance spectroscopy in pediatric neuroradiology: clinical and research applications. Pediatr Radiol. 2010;40(1):3–30.
2. Limperopoulos C. Introduction: Imaging the developing brain. Semin Perinatol. 2010;34(1):1–2.
3. Girard N, Confort-Gouny S, Schneider J, Barberet M, Chapon F, Viola A, et al. MR imaging of brain maturation. J Neuroradiol. 2007;34(5):290–310.
4. Gressens P, Luton D. Fetal MRI: obstetrical and neurological perspectives. Pediatr Radiol. 2004;34(9):682–4.
5. Chau V, Poskitt KJ, McFadden DE, Bowen-Roberts T, Synnes A, Brant R, et al. Effect of chorioamnionitis on brain development and injury in premature newborns. Ann Neurol. 2009;66(2):155–64.
6. Lawrence RK, Inder TE. Anatomic changes and imaging in assessing brain injury in the term infant. Clin Perinatol. 2008;35(4):679–93.
7. Panigrahy A, Bluml S. Advances in magnetic resonance neuroimaging techniques in the evaluation of neonatal encephalopathy. Top Magn Reson Imaging. 2007;18(1):3–29.
8. Barkovich AJ. MR imaging of the neonatal brain. Neuroimaging Clin N Am. 2006;16(1):117–35. viii–ix.
9. Huppi PS. Advances in postnatal neuroimaging: relevance to pathogenesis and treatment of brain injury. Clin Perinatol. 2002;29(4):827–56.
10. Cady EB. Magnetic resonance spectroscopy in neonatal hypoxic-ischaemic insults. Childs Nerv Syst. 2001;17(3):145–9.
11. Xu D, Vigneron D. Magnetic resonance spectroscopy imaging of the newborn brain—a technical review. Semin Perinatol. 2010;34(1):20–7. PMCID: 2842012.
12. Pugash D, Krssak M, Kulemann V, Prayer D. Magnetic resonance spectroscopy of the fetal brain. Prenat Diagn. 2009;29(4):434–41.
13. Vigneron DB. Magnetic resonance spectroscopic imaging of human brain development. Neuroimaging Clin N Am. 2006;16(1):75–85. viii.
14. Dilenge ME, Majnemer A, Shevell MI. Long-term developmental outcome of asphyxiated term neonates. J Child Neurol. 2001;16(11):781–92.
15. Sreenan C, Bhargava R, Robertson CM. Cerebral infarction in the term newborn: clinical presentation and long-term outcome. J Pediatr. 2000;137(3):351–5.
16. Koelfen W, Freund M, Konig S, Varnholt V, Rohr H, Schultze C. Results of parenchymal and angiographic magnetic resonance imaging and neuropsychological testing of children after stroke as neonates. Eur J Pediatr. 1993;152(12):1030–5.
17. Mercuri E, Anker S, Guzzetta A, Barnett A, Haataja L, Rutherford M, et al. Neonatal cerebral infarction and visual function at school age. Arch Dis Child Fetal Neonatal Ed. 2003;88(6):F487–91. PMCID: 1763223.
18. de Vries LS, Cowan FM. Evolving understanding of hypoxic-ischemic encephalopathy in the term infant. Semin Pediatr Neurol. 2009;16(4):216–25.
19. Gonzalez FF, Ferriero DM. Therapeutics for neonatal brain injury. Pharmacol Ther. 2008;120(1):43–53.
20. Scafidi J, Gallo V. New concepts in perinatal hypoxia ischemia encephalopathy. Curr Neurol Neurosci Rep. 2008;8(2):130–8.
21. Shevell MI, Majnemer A, Miller SP. Neonatal neurologic prognostication: the asphyxiated term newborn. Pediatr Neurol. 1999;21(5):776–84.
22. Biagioni E, Mercuri E, Rutherford M, Cowan F, Azzopardi D, Frisone MF, et al. Combined use of electroencephalogram and magnetic resonance imaging in full-term neonates with acute encephalopathy. Pediatrics. 2001;107(3):461–8.
23. Belet N, Belet U, Incesu L, Uysal S, Ozinal S, Keskin T, et al. Hypoxic-ischemic encephalopathy: correlation of serial MRI and outcome. Pediatr Neurol. 2004;31(4):267–74.
24. Rutherford M, Pennock J, Schwieso J, Cowan F, Dubowitz L. Hypoxic-ischaemic encephalopathy: early and late magnetic resonance imaging findings in relation to outcome. Arch Dis Child Fetal Neonatal Ed. 1996;75(3):145–51. PMCID: 1061190.
25. Barnett A, Mercuri E, Rutherford M, Haataja L, Frisone MF, Henderson S, et al. Neurological and perceptual-motor outcome at 5–6 years of age in children with neonatal encephalopathy: relationship with neonatal brain MRI. Neuropediatrics. 2002;33(5):242–8.
26. Kuenzle C, Baenziger O, Martin E, Thun-Hohenstein L, Steinlin M, Good M, et al. Prognostic value of early MR imaging in term infants with severe perinatal asphyxia. Neuropediatrics. 1994;25(4):191–200.
27. Miller SP, Ramaswamy V, Michelson D, Barkovich AJ, Holshouser B, Wycliffe N, et al. Patterns of brain injury in term neonatal encephalopathy. J Pediatr. 2005;146(4):453–60.
28. Barkovich AJ, Hajnal BL, Vigneron D, Sola A, Partridge JC, Allen F, et al. Prediction of neuromotor outcome in perinatal asphyxia: evaluation of MR scoring systems. AJNR Am J Neuroradiol. 1998;19(1):143–9.
29. Rutherford MA, Pennock JM, Counsell SJ, Mercuri E, Cowan FM, Dubowitz LM, et al. Abnormal magnetic resonance signal in the internal capsule predicts poor neurodevelopmental outcome in infants with hypoxic-ischemic encephalopathy. Pediatrics. 1998;102(2 Pt 1):323–8.
30. Mercuri E, Guzzetta A, Haataja L, Cowan F, Rutherford M, Counsell S, et al. Neonatal neurological examination in infants with hypoxic ischaemic encephalopathy: correlation with MRI findings. Neuropediatrics. 1999;30(2):83–9.
31. Govaert P, Matthys E, Zecic A, Roelens F, Oostra A, Vanzieleghem B. Perinatal cortical infarction within middle cerebral artery trunks. Arch Dis Child Fetal Neonatal Ed. 2008;82(1):59–63. PMCID: 1721024.
32. De Vries LS, Van der Grond J, Van Haastert IC, Groenendaal F. Prediction of outcome in new-born infants with arterial ischaemic stroke using diffusion-weighted magnetic resonance imaging. Neuropediatrics. 2005;36(1):12–20.
33. de Vries LS, Groenendaal F, Eken P, van Haastert IC, Rademaker KJ, Meiners LC. Infarcts in the vascular distribution of the middle cerebral artery in preterm and fullterm infants. Neuropediatrics. 1997;28(2):88–96.
34. Golomb MR. The contribution of prothrombotic disorders to peri- and neonatal ischemic stroke. Semin Thromb Hemost. 2003;29(4):415–24.
35. Ramaswamy V, Miller SP, Barkovich AJ, Partridge JC, Ferriero DM. Perinatal stroke in term infants with neonatal encephalopathy. Neurology. 2004;62(11):2088–91.
36. Mercuri E, Cowan F, Gupte G, Manning R, Laffan M, Rutherford M, et al. Prothrombotic disorders and abnormal neurodevelopmental outcome in infants with neonatal cerebral infarction. Pediatrics. 2001;107(6):1400–4.
37. Cady EB. Metabolite concentrations and relaxation in perinatal cerebral hypoxic-ischemic injury. Neurochem Res. 1996;21(9):1043–52.
38. Groenendaal F, Veenhoven RH, van der Grond J, Jansen GH, Witkamp TD, de Vries LS. Cerebral lactate and N-acetyl-aspartate/choline ratios in asphyxiated full-term neonates demonstrated in vivo using proton magnetic resonance spectroscopy. Pediatr Res. 1994;35(2):148–51.
39. Shu SK, Ashwal S, Holshouser BA, Nystrom G, Hinshaw Jr DB. Prognostic value of 1 H-MRS in perinatal CNS insults. Pediatr Neurol. 1997;17(4):309–18.
40. Barkovich AJ, Baranski K, Vigneron D, Partridge JC, Hallam DK, Hajnal BL, et al. Proton MR spectroscopy for the evaluation of

brain injury in asphyxiated, term neonates. AJNR Am J Neuroradiol. 1999;20(8):1399–405.
41. Roelants-van Rijn AM, van der Grond J, de Vries LS, Groenendaal F. Cerebral proton magnetic resonance spectroscopy of neonates after extracorporeal membrane oxygenation. Acta Paediatr. 2001;90(11):1288–91.
42. Hanrahan JD, Sargentoni J, Azzopardi D, Manji K, Cowan FM, Rutherford MA, et al. Cerebral metabolism within 18 hours of birth asphyxia: a proton magnetic resonance spectroscopy study. Pediatr Res. 1996;39(4 Pt 1):584–90.
43. Peden CJ, Rutherford MA, Sargentoni J, Cox IJ, Bryant DJ, Dubowitz LM. Proton spectroscopy of the neonatal brain following hypoxic-ischaemic injury. Dev Med Child Neurol. 1993;35(6):502–10.
44. Cady EB, Amess P, Penrice J, Wylezinska M, Sams V, Wyatt JS. Early cerebral-metabolite quantification in perinatal hypoxic-ischaemic encephalopathy by proton and phosphorus magnetic resonance spectroscopy. Magn Reson Imaging. 1997;15(5):605–11.
45. Miller SP, Newton N, Ferriero DM, Partridge JC, Glidden DV, Barnwell A, et al. Predictors of 30-month outcome after perinatal depression: role of proton MRS and socioeconomic factors. Pediatr Res. 2002;52(1):71–7.
46. Holshouser BA, Ashwal S, Shu S, Hinshaw Jr DB. Proton MR spectroscopy in children with acute brain injury: comparison of short and long echo time acquisitions. J Magn Reson Imaging. 2000;11(1):9–19.
47. Roelants-Van Rijn AM, van der Grond J, de Vries LS, Groenendaal F. Value of (1)H-MRS using different echo times in neonates with cerebral hypoxia-ischemia. Pediatr Res. 2001;49(3):356–62.
48. Robertson NJ, Lewis RH, Cowan FM, Allsop JM, Counsell SJ, Edwards AD, et al. Early increases in brain myo-inositol measured by proton magnetic resonance spectroscopy in term infants with neonatal encephalopathy. Pediatr Res. 2001;50(6):692–700.
49. Fan G, Wu Z, Chen L, Guo Q, Ye B, Mao J. Hypoxia-ischemic encephalopathy in full-term neonate: correlation proton MR spectroscopy with MR imaging. Eur J Radiol. 2003;45(2):91–8.
50. Groenendaal F, Roelants-Van Rijn AM, van Der Grond J, Toet MC, de Vries LS. Glutamate in cerebral tissue of asphyxiated neonates during the first week of life demonstrated in vivo using proton magnetic resonance spectroscopy. Biol Neonate. 2001;79(3–4):254–7.
51. Pu Y, Li QF, Zeng CM, Gao J, Qi J, Luo DX, et al. Increased detectability of alpha brain glutamate/glutamine in neonatal hypoxic-ischemic encephalopathy. AJNR Am J Neuroradiol. 2000;21(1):203–12.
52. Zhu W, Zhong W, Qi J, Yin P, Wang C, Chang L. Proton magnetic resonance spectroscopy in neonates with hypoxic-ischemic injury and its prognostic value. Transl Res. 2008;152(5):225–32.
53. Kadri M, Shu S, Holshouser B, Deming D, Hopper A, Peverini R, et al. Proton magnetic resonance spectroscopy improves outcome prediction in perinatal CNS insults. J Perinatol. 2003;23(3):181–5.
54. Penrice J, Cady EB, Lorek A, Wylezinska M, Amess PN, Aldridge RF, et al. Proton magnetic resonance spectroscopy of the brain in normal preterm and term infants, and early changes after perinatal hypoxia-ischemia. Pediatr Res. 1996;40(1):6–14.
55. Shanmugalingam S, Thornton JS, Iwata O, Bainbridge A, O'Brien FE, Priest AN, et al. Comparative prognostic utilities of early quantitative magnetic resonance imaging spin-spin relaxometry and proton magnetic resonance spectroscopy in neonatal encephalopathy. Pediatrics. 2006;118(4):1467–77.
56. Amess PN, Penrice J, Wylezinska M, Lorek A, Townsend J, Wyatt JS, et al. Early brain proton magnetic resonance spectroscopy and neonatal neurology related to neurodevelopmental outcome at 1 year in term infants after presumed hypoxic-ischaemic brain injury. Dev Med Child Neurol. 1999;41(7):436–45.
57. Hanrahan JD, Cox IJ, Azzopardi D, Cowan FM, Sargentoni J, Bell JD, et al. Relation between proton magnetic resonance spectroscopy within 18 hours of birth asphyxia and neurodevelopment at 1 year of age. Dev Med Child Neurol. 1999;41(2):76–82.
58. Robertson NJ, Cox IJ, Cowan FM, Counsell SJ, Azzopardi D, Edwards AD. Cerebral intracellular lactic alkalosis persisting months after neonatal encephalopathy measured by magnetic resonance spectroscopy. Pediatr Res. 1999;46(3):287–96.
59. Boichot C, Walker PM, Durand C, Grimaldi M, Chapuis S, Gouyon JB, et al. Term neonate prognoses after perinatal asphyxia: contributions of MR imaging, MR spectroscopy, relaxation times, and apparent diffusion coefficients. Radiology. 2006;239(3):839–48.
60. Cheong JL, Cady EB, Penrice J, Wyatt JS, Cox IJ, Robertson NJ. Proton MR spectroscopy in neonates with perinatal cerebral hypoxic-ischemic injury: metabolite peak-area ratios, relaxation times, and absolute concentrations. AJNR Am J Neuroradiol. 2006;27(7):1546–54.
61. Thayyil S, Chandrasekaran M, Taylor A, Bainbridge A, Cady EB, Chong WK, et al. Cerebral magnetic resonance biomarkers in neonatal encephalopathy: a meta-analysis. Pediatrics. 2010;125(2): e382–95.
62. Wilkinson D. MRI and withdrawal of life support from newborn infants with hypoxic-ischemic encephalopathy. Pediatrics. 2010;126(2):e451–8.
63. Vigneron DB, Barkovich AJ, Noworolski SM, von dem Bussche M, Henry RG, Lu Y, et al. Three-dimensional proton MR spectroscopic imaging of premature and term neonates. AJNR Am J Neuroradiol. 2001;22(7):1424–33.
64. Miller SP, Weiss J, Barnwell A, Ferriero DM, Latal-Hajnal B, Ferrer-Rogers A, et al. Seizure-associated brain injury in term newborns with perinatal asphyxia. Neurology. 2002;58(4):542–8.
65. Pu Y, Garg A, Corby R, Gao JH, Zeng CM, Li QF. A positive correlation between alpha-glutamate and glutamine on brain 1 H-MR spectroscopy and neonatal seizures in moderate and severe hypoxic-ischemic encephalopathy. AJNR Am J Neuroradiol. 2008;29(2):216.
66. Barkovich AJ, Westmark KD, Bedi HS, Partridge JC, Ferriero DM, Vigneron DB. Proton spectroscopy and diffusion imaging on the first day of life after perinatal asphyxia: preliminary report. AJNR Am J Neuroradiol. 2001;22(9):1786–94.
67. Hanrahan JD, Cox IJ, Edwards AD, Cowan FM, Sargentoni J, Bell JD, et al. Persistent increases in cerebral lactate concentration after birth asphyxia. Pediatr Res. 1998;44(3):304–11.
68. Holshouser BA, Ashwal S, Luh GY, Shu S, Kahlon S, Auld KL, et al. Proton MR spectroscopy after acute central nervous system injury: outcome prediction in neonates, infants, and children. Radiology. 1997;202(2):487–96.
69. da Silva LF, Hoefel Filho JR, Anes M, Nunes ML. Prognostic value of 1H-MRS in neonatal encephalopathy. Pediatr Neurol. 2006;34(5):360–6.
70. Pavlakis SG, Kingsley PB, Harper R, Buckwald S, Spinazzola R, Frank Y, et al. Correlation of basal ganglia magnetic resonance spectroscopy with Apgar score in perinatal asphyxia. Arch Neurol. 1999;56(12):1476–81.
71. L'Abee C, de Vries LS, van der Grond J, Groenendaal F. Early diffusion-weighted MRI and 1 H-Magnetic Resonance Spectroscopy in asphyxiated full-term neonates. Biol Neonate. 2005;88(4):306–12.
72. Meyer-Witte S, Brissaud O, Brun M, Lamireau D, Bordessoules M, Chateil JF. Prognostic value of MR in term neonates with neonatal hypoxic-ischemic encephalopath: MRI score and spectroscopy. About 26 cases. Arch Pediatr. 2008;15(1):9–23.
73. Zarifi MK, Astrakas LG, Poussaint TY, Zurakowski D, Plessis Ad A, Tzika AA. Prediction of adverse outcome with cerebral lactate level and apparent diffusion coefficient in infants with perinatal asphyxia. Radiology. 2002;225(3):859–70.
74. Angeles DM, Ashwal S, Wycliffe ND, Ebner C, Fayard E, Sowers L, et al. Relationship between opioid therapy, tissue-damaging

procedures, and brain metabolites as measured by proton MRS in asphyxiated term neonates. Pediatr Res. 2007;61(5 Pt 1):614–21.
75. Anand KJ, Scalzo FM. Can adverse neonatal experiences alter brain development and subsequent behavior? Biol Neonate. 2000;77(2):69–82.
76. Porter FL, Wolf CM, Miller JP. Procedural pain in newborn infants: the influence of intensity and development. Pediatrics. 1999;104(1):e13.
77. Kelen D, Robertson NJ. Experimental treatments for hypoxic ischaemic encephalopathy. Early Hum Dev. 2010;86(6):369–77.
78. Corbo ET, Machado S, Merritt T, Wycliffe N, Ashwal S, Bartnik-Olson B. The effect of whole-body cooling on brain metabolism in the thalami following perinatal hypoxic ischemic injury. Pediatr Res. 2012;71(1):85–92.
79. Groenendaal F, van der Grond J, Witkamp TD, de Vries LS. Proton magnetic resonance spectroscopic imaging in neonatal stroke. Neuropediatrics. 1995;26(5):243–8.
80. Venkataraman A, Kingsley PB, Kalina P, Pavlakis SG, Buckwald S, Spinazzola R, et al. Newborn brain infarction: clinical aspects and magnetic resonance imaging. CNS Spectr. 2004;9(6):436–44.
81. Huppi PS, Schuknecht B, Boesch C, Bossi E, Felblinger J, Fusch C, et al. Structural and neurobehavioral delay in postnatal brain development of preterm infants. Pediatr Res. 1996;39(5):895–901.
82. Roelants-van Rijn AM, van der Grond J, Stigter RH, de Vries LS, Groenendaal F. Cerebral structure and metabolism and long-term outcome in small-for-gestational-age preterm neonates. Pediatr Res. 2004;56(2):285–90.
83. Robertson NJ, Kuint J, Counsell TJ, Rutherford TA, Coutts A, Cox IJ, et al. Characterization of cerebral white matter damage in preterm infants using 1 H and 31P magnetic resonance spectroscopy. J Cereb Blood Flow Metab. 2000;20(10):1446–56.
84. Toft PB, Leth H, Peitersen B, Lou HC. Metabolic changes in the striatum after germinal matrix hemorrhage in the preterm infant. Pediatr Res. 1997;41(3):309–16.
85. Wang X, Wu W, Hou BL, Zhang P, Chineah A, Liu F, et al. Studying neonatal bilirubin encephalopathy with conventional MRI, MRS, and DWI. Neuroradiology. 2008;50(10):885–93.
86. Augustine EM, Spielman DM, Barnes PD, Sutcliffe TL, Dermon JD, Mirmiran M, et al. Can magnetic resonance spectroscopy predict neurodevelopmental outcome in very low birth weight preterm infants? J Perinatol. 2008;28(9):611–8. PMCID: 2844764.
87. Gimenez M, Soria-Pastor S, Junque C, Caldu X, Narberhaus A, Botet F, et al. Proton magnetic resonance spectroscopy reveals medial temporal metabolic abnormalities in adolescents with history of preterm birth. Pediatr Res. 2008;64(5):572–7.
88. Johnston MV. Congenital heart disease and brain injury. N Engl J Med. 2007;357(19):1971–3.
89. Sherlock RL, McQuillen PS, Miller SP. Preventing brain injury in newborns with congenital heart disease: brain imaging and innovative trial designs. Stroke. 2009;40(1):327–32.
90. Scallan MJ. Brain injury in children with congenital heart disease. Paediatr Anaesth. 2003;13(4):284–93.
91. Bird GL, Jeffries HE, Licht DJ, Wernovsky G, Weinberg PM, Pizarro C, et al. Neurological complications associated with the treatment of patients with congenital cardiac disease: consensus definitions from the Multi-Societal Database Committee for Pediatric and Congenital Heart Disease. Cardiol Young. 2008;18 Suppl 2:234–9. PMCID: 2742973.
92. Ashwal S, Holshouser BA, Hinshaw Jr DB, Schell RM, Bailey L. Proton magnetic resonance spectroscopy in the evaluation of children with congenital heart disease and acute central nervous system injury. J Thorac Cardiovasc Surg. 1996;112(2):403–14.
93. Mahle WT, Tavani F, Zimmerman RA, Nicolson SC, Galli KK, Gaynor JW, et al. An MRI study of neurological injury before and after congenital heart surgery. Circulation. 2002;106(12 Suppl 1):I109–14.
94. Ashwal S, Holshouser BA, del Rio MJ, Tong KA, Applegate RL, Bailey LL. Serial proton magnetic resonance spectroscopy of the brain in children undergoing cardiac surgery. Pediatr Neurol. 2003;29(2):99–110.
95. Miller SP, McQuillen PS, Vigneron DB, Glidden DV, Barkovich AJ, Ferriero DM, et al. Preoperative brain injury in newborns with transposition of the great arteries. Ann Thorac Surg. 2004;77(5):1698–706.
96. Miller SP, McQuillen PS, Hamrick S, Xu D, Glidden DV, Charlton N, et al. Abnormal brain development in newborns with congenital heart disease. N Engl J Med. 2007;357(19):1928–38.
97. Park IS, Yoon SY, Min JY, Kim YH, Ko JK, Kim KS, et al. Metabolic alterations and neurodevelopmental outcome of infants with transposition of the great arteries. Pediatr Cardiol. 2006;27(5):569–76.
98. Bulas D, Glass P. Neonatal ECMO: neuroimaging and neurodevelopmental outcome. Semin Perinatol. 2005;29(1):58–65.
99. Voet D, Voet J. Biochemistry. 3rd ed. New Jersey: Wiley; 2004.
100. de Graaf RA. In vivo NMR spectroscopy: principles and techniques. 2nd ed. New Jersey: Wiley; 2007.
101. Cerdan S, Subramanian VH, Hilberman M, Cone J, Egan J, Chance B, et al. 31P NMR detection of mobile dog brain phospholipids. Magn Reson Med. 1986;3(3):432–9.
102. Murphy EJ, Rajagopalan B, Brindle KM, Radda GK. Phospholipid bilayer contribution to 31P NMR spectra in vivo. Magn Reson Med. 1989;12(2):282–9.
103. Buchli R, Martin E, Boesiger P, Rumpel H. Developmental changes of phosphorus metabolite concentrations in the human brain: a 31P magnetic resonance spectroscopy study in vivo. Pediatr Res. 1994;35(4 Pt 1):431–5.
104. Cady EB, Costello AM, Dawson MJ, Delpy DT, Hope PL, Reynolds EO, et al. Non-invasive investigation of cerebral metabolism in newborn infants by phosphorus nuclear magnetic resonance spectroscopy. Lancet. 1983;1(8333):1059–62.
105. Hope PL, Costello AM, Cady EB, Delpy DT, Tofts PS, Chu A, et al. Cerebral energy metabolism studied with phosphorus NMR spectroscopy in normal and birth-asphyxiated infants. Lancet. 1984;2(8399):366–70.
106. Azzopardi D, Wyatt JS, Cady EB, Delpy DT, Baudin J, Stewart AL, et al. Prognosis of newborn infants with hypoxic-ischemic brain injury assessed by phosphorus magnetic resonance spectroscopy. Pediatr Res. 1989;25(5):445–51.
107. Roth SC, Edwards AD, Cady EB, Delpy DT, Wyatt JS, Azzopardi D, et al. Relation between cerebral oxidative metabolism following birth asphyxia, and neurodevelopmental outcome and brain growth at one year. Dev Med Child Neurol. 1992;34(4):285–95.
108. Martin E, Buchli R, Ritter S, Schmid R, Largo RH, Boltshauser E, et al. Diagnostic and prognostic value of cerebral 31P magnetic resonance spectroscopy in neonates with perinatal asphyxia. Pediatr Res. 1996;40(5):749–58.
109. Maisels MJ. Neonatal hyperbilirubinemia and kernicterus - not gone but sometimes forgotten. Early Hum Dev. 2009;85(11):727–32.
110. Ahlfors CE. Predicting bilirubin neurotoxicity in jaundiced newborns. Curr Opin Pediatr. 2010;22(2):129–33.
111. Cohen RS, Wong RJ, Stevenson DK. Understanding neonatal jaundice: a perspective on causation. Pediatr Neonatol. 2010;51(3):143–8.
112. Groenendaal F, van der Grond J, de Vries LS. Cerebral metabolism in severe neonatal hyperbilirubinemia. Pediatrics. 2004;114(1):291–4.
113. Oakden WK, Moore AM, Blaser S, Noseworthy MD. 1 H MR spectroscopic characteristics of kernicterus: a possible metabolic signature. AJNR Am J Neuroradiol. 2005;26(6):1571–4.
114. Rozance PJ, Hay Jr WW. Describing hypoglycemia—definition or operational threshold? Early Hum Dev. 2010;86(5):275–80. PMCID: 2900507.

115. Straussman S, Levitsky LL. Neonatal hypoglycemia. Curr Opin Endocrinol Diabetes Obes. 2010;17(1):20–4.
116. Montassir H, Maegaki Y, Ogura K, Kurozawa Y, Nagata I, Kanzaki S, et al. Associated factors in neonatal hypoglycemic brain injury. Brain Dev. 2009;31(9):649–56.
117. Hay Jr WW, Raju TN, Higgins RD, Kalhan SC, Devaskar SU. Knowledge gaps and research needs for understanding and treating neonatal hypoglycemia: workshop report from Eunice Kennedy Shriver National Institute of Child Health and Human Development. J Pediatr. 2009;155(5):612–7.
118. Kim SY, Goo HW, Lim KH, Kim ST, Kim KS. Neonatal hypoglycaemic encephalopathy: diffusion-weighted imaging and proton MR spectroscopy. Pediatr Radiol. 2006;36(2):144–8.
119. Musson RE, Batty R, Mordekar SR, Wilkinson ID, Griffiths PD, Connolly DJ. Diffusion-weighted imaging and magnetic resonance spectroscopy findings in a case of neonatal hypoglycaemia. Dev Med Child Neurol. 2009;51(8):653–4.
120. LaFranchi SH. Newborn screening strategies for congenital hypothyroidism: an update. J Inherit Metab Dis. 2010;33 Suppl 2:S225–33.
121. Shih JL, Agus MS. Thyroid function in the critically ill newborn and child. Curr Opin Pediatr. 2009;21(4):536–40.
122. Akinci A, Sarac K, Gungor S, Mungan I, Aydin O. Brain MR spectroscopy findings in neonates with hypothyroidism born to mothers living in iodine-deficient areas. AJNR Am J Neuroradiol. 2006;27(10):2083–7.
123. Bizzi A, Castelli G, Bugiani M, Barker PB, Herskovits EH, Danesi U, et al. Classification of childhood white matter disorders using proton MR spectroscopic imaging. AJNR Am J Neuroradiol. 2008;29(7):1270–5. PMCID: 2944924.
124. Barkovich AJ. An approach to MRI of metabolic disorders in children. J Neuroradiol. 2007;34(2):75–88.
125. Burlina AP, Aureli T, Bracco F, Conti F, Battistin L. MR spectroscopy: a powerful tool for investigating brain function and neurological diseases. Neurochem Res. 2000;25(9–10):1365–72.
126. Chabrol B, Salvan AM, Confort-Gouny S, Vion-Dury J, Cozzone PJ. Localized proton magnetic resonance spectroscopy of the brain differentiates the inborn metabolic encephalopathies in children. C R Acad Sci III. 1995;318(9):985–92.
127. Barker PB, Horska A. Neuroimaging in leukodystrophies. J Child Neurol. 2004;19(8):559–70.
128. Gulati S, Shah T, Menon S, Jayasundar R, Kalra V. Magnetic resonance spectroscopy in pediatric neurology. Indian J Pediatr. 2003;70(4):317–25.
129. Lin A, Ross BD, Harris K, Wong W. Efficacy of proton magnetic resonance spectroscopy in neurological diagnosis and neurotherapeutic decision making. NeuroRx. 2005;2(2):197–214. PMCID: 1064986.
130. Lin DD, Crawford TO, Barker PB. Proton MR spectroscopy in the diagnostic evaluation of suspected mitochondrial disease. AJNR Am J Neuroradiol. 2003;24(1):33–41.
131. Wang ZJ, Zimmerman RA. Proton MR spectroscopy of pediatric brain metabolic disorders. Neuroimaging Clin N Am. 1998;8(4):781–807.
132. Engelke UF, Liebrand-van Sambeek ML, de Jong JG, Leroy JG, Morava E, Smeitink JA, et al. N-acetylated metabolites in urine: proton nuclear magnetic resonance spectroscopic study on patients with inborn errors of metabolism. Clin Chem. 2004;50(1):58–66.
133. Bamforth FJ, Dorian V, Vallance H, Wishart DS. Diagnosis of inborn errors of metabolism using 1 H NMR spectroscopic analysis of urine. J Inherit Metab Dis. 1999;22(3):297–301.
134. Brown JC, Mills GA, Sadler PJ, Walker V. 1 H NMR studies of urine from premature and sick babies. Magn Reson Med. 1989;11(2):193–201.
135. Trump S, Laudi S, Unruh N, Goelz R, Leibfritz D. 1 H-NMR metabolic profiling of human neonatal urine. MAGMA. 2006;19(6):305–12.
136. Ma S, Shieh LI, Huang CC. High-resolution proton nuclear magnetic resonance studies of urine from asphyxiated newborn infants. Appl Biochem Biotechnol. 1995;53(1):37–51.
137. Coen M, O'Sullivan M, Bubb WA, Kuchel PW, Sorrell T. Proton nuclear magnetic resonance-based metabonomics for rapid diagnosis of meningitis and ventriculitis. Clin Infect Dis. 2005;41(11):1582–90.
138. Oh W, Perritt R, Shankaran S, Merritts M, Donovan EF, Ehrenkranz RA, et al. Association between urinary lactate to creatinine ratio and neurodevelopmental outcome in term infants with hypoxic-ischemic encephalopathy. J Pediatr. 2008;153(3):375–8.
139. Braun KP, Gooskens RH, Vandertop WP, Tulleken CA, van der Grond J. 1 H magnetic resonance spectroscopy in human hydrocephalus. J Magn Reson Imaging. 2003;17(3):291–9.
140. McNatt SA, McComb JG, Nelson MD, Bluml S. Proton magnetic resonance spectroscopy of hydrocephalic infants. Pediatr Neurosurg. 2007;43(6):461–7.
141. Hoon Jr AH, Melhem ER. Neuroimaging: applications in disorders of early brain development. J Dev Behav Pediatr. 2000;21(4):291–302.
142. Groeschel S, Brockmann K, Dechent P, Wilichowski E, Frahm J, Hanefeld F. Magnetic resonance imaging and proton magnetic resonance spectroscopy of megalencephaly and dilated Virchow-Robin spaces. Pediatr Neurol. 2006;34(1):35–40.
143. Azpurua H, Alvarado A, Mayobre F, Salom T, Copel JA, Guevara-Zuloaga F. Metabolic assessment of the brain using proton magnetic resonance spectroscopy in a growth-restricted human fetus: case report. Am J Perinatol. 2008;25(5):305–9.
144. Lee AG, Goldberg MF, Gillard JH, Barker PB, Bryan RN. Intracranial assessment of incontinentia pigmenti using magnetic resonance imaging, angiography, and spectroscopic imaging. Arch Pediatr Adolesc Med. 1995;149(5):573–80.
145. Sutton LN, Lenkinski RE, Cohen BH, Packer RJ, Zimmerman RA. Localized 31P magnetic resonance spectroscopy of large pediatric brain tumors. J Neurosurg. 1990;72(1):65–70.
146. Cutter WJ, Daly EM, Robertson DM, Chitnis XA, van Amelsvoort TA, Simmons A, et al. Influence of X chromosome and hormones on human brain development: a magnetic resonance imaging and proton magnetic resonance spectroscopy study of Turner syndrome. Biol Psychiatry. 2006;59(3):273–83.
147. Sigirci A, Alkan A, Kutlu R, Gulcan H. Multivoxel magnetic resonance spectroscopy in a rhizomelic chondrodysplasia punctata case. J Child Neurol. 2005;20(8):698–701.
148. Viola A, Confort-Gouny S, Ranjeva JP, Chabrol B, Raybaud C, Vintila F, et al. MR imaging and MR spectroscopy in rhizomelic chondrodysplasia punctata. AJNR Am J Neuroradiol. 2002;23(3):480–3.
149. Sijens PE, Reijngoud DJ, Soorani-Lunsing RJ, Oudkerk M, van Spronsen FJ. Cerebral 1 H MR spectroscopy showing elevation of brain guanidinoacetate in argininosuccinate lyase deficiency. Mol Genet Metab. 2006;88(1):100–2.
150. Janson CG, McPhee SW, Francis J, Shera D, Assadi M, Freese A, et al. Natural history of Canavan disease revealed by proton magnetic resonance spectroscopy (1 H-MRS) and diffusion-weighted MRI. Neuropediatrics. 2006;37(4):209–21.
151. Longo D, Fariello G, Dionisi-Vici C, Cannata V, Boenzi S, Genovese E, et al. MRI and 1 H-MRS findings in early-onset cobalamin C/D defect. Neuropediatrics. 2005;36(6):366–72.
152. Cecil KM, DeGrauw TJ, Salomons GS, Jakobs C, Egelhoff JC, Clark JF. Magnetic resonance spectroscopy in a 9-day-old heterozygous female child with creatine transporter deficiency. J Comput Assist Tomogr. 2003;27(1):44–7.
153. Berry GT, Hunter JV, Wang Z, Dreha S, Mazur A, Brooks DG, et al. In vivo evidence of brain galactitol accumulation in an infant with galactosemia and encephalopathy. J Pediatr. 2001;138(2):260–2.

154. Wang ZJ, Berry GT, Dreha SF, Zhao H, Segal S, Zimmerman RA. Proton magnetic resonance spectroscopy of brain metabolites in galactosemia. Ann Neurol. 2001;50(2):266–9.
155. Shevell MI, Didomenicantonio G, Sylvain M, Arnold DL, O'Gorman AM, Scriver CR. Glutaric acidemia type II: neuroimaging and spectroscopy evidence for developmental encephalomyopathy. Pediatr Neurol. 1995;12(4):350–3.
156. Read MH, Bonamy C, Laloum D, Belloy F, Constans JM, Guillois B, et al. Clinical, biochemical, magnetic resonance imaging (MRI) and proton magnetic resonance spectroscopy (1 H MRS) findings in a fourth case of combined D- and L-2 hydroxyglutaric aciduria. J Inherit Metab Dis. 2005;28(6):1149–50.
157. Lorek AK, Penrice JM, Cady EB, Leonard JV, Wyatt JS, Iles RA, et al. Cerebral energy metabolism in isovaleric acidaemia. Arch Dis Child Fetal Neonatal Ed. 1996;74(3):F211–3. PMCID: 2528338.
158. Jan W, Zimmerman RA, Wang ZJ, Berry GT, Kaplan PB, Kaye EM. MR diffusion imaging and MR spectroscopy of maple syrup urine disease during acute metabolic decompensation. Neuroradiology. 2003;45(6):393–9.
159. Al-Essa MA. Al Amir A, Rashed M, Al Jishi E, Abutaleb A, Mobaireek K, et al. Clinical, fluorine-18 labeled 2-fluoro-2-deoxyglucose positron emission tomography of the brain, MR spectroscopy, and therapeutic attempts in methylenetetrahydrofolate reductase deficiency. Brain Dev. 1999;21(5):345–9.
160. Dinopoulos A, Cecil KM, Schapiro MB, Papadimitriou A, Hadjigeorgiou GM, Wong B, et al. Brain MRI and proton MRS findings in infants and children with respiratory chain defects. Neuropediatrics. 2005;36(5):290–301.
161. Boddaert N, Romano S, Funalot B, Rio M, Sarzi E, Lebre AS, et al. 1 H MRS spectroscopy evidence of cerebellar high lactate in mitochondrial respiratory chain deficiency. Mol Genet Metab. 2008;93(1):85–8.
162. Choi CG, Lee HK, Yoon JH. Localized proton MR spectroscopic detection of nonketotic hyperglycinemia in an infant. Korean J Radiol. 2001;2(4):239–42. PMCID: 2718128.
163. Gabis L, Parton P, Roche P, Lenn N, Tudorica A, Huang W. In vivo 1 H magnetic resonance spectroscopic measurement of brain glycine levels in nonketotic hyperglycinemia. J Neuroimaging. 2001;11(2):209–11.
164. Huisman TA, Thiel T, Steinmann B, Zeilinger G, Martin E. Proton magnetic resonance spectroscopy of the brain of a neonate with nonketotic hyperglycinemia: in vivo-in vitro (ex vivo) correlation. Eur Radiol. 2002;12(4):858–61.
165. Manley BJ, Sokol J, Cheong JL. Intracerebral blood and MRS in neonatal nonketotic hyperglycinemia. Pediatr Neurol. 2010;42(3):219–22.
166. Sener RN. Nonketotic hyperglycinemia: diffusion magnetic resonance imaging findings. J Comput Assist Tomogr. 2003;27(4):538–40.
167. Shah DK, Tingay DG, Fink AM, Hunt RW, Dargaville PA. Magnetic resonance imaging in neonatal nonketotic hyperglycinemia. Pediatr Neurol. 2005;33(1):50–2.
168. Bergman AJ, Van der Knaap MS, Smeitink JA, Duran M, Dorland L, Valk J, et al. Magnetic resonance imaging and spectroscopy of the brain in propionic acidemia: clinical and biochemical considerations. Pediatr Res. 1996;40(3):404–9.
169. Chemelli AP, Schocke M, Sperl W, Trieb T, Aichner F, Felber S. Magnetic resonance spectroscopy (MRS) in five patients with treated propionic acidemia. J Magn Reson Imaging. 2000;11(6):596–600.
170. Zand DJ, Simon EM, Pulitzer SB, Wang DJ, Wang ZJ, Rorke LB, et al. In vivo pyruvate detected by MR spectroscopy in neonatal pyruvate dehydrogenase deficiency. AJNR Am J Neuroradiol. 2003;24(7):1471–4.
171. Caruso PA, Poussaint TY, Tzika AA, Zurakowski D, Astrakas LG, Elias ER, et al. MRI and 1 H MRS findings in Smith-Lemli-Opitz syndrome. Neuroradiology. 2004;46(1):3–14.
172. Eichler F, Tan WH, Shih VE, Grant PE, Krishnamoorthy K. Proton magnetic resonance spectroscopy and diffusion-weighted imaging in isolated sulfite oxidase deficiency. J Child Neurol. 2006;21(9):801–5.
173. Hoffmann C, Ben-Zeev B, Anikster Y, Nissenkorn A, Brand N, Kuint J, et al. Magnetic resonance imaging and magnetic resonance spectroscopy in isolated sulfite oxidase deficiency. J Child Neurol. 2007;22(10):1214–21.
174. Choi CG, Yoo HW. Localized proton MR spectroscopy in infants with urea cycle defect. AJNR Am J Neuroradiol. 2001;22(5):834–7.
175. Engelke UF, Sass JO, Van Coster RN, Gerlo E, Olbrich H, Krywawych S, et al. NMR spectroscopy of aminoacylase 1 deficiency, a novel inborn error of metabolism. NMR Biomed. 2008;21(2):138–47.
176. Davies SE, Iles RA, Stacey TE, de Sousa C, Chalmers RA. Carnitine therapy and metabolism in the disorders of propionyl-CoA metabolism studied using 1 H-NMR spectroscopy. Clin Chim Acta. 1991;204(1–3):263–77.
177. Burns SP, Holmes HC, Chalmers RA, Johnson A, Iles RA. Proton NMR spectroscopic analysis of multiple acyl-CoA dehydrogenase deficiency–capacity of the choline oxidation pathway for methylation in vivo. Biochim Biophys Acta. 1998;1406(3):274–82.

Proton Magnetic Resonance Spectroscopy: Application in Non-Accidental Trauma

9

Barbara Holshouser and Stephen Ashwal

Traumatic injury as a result of child abuse is known by several terms including non-accidental trauma (NAT), inflicted injury, shaken baby syndrome or battered child syndrome. The latter term was introduced by C.H. Kempke in a 1962 paper that served as the driving force that established national statutes mandating identification and reporting of all suspected child abuse and neglect to law enforcement and social services. [1] Child abuse is widespread. In 2006, state and local child protective services in the USA investigated 3.6 million reports of children being abused or neglected and classified more than 900,000 (12.1 per 1,000) of these children as victims with approximately 144,000 due to physical abuse. [2] The National Child Abuse and Neglect Data System (NCANDS) data for 2007 demonstrated that children younger than 1 year accounted for 42.2% of fatalities, while children younger than 4 years accounted for more than three-quarters (75.7%) of fatalities [3]. While inflicted trauma to the brain is reported as the leading cause of death in children younger than 2 years of age, the non-fatal injuries can leave the victim with a lifetime of neurologic deficits. [4, 5] Injuries to a younger child's brain are unique from those affecting older children. In younger children, the skull is thinner which allows transfer of force across a subarachnoid space that is shallow into a brain that is still maturing. In addition, the neck muscles are underdeveloped and the head is relatively heavier compared to the body which may cause sudden impacts or rotational movements to result in enough force to produce diffuse axonal injury or other injuries, such as, subdural, subarachnoid, and retinal hemorrhages. Although, the term "shaken baby syndrome" remains controversial, it is generally agreed that blunt force impact as well as vigorous shaking play a role in the pathogenesis of abusive head injuries in children [6]. Neurotrauma from NAT is complex and results from multiple types of axonal injury that occur in the same brain including hypoxic–ischemic injury designated as vascular axonal injury and diffuse traumatic axonal injury resulting from acceleration–deceleration forces [7, 8]. In general, outcomes after non-accidental brain trauma are recognized to be worse than in children with accidental traumatic brain injury (TBI). [9, 10] This is thought to be a result of multiple factors including a higher incidence of ischemic brain injury, skull fractures, and subdural hemorrhages in a situation where presentation for medical care is often delayed until symptoms occur. Even when there is apparent early recovery from inflicted head trauma, long-term developmental follow-up frequently reveals neurocognitive deficits [11]. Thus, brain injury as a result of non-accidental trauma is one of the most important types of injury in terms of long-term disability.

Efforts have been made to develop tools that better assess severity and correlate with outcome. The more commonly used indicators for evaluating TBI include the Glasgow Coma Scale (GCS) score [12, 13], duration of impaired consciousness and posttraumatic amnesia [14], presence of non-reactive pupils [15], standard brain imaging techniques [2, 9], the presence of skull fractures [9, 13], and duration of impaired consciousness [16]. Changes in these variables have been associated with a poor neurodevelopmental outcome. In addition to these indicators, external injuries, retinal hemorrhages, and a wide range of neurological symptoms are commonly used by clinicians when evaluating patients for NAT [17]. Bilateral retinal and vitreous hemorrhage have been associated with poor neurodevelopmental outcome in multiple studies of NAT [13, 18, 19]. Many studies have demonstrated that most children with NAT show developmental delays, motor, cognitive, and emotional deficits [20–24]. Impairments such as learning disabilities might not manifest until a child attends school [11] whereas behavioral problems, reported to be present in 52% of children after NAT, begin to manifest between the second and third years of life [20].

B. Holshouser, Ph.D. (✉)
Department of Radiology, Section of Magnetic Resonance Imaging, Loma Linda University School of Medicine, Loma Linda, CA, USA
e-mail: bholshouser@llu.edu

S. Ashwal, M.D.
Division of Pediatric Neurology, Department of Pediatrics, Loma Linda University School of Medicine, Loma Linda, CA, USA
e-mail: sashwal@llu.edu

S. Blüml and A. Panigrahy (eds.), *MR Spectroscopy of Pediatric Brain Disorders*,
DOI 10.1007/978-1-4419-5864-8_9, © Springer Science+Business Media, LLC 2013

Because deficits in preschool children are often underestimated, sensitive techniques to recognize injury and thus the potential for impairment at an early age are necessary to provide justification for extended follow-up evaluations.

Imaging is essential in the assessment of suspected NAT and plays a role in outcome prognosis. Most infants are initially evaluated with skeletal X-rays and computed tomography (CT) to determine whether fractures are present, the severity of acute injury and the need for urgent neurosurgical intervention. In children with NAT, retinal hemorrhage, metaphyseal fractures, rib fractures, and subdural hemorrhage are more commonly found compared to children with accidental trauma [10]. For neurotrauma, CT and magnetic resonance imaging (MRI) are the imaging modalities of choice to reveal subdural or subarachnoid hemorrhages, contusions, and brain edema [25]. In addition, MRI can show areas of ischemia on diffusion-weighted imaging (DWI) [26, 27] as well as, parenchymal microhemorrhages (MH) on 2D T2* weighted gradient recalled echo (GRE) imaging [28]. A newer imaging technique, susceptibility weighted imaging (SWI), detected MH in 29 of 101 patients (29%) after NAT and showed that the presence of MH on SWI contributed greatest in a logistic regression model for prediction of long-term neurologic outcome followed by the presence of ischemic injury, initial GCS score and age to achieve an overall predictive accuracy of 92.5% [29]. Magnetic resonance spectroscopy (MRS) can also play a role in the evaluation of NAT and outcome prediction.

MRS offers a unique non-invasive method to quantify the magnitude and regional distribution of injury as it is capable of measuring *N*-acetylaspartate (NAA), a marker of neuronal function and integrity [30]. Reduced NAA is commonly used as a marker for neuronal loss after traumatic or hypoxic–ischemic injury. However, since NAA is produced in neuronal mitochondria and relies on ATP for synthesis, mitochondrial dysfunction may contribute to the temporary reduction in NAA seen after TBI. [31–33] It has been postulated that a temporary drop in NAA following brain injury may also be caused by accelerated lipid synthesis involved in myelin repair or because NAA provides a temporary source of cellular energy locally at the site of axonal injury producing a transient drop which could precede any loss of NAA as a result of axonal death. [34] Thus, NAA measurements may serve as a sensitive and specific biomarker of neuronal injury, dysfunction, loss, or repair.

Hypoxic–ischemic injury (HII) is more common after NAT and may be an additional major factor causing poor outcomes. [23, 35, 36] Some studies have shown that infants with NAT are more likely to have HII as measured by metabolic acidosis [37] and reduced cerebral perfusion pressure [38]. A recent study of 30 children with NAT found that 37% had HII on MRI diffusion weighted images compared to only 9% of children with accidental trauma [27]. Production of lactate (Lac), from impaired aerobic glycolysis, is specifically a marker for HII that can be detected along with NAA changes in MR spectra. In one study of 11 NAT victims, 45% had cerebral Lac and all had worse discharge outcomes compared to those without Lac [39]. Lactate presence has been related to multiple factors including: excessive release of glutamate, disordered mitochondrial and oxidative metabolism, and systemic responses to trauma [40–42].

Victims of abuse are usually younger compared to children who suffer TBI from accidental causes. Infants and young children have less mature airway protective reflexes placing them at higher risk of respiratory failure as reflected in the higher rates of intubation after NAT compared to accidental TBI [27]. Animal models have shown that TBI can produce hyperacute central apnea and respiratory dysfunction [43]. Autopsy studies in victims of NAT have shown that injuries to the lower brainstem and spinal cord are associated with apnea and microscopic evidence of HII [44, 45]. Several studies have associated the presence of lactate on MRS with poor outcome [46, 47].

As reported in another chapter, MRS has been used to examine brain metabolites following accidental TBI. MRS is also useful for evaluating brain injury after NAT and provides insights into brain neurometabolism that differ from accidental TBI, possibly because of the age of the patient or the mechanism of injury. Due to the younger age of children with NAT, evaluation of spectra must be carried out with comparisons to age-matched controls because of spectral changes associated with brain maturation that is also discussed in a previous chapter.

MRS in the Evaluation of NAT

Few studies have used MRS to evaluate brain injury after NAT. Factors such as the optimal time after injury to acquire MRS or the best technique or brain location to yield optimal prognostic results have not been determined, therefore, we, as well as, others have applied similar techniques used in studies evaluating children with accidental TBI. The first report examining spectroscopic data in infants with NAT was published in 1997 and addressed the timing issue [48]. In these case studies, follow-up data were available in three infants with confirmed shaking injury, presence of subdural hematomas, and severe bilateral retinal hemorrhages. Serial single voxel MRS using a stimulated echo acquisition mode sequence (STEAM; TR/TE/TM =1500/30/13.7 ms) in parietal white matter was acquired in all three infants at various times after injury (1 day–5 month). Near normal NAA and creatine (Cr) levels were detected in the infant who recovered, whereas in the two infants with poor neurologic outcomes, spectra showed major abnormalities, with greatly decreased NAA, lower Cr, and the appearance of peaks in the lactate/lipid (1.33 ppm) and lipid (0.9 ppm) regions. Of particular interest in this study was the time course of metabolic

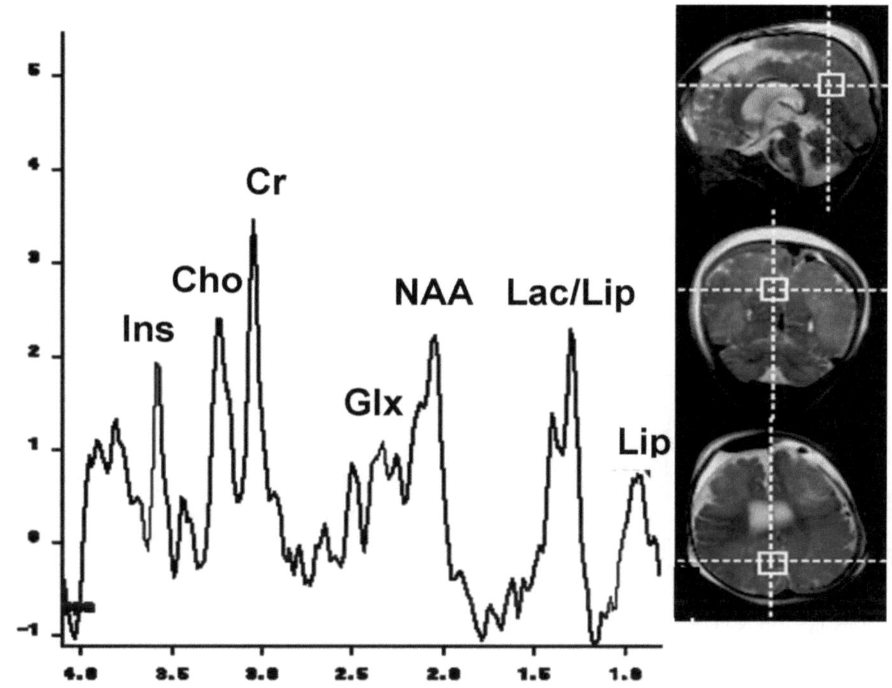

Fig. 9.1 Single voxel MRS (STEAM; TR/TE/TM = 3,000/20/13 ms; 1.5 T) of an 8-month-old confirmed NAT patient. MRI acquired 2 days after injury showed large bilateral subdural hematomas and large bilateral areas of recent infarction in an extensive watershed distribution. MRS (2 days after injury) showed a large lactate doublet at 1.33 ppm, increased lipids at 0.9 ppm, and a marked decrease of NAA, Cr, Cho, and myo-inositol. These spectral findings are consistent with severe hypoxic–ischemic injury. At 2 years after injury, neuropsychologic testing showed significant impairments in functional skills

changes in one infant with a severe outcome. The metabolite levels which were initially near normal at day 5 after injury, decreased to 40% of normal with the appearance of Lac and lipids doubling by day 12 after injury. The authors postulated that these metabolic changes were the first stage in a cascade of metabolic events triggered by the initial injury that may include the release of enzymes that cause accelerated neuronal damage. The effects which may be enhanced by immature brain may explain why the degree of neurological damage suffered in children after NAT is greater than the apparent severity of trauma.

In another study of 53 children, 26 were infants less than 18 months of age and were thus evaluated separately from older children due to developmental MRS changes [49]. Injury in 20 of the 26 infants was due to NAT. In this series of patients, single voxel MRS (STEAM; TR/TE = 3000/20 ms, TM = 13.7 ms, 128 acquisitions, 8 cc volume) was acquired subacutely (5 ± 3 days) in the paramedian mid-occipital gray matter and analyzed for quantitative metabolite levels and ratios. Infants with poor neurological outcomes assessed at 6–12 months after injury were associated with significantly decreased NAA and Cr levels, significantly decreased NAA/Cr and NAA/choline (Cho) ratios and significantly increased Cho/Cr ratios compared to children with good outcomes. In addition, Lac was present in 91% (10 of 11 infants) with poor outcomes and in no infants with good outcomes. Imaging showed evidence of global HII or infarcts in or near the occipital region to explain lactate presence. Overall, the mean NAA and Cr levels were markedly decreased (60 and 40% respectively) in infants with poor outcomes and the presence of lactate and lipids was increased. The marked decrease of NAA and Cr are associated with neuronal energy disruption or failure, while the presence of lipids is associated with cell membrane breakdown leading to the release and solubilization of phospholipids. An example of an NAT patient with global HII illustrating these typical metabolite changes is shown in Fig. 9.1. In this cohort of patients, the presence of lactate used as the only input variable in a discriminant analysis was able to determine long-term neurologic outcome in 96% of the infants. Although this study was not limited to NAT patients only, it illustrated the increased incidence of HII after NAT, the association of HII with poor outcomes and the utility of MRS to detect associated metabolite changes.

In a subsequent retrospective study, MR spectroscopic imaging (MRSI) was acquired after NAT rather than single voxel MRS. This allowed evaluation of a larger area of the brain so that regional comparisons could be made. This study included 44 children with confirmed NAT in whom MRSI was acquired at a mean of 5 days after admission (range 1.30 days) [47] and included correlations between brain regions to clinical and other imaging findings. In these patients, 2D chemical shift imaging (CSI) using a point resolved spectroscopy sequence (PRESS; TR/TE = 3,000/144 ms) was

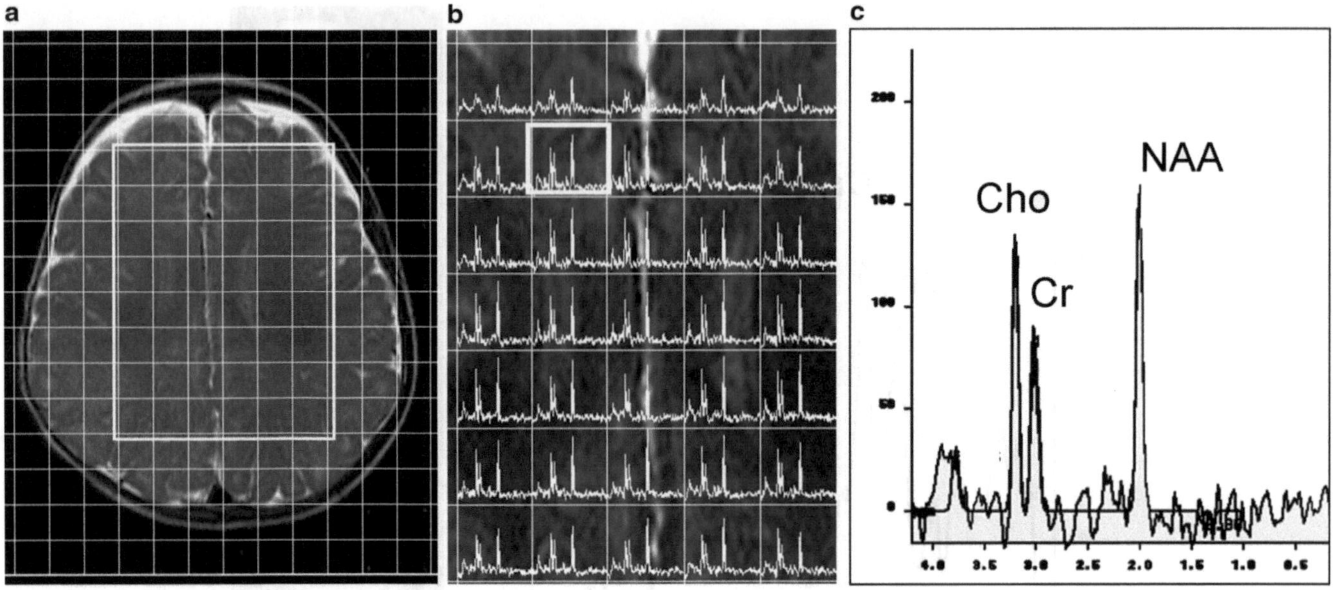

Fig. 9.2 MRI/MRS of a 7-month-old NAT patient done 2 days after injury. (**a**) A T2 weighted image showing extra-axial fluid collection along the bifrontal convexities is overlaid with the MRSI grid. No other MRI abnormalities were noted. (**b**) A spectral map from an MRSI acquisition (PRESS; TR/TE = 3,000/144 ms; 1.5 T) showing normal spectra for age. (**c**) A spectrum from the right frontal white matter is also normal for age. The patient had a normal neurologic evaluation at 7 months after injury

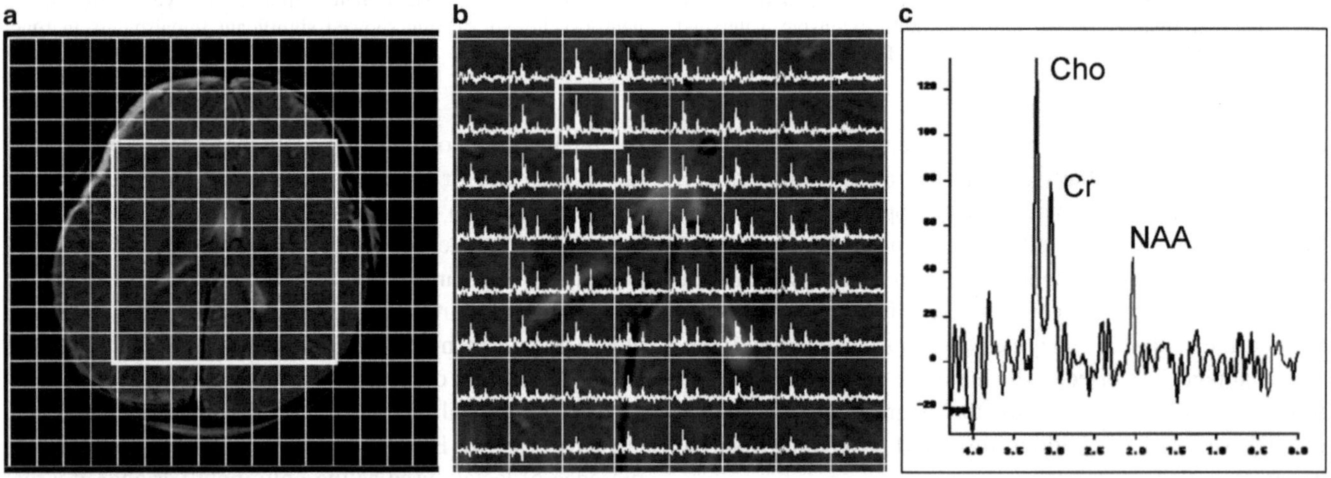

Fig. 9.3 MRI/MRS of a 7-month-old NAT patient done 5 days after injury. (**a**) A T2 weighted image showing a subacute subdural hematoma on the right is overlaid with the MRSI grid. No focal diffusion abnormalities were noted. (**b**) A spectral map from an MRSI acquisition (PRESS; TR/TE = 3,000/144 ms; 1.5 T) shows a marked diffuse decrease of NAA in all spectra. No lactate was detected. (**c**) A spectrum from the right frontal white matter shows a marked decrease in NAA. This spectrum can be compared to a normal spectrum for age in Fig. 9.2c. At 10 years of age, the patient is severely impaired, has spastic quadriplegic cerebral palsy, seizures, and does not respond to or follow commands

acquired through the level of the corpus callosum and included frontal and parieto-occipital gray and white matter. This level was chosen because the callosal region is an area known to be vulnerable to shearing injury as seen with DAI [50, 51]. We found that NAA/Cr and/or NAA/Cho ratios were decreased significantly in children with poor outcomes in four of the five regions analyzed (corpus callosum (CC), frontal white matter (FWM), parieto-occipital white matter (POWM), and parieto-occipital gray matter (POGM). The mean total NAA/Cr and NAA/Cho ratios (an average of ratios from all regions) were also significantly lower in children with poor outcomes. The mean total Cho/Cr ratio tended to be higher in children with poor outcomes but did not reach significance. Figure 9.2 shows imaging and spectral data from a patient with a good outcome and is compared to spectral data from a patient with a poor outcome in Fig. 9.3.

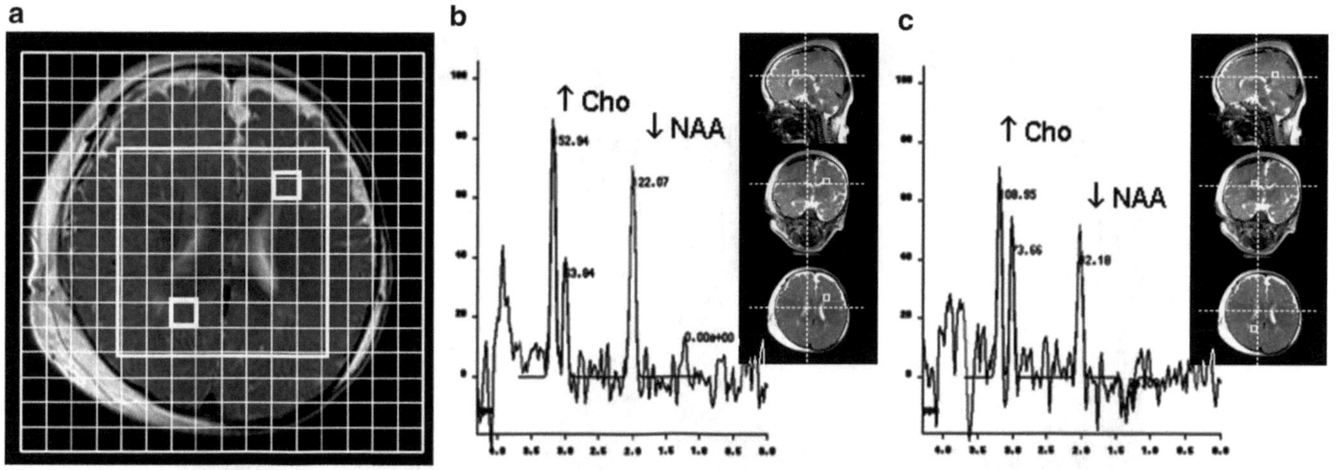

Fig. 9.4 (**a**) CSI (PRESS; TR/TE=3,000/144 ms; 1.5 T) grid overlaid onto a T2 weighted MR image of an 8-month-old NAT patient who presented with an initial GCS score of 6, skull and skeletal fractures, retinal hemorrhages, and seizures. Note the extra-axial fluid collection along the right frontal vertex and the subgaleal fluid collection over the right parietal vertex. MRSI (PRESS; TR/TE=3,000/144 ms; 1.5 T) was acquired 1 day after injury. (**b**) Spectra from the left frontal white matter and (**c**) left parieto-occipital white matter show markedly decreased NAA and increased choline. The neurologic outcome assessed at 30 months after injury showed mild neurologic deficits

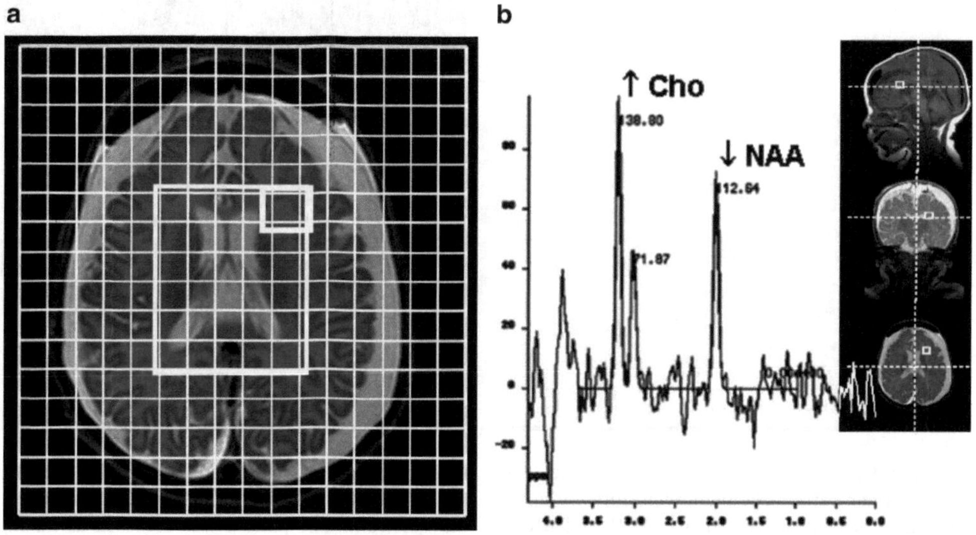

Fig. 9.5 (**a**) CSI grid overlaid onto a T2 weighted MR image of a 4-month-old NAT patient who presented with an initial GCS score of 13, retinal hemorrhages and bilateral large subdural hematomas with hemorrhage of varying ages on MRI acquired 5 days after injury. MRSI (PRESS; TR/TE=3,000/144 ms; 1.5 T) was also acquired 5 days after injury. (**b**) A spectrum from the left frontal white matter shows markedly decreased NAA and increased choline. The neurologic outcome assessed at 3 months after injury showed mild neurologic deficits

It was also observed that NAA ratios from areas susceptible to shaking or impact such as the CC, FWM, and POGM were significantly decreased and correlated with the presence of retinal hemorrhages. In addition, decreased mean total metabolite NAA/Cr and NAA/Cho ratios were significantly correlated with the presence of extra-axial hemorrhage and ischemic injury but not intra-axial hemorrhage, skull fractures, or contusions. The decrease in NAA levels observed in these areas were not always associated with focal injuries and were often in areas of the brain that appeared normal on conventional MR images as shown in two different patients in Figs. 9.4 and 9.5.

Similar to the previous study, many NAT victims had evidence of HII as manifested by elevated lactate and reduced NAA levels. Lactate was present in 10 of 12 (83%) children with poor outcomes compared to 12 of 32 (38%) children with good outcomes and was present in spectra from all children with global injury and children with areas of infarction that were included within the MRSI sampling volume. Also of clinical relevance was that patients with global HII had

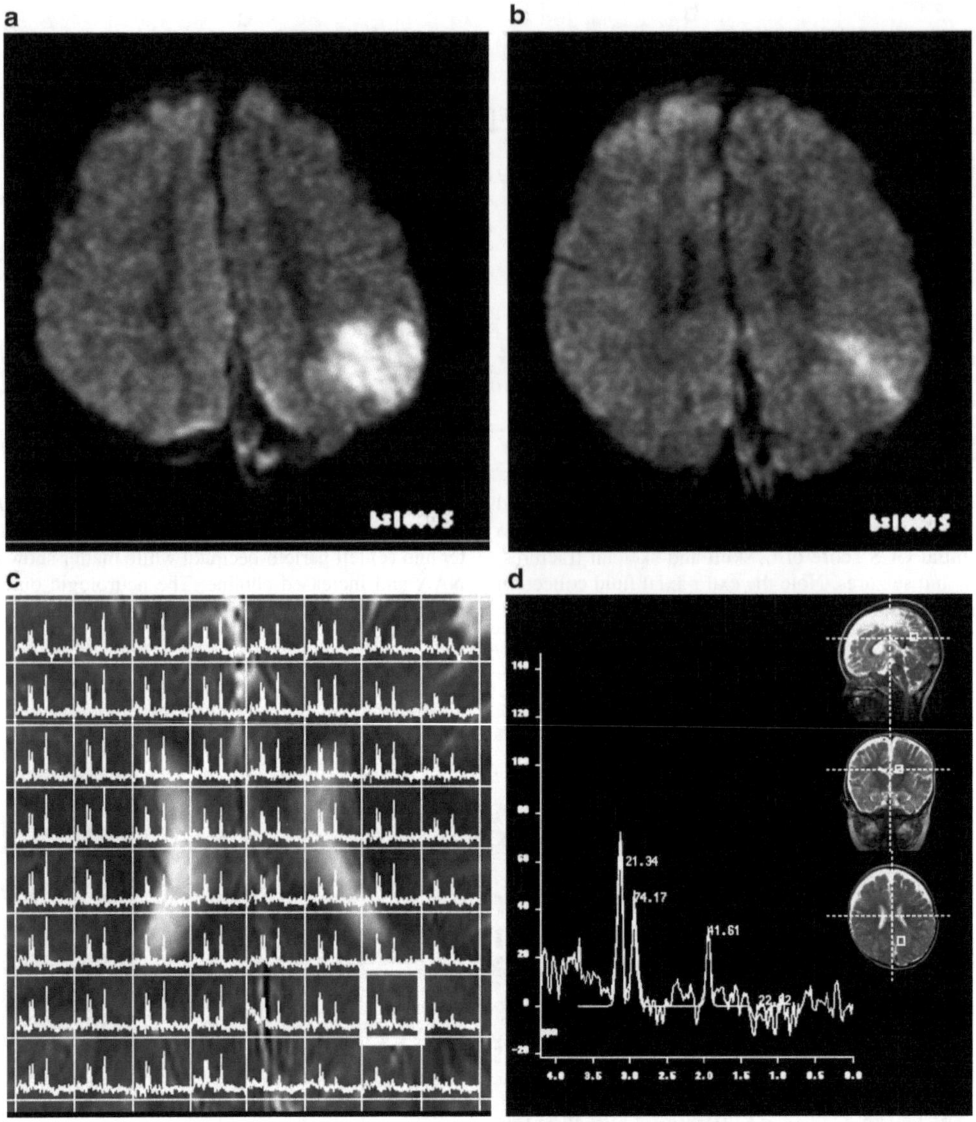

Fig. 9.6 (**a**–**b**) DWI images from a 10-month-old NAT patient taken 6 days after injury showing a left parieto-occipital acute infarction. (**c**) CSI grid overlaid onto a T2 weighted MR image. MRI and MRSI (PRESS; TR/TE=3,000/144 ms; 1.5 T) was acquired 6 days after injury. The patient presented with an initial GCS score of 6, retinal hemorrhages, and seizures. MRI also showed subdural and subarachnoid hemorrhages. (**d**) A spectrum from the left parieto-occipital white matter near the infarction shows markedly decreased NAA levels compared to the contralateral hemisphere. Lactate is not clearly identified in the spectrum. The patient was assessed as having a mild neurologic outcome at 14 months after injury. Neuropsychologic testing performed at 4 years after injury showed that the patient had significant visual and visuospatial deficits and language and cognitive skills ranging from the extremely low to borderline range

significantly lower mean total NAA/Cr and NAA/Cho and higher Cho/Cr ratios than the patients with focal ischemic injury (e.g., infarct) reflecting a significant diffuse injury that led to poorer outcomes. Spectroscopic findings and neurologic outcomes in a patient with a focal infarction (Fig. 9.6) is compared to a patient with diffuse hypoxic–ischemic injury (Fig. 9.7). The presence of lactate in 83% of NAT victims with poor outcome in this study suggests that the presence of lactate (a metabolic marker for HII) along with NAA changes is integral in determining prognosis.

The results of outcome prediction comparing input parameters from MRS, clinical observations, and other radiological imaging findings in this study demonstrated that metabolite changes were more predictive of outcome than other clinical and imaging findings commonly seen in patients after NAT [47]. Results of logistic regression analyses showed that mean total NAA/Cr ratios were more predictive than lactate presence alone for long-term outcome prediction. In this cohort of patients, unlike in the previous study, 38% of children with good outcomes had lactate present. However, in these patients, lactate was confined to smaller areas of focal injury that had less impact on overall outcome than in patients with larger infarcts or global HII. Thus, the extent of HII must be considered in determining outcome in addition to other metabolite

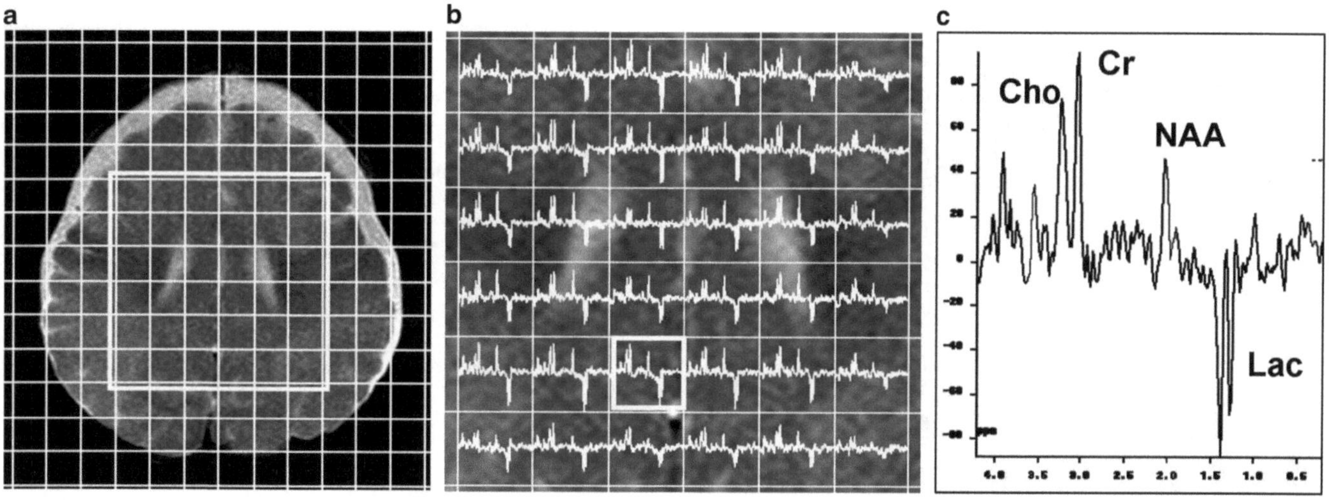

Fig. 9.7 (**a**) CSI grid overlaid onto a T2 weighted MR image of a 3-month-old NAT patient who presented with an initial GCS score of 3, retinal hemorrhages, and diffuse hypoxic–ischemic injury. MRSI (PRESS; TR/TE = 3,000/144 ms; 1.5 T) was acquired 1 day after injury. (**b**). Spectral map shows a diffuse decrease of NAA and large lactate (Lac) peaks (doublet at 1.33 ppm phased down). (**c**). Spectrum from the right parieto-occipital white matter shows markedly decreased NAA and presence of Lac. This patient, assessed at 5 years after injury, had severe neurologic deficits

information. The mean total NAA/Cr ratio reflects neuronal loss or dysfunction over the entire area sampled and was more predictive of outcome compared to measurements from any one region or lactate presence. Furthermore, both ischemic and/or traumatic brain injury can result in decreases of NAA that may not be accompanied by increased lactate; therefore, changes in NAA should better reflect overall injury. As shown in Figs. 9.3 and 9.4, MRS can detect NAA decreases in areas of brain that appear normal on conventional MRI. Reduction of NAA in visibly injured brain is most likely caused by the primary impact, whereas, reduction of NAA in normal-appearing brain may reflect DAI and Wallerian degeneration [52]. Optimal timing of the MRS acquisition has not been determined since serial studies on seriously ill children are difficult to justify and carry out. In addition, it is likely that timing may vary depending on such factors as severity of injury, age of the infant, and type of injury. Our approach has been to acquire the study at least 2–3 days after injury to allow for metabolite concentrations to change enough to be detected but within 2 weeks of injury to allow for early prognosis. This often depends on whether the patient is medically stable or whether there is urgent need for the MRI information. Long-term MRS studies on pediatric accidental TBI patients have shown correlation of early metabolite changes with neurobehavioral measures and initial GCS score [53] and also of presumed neurometabolic recovery [54].

Neuropsychologic Evaluations and NAT

Neuropsychological evidence suggests that there are significant long-term consequences to NAT early in life. Although, studies correlating various NAT related clinical and imaging parameters to neuropsychologic testing have been published [20, 55], there have been no studies relating early MRS findings to long-term neuropsychologic deficits. In our own preliminary work (unpublished), we have evaluated a subset of patients at 2–4 years after injury. All patients were administered measures that assess the full range of functional domains and adaptive skills, as well as, the Parenting Stress Index (i.e., measures parents' child-related and parent-related distress). Two case studies are presented next.

The first case study of a child that was 2 months old at the time of injury, illustrates that mild changes on MRS may be an indication of future deficits. The child presented with skeletal fractures, seizures but no retinal hemorrhages. The initial GCS score was 14. MRI showed a thin left hemispheric convexity subdural hemorrhage, a small right frontal subdural hemorrhage and minimal left parietal subarachnoid hemorrhage. No diffusion abnormalities were seen. The MRSI showed decreased NAA in the left frontal and parietal white matter (Fig. 9.8). The neuropsychological evaluation done 3 years after injury reported average performance on cognitive and language scales; however, on the motor scales the patient's performance was in the low average range. Based on parental reports, the patient showed difficulties in executive functioning skills and behavioral problems were in the clinical range for concern.

The second case study is of a child who was 6 months old at the time of injury and who presented with an initial GCS score of 12, seizures and bilateral retinal hemorrhages. MRI and MRS were acquired 1 day after injury to evaluate worsening right arm and leg weakness. MRI showed a left subdural hemorrhage and a large infarct in the left hemisphere on DWI (Fig. 9.9a). MRSI acquired through the level of the corpus callosum showed a diffuse decrease of all metabolites in the left hemisphere in the area of infarction indicating significant

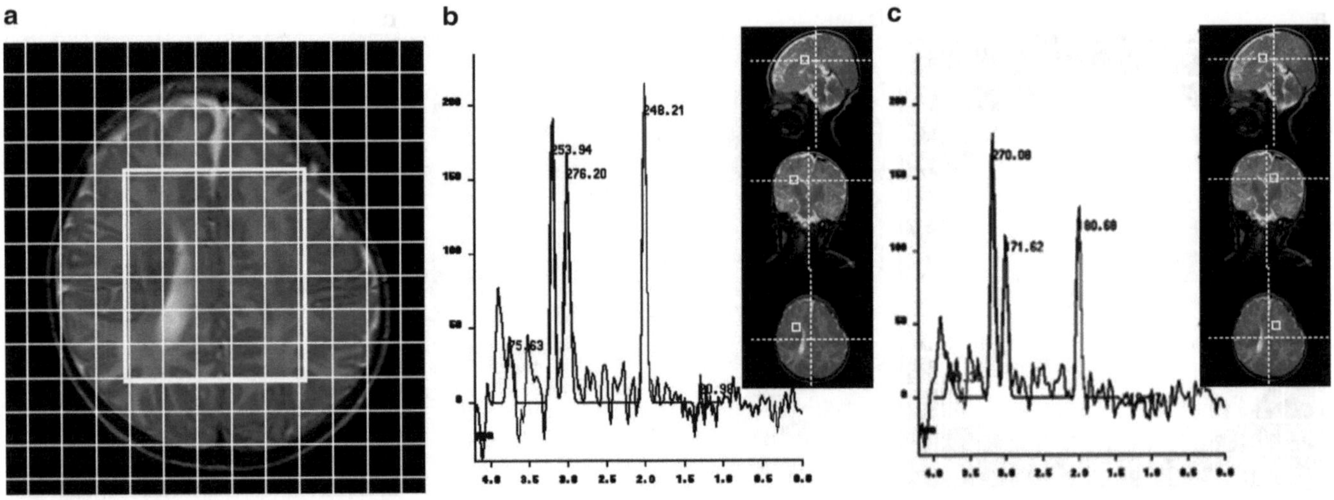

Fig. 9.8 (**a**) CSI grid overlaid onto a T2-weighted MR image of a 2-month-old NAT patient. MRSI (PRESS; TR/TE=3000/144 ms; 1.5 T) was acquired 2 days after injury. (**b**) A spectrum from the left frontal white matter shows normal metabolite ratios. (**c**) A spectrum from the left frontal white matter shows decreased NAA and creatine levels compared to the right

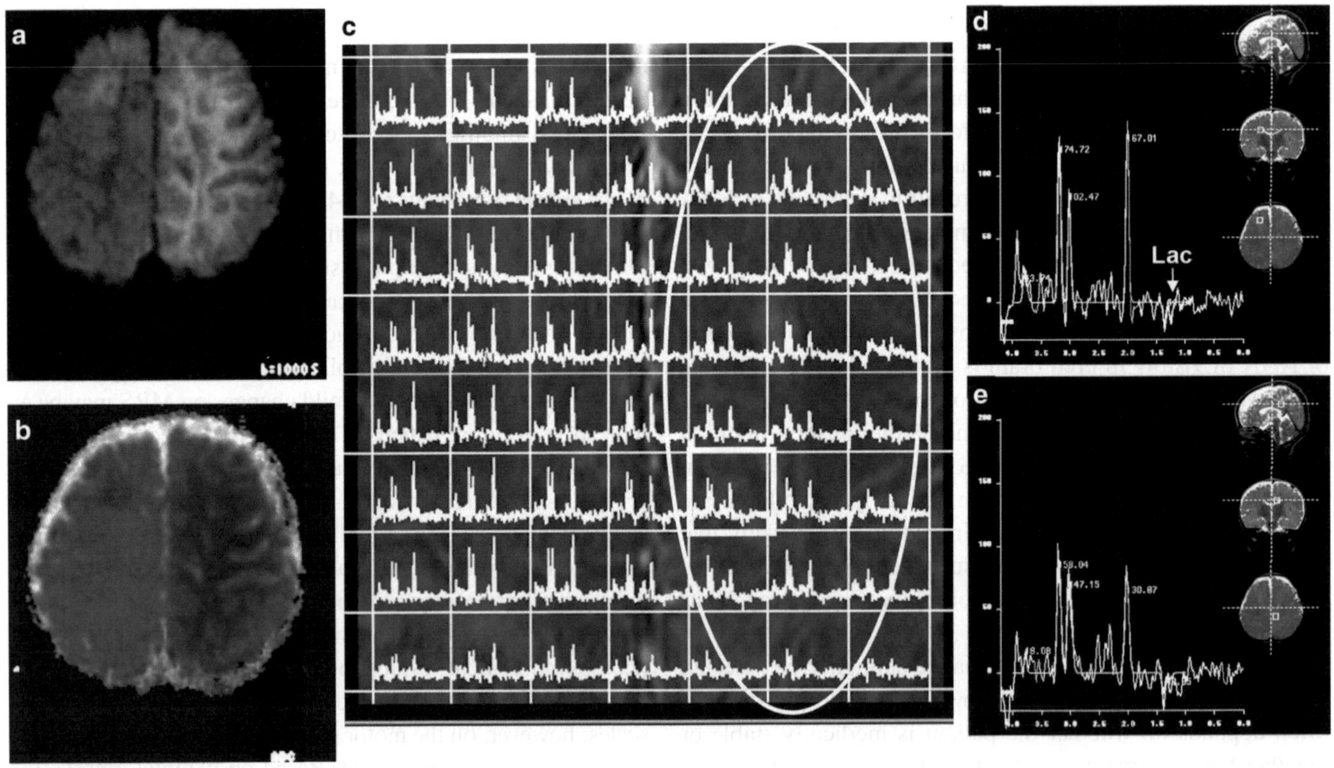

Fig. 9.9 (**a**) DWI image of a 6-month-old NAT patient showing diffuse left hemispheric ischemia and a small right frontal lobe infarct and (**b**) corresponding apparent diffusion coefficient (ADC) map. (**c**). MRSI (PRESS; TR/TE=3,000/144 ms; 1.5 T) spectral map showing diffusely decreased NAA in the left hemisphere (ellipse). (**d**) A spectrum from the right frontal lobe area of infarction shows a small lactate (Lac) peak. **e**) A spectrum from the left hemisphere ischemic area shows a decrease of all metabolites and presence of lactate

neuronal loss or dysfunction. Lactate was detected in a few voxels located in the left posterior white matter (Fig. 9.9b). The fact that lactate was not detected diffusely throughout the left hemisphere may be related to the early timing of the MRS study (1 day after injury). Neuropsychological evaluation done 3 years after injury reported that the patient's visual memory was in the average range, otherwise, all other measures were in the low average to impaired range and the Full Scale IQ was in the borderline range. The patient's behavioral functioning skills were within normal limits as reported by the parents, however, the adaptive (fine motor) and executive functioning skills were in the low average range.

Neuroimaging Mimics of NAT

Conditions such as coagulopathies and several inborn errors of metabolism (IEMs) can present with clinical symptoms, physical findings and neuroimaging abnormalities that can mimic NAT. These conditions should be included in the differential diagnosis when infants present with unexplained subdural hematomas and NAT is suspected. The most common IEM disorders to consider include glutaric aciduria type 1 and Menke's disease. Glutaric aciduria type 1 is an autosomal-recessive disorder caused by a glutatryl-CoA dehydrogenase deficiency which can be mistaken for NAT because of the possible presence of subdural fluid collections, brain atrophy and retinal hemorrhages [56]. Although non-specific, MRS has shown reduced NAA/Cr and elevated Cho/Cr and Ins/Cr in the frontal white matter and right lentiform nuclei [57]. Menke's disease is an X-linked inherited disorder of intestinal copper absorption resulting in copper deficiency [58]. Patients present with brain atrophy, uni- or bilateral subdural hematomas, diffusion abnormalities on MRI and lesions associated with femoral metaphysical spurs that can be mistaken for nonaccidental injury. MRS has shown reduced NAA/Cr that improved with treatment and presence of lactate that resolved with treatment although neurological symptoms did not improve [59].

Summary

Overall, the data from several studies suggest that MRS performed early after injury can be used to evaluate injury severity and more accurately predict long-term prognosis in children with NAT. MRS provides complementary information and frequently detects injury in brain regions that appear normal with conventional MRI and may help better understand the biomechanical forces and tissue changes that cause specific clinical symptoms. A better understanding of these relations is essential if we are to design therapies that might salvage injured brain tissue in these infants and children. All require further study to examine the effects of age, severity and location of injury, gender, and occurrence of ischemia or seizures on long-term neurological, neuropsychological, and behavioral function. MRSI, because it samples a larger area of the brain compared to single voxel MRS, is useful for demonstrating that injury after NAT is much more diffuse than what conventional imaging may show and helps to explain why global neuropsychological deficits are often seen in patients with normal or mild imaging findings. Future studies with higher field strength scanners optimized to acquire 3D MRSI in less time may be extremely useful for evaluating the full extent of brain injury after NAT. It is also likely that the combined use of MRS with newer techniques like diffusion tensor imaging may provide additional information than either method alone and may also provide new insights regarding the evolution of injury over time.

References

1. Kempke C. The battered child syndrome. J Am Med Assoc. 1962;18(1):8.
2. Child Maltreatment 2006. In: U.S. Department of Health and Human Services Administration on Children YaF, editor. US Government Printing Office; Washington, DC2008.
3. Gateway CW. Child Abuse and Neglect Fatalities: Statistics and Interventions, Series: Numbers and Trends. US Dept of Health and Human Services. 2009.
4. Keenan HT, Runyan DK, Marshall SW, Nocera MA, Merten DF, Sinal SH. A population-based study of inflicted traumatic brain injury in young children. JAMA. 2003;290(5):621–6.
5. Theodore AD, Chang JJ, Runyan DK, Hunter WM, Bangdiwala SI, Agans R. Epidemiologic features of the physical and sexual maltreatment of children in the Carolinas. Pediatrics. 2005;115(3):e331–7.
6. Case ME, Graham MA, Handy TC, Jentzen JM, Monteleone JA. Position paper on fatal abusive head injuries in infants and young children. Am J Forensic Med Pathol. 2001;22(2):112–22.
7. Gill JR, Goldfeder LB, Armbrustmacher V, Coleman A, Mena H, Hirsch CS. Fatal head injury in children younger than 2 years in New York City and an overview of the shaken baby syndrome. Arch Pathol Lab Med. 2009;133(4):619–27.
8. Dolinak D, Reichard R. An overview of inflicted head injury in infants and young children, with a review of beta-amyloid precursor protein immunohistochemistry. Arch Pathol Lab Med. 2006;130(5):712–7.
9. Duhaime AC, Alario AJ, Lewander WJ, Schut L, Sutton LN, Seidl TS, et al. Head injury in very young children: mechanisms, injury types, and ophthalmologic findings in 100 hospitalized patients younger than 2 years of age. Pediatrics. 1992;90(2 Pt 1):179–85.
10. Keenan HT, Runyan DK, Marshall SW, Nocera MA, Merten DF. A population-based comparison of clinical and outcome characteristics of young children with serious inflicted and noninflicted traumatic brain injury. Pediatrics. 2004;114(3):633–9.
11. Makaroff KL, Putnam FW. Outcomes of infants and children with inflicted traumatic brain injury. Dev Med Child Neurol. 2003;45(7):497–502.
12. Jennett B, Bond M. Assessment of outcome after severe brain damage. Lancet. 1975;1(7905):480–4.
13. Bonnier C, Nassogne MC, Saint-Martin C, Mesples B, Kadhim H, Sebire G. Neuroimaging of intraparenchymal lesions predicts outcome in shaken baby syndrome. Pediatrics. 2003;112(4):808–14.
14. Broman SH. Traumatic head injury in children. New York: Oxford University Press; 1995.
15. Dashti SR, Decker DD, Razzaq A, Cohen AR. Current patterns of inflicted head injury in children. Pediatr Neurosurg. 1999;31(6):302–6.
16. Prasad MR, Ewing-Cobbs L, Swank PR, Kramer L. Predictors of outcome following traumatic brain injury in young children. Pediatr Neurosurg. 2002;36(2):64–74.
17. Rosas AJ. Medical diagnosis of abuse and neglect. Chap. 3. In: Talley PF, editor. Handbook for the treatment of abused and neglected children. Binghamton, NY: The Haworth Social Work Practice Press; 2005.
18. Wilkinson WS, Han DP, Rappley MD, Owings CL. Retinal hemorrhage predicts neurologic injury in the shaken baby syndrome. Arch Ophthalmol. 1989;107(10):1472–4.
19. Mills M. Funduscopic lesions associated with mortality in shaken baby syndrome. J AAPOS. 1998;2(2):67–71.
20. Barlow KM, Thomson E, Johnson D, Minns RA. Late neurologic and cognitive sequelae of inflicted traumatic brain injury in infancy. Pediatrics. 2005;116(2):e174–85.

21. Ewing-Cobbs L, Kramer L, Prasad M, Canales DN, Louis PT, Fletcher JM, et al. Neuroimaging, physical, and developmental findings after inflicted and noninflicted traumatic brain injury in young children. Pediatrics. 1998;102(2 Pt 1):300–7.
22. Ewing-Cobbs L, Prasad M, Kramer L, Landry S. Inflicted traumatic brain injury: relationship of developmental outcome to severity of injury. Pediatr Neurosurg. 1999;31(5):251–8.
23. Gilles EE, Nelson Jr MD. Cerebral complications of nonaccidental head injury in childhood. Pediatr Neurol. 1998;19(2):119–28.
24. Bonnier C, Nassogne MC, Evrard P. Outcome and prognosis of whiplash shaken infant syndrome; late consequences after a symptom-free interval. Dev Med Child Neurol. 1995;37(11):943–56.
25. Tung GA, Kumar M, Richardson RC, Jenny C, Brown WD. Comparison of accidental and nonaccidental traumatic head injury in children on noncontrast computed tomography. Pediatrics. 2006;118(2):626–33.
26. Suh DY, Davis PC, Hopkins KL, Fajman NN, Mapstone TB. Nonaccidental pediatric head injury: diffusion-weighted imaging findings. Neurosurgery. 2001;49(2):309–18.
27. Ichord RN, Naim M, Pollock AN, Nance ML, Margulies SS, Christian CW. Hypoxic-ischemic injury complicates inflicted and accidental traumatic brain injury in young children: the role of diffusion-weighted imaging. J Neurotrauma. 2007;24(1):106–18.
28. Blitstein MK, Tung GA. MRI of cerebral microhemorrhages. AJR Am J Roentgenol. 2007;189(3):720–5.
29. Colbert CA, Holshouser BA, Aaen GS, Sheridan C, Oyoyo U, Kido D, et al. Value of cerebral microhemorrhages detected with susceptibility-weighted MR Imaging for prediction of long-term outcome in children with nonaccidental trauma. Radiology. 2010;256(3): 898–905.
30. Moffett JR, Ross B, Arun P, Madhavarao CN, Namboodiri AM. N-Acetylaspartate in the CNS: from neurodiagnostics to neurobiology. Prog Neurobiol. 2007;81(2):89–131.
31. Signoretti S, Marmarou A, Fatouros P, Hoyle R, Beaumont A, Sawauchi S, et al. Application of chemical shift imaging for measurement of NAA in head injured patients. Acta Neurochir Suppl. 2002;81:373–5.
32. Demougeot C, Garnier P, Mossiat C, Bertrand N, Giroud M, Beley A, et al. N-Acetylaspartate, a marker of both cellular dysfunction and neuronal loss: its relevance to studies of acute brain injury. J Neurochem. 2001;77(2):408–15.
33. Clark JB. N-acetyl aspartate: a marker for neuronal loss or mitochondrial dysfunction. Dev Neurosci. 1998;20(4–5):271–6.
34. Cecil KM, Hills EC, Sandel ME, Smith DH, McIntosh TK, Mannon LJ, et al. Proton magnetic resonance spectroscopy for detection of axonal injury in the splenium of the corpus callosum of brain-injured patients. J Neurosurg. 1998;88(5):795–801.
35. Biousse V, Suh DY, Newman NJ, Davis PC, Mapstone T, Lambert SR. Diffusion-weighted magnetic resonance imaging in Shaken Baby Syndrome. Am J Ophthalmol. 2002;133(2):249–55.
36. Holshouser BA, Tong KA, Ashwal S. Proton MR spectroscopic imaging depicts diffuse axonal injury in children with traumatic brain injury. AJNR Am J Neuroradiol. 2005;26(5):1276–85.
37. Johnson DL, Boal D, Baule R. Role of apnea in nonaccidental head injury. Pediatr Neurosurg. 1995;23(6):305–10.
38. Barlow KM, Minns RA. The relation between intracranial pressure and outcome in non-accidental head injury. Dev Med Child Neurol. 1999;41(4):220–5.
39. Makoroff KL, Cecil KM, Care M, Ball Jr WS. Elevated lactate as an early marker of brain injury in inflicted traumatic brain injury. Pediatr Radiol. 2005;35(7):668–76.
40. Krishnappa IK, Contant CF, Robertson CS. Regional changes in cerebral extracellular glucose and lactate concentrations following severe cortical impact injury and secondary ischemia in rats. J Neurotrauma. 1999;16(3):213–24.
41. Hovda DA, Becker DP, Katayama Y. Secondary injury and acidosis. J Neurotrauma. 1992;9 Suppl 1:S47–60.
42. Prasad MR, Ramaiah C, McIntosh TK, Dempsey RJ, Hipkens S, Yurek D. Regional levels of lactate and norepinephrine after experimental brain injury. J Neurochem. 1994;63(3):1086–94.
43. Atkinson JL, Anderson RE, Murray MJ. The early critical phase of severe head injury: importance of apnea and dysfunctional respiration. J Trauma. 1998;45(5):941–5.
44. Geddes JF, Vowles GH, Hackshaw AK, Nickols CD, Scott IS, Whitwell HL. Neuropathology of inflicted head injury in children. II. Microscopic brain injury in infants. Brain. 2001;124(Pt 7):1299–306.
45. Geddes JF, Hackshaw AK, Vowles GH, Nickols CD, Whitwell HL. Neuropathology of inflicted head injury in children. I. Patterns of brain damage. Brain. 2001;124(Pt 7):1290–8.
46. Ashwal S, Holshouser BA, Tomasi LG, Shu S, Perkin RM, Nystrom GA, et al. 1 H-magnetic resonance spectroscopy-determined cerebral lactate and poor neurological outcomes in children with central nervous system disease. Ann Neurol. 1997;41(4):470–81.
47. Aaen GS, Holshouser BA, Sheridan C, Colbert C, McKenney M, Kido D, et al. Magnetic resonance spectroscopy predicts outcomes for children with nonaccidental trauma. Pediatrics. 2010;125(2):295–303.
48. Haseler LJ, Arcinue E, Danielsen ER, Bluml S, Ross BD. Evidence from proton magnetic resonance spectroscopy for a metabolic cascade of neuronal damage in shaken baby syndrome. Pediatrics. 1997;99(1):4–14.
49. Ashwal S, Holshouser BA, Shu SK, Simmons PL, Perkin RM, Tomasi LG, et al. Predictive value of proton magnetic resonance spectroscopy in pediatric closed head injury. Pediatr Neurol. 2000;23(2):114–25.
50. Adams JH, Doyle D, Ford I, Gennarelli TA, Graham DI, McLellan DR. Diffuse axonal injury in head injury: definition, diagnosis and grading. Histopathology. 1989;15(1):49–59.
51. Meythaler JM, Peduzzi JD, Eleftheriou E, Novack TA. Current concepts: diffuse axonal injury-associated traumatic brain injury. Arch Phys Med Rehabil. 2001;82(10):1461–71.
52. Garnett MR, Blamire AM, Corkill RG, Cadoux-Hudson TA, Rajagopalan B, Styles P. Early proton magnetic resonance spectroscopy in normal-appearing brain correlates with outcome in patients following traumatic brain injury. Brain. 2000;123(Pt 10):2046–54.
53. Walz NC, Cecil KM, Wade SL, Michaud LJ. Late proton magnetic resonance spectroscopy following traumatic brain injury during early childhood: relationship with neurobehavioral outcomes. J Neurotrauma. 2008;25(2):94–103.
54. Yeo RA, Phillips JP, Jung RE, Brown AJ, Campbell RC, Brooks WM. Magnetic resonance spectroscopy detects brain injury and predicts cognitive functioning in children with brain injuries. J Neurotrauma. 2006;23(10):1427–35.
55. Barlow K, Thompson E, Johnson D, Minns RA. The neurological outcome of non-accidental head injury. Pediatr Rehabil. 2004;7(3):195–203.
56. Bishop FS, Liu JK, McCall TD, Brockmeyer DL. Glutaric aciduria type 1 presenting as bilateral subdural hematomas mimicking non-accidental trauma. Case report and review of the literature. J Neurosurg. 2007;106(3 Suppl):222–6.
57. Kurul S, Cakmakçi H, Dirik E. Glutaric aciduria type 1: proton magnetic resonance spectroscopy findings. Pediatr Neurol. 2004;31(3):228–31.
58. Nassogne MC, Sharrard M, Hertz-Pannier L, Armengaud D, Touati G, Delonlay-Debeney P, Zerah M, Brunelle F, Saudubray JM. Massive subdural haematomas in Menkes disease mimicking shaken baby syndrome. Childs Nerv Syst. 2002;18(12):729–31.
59. Ito H, Mori K, Sakata M, Naito E, Harada M, Kagami S. Transient left temporal lobe lesion in Menkes disease may influence the generation of tonic spasms. Brain Dev. 2011;33(4):345–8.

Leukodystrophies

10

Kim M. Cecil and Diana M. Lindquist

The term "leukodystrophy" is generally reserved for those conditions that are both *progressive* and *genetically determined*. While these conditions may eventually involve and alter gray matter, the primary features impact the white matter. Leukodystrophies arise as a result of a gene defect that manages production or metabolism of exclusively one component of myelin. These defects cause imperfect growth and development or maintenance of myelin sheaths.

For organizational purposes, the disorders described in this chapter can be classified as primary leukodystrophies, perioxisomal disorders producing a leukodystrophy and lysosomal disorders producing leukodystrophies. Table 10.1 summarizes the clinical, spectroscopic, and genetic features of leukodystrophies.

The temporal course of the disease and the normal developmental maturation in children influences not only the clinical and imaging presentations, but also the spectroscopic. As these diseases are progressive, the timing of the spectroscopic evaluation will impact the spectral profile. Metabolic changes within the earliest stages of a disease will often differ significantly from those observed in the latest stages. Early assessment provides important differential diagnosis and prognostic information, while later assessment offers the utility to monitor disease progression and treatment response. Brain development, particularly myelination, may also be proceeding at a normal or near-normal pace in less-affected regions. Interpretation of metabolite changes require consideration of the evolving developmental changes to the metabolic profile occurring in the background in addition to pathologic changes.

A brief definition of additional terms is also necessary for clarity of this discussion. Demyelination, dysmyelination, and hypomyelination are often used haphazardly. Unfortunately, as the literature has relatively few reports of spectroscopy analyses in patients with leukodystrophies, we often include in this chapter the terms used in the original reports in this review. In the absolute sense, these terms describing the state of myelin are pathologic, rather than radiologic as conventional imaging fails to differentiate these entities. The term "demyelination" refers to the breakdown of normal existing myelin or an effect on the ability of the oligodendrocytes to maintain normal myelin structure. In contrast, dysmyelination occurs as a result of an underlying metabolic defect in myelin formation. The term "hypomyelination" is employed to describe a delay in the formation of myelin observed in the pediatric imaging setting as well as the abnormal appearance of myelin with an uncertain etiology. Hypomyelination represents the generic and most accurate *radiological* term to indicate abnormal myelination.

Biochemical Interpretation for the Metabolites of Interest

The interpretation of an MR spectrum primarily relies on variations in chemical concentrations, which alter peak area for the endogenous metabolites, and the appearance of pathologic metabolites (i.e., lactate, alanine, etc.) and exogenous compounds (i.e., propanediol, mannitol). The metabolites commonly observed when acquiring proton MRS of the brain are listed in Table 10.2 accompanied by the chemical shift assignment, which signifies their location on the x-axis relative to an external reference standard. The locations of the metabolites are stable, as the in vivo brain pH does not change sufficiently to result in an alteration in peak assignment. Metabolites with a single resonance, a singlet corresponding to a methyl (CH_3) group, do not change assignment with field strength variations. However, metabolites with methylene (CH_2) and methane (CH) signals may produce a slightly different assignment and splitting pattern at different field strengths. For this chapter, the only metabolite to significantly alter its assignment is myo-inositol (mI). At a field strength of 1.5 Tesla (T), four methine

K.M. Cecil, Ph.D. (✉)
Departments of Radiology, Pediatrics, Neuroscience and Environmental Health, Cincinnati Children's Hospital Medical Center, University of Cincinnati College of Medicine, Cincinnati, OH, USA
e-mail: kim.cecil@chmcc.org

D.M. Lindquist, Ph.D.
Departments of Radiology, Cincinnati Children's Hospital Medical Center, University of Cincinnati College of Medicine, Cincinnati, OH, USA

S. Blüml and A. Panigrahy (eds.), *MR Spectroscopy of Pediatric Brain Disorders*,
DOI 10.1007/978-1-4419-5864-8_10, © Springer Science+Business Media, LLC 2013

Table 10.1 Clinical, spectroscopic, and genetic features of leukodystrophies

Disorder	Gene Name; abbreviation (locus)	OMIM	Mode of inheritance	Primary classification	Primary defect	Metabolic consequence	Key features of brain proton MRS: early stages
Neonatal Adrenoleukodystrophy	*PTS1* and Peroxin genes	202370	Autosomal-recessive	Perioxisomal	Deficiency in oxidizing VLCFA	Accumulation of long-chain fatty acids; infiltration of lipid-laden macrophages	Elevated mI, Cho and lactate; Diminished NAA in white matter
X-linked Adrenoleukodystrophy	Adrenoleukodystrophy; *ALD/ABCD1* (Xq28)	300100	X-linked	Perioxisomal	Inability to oxidize VLCFA into short- chain fatty acids	Accumulation of long-chain fatty acids	Elevated mI, Cho and lactate; Diminished NAA in white matter
Alexander's Disease	Glial fibrillary acidic protein; *GFAP* 17q21	203450	Autosomal-dominant	Leukodystrophy	Presence of Rosenthal fibers, glial fibrillary acid proteins in astrocytes	Failure of myelin deposition due to astrocyte dysfunction	Elevated mI, Cho and lactate; Diminished NAA in affected white matter
Canavan's Disease	Aspartoacylase; *ASPA* (17p13.2)	271900	Autosomal-recessive	Leukodystrophy	Enzyme deficiency-aspartoacylase deficiency-inability to metabolize NAA into aspartate and acetate	NAA accumulation	NAA elevation in white matter
Cerebrotendinous xanthomatosis	27-sterol hydroxylase: *CYP27* 2q35	213700	Autosomal-recessive	Lysosomal	Enzyme deficiency-Sterol 27-hydroxylase	Cholesterol, cholestanol and 7 alpha-hydroxylated bile alcohol accumulations	Decreased NAA, possible elevations of lipids/lactate/macromolecules
Childhood Ataxia with Diffuse CNS Hypomyelination (Vanishing White Matter)	*EIF2B5* (3q27) and other EIF2B genes	603896	Autosomal-recessive	Leukodystrophy	Gene defect in eukaryotic translation initiation factor (mRNA translated into proteins)	Deposition of denatured proteins within oligodendrocytes leading to hypomyelination	Depends on Stage; Decreased NAA and Cho in affected white matter
Globoid cell leukodystrophy (Krabbe's Disease)	Galactocerebrosidase; *GALC* (14q31)	245200	Autosomal-recessive	Lysosomal	Enzyme deficiency-Galactocerebroside beta-galactosidase deficiency	Accumulation of globoid cells in brain tissue	Decreased NAA, elevated mI
Leukoencephalopathy with Brainstem and Spinal Cord Involvement with Elevated Lactate	*DARS2* (1q25.1)	611105	Autosomal-recessive	Leukodystrophy	Mitochondrial aspartyl-tRNA synthetase deficiency	Uncertain	Elevated mI, Cho and lactate; Diminished NAA in white matter
Metachromatic Leukodystrophy	Arylsufatase A; *ARSA* (22q13)	250100, 176801	Autosomal-recessive	Lysosomal	Decreased arylsulfatase A, ARSA activity	Metachromatic sulfatide deposits	Decreased NAA, elevated mI
Pelizaeus-Merzbacher	Proteolipid Protein; *PLP* (Xq22)	312080	X-linked	Leukodystrophy	Duplication or deficiency of PLP gene results in altered myelin	Uncertain	Elevated mI; variable Cho and NAA levels
Refsum Disease	6q23.3, 10p13	266500	Autosomal-recessive	Perioxisomal	Phytanic acid oxidase deficiency	Phytanic acid accumulation	Elevated Cho, lipids; Diminished NAA
Vacuolating megaencephalic leukoencephalopathy	*MLC1* 22q13.33	604004	Autosomal-recessive	Leukodystrophy	Uncertain	Uncertain; vacuolating myelinopathy	All metabolites reduced; ratio pattern diminished NAA, elevated Cho, mI
Zellweger syndrome	Several genes involved in peroxisome biogenesis	214100	Autosomal-recessive	Perioxisomal	Decreased dihydroxyacetone phosphate acyl transferase (DHAP-AT) activity	Elevated long-chain fatty acids, inc phytanic acid, pipecolic acidemia, aminoaciduria, albuminuria	Increased lipid (fatty acid) resonance; decreased NAA

Table 10.2 Metabolite Resonances Observed on Proton MRS

Metabolite	Assignment (ppm)	Functional role
Lipids, macromolecules-Methyl	0.9	Myelin synthesis/degradation
Propanediol	1.1	Solvent for medications
Lipids, macromolecules-Methylene	1.25	Myelin synthesis/degradation
Lactate	1.3	Anerobic glycolysis
Alanine	1.4	Amino acid; Menigioma, Abscess
Acetate	1.9	Lipid, Myelin synthesis, Abscess
N-acetyl aspartate	2	Neuronal, axonal integrity
N-acetyl aspartylglutamate	2.1	Neurotransmitter
Glutamate, glutamine, aspartate, gamma aminobutyric acid	2.1–2.6	Composite of neurotransmitters
Succinate	2.4	Abscess
Pyruvate	2.4	Cellular energetics
Creatine and phosphocreatine	3.0	Energetic buffer
Cholines (glycerolphosphocholine and phosphocholines)	3.2	Myelin synthesis/degradation
Scyllo-inositol, taurine	3.4	Neurotransmitter
Myo-inositol	3.5	Glial marker, osmolytic marker
Glycine	3.5	Neurotransmitter
Glucose	3.6	Cellular energetics
Mannitol	3.8	Medication
Creatine (Methylene)	3.9	Energetic buffer

(CH) protons co-resonate at 3.57 ppm, while at field strength of 3 T, two sets of two protons resonate at 3.5 and 3.6 ppm.

To detect mI levels, a short echo technique (i.e., echo time (TE) ≤35 ms) must be employed for recognizing a resonance appearing at 3.5 ppm. For MRS performed at 1.5 T, the mI resonance normally is distinct with four of the molecule's six methine protons magnetically indistinguishable, thereby co-resonating at the same location (3.5 ppm). However, increased spectral dispersion inherent at higher field strengths (3 T) produces two distinct resonances (3.5 and 3.6 ppm) for the four protons, effectively reducing the signal by half. Normal mI levels visually appear lower at higher field strengths in contrast to 1.5 T. While some reports have found improved detection of mI at high field strength arising from increased signal to noise ratio (SNR), it may be problematic depending on the acquisition conditions. The use of phased array coils and parallel imaging offers tremendous advantages for imaging. Unfortunately in the clinical setting, inadequate methods currently exist for optimally combining the elements of the phased array coil for single-voxel spectroscopy applications. A single coil element with inadequate signal averaging or improper reconstruction (combining channel arrays) can result in low SNR, thereby limiting the ability to detect mI.

The three main metabolite entities, *N*-acetyl aspartate (NAA), the composite of creatine and phosphocreatine (Cr), and the composite of cholines (Cho), are commonly observed independent of echo time (TE) and standard localization technique.

N-acetyl aspartate and *N*-acetyl aspartyl glutamate (NAAG) comprise the resonance at 2 ppm. At higher field strengths, NAAG can be distinguished from NAA, however, for conventional clinical MRS (1.5 T) the two resonances co-resonate. Although originally discovered in 1956 by Tallan [1], the true function of NAA remains uncertain. NAA is one of the most highly abundant free amino acids in the adult human brain with a concentration of approximately 10 mM. NAA synthesis and storage occurs primarily in neurons. Studies [2] indicate many possible roles for NAA:

(a) NAA may serve as a transporter of acetyl groups across the mitochondrial membrane for myelin and lipid synthesis during development
(b) NAA may function as neuronal osmolyte serving as a cotransport substrate for a molecular water pump removing excess water from neurons
(c) NAA supports neuronal energy metabolism of mitochondria and specific brain fatty acids
(d) NAA supplies a reservoir for glutamate [3]
(e) NAA offers a substrate for NAAG biosynthesis

NAAG, a dipeptide derivative of NAA and glutamate, is the most abundant brain peptide. With a concentration of approximately 1 mM, NAAG is found in neurons, oligodendrocytes, and microglia. NAAG signals astrocytes about the state of neurostimulation of the neurons, the changing requirements for vascular energy supplies and metabolic waste removal.

For interpretation of proton MRS, NAA is widely regarded as a marker for neuronal functioning with a contributing role from neuronal and axonal cellular organization. Disorders diminishing neuronal and axonal number and density, impairing neuronal functioning or causing displacement and destruction of neurons demonstrate reduced NAA. The one recognized condition of elevated NAA, Canavan's disease, is described below. White matter disorders that damage myelin such that intra-axonal distances decrease may demonstrate relatively high NAA levels as a simple effect of increased axonal density within the sample, if accompanied by the preservation of axons [4, 5].

Creatine and phosphocreatrine produce a composite resonance at 3.0 and 3.9 ppm upon in vivo proton MRS. For the interested reader, Wyss and Kaddurah-Daouk [6] published a comprehensive review of creatine and creatinine metabolism. These chemicals are involved in the regulation of cellular energy metabolism. The enzyme creatine kinase converts creatine to phosphocreatine using ATP. Phosphocreatine serves as a reserve for high-energy phosphates in the cytosol of neurons and muscle, and it buffers cellular ATP/ADP reservoirs. A recent study of childhood white matter disorders found the Cr concentration the most important MR parameter for classification of the disorder [5]. The implication from this study is that semi-quantitative techniques relying on Cr as an internal standard are inappropriate, especially in white matter disorders.

Trimethylammonium residues comprise the Cho resonance observed on proton MRS at 3.2 ppm. A number of mobile choline-containing compounds contribute to the Cho signal. These primarily include the intracellular pools of the membrane precursor phosphocholine, membrane breakdown product glycerophosphocholine, and a small portion (5%) of free choline for an approximate total observable Cho concentration of 1–2 mM [7]. While phosphatyidylcholine is a major membrane constituent produced in all cells, it does not contribute significantly to the observable Cho signal. For leukodystrophies, elevations of the resonance reflect the precursors of myelin *synthesis* as well as the degradation products upon myelin *degradation and/or destruction*. In contrast to leukodystrophies, increased choline levels observed in tumors arise from increased cellular density and proliferation of membrane phospholipids.

On short echo MRS (TE 35 ms or less) of leukodystrophies, elevations of lipids, macromolecules, neurotransmitters, mI, and lactate levels can be as informative as those for the primary metabolites, NAA, Cr, and Cho. Lipid signals are not usually observed in normal brain parenchyma as they are tightly bound with myelin. However, in select white matter pathologies, elevation of the lipid signal corresponds with myelin membrane degradation. Large macromolecular proteins create a broad set of resonances comprising a large portion of the spectral window (0.9–2.6 ppm) with overlap of lipid signals and the methylene signals of several neurotransmitters. Macromolecular proteins include glutamate moieties. Gamma aminobutyric acid (GABA), glutamate, and glutamine create a composite set of multiple signals appearing around 2.1–2.6 ppm. For many disorders, especially white matter diseases, the mI signals offer information about glial responses, typically increasing in response to injury.

Lactate appears as a doublet resonance at 1.3 ppm. Using long echo times, such as 144 and 288 ms, lactate can be distinguished from lipid signals. Sampling with an echo time of 144 ms inverts the resonance below the baseline due to a property known as spin or "J-coupling". While this distinguishes the resonance from macromolecules and lipids, the signal intensity is diminished, which is especially problematic at low concentrations (on the order of 5 mM or below) and within some technical circumstances (i.e., errors in pulse generation and reception). The doublet resonance emerges above the baseline at an echo time of 288 ms. The appearance of lactate is pathologic as it classically represents anaerobic glycolysis. Lactate signal may also possibly reflect mitochondrial impairment, an inflammatory response or macrophage infiltration depending upon the condition.

Primary Leukodystrophies

Alexander's Disease

The genetic foundation for Alexander's disease arises from heterozygous and dominant, usually de novo, mutations in the genes encoding for glial fibrillary acidic protein (GFAP). The key histologic feature is a considerable amount of Rosenthal fibers within the white matter as these fibers accumulate in astrocytes. In biopsy specimens, Rosenthal fibers label extensively for GFAP upon immunocytochemistry. The current standard for diagnosis now relies on detection of pathogenic mutation in the *GFAP* gene.

Generally, Alexander's disease begins in the periventricular white matter, usually involving the frontal lobes and then extending into the parieto-temporal and finally, the occipital regions. Eventually, there is involvement of the cerebellar white matter and spinal cord.

The most commonly encountered variant of Alexander's disease is the infantile form, presenting in the first 2 years of life. The onset of symptoms appears at birth, with delay in development, hypotonia, seizures, and progressive macrocephaly. Children with the infantile form of disease rarely survive to the second decade. The juvenile form presents after 4 years of age with speech and swallowing difficulties, ataxia, and spasticity. Progression is slower, with a more prolonged survival. Adult onset disease has a more variable clinical and imaging presentation, and is occasionally diagnosed incidentally at autopsy.

Conventional MRI findings for the infantile form demonstrate macrocephaly with hyperintensity on T_2-weighted images involving the white matter areas, commonly seen in the frontal areas with progression posteriorly to involve other parts of the cerebral hemispheres. Van der Knaap et al. [8].

identified five characteristics of Alexander's disease on MR imaging that can be applied to suspected cases in order to make a presumptive diagnosis. These characteristics include extensive cerebral white matter changes with frontal predominance, a periventricular rim with high signal on T_1-weighted images and low signal on T_2-weighted images, signal abnormalities with swelling or volume loss in the basal ganglia and thalami, brain stem signal abnormalities, and contrast enhancement of one or more of the following structures: ventricular lining, periventricular rim of tissue, white matter of the frontal lobes, optic chiasm, fornix, basal ganglia, thalamus, dentate nucleus, or brain stem structures. Although many of these abnormalities may be seen in other leukodystrophies, the association of four or more appears to be relatively specific for Alexander's disease. The extent and pattern of contrast enhancement and the distinctive periventricular rim of abnormal signal are not commonly encountered in other leukodystrophies. This is one of the few leukodystrophies in which the administration of contrast provides specific additional information that can lead to the proper diagnosis by imaging. However, recent reports document patients with Rosenthal fibers upon histological examination yet demonstrating unusual and atypical imaging features and often discrepant with a relatively benign clinical course [9–11].

Brockmann et al. [12]. used localized proton MRS to assess metabolic abnormalities in gray and white matter, basal ganglia, and cerebellum of four patients genetically confirmed with infantile Alexander's disease. Elevated concentrations of mI in concert with normal or increased choline compounds in gray and white matter, basal ganglia, and cerebellum point to astrocytosis and demyelination. Neuroaxonal degeneration, as reflected by a reduction of N-acetylaspartate, was most pronounced in cerebral and cerebellar white matter. The accumulation of lactate in affected white matter supports the presence of infiltrating macrophages. Recently, the linear discriminant analysis approach for disease classification described by van der Voorn [5] was applied to juvenile Alexander's disease. The model predicted demyelination as opposed to hypomyelination. However, sequential MRI studies in juvenile Alexander's disease do not support active demyelination due to the often-discrepant clinical and imaging features. This study suggested that spectral features might play a stronger role in determining the nature of Alexander's disease. The lactate elevation found on proton MRS could arise from non-oxidative glycolysis due to the metabolic disruption of disordered astrocytes. As the Rosenthal fibers accumulate, the astrocytes demonstrate hyperplasia and hypertrophy and produce mI elevations. Further study is required to clarify how *GFAP* mutations, classified as Alexander's disease in infants, juveniles, and adults alter brain white matter. Figure 10.1 provides an example of imaging and spectroscopy findings associated with Alexander's disease.

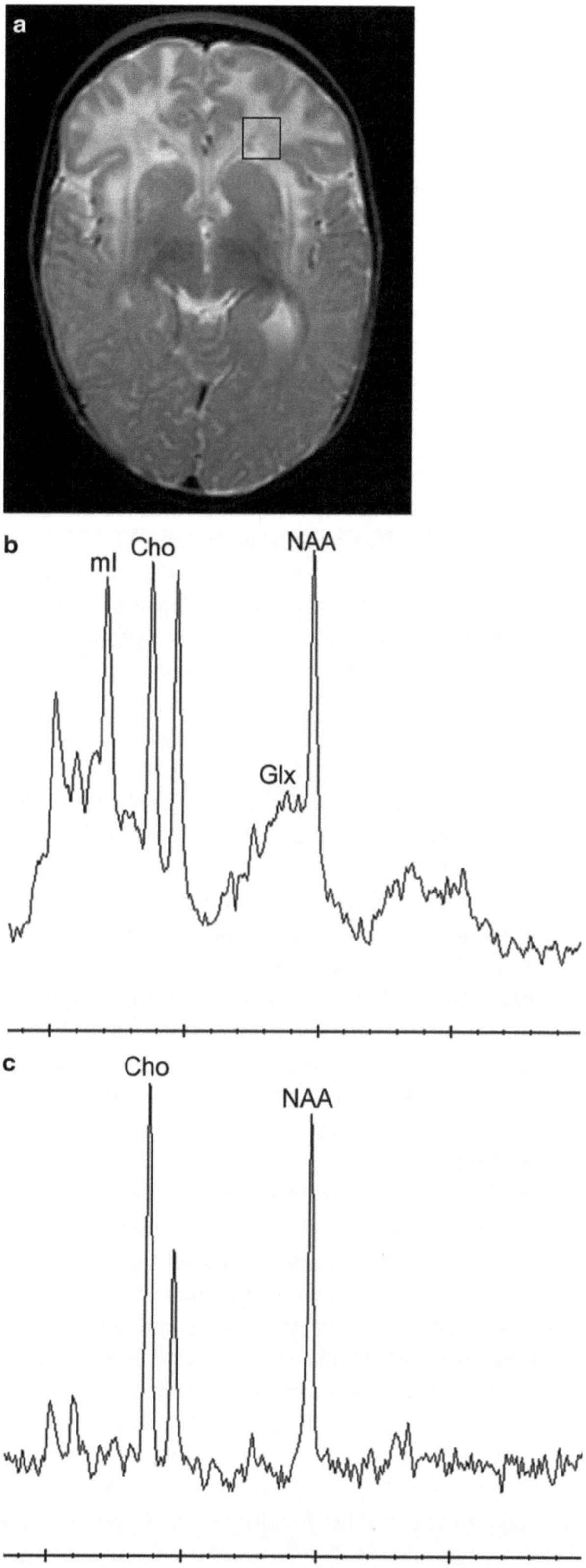

Fig. 10.1 MRI and MRS findings from an 8-month-old female with a novel mutation (A358V) of *GFAP* diagnosed with Alexander's disease. (**a**) Axial T_2-weighted image shows hyperintense signal in the frontal white matter; (**b**) Short echo (35 ms), and (**c**) long echo (288 ms) MR spectra sampling within the left inferior frontal white matter (black voxel on **a**) show reduced NAA/Cr, with elevations of Cho/Cr and mI/Cr. There is also a small lactate peak visible in **c** at 1.3 ppm

Canavan's Disease

Canavan's disease is an autosomal recessive disorder arising from a deficiency of the enzyme aspartoacyclase, a cytosolic enzyme found in oligodendrocytes [13]. Aspartoacylase hydrolyzes NAA to acetate and aspartic acid. With this enzymatic defect, an accumulation of NAA in the brain produces vacuolization in the lower layers of the cerebral cortex and subcortical white matter with intramyelinic swelling and myelin loss [2]. On histologic examination, the disease initiates in a peripheral location, involving the U-fibers of the subcortical white matter of the cerebral hemispheres. Later, the disease progresses and involves the deep white matter structures of both cerebral hemispheres, and eventually it extends to the cerebellum and spinal cord. The involvement of the U-fibers of the white matter is diffuse, with evidence of vacuoles within the subcortical white matter and extending into the adjacent cortex.

Three clinical subtypes, infantile, juvenile, and adult, are also recognized for Canavan's disease. The most common is the infantile type, which usually presents within the first 6 months of life with hypotonia, irritability, and enlarging head size. The symptoms progress and lead to spasticity, blindness, choreoathetoid movement, and myoclonic seizures. There is no cure or standard course for treatment. However, Matalon et al. described the creation of a mouse model to improve understanding of the disease pathophysiology and advance gene therapy for this disorder [14]. Recently, Assadi et al. reported the findings of an open-label trial of lithium citrate to reduce excessive NAA within the brain [15].

The MRI findings parallel the myelin degeneration of the white matter tracts. The first change detected is hyperintensity on T_2-weighted images of the subcortical U-fibers. Eventually, diffuse involvement of the disease occurs in all the white matter fiber tracts for both cerebral hemispheres. In the later stages of the disease, there is volume loss of the cerebral hemispheres.

Figure 10.2 illustrates imaging and spectroscopy findings associated with Canavan's disease. MRS performed within cerebral white matter demonstrates marked elevation of the NAA peak, essentially exclusive for Canavan's disease [16–23]. The NAA elevation is especially pronounced on long echo MRS acquisitions. However, it is important to recognize that on long echo, Cr T_2 relaxation values are much shorter than those for NAA. This results in a significant reduction in signal intensity levels for Cr at long echo times. Hence, an increased NAA/Cr ratio on a 144 ms or 288 ms echo time MRS acquisition is not sufficient alone for diagnosing Canavan's. Short echo MRS acquisitions will also demonstrate a dramatic elevation of NAA/Cr or any NAA/metabolite ratio for Canavan's. Increased amounts of NAA in the brain, confirmed by multiple short and long echo time acquisitions, urine, and plasma can yield a definitive diagnosis for Canavan's disease in accordance with described imaging and clinical findings.

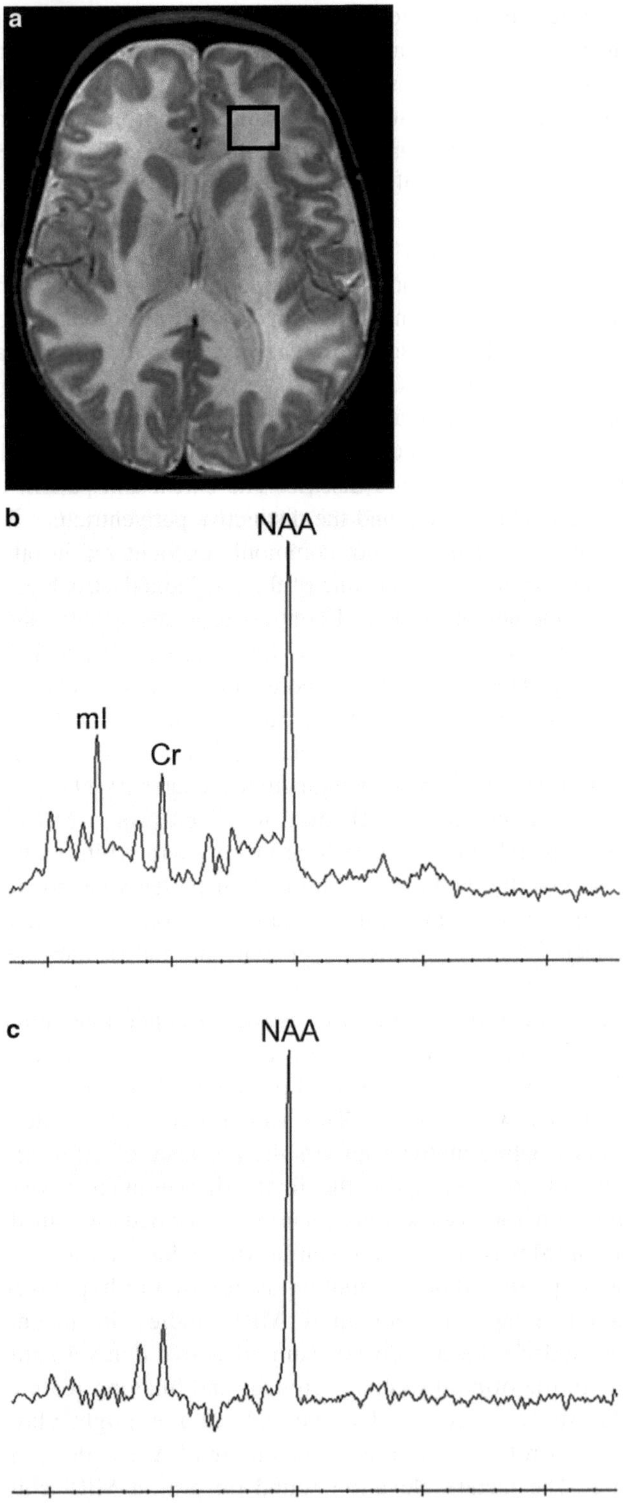

Fig. 10.2 MRI and MRS findings from a 12-month-old female diagnosed with Canavan's disease. (**a**) Axial T_2-weighted image shows hyperintense signal throughout the white matter. (**b**) Short echo (35 ms) and (**c**) long echo (288 ms) MR spectra show significant elevation of NAA sampling within the left frontal white matter (black voxel on **a**) . Myo-inositol also appears elevated in (**b**), which suggests ongoing gliosis. NAA accumulates in the mitochondria due to the deficiency in aspartoacylase, which impairs myelin synthesis, as evidenced in the image

Childhood Ataxia with CNS Hypomyelination or Leukoencephalopathy with Vanishing White Matter

Childhood ataxia with central nervous system hypomyelination (CACH), also referred to as leukoencephalopathy with vanishing white matter disease, is an autosomal recessive disease caused by mutation in any of the five genes-encoding subunits of the eukaryotic translation initiation factor 2B (eIF2B) [24–26]. These genes are essential for initiation of protein synthesis and its regulation in stress response [27, 28]. Patients survive only with residual activity of eI2B, reduced by 20–70% in patient-derived lymphoblasts or fibroblasts [29].

CACH is primarily a brain disorder, with glial vulnerability a key feature. The neuropathological findings consist of severe, cystic white matter degeneration with only small amounts of myelin breakdown products [28, 30]. Foamy oligodendrocytes, dysmorphic astrocytes and oligodendrocytes, oligodendrocytosis, and apoptotic losses of oligodendrocytes are present. The oligodendrocytes undergo apoptosis in response to major neurologic crises with only a subset of oligodendrocytes remaining functional. Selective vulnerability of glia remains unexplained.

CACH is one of the most prevalent inherited leukodystrophies with more than 250 patients recognized [29]. Originally, the disease was recognized only in young children. More recently, adolescent and adult onset of the disorder has been recognized. The age at onset inversely correlates with disease severity. Stresses, such as acute fright, febrile infections, and minor head trauma, can provoke onset of symptoms with rapid and major neurologic deterioration. In childhood onset, CACH can present in such crisis periods with hypotonia, epilepsy, vomiting irritability accompanied by impaired consciousness spanning from somnolence to coma, and in some patients, death. Outside of these periods, the disease can present with cerebellar ataxia, and less frequently, spasticity and optic atrophy with preservation of cognition. While eventually the disease is fatal, the course is slowly progressive outside of episodes of major neurological deterioration. The adolescent and adult forms of the disease have milder but more protracted clinical courses with less prominent episodes of major deterioration. The clinical symptoms in adults feature seizures, complicated migraine, and psychiatric features.

Descriptions of this disease have been reported in the neuropathologic literature since the 1960s; however, the authors of the reports failed to recognize these cases as a single disease entity. CACH is now regarded as an axonopathy rather than a "hypomyelination" or "demyelination" process [27]. The clinical and MRI findings in the classic childhood form were sufficiently specific to enable recognition of this disease as a distinct entity, with subsequent genetic characterization [31]. Clinical diagnosis of the childhood form can be narrowed with recognition of MRI features. CACH appears on imaging as a diffuse cerebral hemispheric leukoencephalopathy, with abnormal white matter progressing over time indicating rarefaction and cystic degeneration. Abnormal white matter demonstrates hyperintense signal on fluid-attenuated inversion recovery (FLAIR), proton density, and T_2-weighted imaging sequences. FLAIR, proton density, and T_1-weighted imaging reveal a radiating, stripe-like pattern with remaining tissue strands. This feature corresponds with widened blood vessels with reactive astrocytes. The U-fibers can be affected; however, the fornix, optic tracts, anterior commissure, the internal capsules, and the outer part of the corpus callosum appear to be less affected. The cortical gray matter, basal ganglia, and brainstem nuclei appear normal [27, 29, 31]. There has been no evidence of contrast enhancement with CACH as the disease lacks inflammatory changes. The correlation between the MRI findings and the detection of the mutations in *eIF2B1-5* genes is very high, but the genotype–phenotype correlation is poor due to wide variations in the phenotype.

The pathological course demonstrates different features upon proton MRS. Initially, a normal spectral profile is remarkably preserved. However, upon rarefaction and cystic degeneration of the white matter, a marked decrease of NAA, Cr, Cho, and lipids in white matter is reported. In the advanced stages, there is a virtual absence of all parenchymal metabolites with only the presence of CSF metabolites, primarily lactate and glucose, described [27, 31–36].

Leukoencephalopathy with Brain-Stem and Spinal Cord Involvement and Elevated White Matter Lactate

Leukoencephalopathy with brain-stem and spinal cord involvement and elevated white matter lactate (LBSL) arises from compound heterozygous mutations on *both* alleles of the *DARS2* gene (1q25.1) [37]. The protein is a mitochondrial enzyme that specifically aminoacylates aspartyl-tRNA. Mutations in the nuclear *DARS2* gene affect only white matter and spare mitochondrial respiratory chain activities.

As a rare inherited disorder, the clinical presentation for LBSL is defined from reports with individuals or small numbers of patients. The disease is slowly progressive. For many, initial child development is normal, with the deterioration of motor skills beginning in childhood, adolescence or for some, not until adulthood. In a few patient reports, independent walking begins late and demonstrates instability from the start. The pattern of involvement includes a slowly progressive cerebellar ataxia, spasticity, and dorsal column dysfunction with more involvement of the legs than the arms. There is decreased position and vibration sense of the legs compared to the arms. Tendon reflexes are maintained. Manual dexterity may become impaired. Eventually, dysarthria can develop. Most patients have normal cognitive function, however, some may develop learning problems, and experience mild cognitive decline. There are reports of treatable epilepsy with some patients.

Since the clinical features resemble a spinocerebellar ataxia, imaging findings can help distinguish LBSL from other entities [38]. The MRI pattern is quite distinct as the progressive white matter abnormalities, spotty or confluent, spread from the periventricular region outward with sparing of the subcortical U-fibers. The corpus callosum is affected with posterior preference. The pyramidal tracts are affected over their entire length from the posterior limb of the internal capsule and brain stem into the lateral corticospinal tracts of the spinal cord. The sensory tracts are involved from the dorsal columns in the spinal cord, the medial lemniscus throughout the brain stem up to the level of the thalamus and the corona radiata above the level of the thalamus. The cerebellar involvement progresses over time to the point of significant volume loss. These patterns suggest that defects in mitochondrial translation related to DARS2 mutation are responsible for dysfunction of long tract-associated glia [39].

Proton MRS studies of affected white matter may demonstrate a highly significant lactate elevation for patients. For a pediatric patient at our institution, the elevated lactate within regions of signal abnormality has been appreciated for several years (Fig. 10.3). However, lactate elevation is not a requirement for diagnosis as several case reports describe adult patients without lactate elevation in affected white matter [40, 41]. Cho and mI elevations with diminished NAA concentrations are also featured within regions of signal abnormality [38, 42–45]. In regions without signal abnormalities on imaging, the spectra can appear remarkably normal.

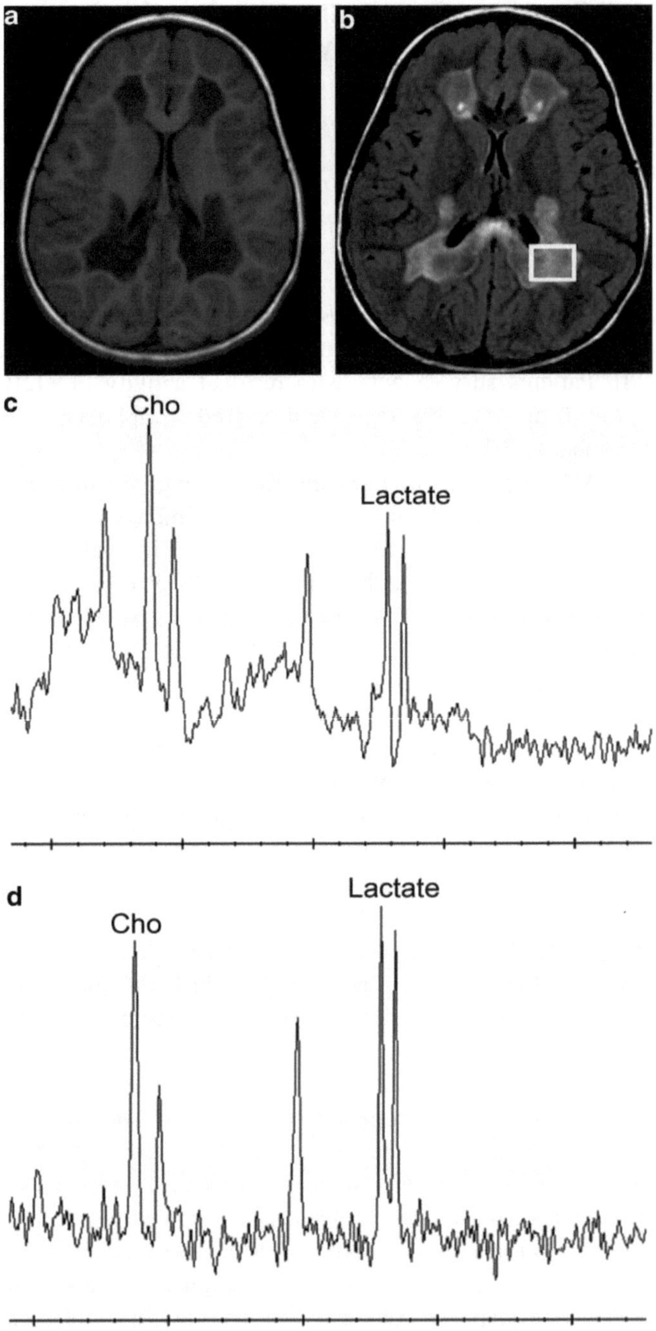

Fig. 10.3 MRI and MRS findings from a 4-year-old girl with two mutations of *DARS2* diagnosed with Leukoencephalopathy with Brain-Stem and Spinal Cord Involvement and Elevated White Matter Lactate (LBSL). (**a**) Axial inversion recovery and (**b**) Axial FLAIR images show significant signal abnormalities in the central white matter, the corpus callosum, and the posterior aspects of the posterior limbs of the internal capsule. (**c**) Short echo (35 ms) and (**d**) long echo (288 ms) MR spectra sampling within the left posterior parietal white matter (white voxel on **b**) show significant reduction of NAA and elevation of Cho. The most striking signals in the spectra are the large lactate resonances

Megalencephalic Leukoencephalopathy with Subcortical Cysts

Megaencephalic Leukoencephalopathy with subcortical cysts (MLC) refers to a leukodystrophy that has been defined by several names:

- Leukoencephalopathy with swelling and discrepantly mild clinical course
- Leukoencephalopathy with swelling and subcortical cysts
- Van der Knaap Disease
- Vaculolating Leukoencephalopathy
- Infantile Leukoencephalopathy

MLC is an autosomal recessive disorder with the primary genetic source of the condition traced to a gene mutation on the long arm of chromosome 22 (22qtel), the *MLC1* gene. *MLC1* encodes a novel protein, MLC1, which is mainly expressed in the brain and leukocytes [46]. Over 50 mutations in the MLC gene have been found in patients diagnosed with the condition. A second gene locus is suspected based upon several reports of patients with clinical, pathologic, and imaging features of MLC with no mutation for MLC1 gene present [47–49]. Histopathologically, MLC features include myelin splitting and intramyelinic vacuole formation.

MLC presents within the first year of life with macrocrania and macrocephaly [50]. Initially, normal mental and motor development occurs with almost all patients having epilepsy at an early age. Epilepsy is usually controlled by medication. Mild mental deterioration occurs late in the disease and is much milder than the motor symptoms. There is a gradual onset of ataxia, spasticity, and extrapyramidal findings. Severity of the disease varies with some patients able to walk into the forties, while others lose their independence after only a few years.

Diagnosis can be established based upon the clinical and MRI findings. MR imaging demonstrates widespread signal abnormalities throughout the white matter, with relative sparing of deep structures [51]. Diffusely abnormal and swollen white matter of the cerebral hemispheres and the presence of subcortical cysts in the anterior-temporal region are strongly suggestive of MLC. Cysts are typically identified in the subcortical temporal lobes, and less frequently in the frontal, parietal, or occipital lobes (see Fig. 10.4). Spectroscopic analyses of affected white matter in patients with MLC revealed marked reduction of N-acetylaspartate, Cr, and Cho with normal values for mI, consistent with axonal loss and astrocytic proliferation, as seen in Fig. 10.4 [5, 52].

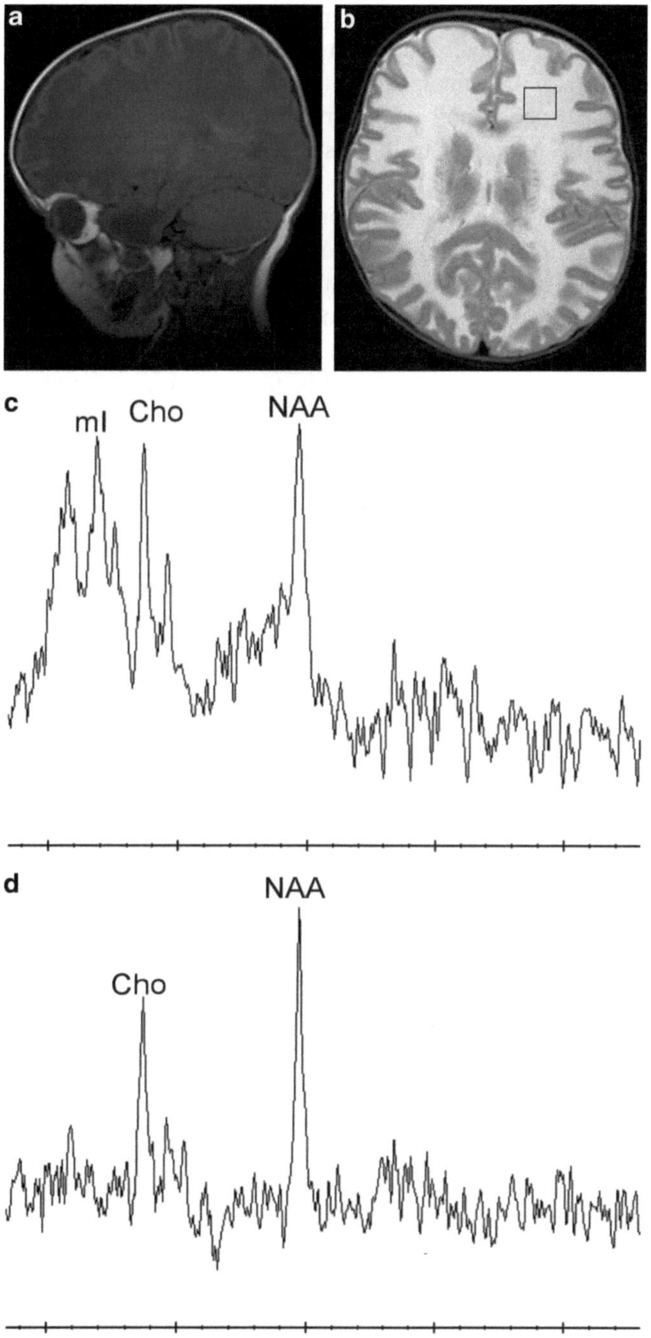

Fig. 10.4 MRI and MRS findings from a 13-month-old male with two heterozygous mutations of intron 3 (C.322-1 G>A) and intron 7 (c.597+1 G>A) of MLC1 diagnosed with Megalencephalic Leukoencephalopathy with Subcortical Cysts (MLC). (**a**) Sagittal T_1-weighted and (**b**) axial T_2-weighted images show diffuse white matter signal abnormalities (hypointense T_1 and hyperintense T_2), decreased sulcation pattern and thinning of cortical gray matter. The formation of temporal cysts within the temporal lobes is noted on the sagittal view. (**c**) Short echo (35 ms) and (**d**) long echo (288 ms) MR spectra sampling within the left frontal white matter (*black* voxel on **b**) show significant reduction of all metabolites as noted by the overall low signal to noise level within the spectrum

Pelizaeus-Merzbacher Disease

Pelizaeus-Merzbacher Disease (PMD) arises from mutations or duplications of the gene-encoding myelin proteolipid protein (*PLP*: Xq22) [53–55]. PMD can exhibit with variable clinical manifestations resulting from alterations in this gene. The more severe phenotypic manifestations have been traditionally characterized as PMD, and result in alterations of multiple functional systems, with symptoms including nystagmus, and compromises in respiratory function, with associated severe disability and morbidity. The most common presentation is that of the slowly progressive "classic" form that presents in infancy with early nystagmus, poor head control, spasticity, ataxia or extrapyramidal movement disorders, and severe developmental delay. These findings slowly progress, usually leading to death in late adolescence or young adulthood. A second pattern of PMD (connatal) begins in the neonatal period and is more rapidly progressive with death typically occurring in the first decade. There are also two other transitional and adult subtypes, respectively. Spastic Paraplegia Type 2 is characterized by lower limb spasticity alone without neurological complications. “Complicated” Spastic Paraplegia Type 2 exhibits cerebellar ataxia, nystagmus, and a pyramidal syndrome.

PMD manifests as a primary defect in myelin formation. It is the prototypical hypomyelination syndrome. The imaging appearance is of an otherwise normal brain, well-conserved neurons and their processes including axons, which is severely delayed in its formation of myelin. Imaging demonstrates a marked delay in myelination from the onset with homogeneous high T_2 signal intensity of cerebral white matter. While many metabolic or neurodegenerative processes are associated with delayed myelination, the absence of other imaging findings is characteristic of the early stages of the *PLP* gene disorders. The characteristic normal progression of myelinaton observed on MR imaging is entirely absent or severely slowed in the *PLP* gene disorders. Patients with the SPG2 phenotype show fewer MRI signal abnormalities. Thus, the levels of myelination assessed by imaging findings obtained after 2 years of age generally correlate with disease severity. Myelination that does occur tends to be patchy, without the characteristic distribution within the white matter tracts. In the later stages of disease, white matter volume may decrease with thinning of the corpus callosum and excess mineralization in the basal ganglia.

Hanefeld et al. [56] evaluated five patients with genetically confirmed duplication of PLP using proton MRS and LCModel [57, 58] quantification. The spectral profile of the affected white matter resembled more closely a pattern consistent with cortical gray matter instead of white matter by demonstrating reduced choline concentrations but increased concentrations of NAA, NAAG, glutamine, mI, and Cr. The spectral profiles within the basal ganglia and parietal gray matter were statistically normal, with a trend toward elevated NAA, NAAG, glutamine, and mI. Enhanced neuroaxonal density, revealed by NAA and NAAG elevations, would occur with the absence of oligodendrocytic tissue and normal myelin sheaths between axons. The absence of myelin sheaths would also produce choline reductions. Reduced signal linewidths were found in the spectra. Since oligodendrocytes possess a significant amount of iron, improved homogeneity can occur in the absence of oligodendrocytes. Finally, elevations of mI, glutamine, and Cr remain consistent with astrogliosis. Takanashi also found increased NAA, Cr, and mI concentrations in the posterior centrum semiovale for pediatric patients with *PLP1* duplications using a similar quantitative approach [59]. In contrast, others have reported decreases in NAA levels [59–61]. Bonavita et al. used proton MRSI to evaluate nine patients with *PLP* mutations [60]. The patients varied in age (range from 6 to 43 years), most had point mutations (8 out of 9) and varied appearance of imaging abnormalities. Clinical scores indicated patients ranged from unaffected to moderately affected (maximum clinical score of 12/25). Compared with age-matched control participants, patients demonstrated significant and widespread (cortex, white matter, and basal ganglia) declines in NAA/Cr and NAA/Cho levels. Garbern et al., examined patients with null *PLP* mutations with single voxel and spectroscopic imaging techniques [62]. Neuropathology from affected relatives of one of the patients examined by MRSI was also performed to extend the significance of the MRS finding of decreased NAA ratio levels in gray and white matter. The absence of *PLP* expression produces axonal degeneration, likely from disruption of oligodendrocyte–axonal interactions, which accounts for the decline of NAA. Pizzini, et al., also found reduced white matter NAA ratios in MRSI studies of three pediatric patients with point mutations of *PLP [61]*.

Differences in the mutation, duplications versus point mutations, and the spectroscopic quantification could potentially account for the discrepant NAA findings. Another potential explanation may be attributed to NAAG elevations. Mochel, et al., reported an elevation of CSF NAAG for patients with hypomyelination disorders, such as PMD, Pelizaeus-Merzbacher-like disease and Canvan’s Disease, obtained with in vitro proton NMR spectroscopy [63, 64]. NAAG was significantly elevated in the CSF of all patients (19/19) with *PLP* duplication; however, for patients (6/7) with *PLP* point mutations, normal NAAG levels were found in the CSF [63]. Unfortunately, no one has specifically examined brain NAAG and its contribution to total NAA levels in PMD.

Lysosomal Disorders Producing Leukodystrophies

Lysosomes are organelles within a cell that contain acid hydrolase enzymes responsible for breaking up waste materials and cellular debris. There are approximately 40 rare inherited disorders affecting metabolism of lipids, glycoproteins, and mucopolysaccharides that result from defects in lysosomal function. This chapter discusses three lysosomal disorders, which can also be classified as leukodystrophies.

Cerebrotendinous Xanthomatosis

Cerebrotendinous Xanthomatosis (CTX) is an autosomal recessive disease that arises from mutations in the gene, *CYP27A1,* on human chromosome 2 at the q35 interval. The mitochondrial enzyme product of this gene, sterol

27-hydroxylase, is important for intestinal fat absorption as it converts cholesterol into bile acids. Abnormal deposition of cholestanol and cholesterol with the CNS and other matter (plasma, urine, feces, etc.) occurs with the disease. The clinical manifestations of the disease are variable, but arise from the abnormal metabolism of cholestanol. The classical triad of the disease includes tendon xanthomas, juvenile cataracts, and progressive neurological impairment. Chronic diarrhea from infancy is one of the earliest manifestations of the disease. In the first decade of life, cataracts appear. The neurologic presentation can include cerebellar ataxia, spasticity of the limbs, seizures, and neurobehavioral disorders. MRI examination can reveal focal or diffuse white matter abnormalities with varying degrees of cerebral and cerebellar atrophy. The findings are often non-specific, but, abnormal signal around the dentate nuclei and adjacent white matter is highly suggestive of the disease [65].

De Stefano used proton MRSI to investigate adult patients with CTX [66]. The findings suggested widespread axonal damage revealed by a decrease in *N*-acetylaspartate and diffuse brain mitochondrial dysfunction with an increase in lactate. A correlation between levels of the putative axonal marker N-acetylaspartate and patients' disability scores suggests that proton MR spectroscopy can provide a useful measure of disease outcome in CTX.

Globoid Cell Leukodystrophy (Krabbe Disease)

Globoid Cell Leukodystrophy (GLD) arises from a deficiency in the enzyme, β-galactocerebrosidase, leading to the accumulation of cerebroside and galactosylsphingosine within the lysosome and inducing apotosis in the oligodendrocyte cell lines. Also known as Krabbe Disease, this autosomal recessive disorder, localized to chromosome 14q31, is seen predominantly in young children with the most common form, infantile, presenting with irritability between 3 and 6 months after birth. The disease progresses with symptoms mimicking encephalitis with motor deterioration, difficulties in feeding and atypical seizures. At the end stage of the disease, the child exists in a vegetative state with decerebrate posturing.

The disease predominantly involves the white matter of the cerebral hemispheres, cerebellum, and spinal cord. Pathologic changes include a marked toxic reduction in the number of oligodendrocytes. Multinucleated globoid appearing cells, as well as reactive macrophages with cerebroside, are scattered throughout the white matter and around blood vessels [67]. Hypomyelination may be extensive leading eventually to gliosis and scarring in the white matter. Gray matter involvement in the basal ganglia region can be found accompanied by punctate calcification.

Delayed myelination may be the first finding noted on MRI in infants with this disease. The appearance features one of two patterns. Patchy hyperintense periventricular signal on T_2-weighted imaging, consistent with hypomyelination, may eventually evolve into a more diffuse pattern in the white matter. In this form, there is often involvement of the thalami with hyperintense T_2-signal as well. A second pattern is patchy low signal on T_2-weighted images representing a paramagnetic effect arising from calcium deposition, which can also be appreciated on brain computed tomography (CT). Additional early changes include abnormal signal in the thalami, cerebellum, caudate heads, and brainstem that may precede the changes in the white matter of the centrum semiovale. Symmetric enlargement of the optic nerves is presumed to reflect accumulation of proteolipid in globoid cells. At times, changes within the cerebellar white matter have also been reported, with hyperintensity noted on T_2-weighted images. The findings within the spinal cord are visualized as atrophic changes. Diffuse volume loss and periventricular white matter abnormalities predominate in the later stages of this disease.

Reduced NAA with elevated Cho and mI have been reported in this disease. Diminished NAA is expected with neuroaxonal loss but spectroscopy has also revealed disturbances in glial cell metabolism associated with hypomyelination. Brockmann [68] found different metabolic profiles dependent upon the presentation (infantile, juvenile, and adult onset) consistent with recognized histopathologic features. For infantile presentation of Krabbe, pronounced Cho and mI elevations in affected white matter reflected demyelination and glial proliferation with reductions in NAA representing neuroaxonal loss, as seen in Fig. 10.5. For juvenile onset patients, the white matter MRS reflected metabolic changes consistent with neuroaxonal loss and astrocytosis. In an adult onset patient, white matter spectroscopy approximated normal metabolic concentrations.

Metachromatic Leukodystrophy

Metachromatic leukodystrophy (MLD) arises from a deficiency in the enzyme arylsulfatase A, which cleaves the sulfate from sulfate-containing lipids, resulting in the accumulation of cerebroside sulfate within the lysosome. This disorder is transmitted in an autosomal-recessive pattern with the arylsulfatase A gene localized to chromosome 22q [67].

There are four subtypes of MLD (1) congenital; (2) late infantile; (3) juvenile; and (4) adult. The most common form, late infantile subtype, presents from around 14 months to 4 years of age. The early presentation begins with an unsteady gait that eventually progresses to severe ataxia and flaccid paralysis, dysarthia, mental retardation, and decerebrate posturing. Genotype–phenotype correlation occurs with the late infantile form homozygous for alleles with no expression of enzyme activity (null allele), heterozygosity for null and non-null alleles in the juvenile form, and homozygosity for non-null alleles in the adult form.

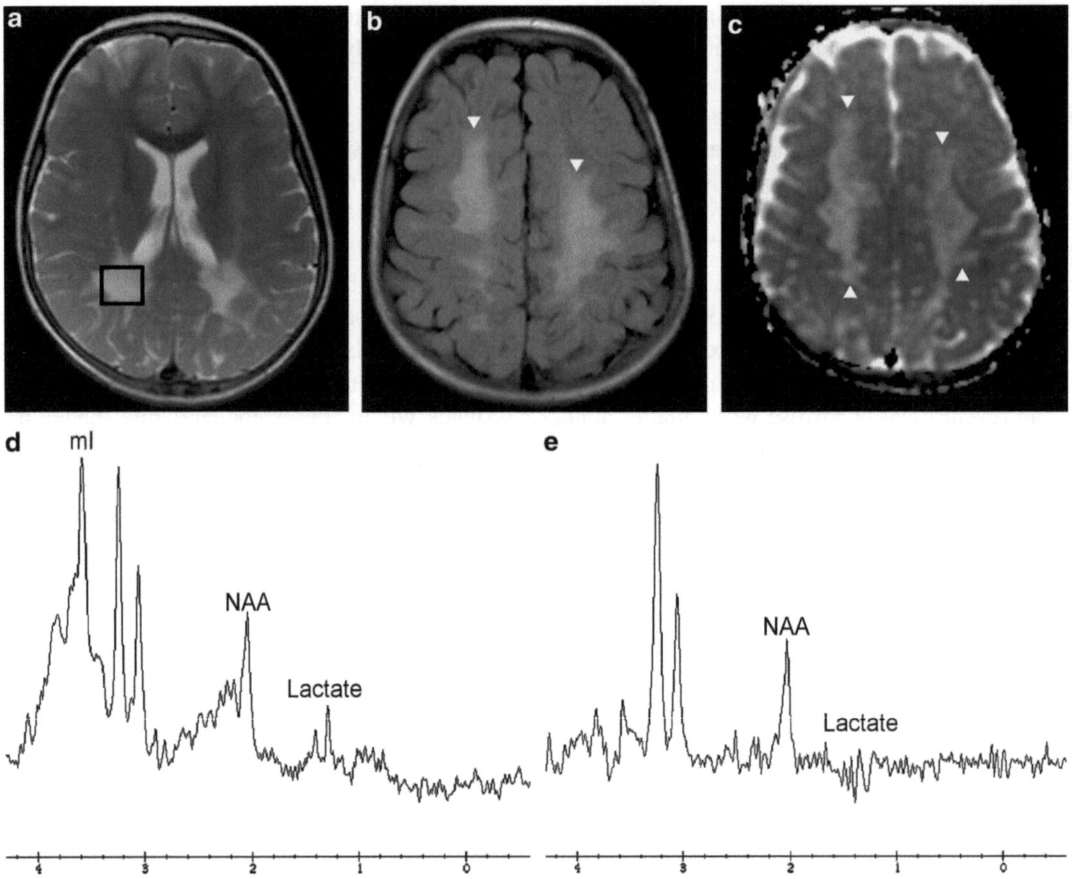

Fig. 10.5 MRI and MRS findings from a 4-year-old girl diagnosed with globoid cell leukodystrophy (Krabbe Disease). (**a**) Axial T_2-weighted image shows hyperintense signal in the parietal white matter; (**b**) Axial FLAIR image shows significant signal abnormalities in the central white matter; (**c**) Axial Apparent Diffusion Coefficient map shows increased diffusion signal (*arrowheads*) within the central white matter; (**d**) Short echo (35 ms) and (**e**) long echo (288 ms) MR spectra sampling within the right parietal white matter (*black* voxel on **a**) show reduced NAA/Cr, with elevations of Cho/Cr and mI/Cr. There is also a small lactate peak visible ind at 1.3 ppm

Histologic analysis of affected white matter demonstrates a complete loss of myelin with evidence of axonal degeneration. Metachromatic granules are reported within engorged lysosomes in white matter, neurons, and on peripheral nerve biopsies. Oligodendrocytes are reduced in number, and areas of demyelination predominate throughout the deep white matter region. Macrophages with vacuolated cytoplasm containing crystalloid sulfatide structures are scattered in the white matter [67]. Early sparing of the subcortical arcuate white matter fibers (U- fibers) occurs until late in the disease process. An inflammatory response is typically absent, which accounts for the lack of contrast enhancement in this disorder, but eventually, myelinated white matter is replaced by astrogliosis and scarring. On T_2-weighted imaging, there is marked hyperintensity of the white matter fiber tracts involving the cerebral hemispheres extending to the cerebellum, brainstem, and spinal cord. The findings are initially focal and patchy, but later develop into diffuse, hyperintense T_2 signal of the centrum semiovale. On T_1-weighted imaging, the white matter fibers may be isointense with or hypointense to gray matter. Over time, a diffuse volume loss of all regions emerges with marked compensatory enlargement of the ventricles and extra-axial fluid spaces. At this end-stage, differentiation of this condition from diffuse hypoxic/ischemic injury or other late-stage neurodegenerative/metabolic diseases is difficult from imaging findings alone.

Proton MRS investigations of patients with MLD have demonstrated reduced NAA as expected from axonal degeneration and neuroaxonal loss, as seen in Fig. 10.6. Disturbances in glial cell metabolism indicated by elevated mI and Cho may reflect the loss of myelin. In one study, Kruse posits that in contrast to other leukodystrophies, late infantile and juvenile MLD patients demonstrate two-to-three fold increases in brain mI. This elevation may reflect a specific aspect of the pathophysiology of demyelination associated with MLD [69]. The study by van der Voorn supports this finding, with highly significant elevations of mI and Cho as useful for classification of demyelinating disorders [5].

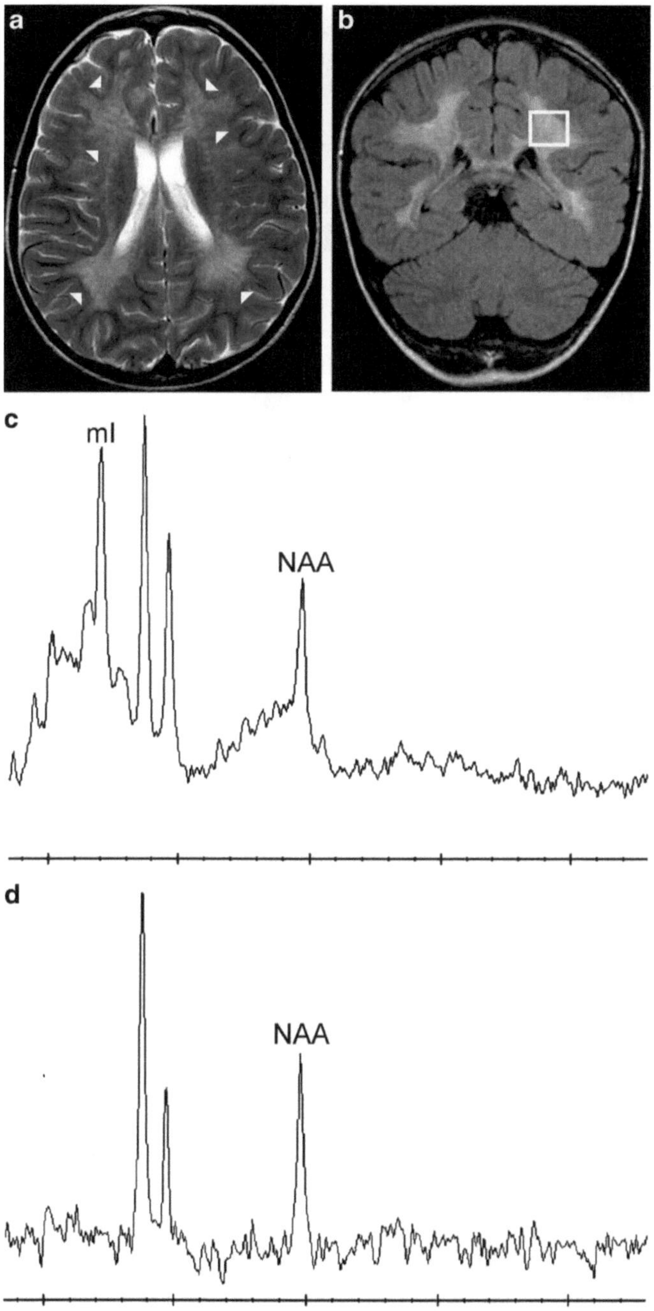

Fig. 10.6 MRI and MRS findings from 7-year-old male diagnosed with metachromatic leukodystrophy. (**a**) Axial T_2-weighted image and (**b**) coronal FLAIR image show hyperintense signal in periventricular white matter with sparing of subcortical U-fibers (*arrowheads* on **a**); (**c**) Short echo (35 ms) and (**d**) long echo (288 ms) sampling within the left posterior parietal white matter (*white* voxel on **b**) feature reduced NAA and Cr, elevated Cho and from the short echo MRS an elevated mI level

Perioxisomal Disorders Producing Leukodystrophies

Peroxisomes are organelles within a cell that contain enzymes responsible for critical cellular processes, including biosynthesis of membrane phospholipids (plasmalogens), cholesterol, and bile acids, conversion of amino acids into glucose, oxidation of fatty acids, reduction of hydrogen peroxide by catalases, and prevention of excess oxalate synthesis. Peroxisomal disorders are subdivided into two major categories (1) biogenesis disorders arising from a failure to form viable peroxisomes, resulting in multiple metabolic abnormalities and (2) disorders resulting from the deficiency of a single peroxisomal enzyme.

Four different disorders comprise the genetically heterogeneous PBD group: Zellweger syndrome (ZS), infantile Refsum's disease (IRD), neonatal adrenoleukodystrophy (NALD), and rhizomelic chondrodysplasia punctata (RCDP). X-linked adrenoleukodystrophy (ALD) is the prototypical peroxisomal disorder in which the morphology of the organelle is found to be normal on electron microscopy, but a single enzyme defect leads to the accumulation of very long-chain fatty acids and progressive CNS deterioration in the form of a chronic progressive encephalopathy.

Zellweger Syndrome

ZS is an autosomal recessive disease characterized by defective peroxisomal functions. Infants are symptomatic early, with hypotonia, seizures, large liver size, and limb and facial anomalies that are easily recognizable at birth. Neuroimaging is relatively specific, correlating well with pathologic appearances of the brain. There is a diffuse lack of myelination throughout the white matter combined with cortical dysplasia. The gyri are broad, with shallow intervening sulci found mainly in the anterior frontal and temporal lobes but also over the convexities in the perirolandic area. Variants of ZS have also been described that do not follow the typical prototype, but demonstrate many common features to ZS. Clinical overlap may occur with other conditions including NALD, IRD, and hyperpipecolic acidemia.

The difference among ZS, NALD, and IRD is one of severity. ZS is the most severe, with death occurring in the first year of life, whereas survival for NALD is limited to childhood, and patients with IRD can survive into adulthood.

MRS performed in older patients with ZS and IRD finds similar features with dramatic lipid and choline elevations, minor mI elevations, and reduced NAA levels for sampled white matter. ZS presents with cortical dysplasia and neuronal heterotopia on imaging. Proton MRS illustrates the neuropathologic aspects of ZS, which include neuronal degeneration, abnormal myelination, and compromised liver function. Bruhn, et al., reported MRS of infants ($N=4$) with impaired peroxisomal function classified as variants of ZS revealed a marked decrease of *N*-acetylaspartate in white and gray matter, thalamus, and cerebellum with two patients also demonstrating an increase of cerebral glutamine and a decrease of the cytosolic mI in gray matter and striatum reflecting impaired hepatic function [70]. Two subjects in the Bruhn study exhibited a notable elevation of mobile lipids and/or cholesterol in white matter. In an unpublished study,

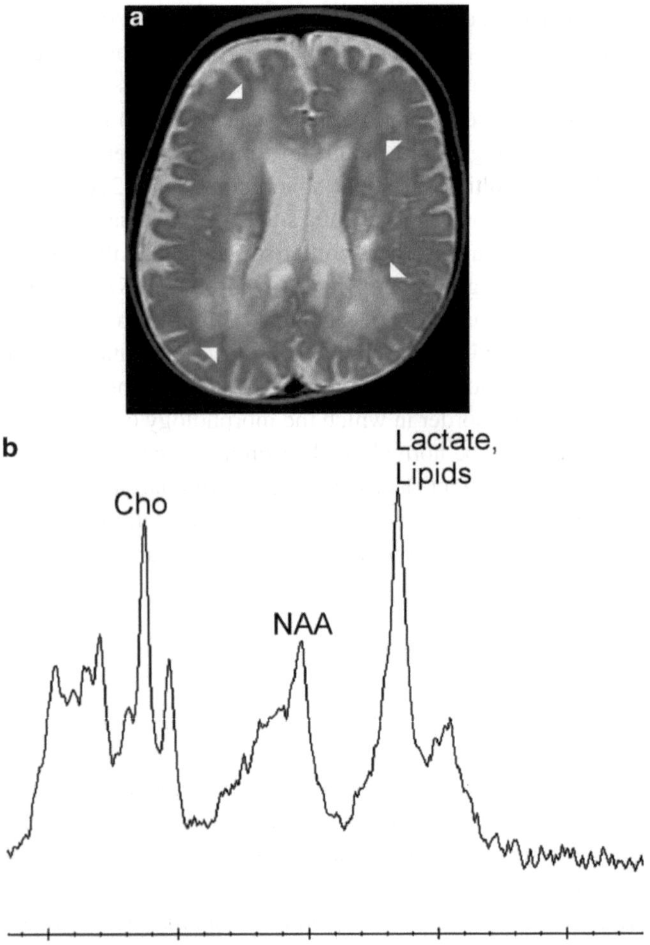

Fig. 10.7 MRI and MRS findings from 3-year-old male diagnosed with Zellweger Syndrome. (**a**) Axial FLAIR shows diffuse periventricular white matter hyperintensities (arrowheads). (**b**) Short echo (35 ms) MR spectrum shows elevated lactate and lipids, as well as increased choline. NAA also appears reduced

MRS performed in older patients with ZS (3 years old) demonstrates similar features with dramatic lipid and choline elevations, minor mI elevations with reduced NAA levels for sampled white matter (Fig. 10.7).

Neonatal Adrenoleukodystrophy

NALD is characterized by the presence of multiple recognizable enzyme deficiencies with grossly normal, but deficient numbers of peroxisomes. Specific conditions include pipecolic and phytanic acidemia and a deficiency of plasmalogen synthetase. This condition also presents with hypotonia in the first months of life, but without many of the facial features of ZS. Cortical abnormalities in the form of a dysplasia can be found in this condition as well with hypomyelination in cerebral white matter. An example of proton MRS in NALD is shown in Fig. 10.8.

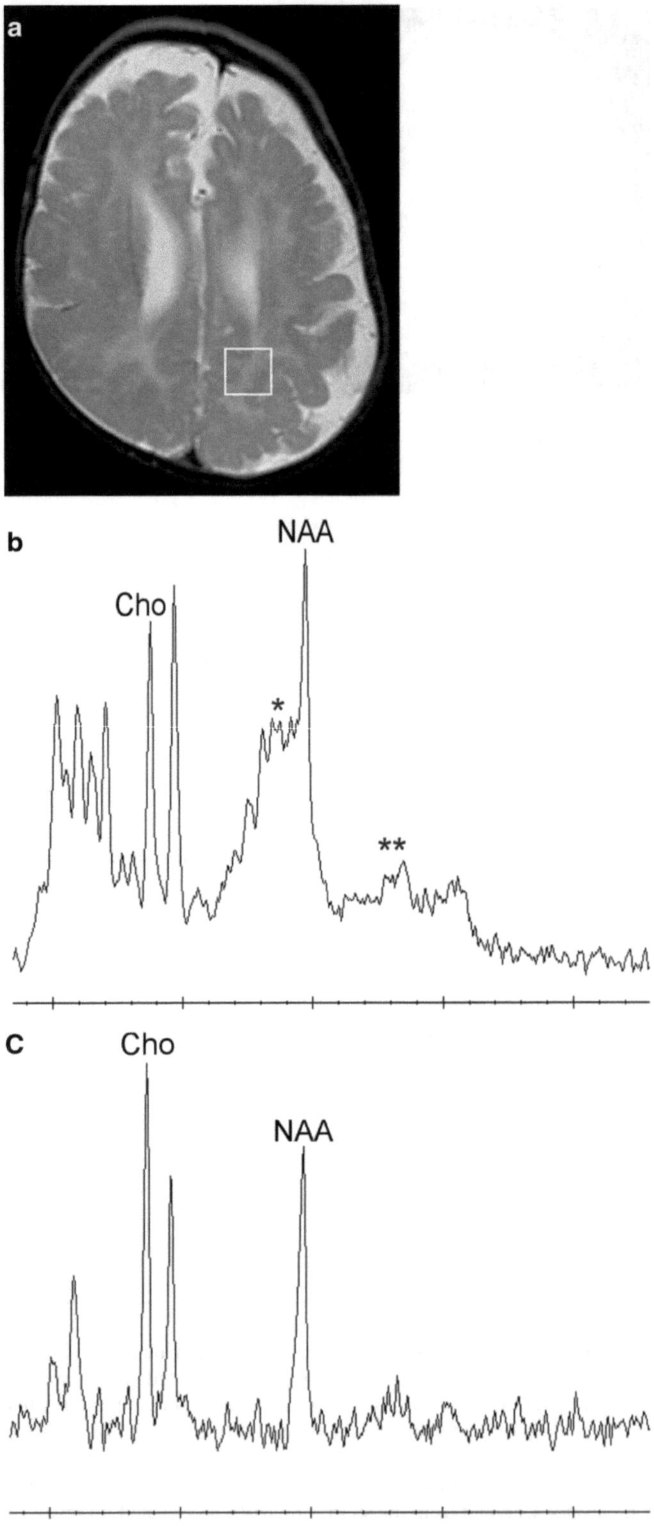

Fig. 10.8 MRI and MRS findings from a 12-month-old male diagnosed with neonatal adrenoleukodystrophy. (**a**) Axial T_2-weighted image shows diffuse white matter signal abnormalities. (**b**) Short echo (35 ms) MR spectrum shows elevated glutamate + glutamine signal (*Asterisk*), as well as a small amount of lipids and lactate (*double asterisk*). (**c**) Long echo (144 ms) MR spectrum clearly shows the reduced NAA and slight elevation of Cho

X-Linked Adrenoleukodystrophy

For X-linked ALD, the morphology of the organelle is found to be normal on electron microscopy; however, a single enzyme defect, acyl-CoA synthetase, and a failure of the incorporation into cholesterol esters for myelin synthesis leads to the accumulation of very long-chain fatty acids and progressive CNS deterioration in the form of a chronic progressive encephalopathy. The "classic" form of ALD is an X-linked disorder (Xq28) with a clinical onset between the ages of 5–7 years, which includes behavioral problems, followed by a rapidly progressive decline in neurologic function, and death within the ensuing 5–8-year period. The first indication of this condition may include mental status changes or a decline in school performance. Clinical symptoms may begin with subtle alterations in neurocognitive function, but eventually progress to severe spasticity and visual deficits, ultimately leading to a vegetative state and death.

X-linked ALD demonstrates a loss of myelin with relative preservation of the subcortical U-fibers along with lymphocytic inflammation and gliosis [67]. It has been described with a typical appearance on MR with predominately posterior involvement that over time progresses from posterior to anterior into the frontal lobes, and from the deep white matter to the peripheral subcortical white matter. The involvement appears symmetrical in a butterfly distribution across the splenium of the corpus callosum, surrounded on its periphery by an enhancing zone. Three zones are readily distinguished on MR: an inner zone of astrogliosis and scarring that appears hypointense on T_1-weighted imaging and hyperintense on T_2-weighted sequences; an intermediate zone of active inflammation that appears isointense on T_1-weighted images and iso- or hypointense on T_2-weighted imaging; and an outer zone of active demyelination that appears minimally hypointense on T_1-weighted images and hyperintense on T_2-weighted imaging. Rarely, involvement can be entirely anterior in a butterfly distribution; however, unilateral and asymmetrical involvement has also been described. Following a bone marrow transplant, the first imaging finding is often the disappearance of gadolinium contrast enhancement within the intermediate zone of inflammation. The progression of disease from posterior to anterior and from deep white matter to the periphery of the brain may be slower compared to its previous course; however, hyperintense signal changes are not significantly reversed.

X-linked ALD patients evaluated with proton MRS demonstrate abnormal spectra within regions of abnormal imaging signal as well as normal appearing white matter (NAWM) (Fig. 10.9) [70–88]. The spectral profile for NAWM of neurologically asymptomatic patients is characterized by slightly elevated concentrations of choline compounds, with an increase of Cho and mI reflecting the onset of demyelination. Markedly elevated concentrations of Cho, mI, and glutamine in affected white matter suggest active demyelination and

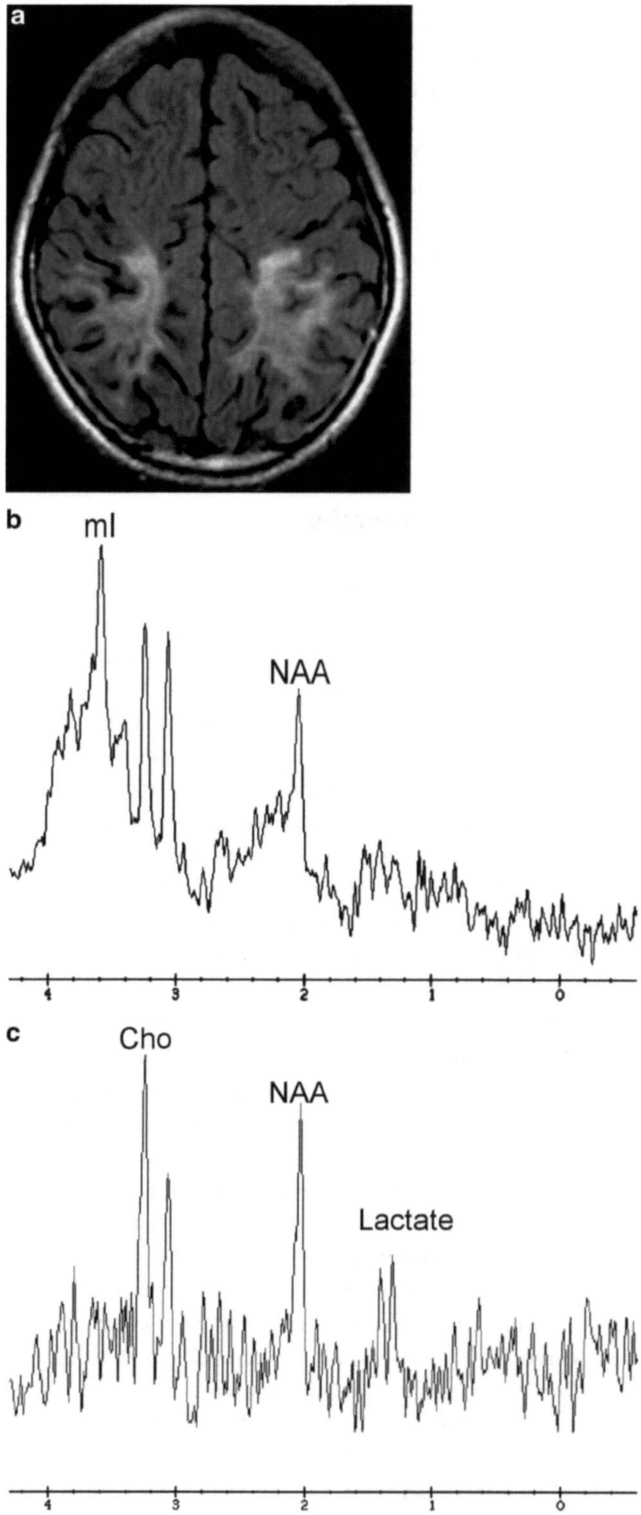

Fig. 10.9 MRI and MRS findings from a 15-year-old diagnosed with X-linked adrenoleukodystrophy, approximately 6 months post-bone marrow transplant. (**a**) Axial FLAIR image shows diffuse signal hyperintensities in the parietal white matter. (**b**) The short echo (35 ms) spectrum reveals decreased NAA associated with neural dysfunction, volume loss, and elevated mI consistent with gliosis. (**c**) The long echo (288 ms) spectrum shows decreased NAA and elevated lactate; however, the low signal to noise reflects contribution of CSF from the adjacent lateral ventricle. The patient imaging was stable, with no abnormal contrast enhancement or abnormal diffusion signal, for at least one year on follow-up studies

glial proliferation. A simultaneous reduction of the concentrations of NAA and glutamate is consistent with neuronal loss and injury. Elevated lactate is consistent with inflammation and/or macrophage infiltration. The more severe metabolic disturbances in ALD correspond to progressive demyelination, neuroaxonal loss, and gliosis leading to clinical deterioration and eventually death. The detection of MRS abnormalities before the onset of neurological symptoms may help in the selection of patients for bone marrow transplantation and stem cell transplant. Stabilization and partial reversal of metabolic abnormalities is demonstrated in some patients after therapies. The spectral profiles can be used to monitor disease evolution and the effects of therapies.

Adrenomyeloneuropathy

A milder form of ALD, known as adrenomyeloneuropathy, occurs in both males and females (heterozygous) that commonly manifests in adulthood. Adrenomyeloneuropathy is thought to represent a form of X-linked ALD or an autosomal recessive form of ALD that does not manifest until later in life. It may arise in families with a previous history of "classic" X-linked ALD. Clinical manifestations include the slow onset of neuromuscular weakness, yet overt CNS manifestations secondary to demyelination are less common, and may not manifest until very late in the disease process. Clinical progression does not necessarily correspond with the severity of imaging findings at the time of initial diagnosis.

For patients with adrenomyeloneuropathy, the MRI is often within normal limits for age. High signal on T_2-weighted imaging representing demyelination can be identified in the corticospinal and spinocerebellar tracts of the brainstem. Abnormal signal may eventually extend into the midbrain and posterior limb of the internal capsule; however, the typical deep white matter involvement as seen in ALD is less common. When present, it is less extensive than in ALD, and is generally only seen very late in the disease process. Demyelination of cerebellar deep white matter can be found, primarily centered about pontocerebellar tracts of the middle cerebellar peduncles, pontocerebral tracts, and the medial lemniscus.

Ratai and colleagues employed MRSI at 7 T in adults with adult cerebral ALD, adrenomyeloneuropathy, and females heterozygous for X-linked ALD [88]. Patients with adrenomyeloneuropathy demonstrated lower NAA/Cr and Glu/Cr ratios compared to healthy controls. No significant differences were found between patients with adrenomyeloneuropathy and female heterozygotes. In NAWM of those with adult cerebral ALD, the mI/Cr and Cho/Cr levels were 46% and 21% higher than patients with adrenomyeloneuropathy, respectively.

Summary

Leukodystrophies are associated with substantial morbidity and mortality in children [89]. In a recent retrospective review of a regional children's hospital in the US over an 8-year period, the incidence of leukodystrophies was estimated at 1 in 7,663 live births. Unfortunately, much of our understanding of these disorders is limited by individual or small case series. Magnetic resonance imaging and spectroscopy have assisted in the diagnosis of leukodystrophies; however, greater clinical and research efforts toward diagnosing these disorders and monitoring therapies is sorely needed.

Acknowledgments The author's efforts were supported by grants from the National Institutes of Health, NIEHS R01 ES015559, NCI R01 CA112182, and NIMH P50 MH077138. The authors have no competing financial or non-financial interests to declare.

References

1. Tallan HH, Moore S, Stein WH. N-Acetyl-L-aspartic acid in brain. J Biol Chem. 1956;219(1):257–64.
2. Moffett JR, Tieman SB, Weinberger DR, Coyle JT, Namboodiri AMA. N-Acetylaspartate A unique neuronal molecule in the central nervous system; 2006, 2004; Bethesda, Maryland, USA.
3. Clark JF, Doepke A, Filosa JA, et al. N-acetylaspartate as a reservoir for glutamate. Med Hypotheses. 2006;67(3):506–12.
4. De Stefano N, Bartolozzi ML, Guidi L, Stromillo ML, Federico A. Magnetic resonance spectroscopy as a measure of brain damage in multiple sclerosis. J Neurol Sci. 2005;233(1–2):203–8.
5. van der Voorn JP, Pouwels PJ, Hart AA, et al. Childhood white matter disorders: quantitative MR imaging and spectroscopy. Radiology. 2006;241(2):510–7.
6. Wyss M, Kaddurah-Daouk R. Creatine and creatinine metabolism. Physiol Rev. 2000;80(3):1107–213.
7. Stork C, Renshaw PF. Mitochondrial dysfunction in bipolar disorder: evidence from magnetic resonance spectroscopy research. Mol Psychiatry. 2005;10(10):900–19.
8. van der Knaap MS, Naidu S, Breiter SN, et al. Alexander disease: diagnosis with MR imaging. AJNR Am J Neuroradiol. 2001;22(3):541–52.
9. van der Knaap MS, Ramesh V, Schiffmann R, et al. Alexander disease: ventricular garlands and abnormalities of the medulla and spinal cord. Neurology. 2006;66(4):494–8.
10. van der Knaap MS, Salomons GS, Li R, et al. Unusual variants of Alexander's disease. Ann Neurol. 2005;57(3):327–38.
11. Dinopoulos A, Gorospe JR, Egelhoff JC, et al. Discrepancy between neuroimaging findings and clinical phenotype in Alexander disease. AJNR Am J Neuroradiol. 2006;27(10):2088–92.
12. Brockmann K, Dechent P, Meins M, et al. Cerebral proton magnetic resonance spectroscopy in infantile Alexander disease. J Neurol. 2003;250(3):300–6.
13. Madhavarao CN, Moffett JR, Moore RA, Viola RE, Namboodiri MA, Jacobowitz DM. Immunohistochemical localization of aspartoacylase in the rat central nervous system. J Comp Neurol. 2004;472(3):318–29.

14. Matalon R, Rady PL, Platt KA, et al. Knock-out mouse for Canavan disease: a model for gene transfer to the central nervous system. J Gene Med. 2000;2(3):165–75.
15. Assadi M, Janson C, Wang DJ, et al. Lithium citrate reduces excessive intra-cerebral N-acetyl aspartate in Canavan disease. Eur J Paediatr Neurol. 2010;14(4):354–9.
16. Krawczyk H, Gradowska W. Characterisation of the 1 H and 13C NMR spectra of N-acetylaspartylglutamate and its detection in urine from patients with Canavan disease. J Pharm Biomed Anal. 2003;31(3):455–63.
17. Gordon N. Canavan disease: a review of recent developments. Eur J Paediatr Neurol. 2001;5(2):65–9.
18. Moreno A, Ross BD, Bluml S. Direct determination of the N-acetyl-L-aspartate synthesis rate in the human brain by (13)C MRS and [1-(13)C]glucose infusion. J Neurochem. 2001;77(1):347–50.
19. Bluml S, Moreno A, Hwang JH, Ross BD. 1-(13)C glucose magnetic resonance spectroscopy of pediatric and adult brain disorders. NMR Biomed. 2001;14(1):19–32.
20. Aydinli N, Caliskan M, Calay M, Ozmen M. Use of localized proton nuclear magnetic resonance spectroscopy in Canavan's disease. Turk J Pediatr. 1998;40(4):549–57.
21. Wittsack HJ, Kugel H, Roth B, Heindel W. Quantitative measurements with localized 1 H MR spectroscopy in children with Canavan's disease. J Magn Reson Imaging. 1996;6(6):889–93.
22. Engelbrecht V, Rassek M, Gartner J, Kahn T, Modder U. Magnetic resonance tomography and localized proton spectroscopy in 2 siblings with Canavan's disease. Rofo. 1995;163(3):238–44.
23. Toft PB, Geiss-Holtorff R, Rolland MO, et al. Magnetic resonance imaging in juvenile Canavan disease. Eur J Pediatr. 1993;152(9):750–3.
24. Leegwater PA, Vermeulen G, Konst AA, et al. Subunits of the translation initiation factor eIF2B are mutant in leukoencephalopathy with vanishing white matter. Nat Genet. 2001;29(4):383–8.
25. van der Knaap MS, Leegwater PA, Konst AA, et al. Mutations in each of the five subunits of translation initiation factor eIF2B can cause leukoencephalopathy with vanishing white matter. Ann Neurol. 2002;51(2):264–70.
26. van der Knaap MS, Breiter SN, Naidu S, Hart AA, Valk J. Defining and categorizing leukoencephalopathies of unknown origin: MR imaging approach. Radiology. 1999;213(1):121–33.
27. van der Knaap MS, Pronk JC, Scheper GC. Vanishing white matter disease. Lancet Neurol. 2006;5(5):413–23.
28. Pronk JC, van Kollenburg B, Scheper GC, van der Knaap MS. Vanishing white matter disease: a review with focus on its genetics. Ment Retard Dev Disabil Res Rev. 2006;12(2):123–8.
29. Bugiani M, Boor I, Powers JM, Scheper GC, van der Knaap MS. Leukoencephalopathy with Vanishing White Matter: A Review. J Neuropathol Exp Neurol. 2010;69(10):987–96.
30. Van Haren K, van der Voorn JP, Peterson DR, van der Knaap MS, Powers JM. The life and death of oligodendrocytes in vanishing white matter disease. J Neuropathol Exp Neurol. 2004;63(6):618–30.
31. van der Knaap MS, Barth PG, Gabreels FJ, et al. A new leukoencephalopathy with vanishing white matter. Neurology. 1997; 48(4):845–55.
32. van der Knaap MS, Kamphorst W, Barth PG, Kraaijeveld CL, Gut E, Valk J. Phenotypic variation in leukoencephalopathy with vanishing white matter. Neurology. 1998;51(2):540–7.
33. Schiffmann R, Moller JR, Trapp BD, et al. Childhood ataxia with diffuse central nervous system hypomyelination. Ann Neurol. 1994;35(3):331–40.
34. Tedeschi G, Schiffmann R, Barton NW, et al. Proton magnetic resonance spectroscopic imaging in childhood ataxia with diffuse central nervous system hypomyelination. Neurology. 1995;45(8):1526–32.
35. Dreha-Kulaczewski SF, Dechent P, Finsterbusch J, et al. Early reduction of total N-acetyl-aspartate-compounds in patients with classical vanishing white matter disease. A long-term follow-up MRS study. Pediatr Res. 2008;63(4):444–9.
36. Hanefeld F, Holzbach U, Kruse B, Wilichowski E, Christen HJ, Frahm J. Diffuse white matter disease in three children: an encephalopathy with unique features on magnetic resonance imaging and proton magnetic resonance spectroscopy. Neuropediatrics. 1993;24(5):244–8.
37. Scheper GC, van der Klok T, van Andel RJ, et al. Mitochondrial aspartyl-tRNA synthetase deficiency causes leukoencephalopathy with brain stem and spinal cord involvement and lactate elevation. Nat Genet. 2007;39(4):534–9.
38. van der Knaap MS, van der Voorn P, Barkhof F, et al. A new leukoencephalopathy with brainstem and spinal cord involvement and high lactate. Ann Neurol. 2003;53(2):252–8.
39. Labauge P, Dorboz I, Eymard-Pierre E, Dereeper O, Boespflug-Tanguy O. Clinically asymptomatic adult patient with extensive LBSL MRI pattern and DARS2 mutation. J Neurol. 2010;258:335–7. doi:10.1007/s00415-010-5755-5.
40. Labauge P, Roullet E, Boespflug-Tanguy O, et al. Familial, adult onset form of leukoencephalopathy with brain stem and spinal cord involvement: inconstant high brain lactate and very slow disease progression. Eur Neurol. 2007;58(1):59–61.
41. Petzold GC, Bohner G, Klingebiel R, Amberger N, van der Knaap MS, Zschenderlein R. Adult onset leucoencephalopathy with brain stem and spinal cord involvement and normal lactate. J Neurol Neurosurg Psychiatry. 2006;77(7):889–91.
42. Uluc K, Baskan O, Yildirim KA, et al. Leukoencephalopathy with brain stem and spinal cord involvement and high lactate: a genetically proven case with distinct MRI findings. J Neurol Sci. 2008;273(1–2):118–22.
43. Tavora DG, Nakayama M, Gama RL, Alvim TC, Portugal D, Comerlato EA. Leukoencephalopathy with brainstem and spinal cord involvement and high brain lactate: report of three Brazilian patients. Arq Neuropsiquiatr. 2007;65(2):506–11.
44. Linnankivi T, Lundbom N, Autti T, et al. Five new cases of a recently described leukoencephalopathy with high brain lactate. Neurology. 2004;63(4):688–92.
45. Serkov SV, Pronin IN, Bykova OV, et al. Five patients with a recently described novel leukoencephalopathy with brainstem and spinal cord involvement and elevated lactate. Neuropediatrics. 2004;35(1):1–5.
46. Boor PK, de Groot K, Waisfisz Q, et al. MLC1: a novel protein in distal astroglial processes. J Neuropathol Exp Neurol. 2005;64(5):412–9.
47. Blattner R, Von Moers A, Leegwater PA, Hanefeld FA, Van Der Knaap MS, Kohler W. Clinical and genetic heterogeneity in megalencephalic leukoencephalopathy with subcortical cysts (MLC). Neuropediatrics. 2003;34(4):215–8.
48. Patrono C, Di Giacinto G, Eymard-Pierre E, et al. Genetic heterogeneity of megalencephalic leukoencephalopathy and subcortical cysts. Neurology. 2003;61(4):534–7.
49. van der Knaap MS, Lai V, Kohler W, et al. Megalencephalic leukoencephalopathy with cysts without MLC1 defect. Ann Neurol. 2010;67(6):834–7.
50. van der Knaap MS, Barth PG, Stroink H, et al. Leukoencephalopathy with swelling and a discrepantly mild clinical course in eight children. Ann Neurol. 1995;37(3):324–34.
51. Leegwater PA, Boor PK, Yuan BQ, et al. Identification of novel mutations in MLC1 responsible for megalencephalic leukoencephalopathy with subcortical cysts. Hum Genet. 2002;110(3):279–83.
52. Brockmann K, Finsterbusch J, Terwey B, Frahm J, Hanefeld F. Megalencephalic leukoencephalopathy with subcortical cysts in an adult: quantitative proton MR spectroscopy and diffusion tensor MRI. Neuroradiology. 2003;45(3):137–42.
53. Hudson LD, Puckett C, Berndt J, Chan J, Gencic S. Mutation of the proteolipid protein gene PLP in a human X chromosome-linked myelin disorder. Proc Natl Acad Sci USA. 1989;86(20):8128–31.

54. Gencic S, Abuelo D, Ambler M, Hudson LD. Pelizaeus-Merzbacher disease: an X-linked neurologic disorder of myelin metabolism with a novel mutation in the gene encoding proteolipid protein. Am J Hum Genet. 1989;45(3):435–42.
55. Garbern JY, Hobson GM. PLP1-Related Disorders. In: Pagon RA, Bird TC, Dolan CR, Stephens K, eds. GeneReviews [Internet]. Seattle: University of Washington; 1999 [updated 2010 Mar 16].
56. Hanefeld FA, Brockmann K, Pouwels PJ, Wilken B, Frahm J, Dechent P. Quantitative proton MRS of Pelizaeus-Merzbacher disease: evidence of dys- and hypomyelination. Neurology. 2005;65(5):701–6.
57. Provencher SW. Automatic quantitation of localized in vivo 1 H spectra with LCModel. NMR Biomed. 2001;14(4):260–4.
58. Provencher SW. Estimation of metabolite concentrations from localized in vivo proton NMR spectra. Magn Reson Med. 1993;30(6):672–9.
59. Takanashi J, Inoue K, Tomita M, et al. Brain N-acetylaspartate is elevated in Pelizaeus-Merzbacher disease with PLP1 duplication. Neurology. 2002;58(2):237–41.
60. Bonavita S, Schiffmann R, Moore DF, et al. Evidence for neuroaxonal injury in patients with proteolipid protein gene mutations. Neurology. 2001;56(6):785–8.
61. Pizzini F, Fatemi AS, Barker PB, et al. Proton MR spectroscopic imaging in Pelizaeus-Merzbacher disease. AJNR Am J Neuroradiol. 2003;24(8):1683–9.
62. Garbern JY, Yool DA, Moore GJ, et al. Patients lacking the major CNS myelin protein, proteolipid protein 1, develop length-dependent axonal degeneration in the absence of demyelination and inflammation. Brain. 2002;125(Pt 3):551–61.
63. Mochel F, Boildieu N, Barritault J, et al. Elevated CSF N-acetylaspartylglutamate suggests specific molecular diagnostic abnormalities in patients with white matter diseases. Biochim Biophys Acta. 2010;1802(11):1112–7.
64. Mochel F, Engelke UF, Barritault J, et al. Elevated CSF N-acetylaspartylglutamate in patients with free sialic acid storage diseases. Neurology. 2010;74(4):302–5.
65. Valk J, van der Knaap MS. Selective vulnerability in toxic encephalopathies and metabolic disorder. Riv Neuroradiol. 1996;9:749–60.
66. De Stefano N, Dotti MT, Mortilla M, Federico A. Magnetic resonance imaging and spectroscopic changes in brains of patients with cerebrotendinous xanthomatosis. Brain. 2001;124(Pt 1):121–31.
67. Kumar V, Abbas AK, Fausto N. Robbins and Cotran pathologic basis of disease. 7th ed. Philadelphia: Elsevier Saunders; 2005.
68. Brockmann K, Dechent P, Wilken B, Rusch O, Frahm J, Hanefeld F. Proton MRS profile of cerebral metabolic abnormalities in Krabbe disease. Neurology. 2003;60(5):819–25.
69. Kruse B, Hanefeld F, Christen HJ, et al. Alterations of brain metabolites in metachromatic leukodystrophy as detected by localized proton magnetic resonance spectroscopy in vivo. J Neurol. 1993;241(2):68–74.
70. Bruhn H, Kruse B, Korenke GC, et al. Proton NMR spectroscopy of cerebral metabolic alterations in infantile peroxisomal disorders. J Comput Assist Tomogr. 1992;16(3):335–44.
71. Confort-Gouny S, Vion-Dury J, Chabrol B, Nicoli F, Cozzone PJ. Localised proton magnetic resonance spectroscopy in X-linked adrenoleukodystrophy. Neuroradiology. 1995;37(7):568–75.
72. Eichler FS, Barker PB, Cox C, et al. Proton MR spectroscopic imaging predicts lesion progression on MRI in X-linked adrenoleukodystrophy. Neurology. 2002;58(6):901–7.
73. Eichler FS, Itoh R, Barker PB, et al. Proton MR spectroscopic and diffusion tensor brain MR imaging in X-linked adrenoleukodystrophy: initial experience. Radiology. 2002;225(1):245–52.
74. Izquierdo M, Adamsbaum C, Benosman A, Aubourg P, Bittoun J. MR spectroscopic imaging of normal-appearing white matter in adrenoleukodystrophy. Pediatr Radiol. 2000;30(9):621–9.
75. Korenke GC, Pouwels PJ, Frahm J, et al. Arrested cerebral adrenoleukodystrophy: a clinical and proton magnetic resonance spectroscopy study in three patients. Pediatr Neurol. 1996;15(2):103–7.
76. Kruse B, Barker PB, van Zijl PC, Duyn JH, Moonen CT, Moser HW. Multislice proton magnetic resonance spectroscopic imaging in X-linked adrenoleukodystrophy. Ann Neurol. 1994;36(4):595–608.
77. Liang JS, Lee WT, Hwu WL, et al. Adrenoleukodystrophy: clinical analysis of 9 Taiwanese children. Acta Paediatr Taiwan. 2004;45(5):272–7.
78. Moser HW, Barker PB. Magnetic resonance spectroscopy: a new guide for the therapy of adrenoleukodystrophy. Neurology. 2005;64(3):406–7.
79. Oz G, Tkac I, Charnas LR, et al. Assessment of adrenoleukodystrophy lesions by high field MRS in non-sedated pediatric patients. Neurology. 2005;64(3):434–41.
80. Pouwels PJ, Kruse B, Korenke GC, Mao X, Hanefeld FA, Frahm J. Quantitative proton magnetic resonance spectroscopy of childhood adrenoleukodystrophy. Neuropediatrics. 1998;29(5):254–64.
81. Rajanayagam V, Balthazor M, Shapiro EG, Krivit W, Lockman L, Stillman AE. Proton MR spectroscopy and neuropsychological testing in adrenoleukodystrophy. AJNR Am J Neuroradiol. 1997;18(10):1909–14.
82. Rajanayagam V, Grad J, Krivit W, et al. Proton MR spectroscopy of childhood adrenoleukodystrophy. AJNR Am J Neuroradiol. 1996;17(6):1013–24.
83. Salvan AM, Confort-Gouny S, Chabrol B, Cozzone PJ, Vion-Dury J. Brain metabolic impairment in non-cerebral and cerebral forms of X-linked adrenoleukodystrophy by proton MRS: identification of metabolic patterns by discriminant analysis. Magn Reson Med. 1999;41(6):1119–26.
84. Tourbah A, Stievenart JL, Iba-Zizen MT, et al. Localized proton magnetic resonance spectroscopy in patients with adult adrenoleukodystrophy. Increase of choline compounds in normal appearing white matter. Arch Neurol. 1997;54(5):586–92.
85. Tzika AA, Ball Jr WS, Vigneron DB, Dunn RS, Kirks DR. Clinical proton MR spectroscopy of neurodegenerative disease in childhood. AJNR Am J Neuroradiol. 1993;14(6):1267–81.
86. Tzika AA, Ball Jr WS, Vigneron DB, Dunn RS, Nelson SJ, Kirks DR. Childhood adrenoleukodystrophy: assessment with proton MR spectroscopy. Radiology. 1993;189(2):467–80.
87. Wilken B, Dechent P, Brockmann K, et al. Quantitative proton magnetic resonance spectroscopy of children with adrenoleukodystrophy before and after hematopoietic stem cell transplantation. Neuropediatrics. 2003;34(5):237–46.
88. Ratai E, Kok T, Wiggins C, et al. Seven-Tesla proton magnetic resonance spectroscopic imaging in adult X-linked adrenoleukodystrophy. Arch Neurol. 2008;65(11):1488–94.
89. Bonkowsky JL, Nelson C, Kingston JL, Filloux FM, Mundorff MB, Srivastava R. The burden of inherited leukodystrophies in children. Neurology. 2010;75(8):718–25.

Metabolic Disorders

11

Kim M. Cecil and Diana M. Lindquist

Magnetic resonance spectroscopy (MRS) provides a powerful tool in narrowing the differential diagnosis in pediatric brain disorders. The foremost utility of MRS should be the recognition of metabolic disorders, especially within the context of early detection, as the specificity of imaging is limited until macroscopic structural changes have occurred. Unfortunately, the literature provides only a limited number of case reports and small patient series employing MRS in the diagnosis and monitoring of metabolic diseases. This is likely because many metabolic disorders are rare, and tend to present during childhood as well as the inherent limitations of MRS, which include the ability to only primarily detect cellular events (neuronal dysfunction, lactic acidemia abnormal myelination, gliosis, etc.) and low signal to noise ratio (SNR). This chapter will describe diseases such as lysosomal storage diseases, mitochondrial disorders, amino acidurias, organic acidurias, urea cycle defects, creatine disorders, and other miscellaneous metabolic disorders. Table 11.1 provides a succinct yet fairly comprehensive summary of the disease features. The goal of the chapter is to introduce the reader to the defect, its genetic origins, common symptoms, treatment options, and findings upon magnetic resonance imaging (MRI) and spectroscopy with an emphasis on the pediatric population. Very few disorders or diseases have an MRS profile that is disease specific. Most disorders require integration of clinical symptoms, family histories, laboratory (metabolic and molecular) test results, MRI interpretation and the now more commonly acquired MRS results to formulate disease diagnosis. Understanding the role that MRS can provide will facilitate patient care and ultimately improve our collective knowledge of pediatric metabolic brain disorders.

K.M. Cecil, Ph.D. (✉)
Departments of Radiology, Pediatrics, Neuroscience and Environmental Health, Cincinnati Children's Hospital Medical Center, University of Cincinnati College of Medicine, Cincinnati, OH, USA
e-mail: kim.cecil@chmcc.org

D.M. Lindquist Ph.D.
Departments of Radiology, Cincinnati Children's Hospital Medical Center, University of Cincinnati College of Medicine, Cincinnati, OH, USA

Lysosomal Storage Diseases

Many neurodegenerative diseases are characterized by the accumulation of nondegradable molecules in cells or at extracellular sites in the brain. One such class of diseases is the lysosomal storage disorders, which arise from defects in lysosomal function. The lysosomes are intracellular organelles responsible for degrading lipids, proteins, and complex carbohydrates. For many lysosomal disorders, the genetic mutation resulting in the absence or partial deficiency of an enzyme or protein is known and functionally understood. For most of the lysosomal diseases, the substrate for the defective enzyme builds up to produce intra-lysosomal storage. While the diseases are complex, mechanical disruption of the cell due to the storage of undegradable material leads to cellular dysfunction. In general, the pathology primarily involves neuronal dysfunction rather than loss, with the exception of differential loss of Purkinje cells that characterize several storage diseases, including Niemann-Pick disease type C (NPC) and the massive cell loss that occurs in the neuronal ceroid lipofuscinoses (NCL). Unknown is whether the storage material affects cellular function only when it begins to accumulate in extra-lysosomal sites or if problems in cell homeostasis are triggered while the material is still confined to the lysosome.

Lysosomal disorders are typically inherited as autosomal recessive traits, usually afflict infants and young children, involve brain pathology and are untreatable. However, adult-onset forms do exist. The collective frequency of lysosomal storage diseases is estimated to be approximately 1 in 8,000 live births, with some occurring at high frequency in select populations. The common biochemical hallmark of these diseases is the storage of macromolecules in the lysosome.

Lysosomal disorders primarily impacting gray matter include the neuronal ceroid lipofuciscinoses, gangliosidoses, and mucopolysaccharidoses. Two of the more common lysosomal disorders, metachromatic leukodystrophy and Krabbe's disease, demonstrate abnormalities in white matter as described in this book's chapter on leukodystrophies.

S. Blüml and A. Panigrahy (eds.), *MR Spectroscopy of Pediatric Brain Disorders*,
DOI 10.1007/978-1-4419-5864-8_11,

Table 11.1 Summary of features of metabolic disorders

General classification	Disorder	Gene Name; abbreviation (locus)	OMIM	Mode of inheritance	Primary defect	Metabolic consequence	Key features of brain proton MRS: early stages
Amino aciduria	Non-ketotic hyperglycinemia	Multiple genes AMT 3p21.31, GCSH 16q23.2, GLDC 9p24.1	605899	Autosomal-recessive	Defective mitochondrial enzyme involved in glycine cleavage	Elevated glycine	Elevated glycine
Amino Aciduria	Phenylketonuria	Phenylalanine hydroxylase (PAH); (12q23.2)	261600	Autosomal-recessive	Phenylalanine hydroxylase deficiency	Hyperphenyl-alaninemia; Phenylpyruvic acidemia	Elevated phenylalanine
Lysosomal	Neuronal Ceroid Lipofuscinosis	CLN3(16p11.2)	204200	Autosomal-recessive	Defects involve lysosomal function	Lipopigment in extraneu-ronal cells	Decreased NAA, elevated mI
Lysosomal	Niemann Pick type C	NPC 1 18q11.2	257220	Autosomal-recessive	Defective cholesterol esterification due to a deficiency of sphingomyelinase	Abnormal Cholesterol Homeostasis	Elevated lipid, Cho/Cr; diminished NAA/Cr
Lysosomal	Salla Disease	SLC17A5 6q13	604369	Autosomal-recessive	Defect in sialic acid transport at the lysosomal membrane	Elevated *N*-acetyl-neuraminic acid	Increased N-acetyl compounds, creatine with decreased choline
Lysosomal	Sandhoff's disease	hexosaminidase; HEXB 5q13.3	268800	Autosomal-recessive	Defect in beta subunit of hexosaminidase A and B isoenzymes	Accumulation of GM2 gangliosides	Decreased NAA, elevated mI
Lysosomal	Sjorgren-Larsson Syndrome	Fatty aldehyde dehydroge-nase (17p11.2)	270200	Autosomal-recessive	Fatty alcohol oxidation failure	Elevated free fatty alcohols	Increased lipid (fatty alcohol) resonance; elevated Cr, Cho, mI associated with myelin abnormalities
Lysosomal	Tay-Sach's	Hexosaminidase A; HEXA 15q23	272800	Autosomal-recessive	Defect in alpha subunit of hexosaminidase A	GM2 ganglioside accumulation	Ballooned neurons-decreased NAA
Mitochondrial	Pyruvate Decarboxylase Deficiency	E1-alpha polypeptide of Pyruvate Dehydrogenase; PDHA1 (Xp22.12)	312170	X-linked	Defect in first of 3 enzymes in PDH-glycolysis and TCA cycle	Elevated lactate, pyruvate, ammonia, alanine	Elevated lactate
Mitochondrial	Pyruvate Dehydrogenase deficiency	Multiple genes of the Pyruvate Dehydrogenase complex	Multiple	Multiple	Defect in enzymes coupling glycolysis and TCA cycle for conversion of pyruvate to acetyl-CoA	Elevated lactate, pyruvate, ammonia, alanine	Elevated lactate
Organic aciduria	Glutaric Aciduria	Type I - glutaryl-CoA-dehydrogenase; GCDH(19p13.2)	231670	Autosomal-recessive	Enzyme deficiency altering metabolism of lysine, hydroxylysine, tryptophan	Elevation of glutaric acid, hypoglycemia	Decreased NAA/Cr, elevated Cho/Cr, mI/Cr
Organic aciduria	Glutaric Aciduria	Type II- multiple acyl CoA dehydrogenase genes;4q32.1, 15q24.2-q24.3, 19q13.41	231680	Autosomal-recessive	Disorder of fatty acid, amino acid and choline metabolism	Elevation of glutaric acid, lactic ethylmalonic, butyric, isobutyric, 2-methyl-butyric and isovaleric acids	no prior studies
Organic aciduria	L-Hydroxyglutaric Aciduria	L2HGDH (14q21.3)	236792	Autosomal-recessive	Toxicity of L-2-hydroxy glutarate	Elevation of L-2-hydroxyglutaric acid and lysine	Decreased NAA, Cho and elevated mI

Organic aciduria	Maple Syrup Urine Disease	Mutations in the catalytic subunit genes of the branched chain alpha keto acid dehydrogenase complex; BCKD (19q13.2, 7q31.1, 6q14.1, 1p21.2)	248600	Autosomal-recessive	Defect in the genes of the branched chain alpha keto acid dehydrogenase blocking oxidative decarboxylation	Elevation of branched-chain amino acids, leucine, isoleucine & valine	Elevated resonances in lipid/lactate range, Cho, mI and diminished NAA
Organic Aciduria	Methylmalonic Aciduria	methylmalonyl-CoA mutase; MUT (6p12.3)	251000	Autosomal-recessive	Defect in methylmalonyl-CoA mutase; disorder of methylmalonate and cobalamin metabolism	Elevation of methyl malonic acid, glycine, ammonia; ketoacidosis, low carnitine	Decreased NAA, mI; elevated GLX, lactate
Organic Aciduria	Proprionic Aciduria	Proprionic-CoA carboxylase; PCCA (13q32.3), PCCB (3q22.3)	232050	Autosomal-recessive	Defect in proprionic-CoA carboxylase	Elevated proprionic acid, glycine	Decreased NAA, mI; elevated GLX, lactate
Urea Cycle	Argininemia (Arginase Deficiency)	arginase; ARG1(6q23.2)	207800	Autosomal-recessive	Defect encoding enzyme-ARG1	Elevated ammonia, arginine & other amino acids	Elevated glutamine; possible elevation mI and lactate
Urea Cycle	Argininosuccinate lysase Deficiency	argininosuccinate lyase; ASL(7q11.21)	207900	Autosomal-recessive	Defect encoding enzyme-ASL	Elevated ammonia, glutamine, & plasma citrulline	Elevated glutamine; possible elevation mI and lactate
Urea Cycle	Carbamoyl Phosphate Synthetase I Deficiency	carbamoyl phosphate synthetase I; CPS1(2q34)	237300	Autosomal-recessive	Defect encoding enzyme-CPS 1 enzyme deficiency-Catalyzes first committed step in the urea cycle	Elevated ammonia; low plasma citrulline, arginine, & urinary orotic acid	Elevated glutamine; possible elevation mI and lactate
Urea Cycle	Citrullinemia, Classic (Argininosuccinate Synthetase Deficiency)	argininosuccinate synthetase; ASS(9q34.11)	215700	Autosomal-recessive	Gene defect encoding enzyme-ASS	Elevated ammonia, glutamine, plasma citrulline	Elevated glutamine; possible elevation mI and lactate
Urea Cycle	Ornithine Transcarbamylase Deficiency	ornithine carbamoyltransferase; OTC(Xp11.4)	311250	X-linked recessive	Gene defect encoding enzyme-OTC	Elevated ammonia, glutamine, & urinary orotic acid; low plasma citrulline	Elevated glutamine; possible elevation mI and lactate
Miscellaneous	Creatine Deficiency-Arginine:Glycine Amidinotransferase Deficiency	GATM (15q21.1)	602360	Autosomal-recessive	Creatine Synthesis impaired	Creatine deficient in brain, blood, urine, muscle; No accumulation of precursors	Diffuse Creatine deficiency
Miscellaneous	Creatine Deficiency-Creatine Transporter Defect	SLC6A8 (Xq28)	300352 300036	X-linked	Creatine transport impaired to the brain	Creatine elevated in blood, urine & CSF yet absent from brain	Diffuse Creatine deficiency
Miscellaneous	Creatine Deficiency-Guanidinoacetate Methyltransferase Deficiency	GAMT (19p13.3)	601240	Autosomal-recessive	Creatine Synthesis impaired	Creatine deficient in brain, blood, urine, muscle; Accumulate GAA	Diffuse Creatine deficiency; GAA elevation
Miscellaneous	Galactosemia	GALT (9p13.3)	230400	Autosomal-recessive	defect encoding galactose-1-phosphate uridyltransferase	Elevated galactitol	Elevated galactitol when untreated
Miscellaneous	Wilson Disease	ATP7B(13q14.3)	277900	Autosomal-recessive	defect in copper transport	Elevated intracellular copper	Hepatic disease features: decreased Cho, mI

However, broader involvement of gray and white matter often occurs in later stages of lysosomal disease progression. The following sections discuss several lysosomal storage disorders with published reports employing MRS.

Neuronal Ceroid Lipofuscinosis

NCL, one of the most common neurodegenerative syndromes, is a disorder or group of disorders characterized by striking volume loss of brain parenchyma. NCL can be divided into six subtypes based upon age at onset. The various subtypes are associated with different mutations in the *CLN* genes, and have similar clinical manifestations occurring at different ages. These include seizures and abnormal eye movements, with subsequent vision loss, dementia, hypotonia, speech and motor deficits. Upon pathology, these disorders are characterized by distinctive granular inclusions in neuronal lysosomes, referred to as granular osmiophilic deposits. Imaging findings lag behind the clinical presentation in all subtypes, with the exception of the infantile form of NCL, and feature progressive cerebral and cerebellar volume loss. Later disease stages are characterized by development of a band of hyperintense signal in the periventricular white matter on T2-weighted images. Proton MRS has shown progressive decreases in *N*-acetyl aspartate (NAA) and relative increases in myo-inositol (mI) in NCL. An example from a 9-month-old patient with NCL is demonstrated in Fig. 11.1.

Confort-Gouny et al. reported MRS findings from the basal ganglia of a 4-year-old patient with infantile NCL demonstrating an unusual increase of mI and taurine levels with a reduction of NAA [1]. The patient demonstrated extensive cerebral atrophy. Brockmann et al. described a series of five patients with NCL using proton MRS [2]. Juvenile NCL demonstrated normal metabolite levels, while infantile NCL was characterized by a complete loss of NAA, marked reductions of creatine (Cr) and cholines (Cho), and increases of mI and lactate in both gray and white matter. Reduced NAA and elevated lactate were also detected in gray and white matter of late-infantile NCL; however, in this case, not only mI but also Cr and Cho were increased in white matter. Sietz et al. sampled predominately parietal lobe white matter in three patients with late-infantile NCL and compared the findings with healthy control participants [3]. Again, reduced NAA with elevated mI levels relative to Cr were reported. Vanhanen et al. examined eight infantile patients with MRI, MRS acquired in the thalamus and parietal-occipital white matter, and perfusion single photon emission computed tomography [4]. The disease presentations varied from preclinical to late stage. While not specific for infantile NCL, MRS revealed cerebral abnormalities before symptoms, structural changes or blood flow changes appeared in the patients. Patients between 3 and 5 months of age, classified as stage 0, demonstrated reduced NAA and elevated Cho levels to Cr. By 17 months, classified as stage 2, decreased NAA and

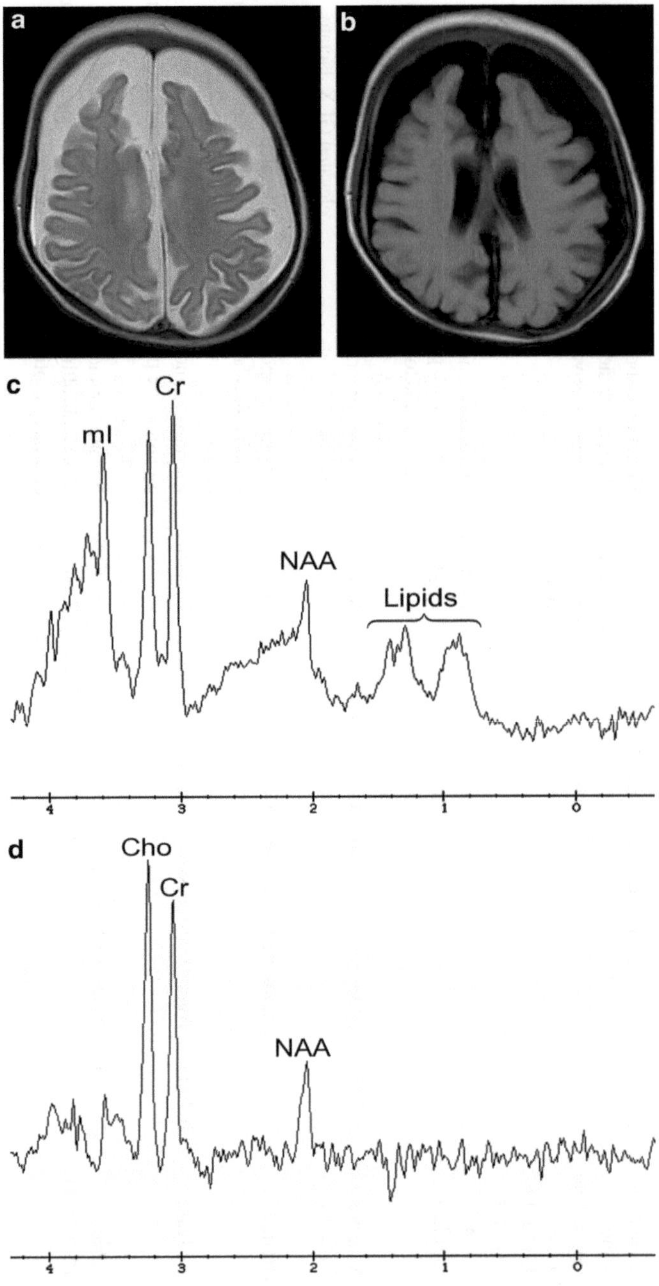

Fig. 11.1 Figures from a 9-month-old twin male followed for a neuropathic form of osteopetrosis who presented with MRI and MRS findings consistent with neuronal ceroid lipofuscinosis. (**a**) Axial T2-weighted image reveals hyperintense signal from CSF-associated supratentorial volume loss; (**b**) Axial FLAIR image confirming volume loss and CSF signal; (**c**) Short echo (35 ms), and (**d**) Intermediate echo (144 ms) MR spectra sampling within the right parietal lobe demonstrate reduced NAA, with elevations of lipids and mI/Cr

Cho were accompanied by increased mI in the thalamus and parietal white matter. By Stage 4, NAA and Cho levels declined significantly with lipids, lactate and mI increased. Reduction of NAA in the thalamus and white matter was thought to reflect neuroaxonal damage or possibly changes in the function of the remaining cells. As Cho mainly represents structural components of the cell membrane, especially myelin sheaths in white matter, an increase of Cho and Cho/Cr reflected demyelination. High Cho and increasing mI indicated progression of demyelination with glial proliferation. Increased levels of mI, lipids, and lactate also indicated gliosis, cell loss and abnormal anaerobic metabolism of the macrophages, and possibly, atrophic thalamic astrocytes filled with abnormal storage material [4]. At the latest stage, the spectrum was dominated by the lipid signals, which could serve as markers of myelin breakdown product. The complete absence of NAA, barely detectable Cho and Cr, and relatively high mI and lipids indicated almost complete neuroaxonal loss, ongoing demyelination, and gliosis.

Sitter et al., employing principal component analysis of ex vivo spectra obtained from infantile NCL autopsy brain tissue found decreased NAA, gamma amino butyric acid (GABA), glutamate and glutamine with increased mI. Ex vivo spectra obtained from juvenile NCL autopsy brain tissue did not differ from controls [5].

Niemann Pick Type C (NPC)

NPC is an autosomal-recessive, neurovisceral, lysosomal lipid storage disorder that results from defective cholesterol esterification and is associated with impaired intracellular lipid trafficking leading to accumulation of cholesterol and glycosphingolipids in the brain, the liver, the spleen, and lung. It is estimated to occur with a minimal incidence of 1 in 120,000 live births [6]. NPC has a very heterogeneous clinical presentation from a neonatal rapidly fatal disorder to an adult-onset chronic neurodegenerative disease. The initial presentation is visceral, with systemic signs of cholestatic jaundice in the neonatal period. Presentation during infancy or childhood can feature isolated splenomegaly or hepatosplenomegaly. In the early-infantile, late-infantile and juvenile period, a wide range of nonspecific and progressive neurologic symptoms varies according to the age at onset. The first neurologic symptoms may include delay in developmental motor milestones (early infantile period), falls, clumsiness, cataplexy, and academic difficulties (late infantile and juvenile period). Seizures, dysarthria, dysphagia, ataxia, and psychiatric disturbances can occur within the disease course. The most characteristic sign is vertical supranuclear gaze palsy. The prognosis largely correlates with the age at onset of the neurological manifestations. NPC is transmitted in an autosomal recessive manner and is caused by mutations of either the *NPC1* (95% of families) or the *NPC2* genes. Confirmation of the diagnosis requires molecular genetic testing of *NPC1* and *NPC2* genes from living skin fibroblasts to demonstrate accumulation of unesterified cholesterol in perinuclear vesicles (lysosomes) after staining with filipin [6]. NPC is currently described as a cellular cholesterol trafficking defect, but in the brain, the prominently stored lipids are gangliosides.

Tedeschi et al. evaluated ten patients with NPC using proton spectroscopic imaging (MRSI) and compared the findings with those obtained from 15 healthy controls [7]. NAA/Cr levels were significantly decreased in the frontal and parietal cortices, centrum semiovale, and caudate nucleus. Cho/Cr levels were significantly increased in the frontal cortex and centrum semiovale. Significant correlations were found between clinical staging scale scores and MRSI abnormalities.

Cholesterol-lowering agents effectively decrease *hepatic* lipids in NPC patients. Sylvain et al. described the effects of such agents on *neurologic features* using proton MRS in a 9-month-old boy with progressive hepatosplenomegaly and neurodevelopmental delay [8]. MRS acquired within a supraventricular volume of central white and gray matter revealed an abnormal lipid signal. The patient was treated with cholesterol-lowering agents (i.e., cholestyramine, lovastatin). Repeat standardized neurodevelopmental assessments (Peabody and Griffith scales) at 13 and 19 months were normal. The MRS no longer detected the previously observed abnormally elevated lipid resonance.

Miglustat (*N*-butyl-deoxynojirimycin), an inhibitor of glycosphingolipid synthesis, has been approved to treat patients in the USA and Europe, but questions remain regarding its efficacy. Galanaud et al. acquired proton MRS in three locations (centrum semiovale, basal ganglia, and cerebellum) for three adults with NPC treated with Miglustat for 24 months [9]. All patients reported mild clinical improvement or stabilization. With multiple timepoints assessed, the Cho/Cr levels within the parietal white matter (centrum semiovale) were observed in all three patients to decrease over time. Although these results were preliminary, there was evidence that Miglustat had some beneficial effect on brain dysfunction in NPC.

Salla Disease

Mutations in the *SLC17A5* gene encoding the lysosomal transport protein, sialin, result in defective free sialic acid transport out of lysosomes. The resulting increased lysosomal storage of free sialic acid produces a neurodegenerative disorder with varying phenotypes: Salla Disease, Intermediate-severe Salla disease or Infantile free sialic acid storage disease.

Salla disease, the mildest phenotype, is characterized by normal appearance and neurologic findings at birth followed by slowly progressive neurologic deterioration resulting in mild-to-moderate psychomotor retardation, spasticity, athetosis, and epileptic seizures. Varho et al. examined eight pediatric and adult patients with Salla disease using quantitative single voxel MRS [10]. The study found 34% higher NAA, 47% higher Cr, and 35% lower Cho concentrations in the parietal white matter and 53% higher Cr in the basal ganglia of patients with Salla disease compared with the age-matched control subjects. The patients had 22% higher water content in their parietal white matter, whereas in the basal ganglia, the water concentrations did not differ significantly. The authors attributed the high NAA signal from accumulated lysosomal *N*-acetylneuraminic acid, which offsets the possible loss of NAA. The high Cr agrees with an increased glucose uptake found in their earlier 2-fluoro-2-deoxy-D-glucose-positron emission tomography study, reflecting increased energy demand [11].

Gangliosidoses

Gangliosides are glycolipids within the central nervous system (CNS), which are key components of the neuronal cell membranes and myelin, and are responsible in part for cellular recognition and communication. The gangliosidoses are divided into two groups referred to as the GM_1 and GM_2. In GM_1, the primary enzyme deficiency is that of β-galactosidase. For GM_2 an abnormal accumulation of gangliosides results from a hexosaminidase deficiency. The most common forms of *GM2* gangliosidoses are autosomal recessive and include Tay-Sachs disease and Sandoff disease. Affected individuals undergo progressive neurodegeneration in response to the glycosphingolipid storage.

Tay-Sachs Disease

Tay-Sachs disease arises with β–*N*-acetylhexosaminidase-A isoenzyme deficiency (*HEXA*, chromosomal locus 15q23-q24). Several phenotypes exist depending on age at presentation (acute infantile, juvenile, chronic, and adult-onset) and activity of hexosaminidase A. Infantile onset occurs usually before 6 months of age and typically includes developmental regression, especially motor skills, weakness, increased startle response, decreased attentiveness, blindness, and bilateral cherry-red spots on the macula in 90% of patients, but may also feature irritability, hypotonia, myoclonic seizures, and macrocephaly. Death usually results by 3 years of age. Juvenile Tay-Sachs can begin between 2 and 10 years of age. Symptoms manifest as ataxia, loss of coordination, cognitive decline, with seizures and spasticity by the end of the first decade of life. By 15 years, patients are usually in a vegetative state. Although this disease is often associated with Ashkenazi Jewish heritage, Tay-Sachs disease has been reported in all ethnic, racial, and religious groups. Populations that are relatively isolated genetically have been found to carry HEXA mutations. Carrier screening programs in persons with Ashkenazi Jewish heritage in North America have reduced the incidence of the disease by over 90% [12, 13].

Aydin et al. employed MRI with MRS within the basal ganglia three children aged 10, 20, and 21 months diagnosed with Tay-Sachs disease [14]. On T2-weighted MR images, abnormal hyperintense signal changes in the basal ganglia and cerebral white matter were appreciated. Compared with healthy controls, an increase in mI/Cr and Cho/Cr levels was found with a decrease in the NAA/Cr level.

Imamura et al. reported the clinical findings and proton MRS of 4-year-old monozygotic female twins with a mild presentation of early onset Tay-Sachs disease [15]. The young twins demonstrated similar, slowly progressive clinical symptoms and deterioration; however, the younger sister also demonstrated intractable myoclonus in the right leg. Serial MR images showed abnormal hyperintensity on T2-weighted images in bilateral white matter, but no signal changes in the basal ganglia and thalamus during any of the phases of the disease. NAA/Cr levels were decreased in the both white matter lesions and the basal ganglia, with elevated mI/Cr levels in regions of signal abnormality. An elevated resonance, described as lactate, was appreciated in the basal ganglia of the younger twin with myoclonus; however, its appearance is more suggestive of lipids with an uncertain lactate contribution. These features would be consistent with a process of demyelination with breakdown products or possibly fatty acid chains of accumulated sphingosine.

The juvenile phenotype of Tay-Sachs disease is mainly characterized by motor neuron and spinocerebellar dysfunction as gangliosides accumulate in the neurons, axons and glia. Felderhoff-Muesser et al. used phosphorus MRS to examine the metabolic changes of a 16-year-old patient with juvenile Tay-Sachs disease [16]. A decreased amount of phosphodiesters and membrane-bound phosphates was demonstrated, suggesting an activation of phosphodiesterases by accumulating gangliosides. Severe changes in phosphorus metabolism corresponded well with clinical findings.

Sandhoff's Disease

Sandhoff's disease is due to a deficiency of A and B isoenzymes of hexosaminidase. The clinical course is similar to Tay-Sachs disease. There is visceral involvement, including hepatomegaly, cardiac and renal tubular abnormalities. Cerebral MRI in the early stages demonstrates increased T_2 signal in the basal ganglia, particularly with the enlarged caudate nuclei. Later, cortical and deep gray matter volume loss occurs with patchy increases in T_2 signal in the white matter. Thalamic involvement is more indicative of Sandhoff's disease.

Wilken et al. described MRI and quantitative proton MRS findings for a girl with an enzymatically established diagnosis of Sandhoff's disease [17]. MRI of the brain showed signal changes in the periventricular white matter, pyramidal tract, basal ganglia, and cerebellar hemispheres. Proton MRS at the age of 13 months revealed a reduction of total NAA, with elevated mI and scyllo-inositol in white matter, gray matter, and thalamus. Cr was elevated in the white matter, but reduced in the basal ganglia. Cho concentrations were normal for all regions. A new resonance at 2.07 ppm was detected in all regions and ascribed to *N*-acetylhexosamine with the highest regional concentrations obtained in white matter and thalamus. While conventional MRS findings correspond with neuroaxonal damage and pronounced astrocytosis, the observation of *N*-acetylhexosamine appears as a specific marker of Sandhoff's disease indicating accumulation of hexosamine-containing oligosaccharides. Support for the interpretation of this novel resonance was obtained by an in vitro MRS study of a Sandhoff mouse model. Lowe et al. found that perchloric acid extracts of the Sandhoff mouse brain exhibited several resonances around 2.07 ppm on spectra that were not present in the corresponding spectra from extracts of wild-type mouse brain [18]. Ex vivo MRS of intact brain tissue with magic angle spinning also showed additional resonances around 2.07 ppm. High-performance liquid chromatography and mass spectrometry of Sandhoff extracts after MRS analyses identified the presence of *N*-acetylhexosamine-containing oligosaccharides. These resonances appeared to increase with disease progression and are likely to arise from the stored glycosphingolipids.

Sjorgen-Larsson Syndrome

Sjorgen-Larsson Syndrome (SLS) is an autosomal recessively inherited neurocutaneous disorder caused by a deficiency of the microsomal enzyme fatty aldehyde dehydrogenase (FALDH) arising from mutations in the *ALDH3A2* gene on chromosome 17 (17p11.2). The deficiency of the enzyme impairs the oxidation of medium and long-chain fatty aldehydes. The classical triad of severe clinical abnormalities includes ichthyosis, mental retardation, and spasticity. MRI of the brain shows hypomyelination, with a zone of periventricular signal abnormalities consistent with gliosis in white matter and mild ventricular enlargement.

Miyanomae et al. first described the proton MRS (single voxel and MRSI) findings in a 25-year-old male with confirmed SLS [19]. An elevated lipid resonance appearing at 1.3 ppm was accompanied by reduced NAA/Cr level. Mano et al. extended this finding by employing short echo time (18 ms) stimulated echo acquisition mode (STEAM) MRS localization in two patients, a 6-year-old female and 5-year-old male, homozygous for SLS, noting two lipids resonances at 1.3 and 0.9 ppm within abnormal signal intensity white matter and normal appearing basal ganglia [20]. These lipid resonances could represent accumulated fatty alcohols or their metabolites. Williamsen et al. conducted quantitative MRS in 18 SLS patients, ranges 5 months to 45 years, with 14 returning for follow-up [21]. Upon comparison with healthy controls, proton MRS of gray matter was normal. Proton MRS of white matter revealed a prominent peak at 1.3 ppm, normal levels of NAA, and elevated levels of Cr (+14%), Cho (+18%), and mI (+54%). Abnormalities on MR imaging and proton MR spectroscopy emerge during the first years of life and then stabilize such that they were similar in all patients with SLS, but with varying severity. The changes are confined to cerebral white matter and suggest an accumulation of lipids, periventricular gliosis, delayed myelination, and a mild permanent myelin deficit. Several other articles replicating the MRS findings and monitoring lipid resonance levels upon therapeutic intervention have been reported [22–27].

Kaminaga et al., subsequently examined four, asymptomatic, heterozygous SLS parents of homozygous SLS children [28]. An abnormal lipid resonance, centered at 0.9 ppm, was present on the spectra for each heterozygote. A moderate decrease in fatty alcohol:NAD1 oxidoreductase complex activity has been reported in persons heterozygotic for SLS. While the significance of the resonance in SLS heterozygotes is uncertain, the breakdown of myelin and accumulation of branched-chain fatty alcohol, possibly phytol, in cerebral parenchyma may also be possible.

Mitochondrial Diseases

Mitochondrial diseases arise from mutations in nuclear and mitochondrial DNA, which alter the functions of proteins (~20,000 distinct) or RNA molecules within the mitochondria. This heterogeneous group of genetic disorders (>150 recognized pathogenic mutations for maternally inherited syndromes) can produce a variety of complicated clinical presentations and can present at any age with a minimum prevalence estimated at 1 in 5000 [29]. Common neurological features described for patients include developmental delays, seizures, encephalopathy, ataxia, spasticity, migraine, and stroke-like episodes. Liver failure, gastrointestinal disorders, cardiac disease, ptosis, external ophthalmoplegia, proximal myopathy, and exercise intolerance are also found in some patients. Patients with the same genetic mutation can give rise to multiple clinical phenotypes. Alternatively, an identical clinical phenotype can result from diverse genetic mutations within nuclear or mitochondrial genes. Mitochondria have many roles in cellular maintenance. The classic role is to generate cellular energy in the form of adenosine triphosphate (ATP) via a process known as oxidative phosphorylation. Dozens of metabolic pathways are housed within the mitochondria including the citric acid cycle, heme biosynthesis, calcium homeostasis, fatty acid/amino acid oxidation, pyrimidine biosynthesis, and apoptosis. Tissues heavily reliant on aerobic metabolism, such as the CNS, heart, liver, skeletal muscle, kidney and the endocrine and respiratory systems are sensitive to mitochondrial defects.

While mitochondrial diseases are not curable, treatment to alleviate symptoms and slow down disease progression may be beneficial to patients.

Some of the more commonly recognized and described mitochondrial diseases include MELAS (mitochondrial myopathy, encephalopathy lactic acidosis, and stroke-like episodes), Leigh Syndrome, Kearns-Sayre Syndrome, Pearson syndrome, MNGIE (mitochondrial neurogastrointestinal encephalomyopathy), Alpers Syndrome, and the respiratory chain disorders. The respiratory chain disorders are characterized biochemically by defective oxidative phosphorylation. These disorders as a group are among the most common inborn errors of metabolism. The mitochondrial respiratory chain is composed of five macromolecular complexes, encoded by 13 mtDNA and ~77 nuclear genes. It is the only metabolic pathway in the cell that is under dual control of both the mtDNA and nDNA. By convention, mitochondrial disorders refer only to respiratory chain disorders. However, given the larger role of mitochondria beyond "energy factories," newer published literature now makes reference to mitochondrial diseases in broader terms to reflect dysfunction in other metabolic pathways located in the mitochondria. Many of the disorders described elsewhere in this chapter (i.e., organic acidurias), and other chapters within this book (i.e., Leukoencephalopathy with Brain-Stem and Spinal Cord Involvement and Elevated White Matter Lactate (LBSL in the Leukodystrophy chapter)) could now be considered mitochondrial-based disorders. While most neuroimaging abnormalities in patients with mitochondrial diseases are nonspecific, MRI and MRS can play an important supporting role aiding diagnosis of a mitochondrial disease, and directing additional workup. There are numerous case reports and series of heterogeneous patients with mitochondrial diseases described within the literature [30–37]. Key neuroimaging features for respiratory chain disorders can include cerebral and cerebellar volume loss, focal lesions in deep gray matter structures, delay in myelination and leukodystrophy. These features are consistent with findings from pathology which indicate a gray matter pattern with neuronal loss and vasculo-necrotic multifocal lesions and a white matter pattern consisting of spongy degeneration and demyelination with gliosis present; both patterns in varying severity within gray and white matter [38]. Analogous to blood lactate levels, not all patients with mitochondrial disease demonstrate lactate elevations in the CNS. Proton MRS often reveals an elevation of lactic acid especially within acute or sub-acute focal lesions, CSF and during a period of clinical exacerbation, such as an infection. This is illustrated in Fig. 11.2. Chronic lesions and normal appearing brain parenchyma do not necessarily reveal elevated lactate for most patients with mitochondrial diseases. Care must also be taken not to confuse signals originating from the propanediol solvent used in seizure medication, especially when incorporated with large doses of phenobarbital. The solvent appears as a doublet resonance located at 1.1. ppm, to the right just upfield of the lactate signal. There is evidence propanediol itself metabolizes to lactate.

Deficient activity in a macromolecular complex can be measured, but may produce different clinical and imaging presentations arising from distinct defects in sub-components. This is illustrated upon comparing the MRI and MRS findings of two patients both diagnosed with deficient Complex I activity in Figs. 11.2 and 11.3.

Reduction of NAA/Cr levels has been reported in the literature for respiratory chain disorders, with some demonstrating a measure of reversibility. For patients with complex II deficiency, deficient electron transport chain activity results in significant increases in succinate. Succinate is normally not appreciated on proton MRS as it arises at 2.4 ppm with the methylene resonances of glutamate and other amino acids. However, Brockmann reported a very large succinate resonance accompanied by elevated lactate and reduced NAA/Cr within the white matter of three patients diagnosed with complex II deficiency [39].

Amino Acidurias

Nonketotic hyperglycinemia (NKH), also referred to as glycine encephalopathy, is an autosomal recessive disorder of glycine metabolism. The defective glycine cleavage enzyme produces elevated concentrations of glycine in plasma, urine, CSF, and CNS, instead of the normal conversion to serine. Confined to the mitochondria, the glycine cleavage enzyme is composed of four protein components: P protein (a pyridoxal phosphate-dependent glycine decarboxylase, chromosome 9p22), H protein (a lipoic acid-containing protein, chromosome 16q24), T protein (a tetrahydrofolate-requiring enzyme, aminomethyltransferase, chromosome 3p21.2-p21.1), and L protein (a dihydrolipoamide dehydrogenase, chromosome 7q31-q32). Mutations in the P, H, and T proteins are known to produce glycine encephalopathy, with a majority (70–80%) arising from glycine decarboxylase defects. Historically, NKH was biochemically diagnosed from an elevated glycine CSF-to-plasma ratio. Confirmation with an enzyme assay of liver tissue or mutational analysis can be definitive for diagnosis.

The toxic effects of glycine accumulation become clinically apparent quickly, with the majority of patients presenting in the neonatal period. Approximately 85% of NKH patients have the severe neonatal form of the disorder. Patients can present with hiccups, poor feeding, lethargy, severe hypotonia, and early infantile seizures with myoclonic jerks associated with burst-suppression pattern on electroencephalography. Most will have repeated episodes of severe and prolonged apnea that can lead to death. Surviving

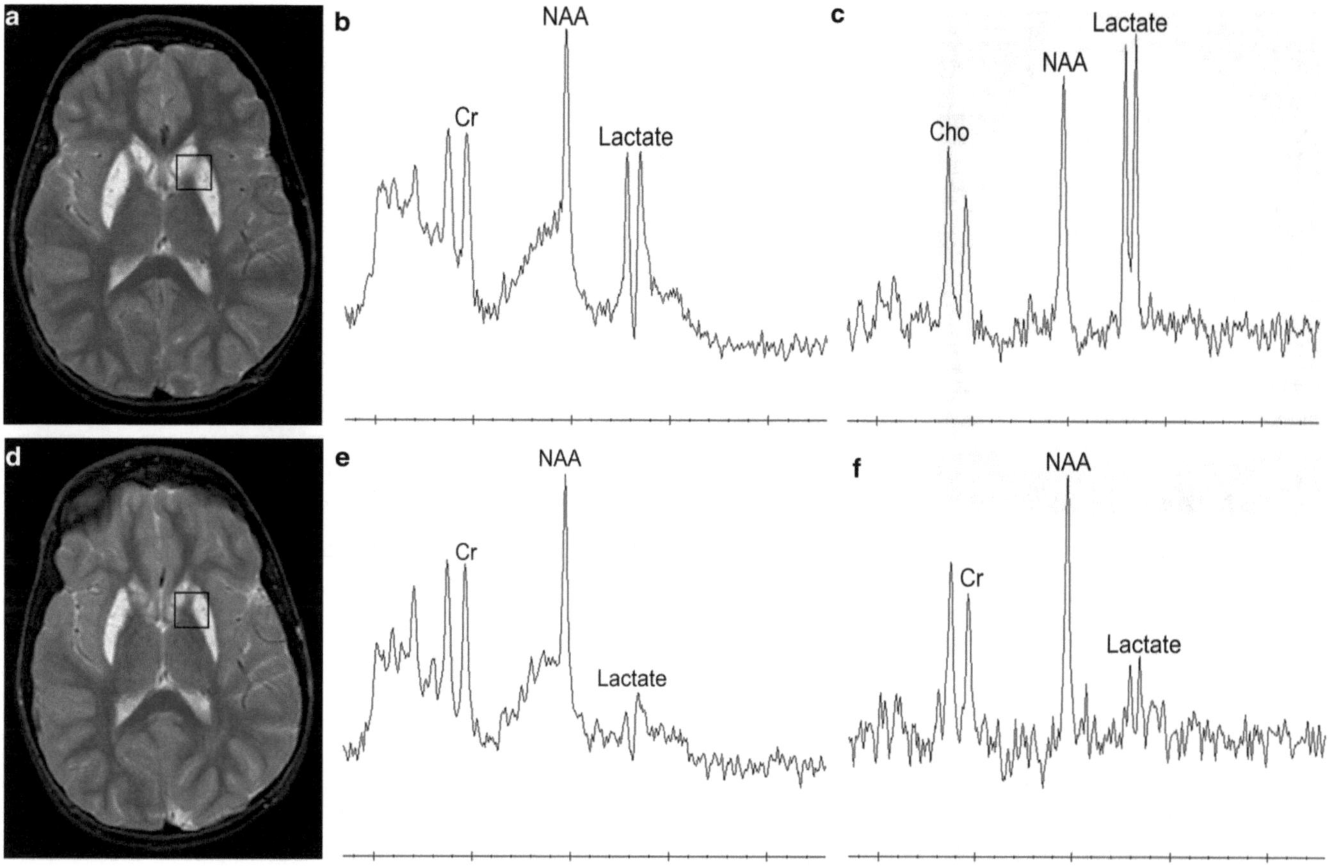

Fig. 11.2 MRI and MRS findings obtained from an 8-year-old female with Complex I deficiency presenting during a period of febrile illness. (**a**) Axial T2-weighted image shows hyperintense signal bilaterally within the caudate and putamen in the pattern characteristic of Leigh syndrome. (**b**) Short echo (35 ms) and (**c**) long echo (288 ms) MR spectra show significant elevation of lactate sampling within the left basal ganglia. Three months later, upon returning to baseline, (**d**) axial T2-weighted image shows no change, however, the lactate levels returned to the patient's baseline status as shown in the (**e**) short echo (35 ms) and (**f**) long echo (288 ms) MR spectra

infants usually have profound intellectual disabilities and intractable seizures. Some patients can present with atypical, milder forms of the disorder if residual enzyme activity remains present. Patients are treated with sodium benzoate to reduce glycine levels in the blood and CSF, and with dextromethorphan to counteract the neurostimulatory effect of high glycine levels on *N*-methyl-**D**-aspartate (NMDA) receptors. Unfortunately, these pharmacologic therapies often fail suggesting that irreversible glycine-induced brain damage occurs in utero.

The glycine cleavage enzyme maintains extracellular glycine concentrations as glycine serves as an excitation modulator of NMDA receptors in the brain. The excessive activation of these receptors produces neuronal and axonal injury. NMDA receptors also play an important role in neurogenesis. Thus, the excess glycine concentration can potentially impair neurogenesis and produce cellular neurotoxicity.

Imaging features support this notion of fetal injury with abnormalities demonstrated on neonatal MRI, which generally include thinning or agenesis of the corpus callosum with hypomyelination. Pathology in nonketotic hyperglycinemia is characterized by vacuolation, astrocytosis, and demyelination, also called vacuolating myelinopathy. Because these changes only occur in *myelinated* white matter, in the neonate they are restricted to the dorsal limbs of the internal capsule, dorsal brainstem, pyramidal tracts in the coronal radiata, and lateral thalamus. Significant volume loss is also appreciated with enlarged ventricles and prominent sulci.

Heindel et al. first employed proton MRS to describe the findings from two children suffering from nonketotic hyperglycinemia [40]. In a 2-month-old female, the signal of the inhibitory neurotransmitter glycine was present with equal signal intensity and prominence in the parieto occipital white matter and in the basal ganglia region. In a 10-day-old female with follow-up studies performed within the first 4 months of life, a reduction of glycine in brain tissue corresponded more reliably with clinical findings than the stable values in plasma and cerebrospinal fluid. Gabis et al. monitored the course of treatment with sodium benzoate and detromethophan in a male child at 10 and 13 months of age [41]. Over the period, a small increase in glycine coupled with a dramatic elevation of the composite glutamate and glutamine (Glx) was observed.

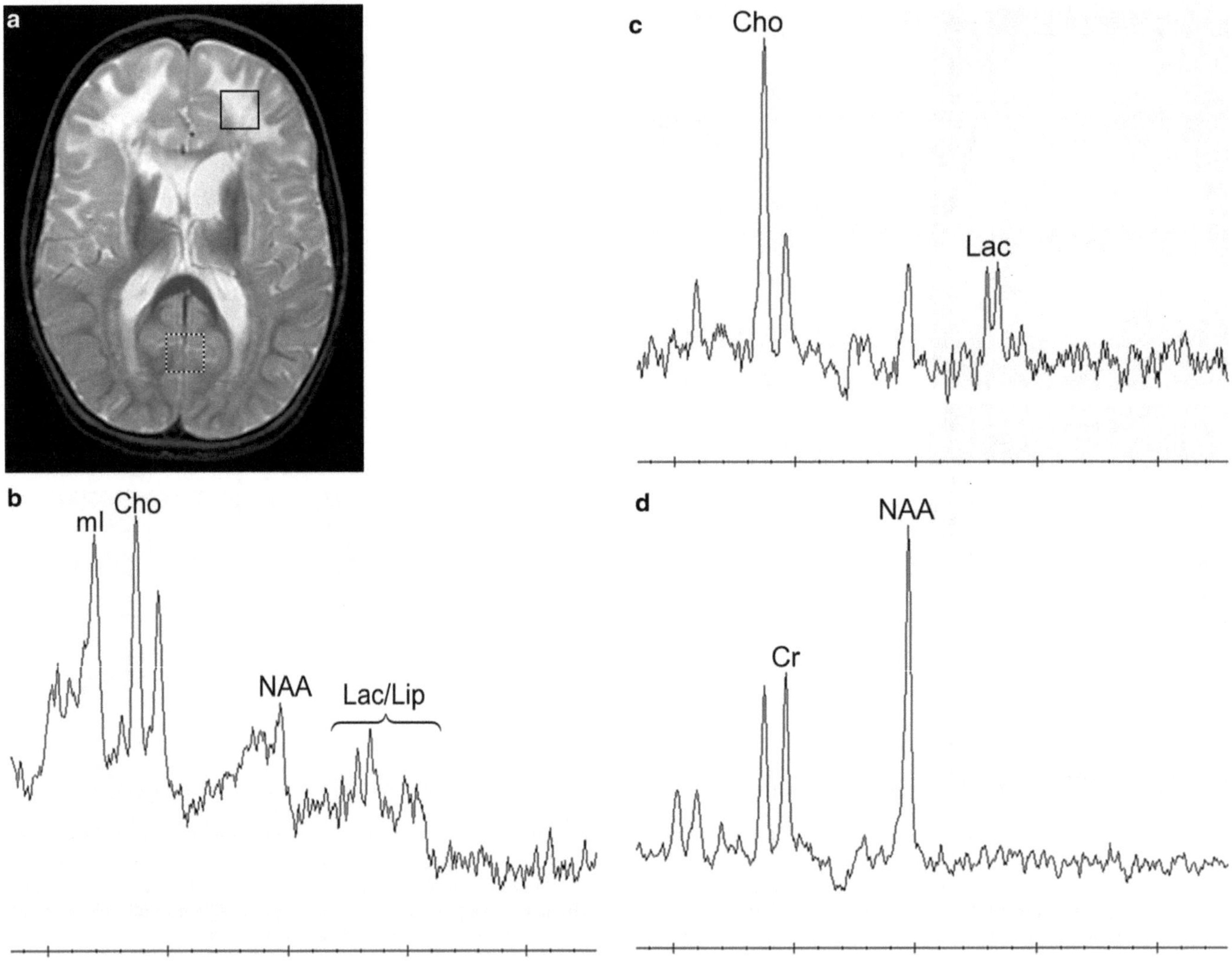

Fig. 11.3 MRI and MRS findings obtained from a 4-year-old female with Complex I deficiency presenting with encephalomyopathy and choreoathetosis. (**a**) Axial T2-weighted images reveal abnormal hyperintense signal with U fiber involvement and sparing the internal capsule. (**b**) Short echo (35 ms), and (**c**) long echo (288 ms) reveal significant lactate, mI and Cho elevations with low NAA within the affected frontal white matter. (**d**) Long echo MR spectra sampling within unaffected the calcarine fissure

These findings were in agreement with glycine and glutamine levels monitored in the blood. Choi et al. monitored a patient with neonatal presentation of NKH at 6, 12, and 17 days of life before expiration at 20 days. Proton MRS aided initial diagnosis with the prominent glycine resonance, reflected improvement at 12 days with reduced glycine, and indicated distress with the appearance of a lactate resonance at 17 days. These three studies described elevated glycine in terms of a ratio to brain Cr. Huisman et al. employed quantitative proton MRS approach which allowed for the determination of elevated glycine concentrations in the basal ganglia, cerebellar, parietal–occipital, and frontal white matter for a male at 7 days of life [42]. Results were in agreement with findings obtained at day 9 upon autopsy conducted 12 h postmortem. Other metabolite concentrations were within normal limits for the site. This contrasts an in vitro study of the blood, CSF and in vivo brain from patients with NKH. Viola et al. reported elevated Cr levels in addition to elevations of glycine for blood, fluids, and brain [43]. Increased lactate, pyruvate, alanine, proline, and sulfur amino acids were also observed in the blood and CSF. These elevations were thought to represent the consequence of glycine disposal via several metabolic pathways. With longitudinal monitoring of two patients, the in vivo elevation of creatine was noted by comparing the individual metabolite area with the total area of all measured metabolites. Comparing two patients with in vivo MRS acquired, a low NAA/glycine level was found in the fatal case suggesting it may represent a prognostic marker for poorer outcomes. For these two patients, vigabatrin was part of a medication regimen to control seizures. However, Tekgul et al. reported vigabatrin-associated deterioration in two infants with NKH [44].

Figure 11.4 illustrates the MRI and MRS findings in a patient with a neonatal NKH presentation. On short echo proton MRS performed at 1.5 T, mI and glycine co-resonate at

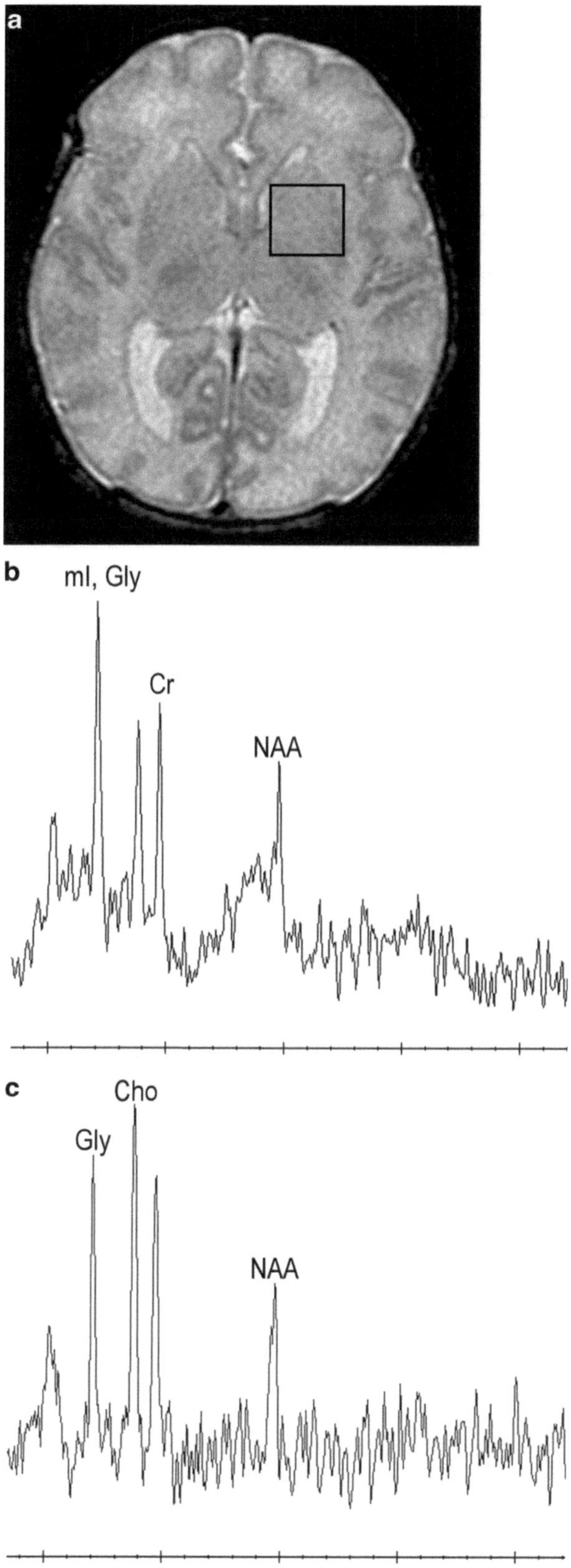

Fig. 11.4 MRI and MRS findings from a neonate diagnosed with nonketotic hyperglycinemia. (**a**) Axial T2-weighted image, (**b**) Short Echo MRS and (**c**) Intermediate Echo (144 ms) MRS. The short echo spectrum demonstrates a composite myo-inositol and glycine resonance at 3.5 ppm. The intermediate echo spectrum demonstrates the elevated signal at 3.5 arises from glycine. (Imaging and spectroscopy courtesy of Dr. Charles Glasier)

3.5 ppm as 4 of the 6 mI methine protons contribute to the resonance signal. In adults, the resonance at 3.5 ppm is composed of approximately mI (75%), mI-monophosphate (15%), and the α-protons of glycine (15%). At 3 T, the spectral pattern for mI complicates as only two methine protons contribute to the resonance at 3.5 ppm. (Since glycine is a singlet, there is no change in the chemical shift or pattern.) Thus, the apparent signal intensity drops upon qualitative assessment due to the mI contribution at 3 T. Estimates for adults indicate normal levels of glycine range from 0.4 to 1 mM in the brain. On short echo MRS, the resonance at 3.5 ppm is one of the most prominent in neonates. The contribution of mI and glycine components to the resonance varies with age, particularly in the first months and years of life. High quality, normative proton MRS data obtained from a range of neonates, infants and children is required for discrimination of mI and glycine in vivo. Normally, the resonance at 3.5 ppm on short echo MRS declines to near adult values by 4–6 months of age. Clinically, by sampling a combination of short (echo times less than 35) and long echo (echo times of 135, 144, 270, 288 ms), one can discriminate mI from glycine [45, 46]. The difference in T2 relaxation times can be exploited to discriminate these two amino acids as the multiplet mI has a shorter T2 value compared to that of the glycine singlet. For research purposes, advanced echo time averaging sequences can be employed for discrimination of glycine [47]. Care must be taken to avoid confusion with other metabolites, some as complex multiplets with relatively low concentrations, which occur between 3.5 and 4.0 ppm. For example, Manley et al. erroneously reported an elevation of glycine arising from intracerebral blood in a female patient with an apparent transient form of NKH [48]. Proton MRS sampling of parenchyma with blood or blood products is plagued with artifacts. Thus, the water suppression and spectral localization would have likely failed to distortions of the local magnetic field due to iron products. The short echo spectrum presented in the study may suggest an elevation of mI-Gly, if not corrected for age and location. The assigned glycine resonance on the good quality long echo (echo time 270 ms) spectrum was incorrect as the location of the prominent resonance was further downfield (to the left of the spectrum) from the 3.5 ppm resonance location of glycine.

Organic Acidurias

Glutaric Acidurias

Glutaric Aciduria type 1 (GA-I), an autosomal recessive inborn error of lysine, hydroxylysine and tryptophan metabolism, occurs as a result of glutaryl-CoA dehydrogenase deficiency, with the responsible gene, *GCDH*, located at chromosome 19p13.2. The disorder usually manifests between birth and 18 months of life with acute striatal degeneration with neurologic dysfunction characterized by encephalopathy, subtle neurologic signs in infancy (irritability or hypotonia), to dystonia, choreoathetosis, loss of milestones and seizures. The diagnosis of GA-I is made by the presence of increased urinary glutaric acid and 3-hydroxyglutaric acid. The disorder is confirmed by a deficiency or absence of glutaryl-CoA dehydrogenase in cultured fibroblasts. Hoffman et al. found that 20–30% of patients had "chronic" subdural effusions and hematomas identified on neuroimaging studies [49]. The presence of subdural effusions on imaging in GA-I can mimic abusive head trauma; however, appropriate biochemical and imaging can usually distinguish the two entities. Another prominent clinical feature of infants and children with GA-I is macrocephaly, but not megaencephaly. Hoffman et al. found that 70% of the patients with GA-I studied had either macrocephaly or increasing head circumference past the 97th percentile [49]. Common features on neuroimaging include widened or enlarged Sylvian fissures, increased spaces anterior to the frontotemporal lobes but no evidence of frontotemporal atrophy. Enlargement of the Sylvian fissure has been correlated with severity of the enzyme deficiency. Basal ganglia and white matter signal abnormalities have also been noted.

Early case reports employing proton and phosphorus MRS in GA-I were discrepant in their findings. Several reported cases with no spectral abnormalities. [50–52] However, the lack of rigorous quantification and appropriate control groups or the examinations conducted during stable periods could explain the discrepancy with later case reports and series. Kurul, Cakmakci and Dirik [53] reported findings in a 19-month-old male with GA-I. Short echo MRS of right frontal white matter and right lentiform nuclei revealed decreased NAA/Cr levels, slightly increased Cho/Cr levels, and increased mI/Cr levels, compared with the age-matched control patients. Oguz, Ozturk and Cila [54] described widespread restricted diffusion in the white matter and increased diffusion in bilateral putamen in a 11-month-old male diagnosed with GA-I. The MRS showed decreased NAA/Cr levels found on MRSI performed with a TE of 135 ms compared with a sex- and age-matched control with no significant change in Cho/Cr levels. Elevated lactate levels were noted in affected basal ganglia and in normal appearing regions of brain parenchyma. Sijens et al [55]. employed a MRSI approach in two patients with GA-I and reported reductions in the white matter NAA signal, in the more severe case accompanied by a loss of glutamate and the appearance of lactate signals. In the largest case series to date, Perez-Duenas [150] examined symptomatic pediatric patients and asymptomatic siblings with GA-I with proton MRS at an echo time of 135 ms. For the symptomatic patients, the MRI and MRS were performed between three and 8 days after the onset of acute encephalopathic crisis. For the encephalopathic patients, isotropic diffusion images showed high signal changes with corresponding low apparent diffusion coefficient (ADC) values within the putamen, caudate nuclei and globus pallidus, and for one patient, the cerebral peduncles including the substantia nigra. The imaging for the asymptomatic siblings appeared normal. MRS showed decreased NAA/Cr levels at the basal ganglia in encephalopathic patients when compared to a group of sex- and age-matched controls.

Glutaric aciduria type II (GA-II), also referred to as multiple acyl CoA dehydrogenase deficiency, is an autosomal recessive, mitochondrial electron transport chain disorder that impairs electron transfer flavoprotein (ETF) or electron transfer flavoprotein-ubiquinone oxidoreductase (at coenzyme Q). Three genes, *ETFA (*alpha polypeptide), *ETFB* (beta polypeptide), and *ETFDH* (dehydrogenase), provide instructions for generating two enzymes. These enzymes are normally active in the mitochondria and assist in metabolizing proteins and fats to provide energy for the body. If an enzyme is defective, absent, or partially functioning, then the unprocessed nutrients accumulate and damage cells, causing the signs and symptoms of GA-II. The complete loss of either enzyme produced from the *ETFA*, *ETFB*, or *ETFDH* genes generally produce the most severe symptoms in patients. Mutations that allow the enzyme to retain some activity may result in milder forms of the disorder. The brain involvement is often revealed with abnormal T2 prolongation within the basal ganglia, periventricular white matter and the splenium of the corpus callosum. Firat et al [56]. examined a 12-year-old female patient with GA-II and compared her results with data obtained from four healthy age- and sex-matched volunteers. During clinical exacerbation, frontal lobe Cho/Cr level was greater than the levels reported for the comparison participants. The NAA/Cr level was lower than normal limits. After successful riboflavin treatment and dietary restriction for proteins, the NAA/Cr level normalized, however, the Cho/Cr level remained below the normal range, suggesting riboflavin-responsive multiple acyl-coA dehydrogenase deficiency. An elevated Cho/Cr ratio and decreased NAA/Cr ratio appeared consistent with a demyelinating process in the active phase of glutaric aciduria type II. MRS aided in monitoring the progress of the disease and the efficacy of treatment by demonstrating changes in NAA/Cr and Cho/Cr levels.

L-Hydroxyglutaric Aciduria

L-2-Hydroxyglutaric aciduria (LHG) arises from mutations in L-2-hydroxyglutarate dehydrogenase gene (*L2HGDH*) localized on chromosome 14q21.3. Two independent groups simultaneously identified the first pathogenic mutations [57, 58]. Elevated levels of L-2-hydroxyglutaric acid (L2HG) in urine, CSF and to a lesser extent, plasma, are found in patients with the disorder. Most patients experience a slowly progressive clinical course. The most common presenting signs include developmental delay, hypotonia, epilepsy, hypotonia, spascticity, extrapyramidal symptoms, behavioral problems, and cerebellar ataxia. Hypotonia and spasticity may be dependent on disease duration, with hypotonia in the earlier stages and spasticity in the later stages.

Accumulation of L2HG is toxic to the human brain, producing an appearance similar to a leukoencephalopathy and increasing the susceptibility of a patient to develop tumors. The MRI pattern of signal abnormalities of the subcortical cerebral white matter, putamen, caudate nucleus, globus pallidus, and dentate nucleus has been described [59–62]. Hanefeld et al. first described the spectroscopic findings in LHG with a case report of a 16-year-old female [63]. Using quantitative, short echo proton MRS, the study found 50% decrease of NAA, a 75% increase of mI and a 40% decrease of Cho in white matter relative to age-matched controls. MRS findings upon follow-up 2 years later demonstrated further declines in NAA and increases in mI. Sener et al. reported the detection of a singlet resonance at 2.50 ppm, suspected to represent L2HG, in a 10-month-old male with urinary levels of L2HG greater than 80 times normal [64]. Aydin reported a multiplet within the region of 2.1 and 2.5 ppm, for two male siblings (ages 10 and 12 years), which potentially could represent L2HG, coupled by the commonly observed Glx resonances [65]. Further study is needed to clarify these findings.

Branched Chain Organic Acidurias

Branched chain organic acidurias are disorders that arise due to abnormal enzymes primarily involving the catabolism of branched-chain amino acids. These enzymes are necessary for the proper metabolism of the amino acids leucine, isoleucine, and valine. The most commonly encountered disorders include maple syrup urine disease, propionic aciduria, and methylmalonic aciduria.

Maple Syrup Urine Disease

Maple syrup urine disease (MSUD) is a rare autosomal recessive disorder caused by defective oxidative decarboxylation of the branched-chain amino acids valine, isoleucine, and leucine. The accumulation of metabolites in the urine leads to the characteristic odor resembling maple syrup. While cerebral imaging may initially be unremarkable, diffuse cerebral edema develops in the deep cerebellar white matter, posterior limb of the internal capsule, periorlandic white matter, dorsal brainstem and pons. Imaging studies have shown reversible brain edema during acute metabolic decompensation.

Proton MRS of the brain appears to be useful for examining patients suffering from MSUD in different metabolic states. Felber et al. demonstrated the appearance of a previously unassigned resonance in a 3-year-old male with MSUD [66]. This peak disappeared with normalization of branched-chain amino acids and oxoacids in the plasma and cerebrospinal fluid. In vitro spectroscopy of these acids at 1.5 T confirmed the chemical shift position of the acid methyl components. The duration of lactate elevation correlated with the presence of brain edema and coma. Heindel et al. replicated the finding of accumulation of branched-chain amino acids and their corresponding 2-oxo acids in the brain of a 9-year-old girl suffering from classical MSUD [67]. During acute metabolic decompensation, the compounds appeared as a resonance located at 0.9 ppm. The brain tissue concentration of these acids could be estimated as 0.9 mmol/l. Six patients with MSUD were evaluated by Jan et al., during acute presentation with metabolic decompensation [68]. Follow-up examinations were performed after clinical and metabolic recovery. Diffusion-weighted imaging (DWI) demonstrated marked diffusion restriction compatible with cytotoxic or intramyelinic sheath edema in the brainstem, basal ganglia, thalami, cerebellar and periventricular white matter and the cerebral cortex. Long echo MRS was performed in four of the six patients revealing the abnormal branched-chain amino acids and branched-chain alpha-keto acids peak at 0.9 ppm as well as elevated lactate on proton MRS. The changes were reversed with treatment without evidence of volume loss or persistent tissue damage. The presence of cytotoxic or intramyelinic edema as evidenced by restricted water diffusion on DWI, with the presence of lactate on spectroscopy, appear worrisome for irreversible injury, however, in the context of metabolic decompensation in MSUD, it appears that changes in cell osmolarity and metabolism can reverse completely after metabolic correction. An example of MRI and MRS findings in an infant diagnosed with MSUD is shown in Fig. 11.5.

Propionic Aciduria

Propionic aciduria occurs due to a mutation in the genes encoding proprionyl-CoA carboxylase, a mitochondrial biotin-dependent enzyme. Untreated, propionic aciduria leads to metabolic decompensation and toxic encephalopathy. Chemelli et al. described MRS findings for four children, who diagnosed early in life, suffered at most one period of metabolic decompensation and were properly treated by protein restriction and carnitine supplementation, during a phase of clinically and metabolically stable conditions [69]. Two children with the longest delay before onset of therapy showed cerebral volume loss. MRS yielded elevated lactate peaks in all of the children. The presence of lactate could arise from aerobic oxidation within the citric acid cycle due to elevated intracellular propionic metabolites. Bergman et al. studied three patients with elevated urinary 3-hydroxy-propionic acid concentrations diagnosed with propionic aciduria using a short echo single voxel STEAM approach [70]. While not appropriate for lactate quantification, the STEAM method allowed for quantification of the key metabolites. The study found decreased NAA, decreased mI, and elevated Glx levels. Cho levels were elevated for one patient.

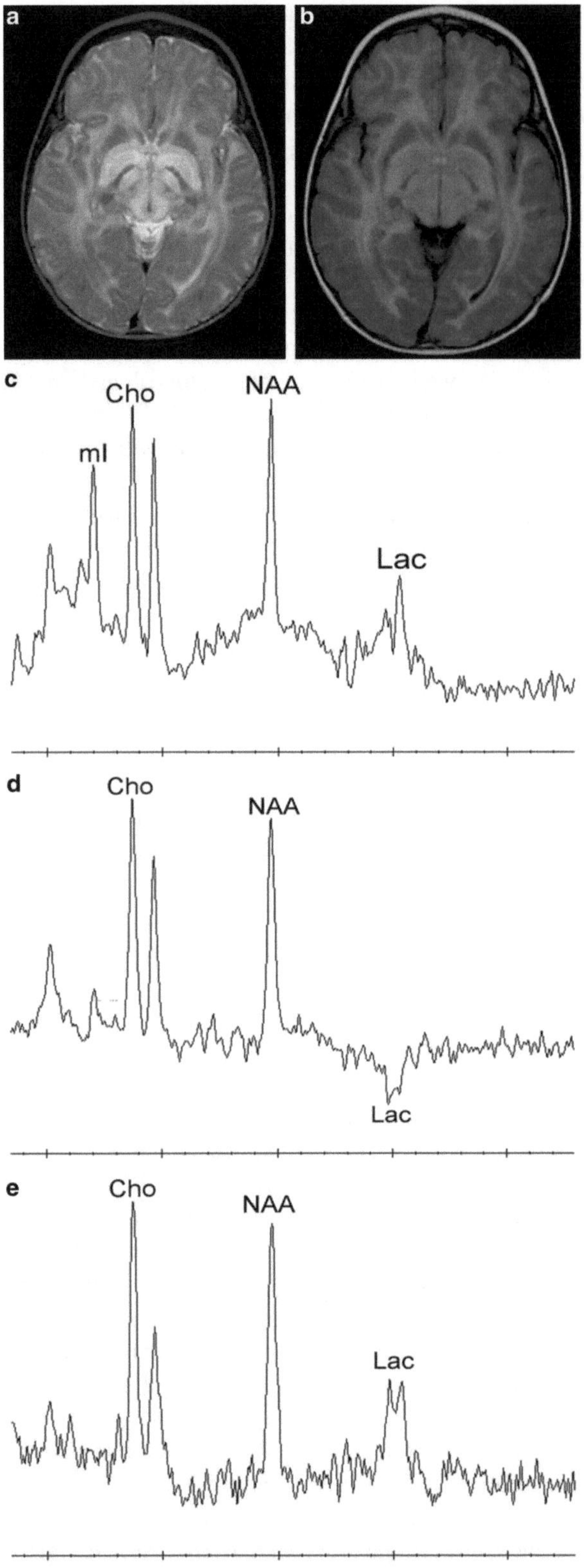

Fig. 11.5 MRI and MRS findings from an infant diagnosed with Maple Syrup Urine Disease. (**a**) Axial T2-weighted image, (**b**) Axial FLAIR, (**c**) Short Echo MRS (**d**) Intermediate Echo (144 ms) MRS and (**e**) Long Echo (288 ms). On short echo MRS, a composite of branched chain amino acids (0.9 ppm) with lactate (1.35 ppm). The lactate resonance becomes inverted on intermediate echo and upright on long echo MRS. A reduction in lactate signal intensity is found with the inversion at TE 144 with partial restoration of the signal intensity at TE 288

Methylmalonic Aciduria

In all forms of methylmalonic aciduria, the conversion of methylmalonate-CoA to succinyl-CoA is impaired which causes an accumulation of methylmalonic acid. Methylmalonic aciduria can arise from a genetically heterogeneous group of autosomal recessively inherited metabolic disorders affecting methylmalonate and cobalamin (cbl) (Vitamin B_{12}) metabolism. While methylmalonic aciduria is classified as a relatively rare disorder, it remains important to recognize genetic distinctions for imaging and MRS as small case series typically combine data from small numbers of patients, as the clinical presentations are similar.

"Isolated" methylmalonic aciduria arises from one of three causes:

1. Mutations in the gene located on chromosome 6p12.3, *MUT*, which produces a complete (MUT^{0}) or partial (MUT^{-}) deficiency of the enzyme methylmalonyl-CoA mutase;
2. Mutations in adenosyl-cobalamin (AdoCbl), a coenzyme form of vitamin B_{12} that produce a defect in the synthesis or transport.
   (a) *MMAA* on chromosome 4q31.21; complementation group cblA
   (b) *MMAB* on chromosome 12q24.11; complementation group cblB
3. mutations in the gene located on chromosome 2p13.3, *MCEE*, responsible for deficiency of the enzyme methylmalonyl-Co epimerase

Phenotype varies from severe neonatal-onset forms with poor outcome and high mortality to milder forms with infant and adult onset. All phenotypes demonstrate periods of relative health and intermittent metabolic decompensation associated with intercurrent infections, stress, etc. Disease features within the neonatal period include recurrent vomiting, dehydration, respiratory distress, hypotonia, progressive lethargy, seizures and coma, leading to death if not promptly treated. In the later-onset forms, the clinical picture is more variable, ranging from acute life-threatening encephalopathy to intermittent or chronic symptoms of various degrees.

The diagnosis of MMAs relies on the detection of characteristic compounds in body fluids employing urine organic acid analysis and blood acylcarnitine profiling. Patients demonstrate significantly increased urinary excretion of methylmalonic acid accompanied by increased excretion of methylcitric acid, 3-hydroxypropionic acid, and other derivatives of propionyl-CoA. In blood, propionyl and methylmalonyl carnitine are the key abnormal carnitine esters. Treatment currently relies on patients maintaining a low-protein high-energy diet, carnitine supplementation, and metronidazole. Patients with a B_{12}-responsive phenotype respond favorably to pharmacological doses of vitamin B_{12}.

Neurologic signs arise from the accumulation of toxic compounds proximal to the metabolic block. Methylmalonic aciduria acts as a competitive inhibitor to succinate dehydrogenase, a key enzyme in mitochondrial aerobic oxidation. As energy is depleted, anaerobic and lactic acid production proceeds to compensate, but produces injury to the basal ganglia. The neurological picture includes an acute and progressive dystonic syndrome resulting from basal ganglia lesions. These are localized bilaterally in the globus pallidus and usually occur following acute episodes of metabolic decompensation.

Radmanesh et al. described the imaging findings of 52 Iranian children (37 males, age at scanning 1 month--11 years) diagnosed with methylmalonic aciduria and 33 of 52 treated with standard therapy [71]. Diagnosis of methylmalonic aciduria was confirmed from increased plasma methylmalonyl carnitine or increased urine methylmalonic acid as detected by gas chromatography–mass spectrometry and the propionate incorporation test. Fourteen children had unremarkable imaging. Among the 38 with findings, ventricular dilation (17 studies), cortical atrophy (15), periventricular white matter abnormal signal (12), thinning of the corpus callosum (8), subcortical white matter abnormal signal (6), cerebellar volume loss (4), calcification of the basal ganglia (3), and delay in myelination (3) were noted. Harting et al. noted in four children with isolated methylmalonic aciduria demonstrated a complex spectrum of pallidal lesions, delay in myelination, incomplete opercularization, immature gyral pattern, white matter abnormalities, brainstem and cerebellar changes [72].

In 1998, Lam et al. published as a compilation the findings of early MRS studies in children with metabolic disorders [73]. Examining the basal ganglia with a single voxel short echo STEAM approach, three patients with either methylmalonic aciduria (5 y male), cblC (2.3 month female) or cobalamin deficiency with methylmalonic aciduria and homocysturina (1.7 y female) are described. While not appropriate for lactate quantification, the STEAM method allowed for quantification of the key metabolites. For the patients with methylmalonic aciduria and cblC, NAA was significantly reduced compared to control patients. In 2001, Trinh et al. employed a MRSI approach to evaluate a 14-year-old male with a *MUT* mutation and a 16-month-old female with a cobalamin synthesis defect during an episode of metabolic decompensation [74]. The male patient with partial enzyme deficiency demonstrated normal metabolite levels within the brain parenchyma, however, dramatic elevations of lactate levels were appreciated within the lateral ventricles and other prominent CSF filled spaces. The female patient during the period of illness exacerbation demonstrated reduced levels of NAA and elevated lactate within lesions, which were confirmed on single voxel short echo MRS. However, normal metabolite levels were appreciated on normal appearing brain parenchyma. Takeuchi et al. employed MRI, including DWI, and single voxel PRESS MRS to monitor carnitine and vitamin B12 therapy on a 13-month-old male with methylmalonic aciduria described by high levels of methylmalonic acid, however, the specific defect was not reported [75]. At baseline, imaging revealed abnormal hyperintense signal on T2, DWI (ADC hypointense) bilaterally within the caudate, putamen, and globus pallidus with elevated lactate and diminished NAA/Cr levels. At 2 weeks, 1 month, 4 months and 9 months, repeat imaging and MRS monitored improvement of signal abnormalities within the basal ganglia and normalization of metabolite levels. Michel et al. describes a 5-year-old child with B12 responsive methylmalonic aciduria who presented during a metabolic crisis despite maintenance on a low protein and carnitine-supplemented diet [76]. MRI demonstrated abnormal signal (hyperintense T2, FLAIR, DWI, hypointense ADC) within the globus pallidus bilaterally. Single voxel MRS within the globus pallidus demonstrated reduced NAA and elevated lactate (details not specified in the report). Ten weeks later, when the child was asymptomatic, follow-up MRI and MRS indicated interval improvement.

Longo et al. described MRI and MRS findings in patients with early onset cbl-C/D deficiency determined based upon urinary methylmalonic acid and plasma homocysturina levels [77]. The cbl-C/D deficiency varies from classical, isolated methylmalonic aciduria. Vitamin B12 is a co-factor required by two enzymes, MUT and methinone synthase. Patients with cblC/D deficiency exhibited methylmalonic aciduria and homocysturina. Proton MRS was performed in five patients, using CSI in three patients and single voxel MRS for two. There were no MRS abnormalities appreciated in the spectra for two patients evaluated at 4 years of age. However, for two patients (ages 7 month and 28 month) lactate elevations within the basal ganglia were detected and for one patient (17 month) lactate elevations were noted in the periventricular white matter.

Mitochondrial Encephalomyopathy with Elevated Methylmalonic Aciduria

Mild methylmalonic aciduria has been described in cases of succinate-ligase alpha subunit (*SUCLG1* mutations) and succinate-ligase ADP-forming beta subunit (*SUCLA2* mutations) associated with mitochondrial DNA depletion presenting with severe lactic acidosis and encephalomyopathy. Patient characteristics include hypotonia, muscle atrophy, dystonia, a "Leigh-like" syndrome, mitochondrial DNA depletion in muscle, and a decreased life span surviving usually up to 21 years. This disorder needs to be distinguished from the classic, isolated methylmalonic aciduria despite common shared features. Valayannopoulos et al. described elevated lactate levels and decreased NAA within the basal ganglia of two out of three patients with *SUCLG1* mutations [78]. Carrozzo et al. noted increased lactate in the basal ganglia of one patient with a *SUCLA2* mutation [79].

Table 11.2 Brief summary of urea cycle nomenclature and genetics

Urea cycle	Disease name	Gene symbol	Chromosomal locus	Mode of inheritance
Enzymes				
Ornithine Carbamoyl-transcarboxylase	Ornithine Transcarboxylase Deficiency	OTC	Xp11.4	X-linked
Carbamoylphosphate Synthetase I	Carbamoylphosphate Synthetase I Deficiency	CPS1	2q34	Autosomal recessive
Argininosuccinate Synthase	Citrullinemia Type I	ASS	9q34.11	Autosomal recessive
Argininosuccinate Lyase	Argininosuccinicaciduria	ASL	7q11.21	Autosomal recessive
Arginase	Arginase deficiency	ARG1	6q23.2	Autosomal recessive
CoFactor				
N-acetyl glutamatesynthetase	NAGS Deficiency	NAGS	17q21.31	Autosomal recessive
Transporters[a]				
Citrin	Citrin deficiency-Citrullinemia Type II	SLC25A13	7q21.3	Autosomal recessive
Ornithine Transporter	HHH (hyperornithine, hyperammonemia, homocitrullinuria) syndrome	ORNT1 (SLC25A15)	13q14.11	Autosomal recessive

[a]Defects in the transporter proteins are clinically distinct from the classic urea cycle diseases.

Urea Cycle Defects

The urea cycle is responsible for the clearance of nitrogen, a waste product arising from protein metabolism. Normally nitrogen, accumulated in the form of ammonia, is removed from the blood and converted to urea. Urea is then transferred into the urine and excreted. Five catalytic enzymes, a cofactor, and at least two transport proteins comprise the urea cycle. This cycle is also responsible for endogenous synthesis of arginine. Inherited molecular defects compromising the clearance of nitrogen are listed in Table 11.2.

Severe deficiency or the complete absence of an enzyme or cofactor activity results in the accumulation of ammonia and other precursor metabolites within the first days of life. Initially, infants with a urea cycle disorder are born without disease symptoms. However, a rapid deterioration occurs with acute onset of cerebral edema, lethargy, seizures, neurologic posturing, hyper- or hypoventilation, coma and potentially death. In persons with partial enzyme deficiencies, a milder form can manifest later with less severe hyperammonemia and subtle symptoms (psychiatric symptoms-hyperactive, self-injurious behaviors, autistic features; vomiting, learning disorders, stroke-like episodes, etc.). Hyperammonemia can be exacerbated by illness or stress. Treatment regimes for patients with urea cycle defects include many approaches (dialysis, low protein-dietary restrictions, IV administration of glucose, arginine chloride, and nitrogen scavengers) for reducing ammonia concentrations and minimizing neurologic damage. Diagnosis relies on clinical, biochemical, and molecular genetic analyses. As with all disorders, early diagnosis is important as late-onset urea cycle diseases carry the risk of neurological damage and encephalopathy.

The acute and sub-acute imaging appearances of these disorders mimic hypoxic—ischemic encephalopathy with edema. The insular cortex, perirolandic cortex, basal ganglia, especially the globus pallidi and putamina, demonstrate swelling and abnormal signals with T1 and T2 prolongation. The subcortical white matter, including the U-fibers, is also involved. With prolonged durations of hyperammonemia, cortical volume loss and cystic changes are also appreciated.

Connelly et al. first reported in 1993 an elevation of glutamine with reduction of NAA, Cr, and Cho levels found upon long echo proton MRS examinations within the white matter of two female infants partial ornithine transcarboxylase (OTC) defects hospitalized with encephalopathy associated with hyperammonemia [80]. Elevated glutamine had been described by Kreis et al. in patients with chronic hepatic encephalopathy [81]. Ross et al. reported reduced mI levels in a 14-year-old male patient with partial OTC effectively treated with oral benzoate [82]. Takanashi et al. later expanded the findings in OTC with a study of six patients with late-onset OTC using a short echo MRS approach [83]. Upon comparison with age-matched controls, glutamate and glutamine levels within the centrum semiovale were increased in four patients, proportionally to clinical stage of the disease; choline levels were reduced in the two patients with more severe disease; mI levels were reduced in five of six patients to undetectable levels for five symptomatic patients. NAA and Cr levels were normal for all four patients.

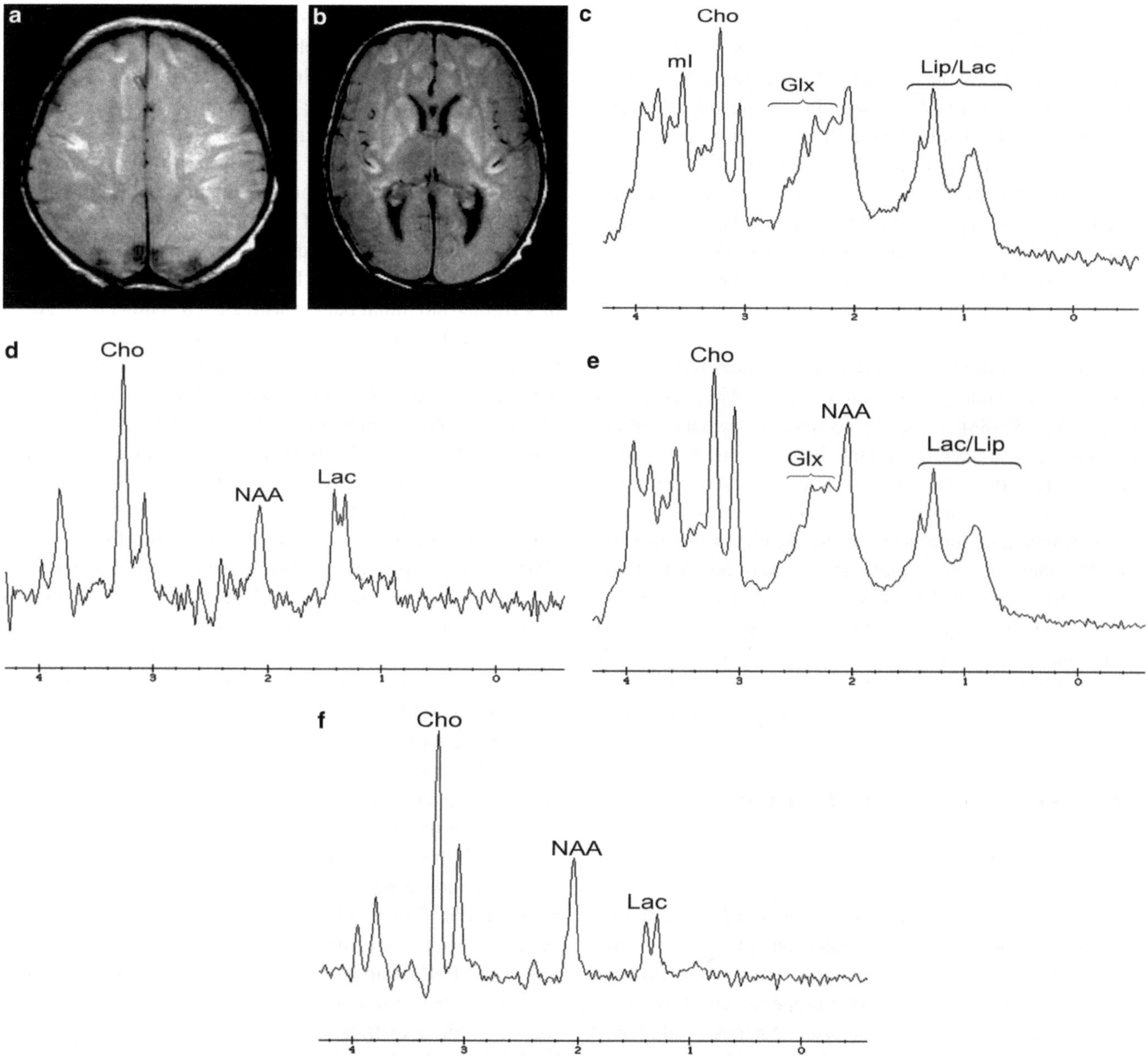

Fig. 11.6 MRI and MRS findings from a 10-day-old female diagnosed with carbamoylphosphate synthetase I. (**a** and **b**) Axial proton density weighted images at two levels demonstrate hyperintense signal and swelling within the cortex and deep gray matter, (**c**) Short Echo and (**d**) Long Echo MRS acquired from the frontal white matter, (**e**) Short Echo and (**f**) Long Echo MRS acquired from the basal ganglia. The short echo MRS demonstrates elevated glutamine, lactate and lipids with reduced NAA. The long echo confirms the lactate elevation and NAA declines

Takanashi et al. suggested a spectroscopic pattern of disease involvement with mI depletion, glutamine accumulation, followed by choline depletion.

Kojic et al. described a 16-year-old female patient with well-controlled CPSI who presented with hyperammonemia, which was corrected over 2 days [84]. Despite maintenance of near normal ammonia levels, the patient suffered further neurologic deterioration. After being comatose for 5 days, short echo proton MRS was acquired within the occipital gray and parietal white matter. The resonances within alpha (3.65–3.8 ppm), beta and gamma (2.02–2.5 ppm) regions corresponding to glutamate and glutamine levels were elevated, especially in gray matter. After 5 weeks and therapeutic efforts to reduce glutamine levels, the patient emerged from the coma. Five months after presentation, when the patient had made an essentially complete recovery, a repeat MRS study indicated a decrease of glutamate and glutamine levels, but without normalization of the levels (Fig. 11.6).

Three urea cycle defects are based within the mitochondria: OTC, carbamoylphosphate synthetase I (CPSI), and N-acetyl glutamate synthetase (NAGS). Other enzymatic defects, argininosuccinate synthase (ASS), argininosuccinate lyase (ASL) and arginase (ARG), plus the ornithine and citrin transporters, function within the cytosol. OTC and CPSI tend to present with the highest risk for acute neurological injury, thought to arise from severe hyperammonemia. ARG and hyperornithine, hyperammonemia and homocitrullinuria (HHH) syndrome (from the ornithine transporter) tend not to have as dramatic elevations of ammonia. However, the major neurological symptoms for ARG and HHH are spastic diplegia/quadriplegia. There are a limited number of case studies reporting the proton MRS findings in patients with ARG and ASL deficiencies [85–88]. These reports have somewhat contradictory findings and uncertain metabolite assignments for arginine and guanidinoacetate (GAA), but raise interesting points about neurological injury arising from entities other than hyperammonemia, such as secondary creatine deficiency with possibly abnormal concentrations of GAA and Cr that may relate to the synthesis defects occurring within the brain.

MRS studies using [13]C- and ^{15}N-labeled compounds in animal models have revealed mechanistically how the brain detoxifies ammonia and synthesize glutamate, glutamine and GABA via neurotransmitter cycling [89–101].

Miscellaneous Metabolic Disorders

Galactosemia

Galactosemia is an autosomal recessive disorder arising from mutations in the *GALT* gene located on chromosome 9p13. Defects in the gene alter the galactose-1-phosphate uridylyltransferase protein responsible for proper metabolism of carbohydrates, specifically galactose. Diagnosis of GALT enzyme activity is necessary to differentiate classic galactosemia (<5% controls) from Duarte variant galactosemia (5–25% control values). Infants with classic galactosemia have no GALT enzyme activity and cannot oxidize galactose to CO_2. Within days of ingesting breast milk or lactose-containing formulas, affected infants develop life-threatening complications including poor feeding, hypoglycemia, jaundice, hepatocellular damage, failure to thrive, bleeding diathesis, and hyperammonemia. If untreated, a bulging anterior fontanel and pseudotumor cerebri have been described. Also, sepsis with *Escherichia coli*, shock and death may occur. During the first 3–10 days of life, if a lactose-galactose-restricted diet is initiated, the symptoms resolve quickly and prognosis is good for prevention of liver failure, *Escherichia coli* sepsis, neonatal death, and intellectual disability. If treatment is delayed, complications such as intellectual disability, speech abnormalities, ocular cataracts, growth retardation, and primary ovarian failure in females are likely [102]. Due to the failure of the primary galactose metabolic pathway, an alternative enzyme activates in which aldose reductase catalyzes the conversion of galactose to galactitol. Excretion of abnormal quantities of galactitol in the urine is characteristic of galactosemia.

Berry et al. first reported detection of galactitol with in vivo proton MRS acquired in the basal ganglia and occipital cortex of a 10-day-old infant patient with galactosemia [103]. At 1.5 Tesla, galactitol resonates with two resonance peaks were located at 3.67 and 3.74 ppm. NAA, Cho and mI/Cr levels were reduced in both regions upon comparison with metabolite levels from age-matched healthy control participants. In a subsequent study of 12 patients diagnosed with galactosemia, Wang et al. demonstrated a correlation existed between the MRS-detected galactitol/Cr level acquired within the basal ganglia and the urine galactitol levels for the four neonates [104]. For eight patients (ages 1.3–47 years) who had been on galactose-restricted diets since the neonatal period, cerebral galactitol was undetectable by proton MRS for six of the patients, with a small elevation observed for the remaining two. This suggested that in order to detect galactitol on in vivo brain proton MRS examination, high galactitol levels are requisite in the patient's urine. Galactosemic patients, who have been following a restricted diet for several years and maintain controlled levels of galactitol in the urine, do not demonstrate galactitol in the brain by in vivo MRS. Otaduy et al. further confirmed this with proton MRS revealing a doublet at 3.7 ppm indicating elevated galactitol in an undiagnosed 6-month-old female [105]. In vitro proton MRS of the patient's urine confirmed the elevations of galactose and galactitol. Follow-up MRS performed at 2 years was within normal limits and did not reveal galactitol as the patient was treated with a restricted lactose-free diet. These findings explains the early negative MRS findings in controlled patients described by Moller et al. in 1995 [106].

Wilson's Disease

Wilson's disease, also known as hepatolenticular degeneration, is an autosomal recessive disorder arising from mutations in the ATPase Copper (2+) Transporting, Beta Polypeptide, *ATP7B* gene located on chromosome 13q14.3. Defects in the gene alter the protein responsible for the transport of copper from the liver to other parts of the body. This protein regulates the elimination of excess copper from the body. With its dysfunction, copper accumulates in the liver, eyes, and brain, particularly the globus pallidus. Signs and symptoms usually begin between 3 and 40 years of age, with liver disease occurring first, and most beginning after puberty. Neurologic dysfunction includes movement disorders, rigid dystonia, and psychiatric disturbances such as depression, anxiety and mood disorders. Diagnosis depends upon the detection of low serum copper and ceruloplasmin concentrations, increased urinary copper excretion, the presence of Kayser-Fleisher rings in the cornea, and/or increased hepatic copper concentration. Lifelong treatment with chelating agents is initiated with symptomatic diagnosis. Copper chelating agents (penicillamine or trientine) increase urinary excretion of copper. High-dose oral zinc reduces with absorption of copper from the gastrointestinal tract and is most effective after initial treatment with a chelating agent. Antioxidants, such as vitamin E, may be used with a chelator or zinc to prevent tissue damage, particularly to the liver. Foods high in copper are also restricted. Orthotopic liver transplantation can be performed for individuals who fail to respond or are unable to tolerate medical therapy.

Pathologic changes noted in the brain include atrophy, cavitations, spongy softening, neuron loss, and the presence of Opalski cells [107, 108]. On MRI, brain involvement with Wilson's disease usually presents with bilateral and symmetric lesions within the globus pallidus, putamen, thalamus, mesencephalon, pons, and dentate nucleus. The basal ganglia are hyperintense on T1-weighted images and the first echo of the T2-weighted sequence, as seen in other causes of hepatic dysfunction. The same areas are typically hyperintense on T2 weighted and FLAIR images early in the course of the disease, but the hyperintense signal may decrease late in the disease associated with an increase in signal on the T1-weighted images. White matter abnormalities are also detected including abnormal signal within the splenium of the corpus callosum [108]. The white matter demonstrates progressive increase in T2 signal due to demyelination and gliosis. Cerebral cortical, and brainstem volume loss have also been described.

Van den Heuvel et al. was the first to explore metabolic changes caused by portosystemic shunting via proton MRS in a study of patients with Wilson's disease [109]. Twenty-two adult patients with biochemically proven Wilson's disease and 13 age-matched adult control subjects underwent MRI and short echo, single voxel MRS sampling within the right and left globi pallidus. NAA/Cr and Cho/Cr levels were decreased in patients with Wilson's disease compared with control subjects. The patients with portosystemic shunting demonstrated lower mI/Cr levels than did patients without portosystemic shunting. Several MRS studies reported in *adults* with Wilson's disease found no differences upon comparison with control participants [110, 111]. However, these reports often employed large volumes of interest in different locations within the brain, conducted different stages of the disease with variability in the periods of treatment, and in patient populations with and without liver dysfunction. Recent studies in adults have improved the characterization of patients and conditions for spectral acquisition. Page et al. employed short echo single voxel proton MRS within the striatum of patients with Wilson's disease [112]. Upon determining metabolite concentrations, reductions of NAA and *N*-acetylaspartylglutamate were found in those patients with neurologic features but not in patients without clinical neurologic involvement upon comparison with age-matched normal control subjects. Choline was also reduced in both patient groups compared with age-matched controls. Lucato et al. recognized the effects of metals (iron, copper) on spectral linewidths by altering metabolite relaxation times [113]. Copper deposition within the brain, especially the globus pallidus, can produce distortions in the linewidths of the metabolites within the spectrum due to the paramagnetic properties of the copper (2+) ion. Compared with control subjects, treated patients with Wilson's disease (mean age 25 years with mean duration of treatment 5 years) had significantly decreased NAA/Cr levels in the basal ganglia, frontal white matter and the parietal–occipital cortex and increased mI/Cr levels in the basal ganglia obtained using a short echo single voxel approach. Cho/Cr and Glx/Cr did not differ between the groups in any location. Using a long echo single voxel approach, Algin et al. examined frontal white matter, thalamus and pons in treated patients with Wilson's disease (mean age 29 years with mean disease duration of 7.9 years) [114]. Measurements in the thalamus and pons showed significantly lower NAA/Cho and NAA/Cr levels in the Wilson's disease group than in the control group. Thalamic and pontine Cho/Cr levels in the patient group were significantly higher than those of the control group. There was no significant difference between treated patients and controls for any metabolite in the frontal white matter. In a series of articles, Tarnacka and colleagues have examined newly diagnosed patients with Wilson's disease, those treated for 1 year and even heterozygote carriers of the disease with proton MRS [115–118]. The patients were classified based on symptoms (neurologic and hepatic involvement) and the response when treated.

Reported within the first article, the globus pallidus and thalamus of 37 patients newly diagnosed with Wilson's disease were examined bilaterally with MRS [117]. Patients demonstrated decreased mI/Cr and NAA/Cr levels and an increased Lip/Cr level in the pallidum. In the pallidum of neurologically impaired patients, Cho/Cr, Glx/Cr and Lip/Cr levels were higher than in control subjects, and the NAA/Cr was significantly lower. In hepatic patients, the mI/Cr, Cho/Cr and NAA/Cr levels were lower than in controls.

In the thalamus, increased Glx/Cr and Lip/Cr levels were observed. The Cho/Cr and Lip/Cr levels were higher in the thalami of neurologically impaired patients, and Lip/Cr levels were higher than controls in hepatic patients.

Tarnacka et al. then followed 17 newly diagnosed patients with Wilson's disease for a 1-year period [118]. During this observation period, six neurological and 9nine hepatic patients improved, while two neurological patients deteriorated. The baseline pretreatment MRS examination found lower mI/Cr, NAA/Cr, and higher Lip/Cr levels in all patients with improvement compared with controls. In patients with hepatic signs, an increase of mI/Cr and Glx/Cr was observed 1 year post-treatment. In patients with neurological improvement after treatment, an increase of NAA/Cr levels was noted. During neurological deterioration, a decrease of Glx/Cr and NAA/Cr levels was observed. However, in a neurologically impaired patient with liver failure exacerbation, a decrease of mI/Cr and increase of Glx/Cr levels was observed.

Tarnacka et al. also examined 27 Wilson's disease patients treated more than 6 years [115]. All patients with marked improvement demonstrated higher levels of Cho/Cr, Glx/Cr, and Lip/Cr levels compared with control participants. No abnormalities with respect to NAA/Cr levels were observed for patients with marked improvement. All patients without marked improvement had lower NAA/Cr and higher Lip/Cr levels compared to controls. Summarizing, the alternations of NAA/Cr levels in neurologically impaired patients and mI/Cr and Glx/Cr levels in patients with liver failure appear to be sensitive markers of the clinical recovery and deterioration in Wilson's disease patients. Asymptomatic, heterozygote carriers demonstrated higher mean ratio levels of Glx/Cr and Lip/Cr in both the pallidum and thalami compared to control subjects suggesting abnormal copper metabolism as well [116].

Proton MRSI and image selected in vivo spectroscopy (ISIS) phosphorus MRS was performed with 40 patients diagnosed with Wilson's disease (treated, 29; untreated, 11) and 30 controls [119]. The mean durations of illness and treatment were 6.2 ± 7.4 and 4.8 ± 5.9 years, respectively. Proton MRS revealed a reduction of NAA/Cho and NAA/Cr levels in striatum of treated patients compared to controls. The mean values of phosphomonoesters (PME), phosphodiesters (PDE), and total phosphorus (TPh) were elevated in patients compared to controls. Elevated levels of PME/PDE observed in the striatum were noted in treated patients as compared to controls in the phosphorus MRS study. The PME/PDE ratio was elevated in the treated group compared to untreated group. The increased duration of illness correlated with increased PME/PDE PME/TPh, and PDE/TPh, and decreased NAA/Cho levels. NAA/Cho levels also correlated with measures of disease severity.

Only two groups have reported proton MRS findings in a total of four children with Wilson's disease. Jayasundar et al. compared the spectral findings of three treated children, ages 8, 12, and 16 years with the oldest child having only 5 days of treatment before demise [120]. Juan et al. reported on a 12-year-old male diagnosed with Wilson's disease without hepatic dysfunction or corneal copper deposition that presented with hemichorea and subnormal copper metabolism [121]. Within the unusual presentation of asymmetrical edematous putaminal lesions, long echo MRS demonstrated lactate accumulation and decrease of the NAA/Cr levels with a markedly increased ADC value on diffusion imaging. For a child in the early stage of Wilson's disease, these findings were suggestive of acute necrosis with anaerobic metabolism of glucose leading suggesting a poor clinical outcome later confirmed at follow-up.

Inborn Errors of Creatine Metabolism: Cerebral Creatine Deficiency Syndromes

Creatine (α-methyl-guanidinoacetic acid) plays an important role in energy metabolism. In humans, Cr is synthesized in the liver, kidney, and pancreas where it is taken up via a sodium- and chloride-dependent Cr transporter (SLC6A8 protein) and ultimately transported via the blood to the muscles, heart, and nervous system, which are rich in creatine kinase. Creatine kinase is an essential enzyme to catalyze phosphorylation of Cr to provide a high-energy phosphate buffer system.

Creatine deficiency syndromes arise from one of three distinct defects, two involving Cr biosynthesis and one involving Cr transport. On proton MRS within the brain, all three disorders demonstrate a severely diminished or completely absent signal at 3.0 ppm for the composite resonance of creatine and phosphocreatine. Some degree of discrimination between synthesis and transporter defects could potentially be afforded from the MRS determination of Cr levels within skeletal muscle. Cr levels in the muscle of some patients with Cr biosynthesis defects are low. However, evidence suggests additional Cr transport mechanisms exist allowing passage of dietary sources of Cr (foods rich in Cr, creatine monohydrate supplements) into the muscle. Cr levels were described within normal limits for muscle in one patient with a transporter defect [122, 123]. However, the urine and plasma measurement of guanidinoacetic acid (GAA), Cr and the excreted form creatinine are the most cost-efficient approaches for narrowing the diagnostic differential. The next tier of testing includes molecular genetic testing; however, it too can be inconclusive. Finally, enzyme activity and Cr uptake can discriminate among the three disorders. Diagnosis remains important as patients with synthesis defects can benefit from dietary Cr supplementation.

Creatine biosynthesis relies on two enzymatic reactions:

1. Arginine glycine amidino transferase (AGAT). The *GATM* gene located on chromosome 15q21.1 15q15.3 catalyzes the transfer of the amidino group from arginine to glycine yielding ornithine and GAA;
2. Guanidinoacetate methyl transferase (GAMT). The *GAMT* gene located on chromosome 19p13.3 catalyzes the methylation of the amidino group in GAA yielding Cr.

Creatine Synthesis Defect: Arginine:Glycine Amidinotransferase Deficiency

AGAT deficiency has been described in seven individuals: three from one Italian family, two from a family of Chinese descent within the USA, and two from Yemenite Jewish descent [124–127]. This autosomal recessive disorder can present with mild-to-moderate intellectual disability, psychomotor delay, language delay, failure-to-thrive and autistic-like behavioral features. Patients with AGAT deficiency appear to respond favorably to creatine monohydrate dietary supplementation with dramatic improvement in neurological abnormalities [128].

Creatine Synthesis Defect: Guanidinoacetate Methyltransferase Deficiency

GAMT deficiency was the first creatine deficiency syndrome recognized and now reportedly affects about 40 individuals worldwide [128, 129]. This autosomal recessive disorder can present with variable clinical features and include mental retardation, language and developmental delay, muscular hypotonia, weakness, extra-pyramidal signs, epilepsy, autistic and in some, hyperactivity and self-aggressive behavior [128]. In many patients, but not all with GAMT deficiency, abnormal hyperintense T2 signal appears within the globus pallidus, which is thought to reflect neuronal injury from GAA accumulation.

If early treatment is implemented, especially in the neonatal period, patients with GAMT defects demonstrate favorable response to creatine monohydrate dietary supplementation (Fig. 11.7). A dietary restriction of arginine in combination with ornithine supplementation reduces the accumulation of GAA by competitive inhibition of AGAT activity. In older patients, the prolonged accumulation of neurotoxic GAA limits the neurological benefits of Cr supplementation [130–135].

Creatine Transporter Defect: SLC6A8 Deficiency

The discovery of the X-linked creatine transporter defect began with the absence of Cr resonance noticed upon proton MRS acquired within the basal ganglia and frontal lobes of a 6-year-old male being evaluated for language delay and a head circumference at the 95th percentile [136]. Imaging was unremarkable (Fig. 11.7). Metabolic testing revealed elevated serum and urine Cr levels with normal substrates and products involved in Cr synthesis and excretion (glycine, ornithine, GAA, and creatinine). Upon exclusion of a synthesis defect, a novel mutation in the human Cr transporter gene, *SLC6A8*, located on Xq28 was hypothesized. Fibroblast from the 6-year-old male confirmed a hemizygous nonsense mutation (R514X) [137]. The maternal female relatives were heterozygous for the mutation. The nonsense mutation most likely results in an unstable and/or inappropriately folded protein that is completely inactive, thereby inhibiting transport of Cr. Reports indicate that over 150 patients have been diagnosed with this disorder. It is now estimated that an incidence of creatine transporter deficiency ranges from 0.25 to 3.5%, making its diagnosis frequency second only to Fragile X syndrome in X-linked mental retardation syndromes [126, 138–146]. There is variability in the clinical presentation; however, common features include speech delay, intellectual disabilities and epilepsy. Epilepsy can usually be controlled with medication. Some patients with creatine transporter deficiency, especially older ones, demonstrate volume loss on MR imaging. At this time, there is no definitive therapy that can allow passage of Cr across the blood–brain barrier to restore brain Cr for patients with creatine transporter deficiency. Chilosi et al. reported neurological improvement in two patients with Cr transporter deficiency treated with arginine supplementation to promote cerebral Cr synthesis [147]. However, this finding was not replicated in four patients supplemented with arginine [148].

Secondary Creatine Transporter Deficiency

Ornithine delta-aminotransferase (OAT) deficiency causes gyrate atrophy of the retina due to high plasma ornithine concentrations. Since Cr synthesis requires the conversion of arginine and glycine into ornithine and guanidinoacetate, high ornithine concentration inhibits this reaction thereby producing a secondary Cr deficiency. Valayannopoulos et al. evaluated with proton MRS seven patients with OAT deficiency [149]. All patients demonstrated profound cerebral Cr deficiency, which was further accompanied with decreased levels of Cr and/or GAA in plasma and urine.

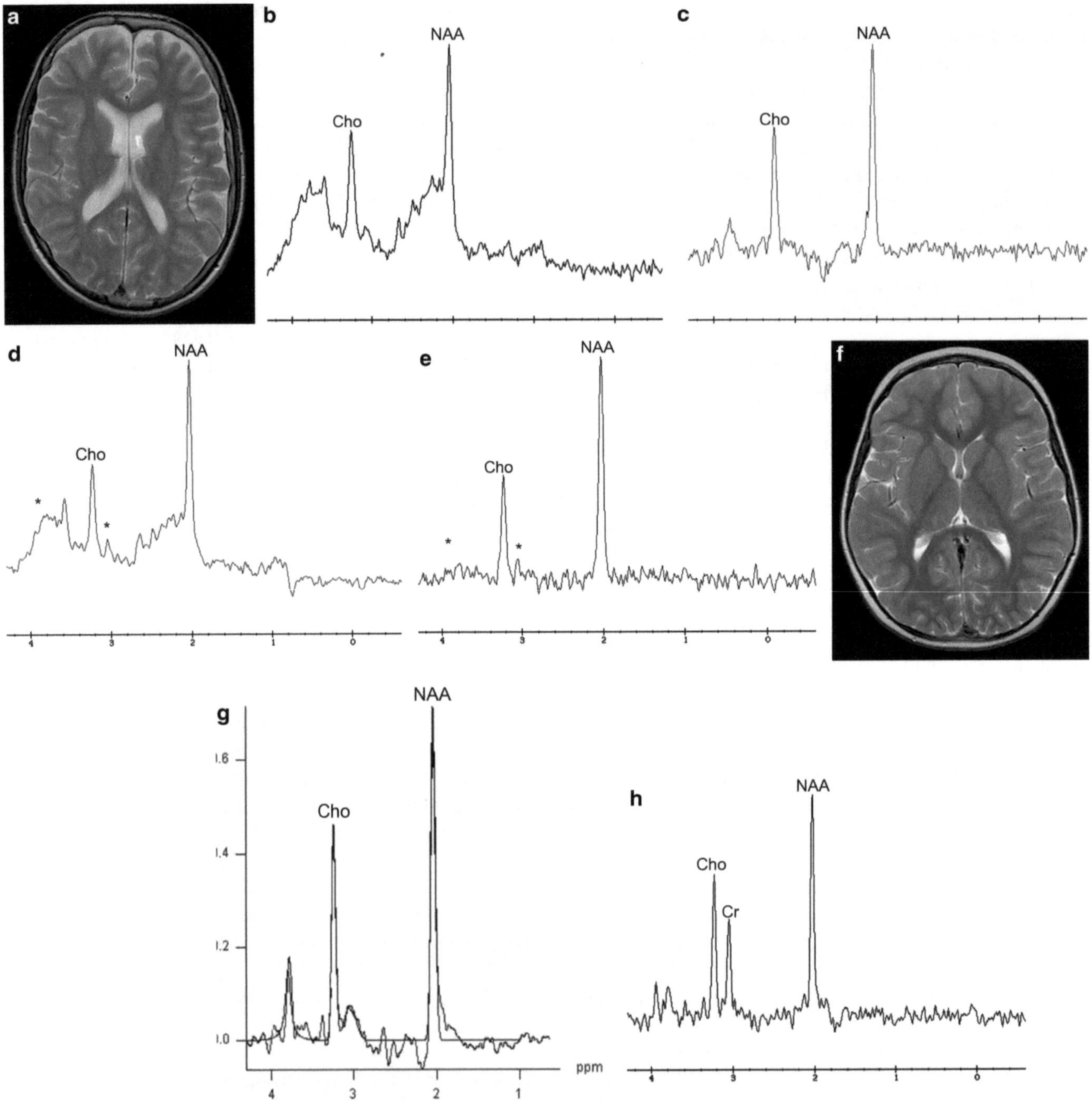

Fig. 11.7 MRI and MRS findings obtained from two patients with creatine deficiency syndromes. The first patient (images **a**–**e**) suffers from a creatine transporter deficiency. (**a**) Axial T2-weighted image obtained at 15 years of age is unremarkable. (**b**) Short and (**c**) Long echo MRS obtained from the left frontal white matter demonstrates the absence of creatine signal at 3.0 and 3.9 ppm. (**d**) Short and (**e**) Long echo MRS were obtained after the male patient suffered an increase in seizure frequency at 15 years of age. A depletion of creatine is again appreciated. The second patient (images (**f**–**h**) suffers from a creatine synthesis defect known as GAMT deficiency. (**f**) Axial T2-weighted imaging demonstrates no signal abnormality with the globus pallidus. The patient was diagnosed after a female sibling was diagnosed at 7 years of age. The presented at 18 months of age with creatine deficiency diagnosed from the long echo MRS acquired within the basal ganglia on a 3 Tesla MR system shown in (**g**). Figure **h** demonstrates long echo MRS acquired on a 1.5 T MR system at 2 years of age following dietary supplementation of creatine

Conclusions

Examples of several metabolic disorders have been presented in this chapter. In determining a differential diagnosis, it is critical to integrate the information obtained from the MRS examination with clinical symptoms, family history, results from MRI and any other imaging, laboratory, metabolic and genetic testing. Because the MRS presentation of these diseases varies with age at onset, the progression of the illness, and effects from treatment, it is crucial that the MRS data be interpreted with this timing-specific information in mind. Thus, the descriptions and data shown in this chapter are intended to be illustrative rather than definitive. It is our intention that the information presented here will serve to guide the reader in interpreting the MR spectra from these and other metabolic disorders.

Acknowledgments This work was supported by grants from the National Institutes of Health, NIEHS R01 ES015559, NCI R01 CA112182, and NIMH P50 MH077138. The authors have no competing financial or non-financial interests to declare.

References

1. Confort-Gouny S, Chabrol B, Vion-Dury J, Mancini J, Cozzone PJ. MRI and localized proton MRS in early infantile form of neuronal ceroid-lipofuscinosis. Pediatr Neurol. 1993;9(1):57–60.
2. Brockmann K, Pouwels PJ, Christen HJ, Frahm J, Hanefeld F. Localized proton magnetic resonance spectroscopy of cerebral metabolic disturbances in children with neuronal ceroid lipofuscinosis. Neuropediatrics. 1996;27(5):242–8.
3. Seitz D, Grodd W, Schwab A, Seeger U, Klose U, Nagele T. MR imaging and localized proton MR spectroscopy in late infantile neuronal ceroid lipofuscinosis. AJNR Am J Neuroradiol. 1998;19(7):1373–7.
4. Vanhanen SL, Puranen J, Autti T, et al. Neuroradiological findings (MRS, MRI, SPECT) in infantile neuronal ceroid-lipofuscinosis (infantile CLN1) at different stages of the disease. Neuropediatrics. 2004;35(1):27–35.
5. Sitter B, Autti T, Tyynela J, et al. High-resolution magic angle spinning and 1 H magnetic resonance spectroscopy reveal significantly altered neuronal metabolite profiles in CLN1 but not in CLN3. J Neurosci Res. 2004;77(5):762–9.
6. Vanier MT. Niemann-Pick disease type C. Orphanet J Rare Dis. 2010;5:16.
7. Tedeschi G, Bonavita S, Barton NW, et al. Proton magnetic resonance spectroscopic imaging in the clinical evaluation of patients with Niemann-Pick type C disease. J Neurol Neurosurg Psychiatry. 1998;65(1):72–9.
8. Sylvain M, Arnold DL, Scriver CR, Schreiber R, Shevell MI. Magnetic resonance spectroscopy in Niemann-Pick disease type C: correlation with diagnosis and clinical response to cholestyramine and lovastatin. Pediatr Neurol. 1994;10(3):228–32.
9. Galanaud D, Tourbah A, Lehericy S, et al. 24 month-treatment with miglustat of three patients with Niemann-Pick disease type C: follow up using brain spectroscopy. Mol Genet Metab. 2009;96(2):55–8.
10. Varho T, Komu M, Sonninen P, et al. A new metabolite contributing to N-acetyl signal in 1 H MRS of the brain in Salla disease. Neurology. 1999;52(8):1668–72.
11. Suhonen-Polvi H, Varho T, Metsahonkala L, et al. Increased brain glucose utilization in Salla disease (free sialic acid storage disorder). J Nucl Med. 1999;40(1):12–8.
12. Kaback M, Lim-Steele J, Dabholkar D, Brown D, Levy N, Zeiger K. Tay-Sachs disease—carrier screening, prenatal diagnosis, and the molecular era. An international perspective, 1970 to 1993. The International TSD Data Collection Network. JAMA. 1993;270(19):2307–15.
13. Kaback MM. Population-based genetic screening for reproductive counseling: the Tay-Sachs disease model. Eur J Pediatr. 2000;159 Suppl 3:S192–195.
14. Aydin K, Bakir B, Tatli B, Terzibasioglu E, Ozmen M. Proton MR spectroscopy in three children with Tay-Sachs disease. Pediatr Radiol. 2005;35(11):1081–5.
15. Imamura A, Miyajima H, Ito R, Orii KO. Serial MR imaging and 1 H-MR spectroscopy in monozygotic twins with Tay-Sachs disease. Neuropediatrics. 2008;39(5):259–63.
16. Felderhoff-Mueser U, Sperner J, Konstanzcak P, Navon R, Weschke B. 31Phosphorus magnetic resonance spectroscopy in late-onset Tay-Sachs disease. J Child Neurol. 2001;16(5):377–80.
17. Wilken B, Dechent P, Hanefeld F, Frahm J. Proton MRS of a child with Sandhoff disease reveals elevated brain hexosamine. Eur J Paediatr Neurol. 2008;12(1):56–60.
18. Lowe JP, Stuckey DJ, Awan FR, et al. MRS reveals additional hexose N-acetyl resonances in the brain of a mouse model for Sandhoff disease. NMR Biomed. 2005;18(8):517–26.
19. Miyanomae Y, Ochi M, Yoshioka H, et al. Cerebral MRI and spectroscopy in Sjogren-Larsson syndrome: case report. Neuroradiology. 1995;37(3):225–8.
20. Mano T, Ono J, Kaminaga T, et al. Proton MR spectroscopy of Sjogren-Larsson's syndrome. AJNR Am J Neuroradiol. 1999;20(9):1671–3.
21. Willemsen MA, Van Der Graaf M, Van Der Knaap MS, et al. MR imaging and proton MR spectroscopic studies in Sjogren-Larsson syndrome: characterization of the leukoencephalopathy. AJNR Am J Neuroradiol. 2004;25(4):649–57.
22. Willemsen MA, Lutt MA, Steijlen PM, et al. Clinical and biochemical effects of zileuton in patients with the Sjogren-Larsson syndrome. Eur J Pediatr. 2001;160(12):711–7.
23. Willemsen MA, Ijlst L, Steijlen PM, et al. Clinical, biochemical and molecular genetic characteristics of 19 patients with the Sjogren-Larsson syndrome. Brain. 2001;124(Pt 7):1426–37.
24. Willemsen MA, Rotteveel JJ, Steijlen PM, Heerschap A, Mayatepek E. 5-Lipoxygenase inhibition: a new treatment strategy for Sjogren-Larsson syndrome. Neuropediatrics. 2000;31(1):1–3.
25. Nakayama M, Tavora DG, Alvim TC, Araujo AC, Gama RL. MRI and 1H-MRS findings of three patients with Sjogren-Larsson syndrome. Arq Neuropsiquiatr. 2006;64(2B):398–401.
26. Lossos A, Khoury M, Rizzo WB, et al. Phenotypic variability among adult siblings with Sjogren-Larsson syndrome. Arch Neurol. 2006;63(2):278–80.
27. Pirgon O, Aydin K, Atabek ME. Proton magnetic resonance spectroscopy findings and clinical effects of montelukast sodium in a case with Sjogren-Larsson syndrome. J Child Neurol. 2006;21(12):1092–5.
28. Kaminaga T, Mano T, Ono J, Kusuoka H, Nakamura H, Nishimura T. Proton magnetic resonance spectroscopy of Sjogren-Larsson syndrome heterozygotes. Magn Reson Med. 2001;45(6):1112–5.
29. DiMauro S. Mitochondrial DNA medicine. Biosci Rep. 2007;27(1–3):5–9.
30. Pavlakis SG, Kingsley PB, Kaplan GP, Stacpoole PW, O'Shea M, Lustbader D. Magnetic resonance spectroscopy: use in monitoring MELAS treatment. Arch Neurol. 1998;55(6):849–52.

31. Wilichowski E, Pouwels PJ, Frahm J, Hanefeld F. Quantitative proton magnetic resonance spectroscopy of cerebral metabolic disturbances in patients with MELAS. Neuropediatrics. 1999;30(5):256–63.
32. Castillo M, Kwock L, Green C. MELAS syndrome: imaging and proton MR spectroscopic findings. AJNR Am J Neuroradiol. 1995;16(2):233–9.
33. Dinopoulos A, Cecil KM, Schapiro MB, et al. Brain MRI and proton MRS findings in infants and children with respiratory chain defects. Neuropediatrics. 2005;36(5):290–301.
34. Bianchi MC, Sgandurra G, Tosetti M, Battini R, Cioni G. Brain magnetic resonance in the diagnostic evaluation of mitochondrial encephalopathies. Biosci Rep. 2007;27(1–3):69–85.
35. Lin DD, Crawford TO, Barker PB. Proton MR spectroscopy in the diagnostic evaluation of suspected mitochondrial disease. AJNR Am J Neuroradiol. 2003;24(1):33–41.
36. Barkovich AJ, Good WV, Koch TK, Berg BO. Mitochondrial disorders: analysis of their clinical and imaging characteristics. AJNR Am J Neuroradiol. 1993;14(5):1119–37.
37. Boddaert N, Romano S, Funalot B, et al. 1 H MRS spectroscopy evidence of cerebellar high lactate in mitochondrial respiratory chain deficiency. Mol Genet Metab. 2008;93(1):85–8.
38. Filosto M, Tomelleri G, Tonin P, et al. Neuropathology of mitochondrial diseases. Biosci Rep. 2007;27(1–3):23–30.
39. Brockmann K, Bjornstad A, Dechent P, et al. Succinate in dystrophic white matter: a proton magnetic resonance spectroscopy finding characteristic for complex II deficiency. Ann Neurol. 2002;52(1):38–46.
40. Heindel W, Kugel H, Roth B. Noninvasive detection of increased glycine content by proton MR spectroscopy in the brains of two infants with nonketotic hyperglycinemia. AJNR Am J Neuroradiol. 1993;14(3):629–35.
41. Gabis L, Parton P, Roche P, Lenn N, Tudorica A, Huang W. In vivo 1 H magnetic resonance spectroscopic measurement of brain glycine levels in nonketotic hyperglycinemia. J Neuroimaging. 2001;11(2):209–11.
42. Huisman TA, Thiel T, Steinmann B, Zeilinger G, Martin E. Proton magnetic resonance spectroscopy of the brain of a neonate with nonketotic hyperglycinemia: in vivo-in vitro (ex vivo) correlation. Eur Radiol. 2002;12(4):858–61.
43. Viola A, Chabrol B, Nicoli F, Confort-Gouny S, Viout P, Cozzone PJ. Magnetic resonance spectroscopy study of glycine pathways in nonketotic hyperglycinemia. Pediatr Res. 2002;52(2):292–300.
44. Tekgul H, Serdaroglu G, Karapinar B, et al. Vigabatrin caused rapidly progressive deterioration in two cases with early myoclonic encephalopathy associated with nonketotic hyperglycinemia. J Child Neurol. 2006;21(1):82–4.
45. Kugel H, Roth B, Pillekamp F, et al. Proton spectroscopic metabolite signal relaxation times in preterm infants: a prerequisite for quantitative spectroscopy in infant brain. J Magn Reson Imaging. 2003;17(6):634–40.
46. Kreis R, Ernst T, Ross BD. Development of the human brain: in vivo quantification of metabolite and water content with proton magnetic resonance spectroscopy. Magn Reson Med. 1993; 30(4):424–37.
47. Prescot AP, de B Frederick B, Wang L, et al. In vivo detection of brain glycine with echo-time-averaged (1)H magnetic resonance spectroscopy at 4.0 T. Magn Reson Med. 2006;55(3):681–6.
48. Manley BJ, Sokol J, Cheong JL. Intracerebral blood and MRS in neonatal nonketotic hyperglycinemia. Pediatr Neurol. 2010; 42(3):219–22.
49. Hoffmann GF, Athanassopoulos S, Burlina AB, et al. Clinical course, early diagnosis, treatment, and prevention of disease in glutaryl-CoA dehydrogenase deficiency. Neuropediatrics. 1996;27(3):115–23.
50. Moller HE, Koch HG, Weglage J, Freudenberg F, Ullrich K. Investigation of the cerebral energy status in patients with glutaric aciduria type I by 31P magnetic resonance spectroscopy. Neuropediatrics. 2003;34(2):57–60.
51. Elster AW. Glutaric aciduria type I: value of diffusion-weighted magnetic resonance imaging for diagnosing acute striatal necrosis. J Comput Assist Tomogr. 2004;28(1):98–100.
52. Santos CC, Roach ES. Glutaric aciduria type I: a neuroimaging diagnosis? J Child Neurol. 2005;20(7):588–90.
53. Kurul S, Cakmakci H, Dirik E. Glutaric aciduria type 1: proton magnetic resonance spectroscopy findings. Pediatr Neurol. 2004;31(3):228–31.
54. Oguz KK, Ozturk A, Cila A. Diffusion-weighted MR imaging and MR spectroscopy in glutaric aciduria type 1. Neuroradiology. 2005;47(3):229–34.
55. Sijens PE, Smit GP, Meiners LC, Oudkerk M, van Spronsen FJ. Cerebral 1 H MR spectroscopy revealing white matter NAA decreases in glutaric aciduria type I. Mol Genet Metab. 2006;88(3):285–9.
56. Firat AK, Karakas HM, Yakinci C. Magnetic resonance spectroscopic characteristics of glutaric aciduria type II. Dev Med Child Neurol. 2006;48(10):847–50.
57. Rzem R, Veiga-da-Cunha M, Noel G, et al. A gene encoding a putative FAD-dependent L-2-hydroxyglutarate dehydrogenase is mutated in L-2-hydroxyglutaric aciduria. Proc Natl Acad Sci USA. 2004;101(48):16849–54.
58. Topcu M, Jobard F, Halliez S, et al. L-2-Hydroxyglutaric aciduria: identification of a mutant gene C14orf160, localized on chromosome 14q22.1. Hum Mol Genet. 2004;13(22):2803–11.
59. D'Incerti L, Farina L, Moroni I, Uziel G, Savoiardo M. L-2-Hydroxyglutaric aciduria: MRI in seven cases. Neuroradiology. 1998;40(11):727–33.
60. Seijo-Martinez M, Navarro C, Castro del Rio M, et al. L-2-hydroxyglutaric aciduria: clinical, neuroimaging, and neuropathological findings. Arch Neurol. 2005;62(4):666–70.
61. Steenweg ME, Salomons GS, Yapici Z, et al. L-2-Hydroxyglutaric aciduria: pattern of MR imaging abnormalities in 56 patients. Radiology. 2009;251(3):856–65.
62. Topcu M, Aydin OF, Yalcinkaya C, et al. L-2-hydroxyglutaric aciduria: a report of 29 patients. Turk J Pediatr. 2005;47(1):1–7.
63. Hanefeld F, Kruse B, Bruhn H, Frahm J. In vivo proton magnetic resonance spectroscopy of the brain in a patient with L-2-hydroxyglutaric acidemia. Pediatr Res. 1994;35(5):614–6.
64. Sener RN. L-2 hydroxyglutaric aciduria: proton magnetic resonance spectroscopy and diffusion magnetic resonance imaging findings. J Comput Assist Tomogr. 2003;27(1):38–43.
65. Aydin K, Ozmen M, Tatli B, Sencer S. Single-voxel MR spectroscopy and diffusion-weighted MRI in two patients with l-2-hydroxyglutaric aciduria. Pediatr Radiol. 2003;33(12):872–6.
66. Felber SR, Sperl W, Chemelli A, Murr C, Wendel U. Maple syrup urine disease: metabolic decompensation monitored by proton magnetic resonance imaging and spectroscopy. Ann Neurol. 1993;33(4):396–401.
67. Heindel W, Kugel H, Wendel U, Roth B, Benz-Bohm G. Proton magnetic resonance spectroscopy reflects metabolic decompensation in maple syrup urine disease. Pediatr Radiol. 1995;25(4):296–9.
68. Jan W, Zimmerman RA, Wang ZJ, Berry GT, Kaplan PB, Kaye EM. MR diffusion imaging and MR spectroscopy of maple syrup urine disease during acute metabolic decompensation. Neuroradiology. 2003;45(6):393–9.
69. Chemelli AP, Schocke M, Sperl W, Trieb T, Aichner F, Felber S. Magnetic resonance spectroscopy (MRS) in five patients with treated propionic acidemia. J Magn Reson Imaging. 2000;11(6):596–600.
70. Bergman AJ, Van der Knaap MS, Smeitink JA, et al. Magnetic resonance imaging and spectroscopy of the brain in propionic acidemia: clinical and biochemical considerations. Pediatr Res. 1996;40(3):404–9.

71. Radmanesh A, Zaman T, Ghanaati H, Molaei S, Robertson RL, Zamani AA. Methylmalonic acidemia: brain imaging findings in 52 children and a review of the literature. Pediatr Radiol. 2008;38(10):1054–61.
72. Harting I, Seitz A, Geb S, et al. Looking beyond the basal ganglia: the spectrum of MRI changes in methylmalonic acidaemia. J Inherit Metab Dis. 2008;31(3):368–78.
73. Lam WW, Wang ZJ, Zhao H, et al. 1 H MR spectroscopy of the basal ganglia in childhood: a semiquantitative analysis. Neuroradiology. 1998;40(5):315–23.
74. Trinh BC, Melhem ER, Barker PB. Multi-slice proton MR spectroscopy and diffusion-weighted imaging in methylmalonic acidemia: report of two cases and review of the literature. AJNR Am J Neuroradiol. 2001;22(5):831–3.
75. Takeuchi M, Harada M, Matsuzaki K, Hisaoka S, Nishitani H, Mori K. Magnetic resonance imaging and spectroscopy in a patient with treated methylmalonic acidemia. J Comput Assist Tomogr. 2003;27(4):547–51.
76. Michel SJ, Given 2nd CA, Robertson Jr WC. Imaging of the brain, including diffusion-weighted imaging in methylmalonic acidemia. Pediatr Radiol. 2004;34(7):580–2.
77. Longo D, Fariello G, Dionisi-Vici C, et al. MRI and 1 H-MRS findings in early-onset cobalamin C/D defect. Neuropediatrics. 2005;36(6):366–72.
78. Valayannopoulos V, Haudry C, Serre V, et al. New SUCLG1 patients expanding the phenotypic spectrum of this rare cause of mild methylmalonic aciduria. Mitochondrion. 2010;10(4):335–41.
79. Carrozzo R, Dionisi-Vici C, Steuerwald U, et al. SUCLA2 mutations are associated with mild methylmalonic aciduria, Leigh-like encephalomyopathy, dystonia and deafness. Brain. 2007;130(Pt 3):862–74.
80. Connelly A, Cross JH, Gadian DG, Hunter JV, Kirkham FJ, Leonard JV. Magnetic resonance spectroscopy shows increased brain glutamine in ornithine carbamoyl transferase deficiency. Pediatr Res. 1993;33(1):77–81.
81. Kreis R, Ross BD, Farrow NA, Ackerman Z. Metabolic disorders of the brain in chronic hepatic encephalopathy detected with H-1 MR spectroscopy. Radiology. 1992;182(1):19–27.
82. Ross B, Kreis R, Ernst T. Clinical tools for the 90s: magnetic resonance spectroscopy and metabolite imaging. Eur J Radiol. 1992;14(2):128–40.
83. Takanashi J, Kurihara A, Tomita M, et al. Distinctly abnormal brain metabolism in late-onset ornithine transcarbamylase deficiency. Neurology. 2002;59(2):210–4.
84. Kojic J, Robertson PL, Quint DJ, Martin DM, Pang Y, Sundgren PC. Brain glutamine by MRS in a patient with urea cycle disorder and coma. Pediatr Neurol. 2005;32(2):143–6.
85. Gungor S, Akinci A, Firat AK, Tabel Y, Alkan A. Neuroimaging findings in hyperargininemia. J Neuroimaging. 2008;18(4):457–62.
86. Sijens PE, Reijngoud DJ, Soorani-Lunsing RJ, Oudkerk M, van Spronsen FJ. Cerebral 1 H MR spectroscopy showing elevation of brain guanidinoacetate in argininosuccinate lyase deficiency. Mol Genet Metab. May 2006;88(1):100–2.
87. Roze E, Azuar C, Menuel C, Haberle J, Guillevin R. Usefulness of magnetic resonance spectroscopy in urea cycle disorders. Pediatr Neurol. 2007;37(3):222–5.
88. Newnham T, Hardikar W, Allen K, et al. Liver transplantation for argininosuccinic aciduria: clinical, biochemical, and metabolic outcome. Liver Transpl. 2008;14(1):41–5.
89. Kanamori K, Ross BD. Glial alkalinization detected in vivo by 1 H-15 N heteronuclear multiple-quantum coherence-transfer NMR in severely hyperammonemic rat. J Neurochem. 1997;68(3):1209–20.
90. Kanamori K, Bluml S, Ross B. Magnetic resonance spectroscopy in the study of hyperammonemia and hepatic encephalopathy. Adv Exp Med Biol. 1997;420:185–94.
91. Kanamori K, Ross BD, Chung JC, Kuo EL. Severity of hyperammonemic encephalopathy correlates with brain ammonia level and saturation of glutamine synthetase in vivo. J Neurochem. 1996;67(4):1584–94.
92. Kanamori K, Ross BD. In vivo activity of glutaminase in the brain of hyperammonaemic rats measured by 15 N nuclear magnetic resonance. Biochem J. 1995;305(Pt 1):329–36.
93. Kanamori K, Ross BD. 15 N n.m.r. measurement of the in vivo rate of glutamine synthesis and utilization at steady state in the brain of the hyperammonaemic rat. Biochem J. 1993;293(Pt 2):461–8.
94. Kanamori K, Parivar F, Ross BD. A 15 N NMR study of in vivo cerebral glutamine synthesis in hyperammonemic rats. NMR Biomed. 1993;6(1):21–6.
95. Geissler A, Kanamori K, Ross BD. Real-time study of the urea cycle using 15N n.m.r. in the isolated perfused rat liver. Biochem J. 1992;287(Pt 3):813–20.
96. Kanamori K, Ross BD, Farrow NA, Parivar F. A 15 N-NMR study of isolated brain in portacaval-shunted rats after acute hyperammonemia. Biochim Biophys Acta. 1991;1096(4):270–6.
97. Farrow NA, Kanamori K, Ross BD, Parivar F. A 15 N-n.m.r. study of cerebral, hepatic and renal nitrogen metabolism in hyperammonaemic rats. Biochem J. 1990;270(2):473–81.
98. Sibson NR, Mason GF, Shen J, et al. In vivo (13)C NMR measurement of neurotransmitter glutamate cycling, anaplerosis and TCA cycle flux in rat brain during. J Neurochem. 2001;76(4):975–89.
99. Sibson NR, Dhankhar A, Mason GF, Behar KL, Rothman DL, Shulman RG. In vivo 13C NMR measurements of cerebral glutamine synthesis as evidence for glutamate-glutamine cycling. Proc Natl Acad Sci USA. 1997;94(6):2699–704.
100. Shen J, Sibson NR, Cline G, Behar KL, Rothman DL, Shulman RG. 15 N-NMR spectroscopy studies of ammonia transport and glutamine synthesis in the hyperammonemic rat brain. Dev Neurosci. 1998;20(4–5):434–43.
101. Sibson NR, Shen J, Mason GF, Rothman DL, Behar KL, Shulman RG. Functional energy metabolism: in vivo 13C-NMR spectroscopy evidence for coupling of cerebral glucose consumption and glutamatergic neuronalactivity. Dev Neurosci. 1998;20(4–5):321–30.
102. Elsas LJ. Galactosemia. In: Pagon RA, Bird TC, Dolan CR, eds. *GeneReviews [Internet]*. October 26, 2010 ed. Seattle, WA: University of Washington; 1993.
103. Berry GT, Hunter JV, Wang Z, et al. In vivo evidence of brain galactitol accumulation in an infant with galactosemia and encephalopathy. J Pediatr. 2001;138(2):260–2.
104. Wang ZJ, Berry GT, Dreha SF, Zhao H, Segal S, Zimmerman RA. Proton magnetic resonance spectroscopy of brain metabolites in galactosemia. Ann Neurol. 2001;50(2):266–9.
105. Otaduy MC, Leite CC, Lacerda MT, et al. Proton MR spectroscopy and imaging of a galactosemic patient before and after dietary treatment. AJNR Am J Neuroradiol. 2006;27(1):204–7.
106. Moller HE, Ullrich K, Vermathen P, Schuierer G, Koch HG. In vivo study of brain metabolism in galactosemia by 1 H and 31P magnetic resonance spectroscopy. Eur J Pediatr. 1995;154(7 Suppl 2):S8–13.
107. Mikol J, Vital C, Wassef M, et al. Extensive cortico-subcortical lesions in Wilson's disease: clinico-pathological study of two cases. Acta Neuropathol. 2005;110(5):451–8.
108. Trocello JM, Guichard JP, Leyendecker A, et al. Corpus callosum abnormalities in Wilson's disease. J Neurol Neurosurg Psychiatry. 2010;82:1119–21.
109. Van Den Heuvel AG, Van der Grond J, Van Rooij LG, Van Wassenaer-van Hall HN, Hoogenraad TU, Mali WP. Differentiation between portal-systemic encephalopathy and neurodegenerative disorders in patients with Wilson disease: H-1 MR spectroscopy. Radiology. May 1997;203(2):539–43.
110. Alanen A, Komu M, Penttinen M, Leino R. Magnetic resonance imaging and proton MR spectroscopy in Wilson's disease. Br J Radiol. 1999;72(860):749–56.

111. Kraft E, Trenkwalder C, Then Bergh F, Auer DP. Magnetic resonance proton spectroscopy of the brain in Wilson's disease. J Neurol. 1999;246(8):693–9.
112. Page RA, Davie CA, MacManus D, et al. Clinical correlation of brain MRI and MRS abnormalities in patients with Wilson disease. Neurology. 2004;63(4):638–43.
113. Lucato LT, Otaduy MC, Barbosa ER, et al. Proton MR spectroscopy in Wilson disease: analysis of 36 cases. AJNR Am J Neuroradiol. 2005;26(5):1066–71.
114. Algin O, Taskapilioglu O, Hakyemez B, et al. Structural and neurochemical evaluation of the brain and pons in patients with Wilson's disease. Jpn J Radiol. 2010;28(9):663–71.
115. Tarnacka B, Szeszkowski W, Golebiowski M, Czlonkowska A. Brain proton magnetic spectroscopy in long-term treatment of Wilson's disease patients. Metab Brain Dis. 2010;25(3):325–9.
116. Tarnacka B, Szeszkowski W, Buettner J, Golebiowski M, Gromadzka G, Czlonkowska A. Heterozygous carriers for Wilson's disease–magnetic spectroscopy changes in the brain. Metab Brain Dis. 2009;24(3):463–8.
117. Tarnacka B, Szeszkowski W, Golebiowski M, Czlonkowska A. Metabolic changes in 37 newly diagnosed Wilson's disease patients assessed by magnetic resonance spectroscopy. Parkinsonism Relat Disord. 2009;15(8):582–6.
118. Tarnacka B, Szeszkowski W, Golebiowski M, Czlonkowska A. MR spectroscopy in monitoring the treatment of Wilson's disease patients. Mov Disord. 2008;23(11):1560–6.
119. Sinha S, Taly AB, Ravishankar S, Prashanth LK, Vasudev MK. Wilson's disease: (31)P and (1)H MR spectroscopy and clinical correlation. Neuroradiology. 2010;52(11):977–85.
120. Jayasundar R, Sahani AK, Gaikwad S, Singh S, Behari M. Proton MR spectroscopy of basal ganglia in Wilson's disease: case report and review of literature. Magn Reson Imaging. 2002;20(1):131–5.
121. Juan CJ, Chen CY, Liu YJ, et al. Acute putaminal necrosis and white matter demyelination in a child with subnormal copper metabolism in Wilson disease: MR imaging and spectroscopic findings. Neuroradiology. 2005;47(6):401–5.
122. Pyne-Geithman GJ, deGrauw TJ, Cecil KM, et al. Presence of normal creatine in the muscle of a patient with a mutation in the creatine transporter: a case study. Mol Cell Biochem. 2004;262(1–2):35–9.
123. deGrauw TJ, Cecil KM, Byars AW, Salomons GS, Ball WS, Jakobs C. The clinical syndrome of creatine transporter deficiency. Mol Cell Biochem. 2003;244(1–2):45–8.
124. Item CB, Stockler-Ipsiroglu S, Stromberger C, et al. Arginine:glycine amidinotransferase deficiency: the third inborn error of creatine metabolism in humans. Am J Hum Genet. 2001;69(5):1127–33.
125. Battini R, Leuzzi V, Carducci C, et al. Creatine depletion in a new case with AGAT deficiency: clinical and genetic study in a large pedigree. Mol Genet Metab. 2002;77(4):326–31.
126. Edvardson S, Korman SH, Livne A, et al. l-arginine:glycine amidinotransferase (AGAT) deficiency: clinical presentation and response to treatment in two patients with a novel mutation. Mol Genet Metab. 2010;101(2–3):228–32.
127. Johnston K, Plawner L, Cooper L, et al. The second family with AGAT deficiency (Creatine biosynthesis defect): diagnosis, treatment and first prenatal diagnosis. *American Society of Human Genetics.* Vol Salt Lake City, Utah USA2005:58.
128. Mercimek-Mahmutoglu S, Stockler-Ipsiroglu S. Creatine deficiency syndromes. In: Pagon RA, Bird TC, Dolan CR, (eds) *GeneReviews [Internet].* Jan. 15, 2009 ed. Seattle, WA: University of Washington; 1993.
129. Stockler S, Holzbach U, Hanefeld F, et al. Creatine deficiency in the brain: a new, treatable inborn error of metabolism. Pediatr Res. 1994;36(3):409–13.
130. Ensenauer R, Thiel T, Schwab KO, et al. Guanidinoacetate methyltransferase deficiency: differences of creatine uptake in human brain and muscle. Mol Genet Metab. 2004;82(3):208–13.
131. Leuzzi V, Bianchi MC, Tosetti M, et al. Brain creatine depletion: guanidinoacetate methyltransferase deficiency (improving with creatine supplementation). Neurology. 2000;55(9):1407–9.
132. Mercimek-Mahmutoglu S, Stoeckler-Ipsiroglu S, Adami A, et al. GAMT deficiency: features, treatment, and outcome in an inborn error of creatine synthesis. Neurology. 2006;67(3):480–4.
133. Schulze A, Mayatepek E, Bachert P, Marescau B, De Deyn PP, Rating D. Therapeutic trial of arginine restriction in creatine deficiency syndrome. Eur J Pediatr. 1998;157(7):606–7.
134. Schulze A, Ebinger F, Rating D, Mayatepek E. Improving treatment of guanidinoacetate methyltransferase deficiency: reduction of guanidinoacetic acid in body fluids by arginine restriction and ornithine supplementation. Mol Genet Metab. 2001;74(4):413–9.
135. Schulze A, Hoffmann GF, Bachert P, et al. Presymptomatic treatment of neonatal guanidinoacetate methyltransferase deficiency. Neurology. 2006;67(4):719–21.
136. Cecil KM, Salomons GS, Ball Jr WS, et al. Irreversible brain creatine deficiency with elevated serum and urine creatine: a creatine transporter defect? Ann Neurol. 2001;49(3):401–4.
137. Salomons GS, van Dooren SJ, Verhoeven NM, et al. X-linked creatine-transporter gene (SLC6A8) defect: a new creatine-deficiency syndrome. Am J Hum Genet. 2001;68(6):1497–500.
138. Puusepp H, Kall K, Salomons GS, et al. The screening of SLC6A8 deficiency among Estonian families with X-linked mental retardation. J Inherit Metab Dis. Jan 10 2009.
139. Arias A, Corbella M, Fons C, et al. Creatine transporter deficiency: prevalence among patients with mental retardation and pitfalls in metabolite screening. Clin Biochem. 2007;40(16–17):1328–31.
140. Betsalel OT, van de Kamp JM, Martinez-Munoz C, et al. Detection of low-level somatic and germline mosaicism by denaturing high-performance liquid chromatography in a EURO-MRX family with SLC6A8 deficiency. Neurogenetics. 2008;9(3):183–90.
141. Newmeyer A, Cecil KM, Schapiro M, Clark JF, Degrauw TJ. Incidence of brain creatine transporter deficiency in males with developmental delay referred for brain magnetic resonance imaging. J Dev Behav Pediatr. 2005;26(4):276–82.
142. Rosenberg EH, Almeida LS, Kleefstra T, et al. High prevalence of SLC6A8 deficiency in X-linked mental retardation. Am J Hum Genet. 2004;75(1):97–105.
143. Lion-Francois L, Cheillan D, Pitelet G, et al. High frequency of creatine deficiency syndromes in patients with unexplained mental retardation. Neurology. 2006;67(9):1713–4.
144. Almeida LS, Rosenberg EH, Martinez-Munoz C, et al. Overexpression of GAMT restores GAMT activity in primary GAMT-deficient fibroblasts. Mol Genet Metab. 2006;89(4):392–4.
145. Rosenberg EH, Munoz CM, Degrauw TJ, Jakobs C, Salomons GS. Overexpression of wild-type creatine transporter (SLC6A8) restores creatine uptake in primary SLC6A8-deficient fibroblasts. J Inherit Metab Dis. 2006;29(2–3):345–6.
146. Clark AJ, Rosenberg EH, Almeida LS, et al. X-linked creatine transporter (SLC6A8) mutations in about 1% of males with mental retardation of unknown etiology. Hum Genet. 2006;119(6):604–10.
147. Pagon RA. GeneTests: an online genetic information resource for health care providers. J Med Libr Assoc. 2006;94(3):343–8.
148. Fons C, Sempere A, Arias A, et al. Arginine supplementation in four patients with X-linked creatine transporter defect. J Inherit Metab Dis. 2008;31(6):724–8.
149. Valayannopoulos V, Boddaert N, Mention K, et al. Secondary creatine deficiency in ornithine delta-aminotransferase deficiency. Mol Genet Metab. 2009;97(2):109–13.
150. Pérez-Dueñas B, De La Osa A, Capdevila A, Navarro-Sastre A, Leist A, Ribes A, García-Cazorla A, Serrano M, Pineda M, Campistol J. (2009). Brain injury in glutaric aciduria type I: the value of functional techniques in magnetic resonance imaging. *Eur J Paediatr Neurol, 13*(6), 534–540.

Phenylketonuria

12

Arabhi Nagasunder and Richard Koch

Phenylketonuria (PKU) is an autosomal recessive genetic disorder caused by a defect in the hepatic enzyme phenylalanine hydroxylase (PAH) characterized by elevated levels of blood phenylalanine (Phe) leading to severely impaired brain development. In addition to poor neurological outcomes, untreated PKU can lead to microcephaly, tremor of hands, epilepsy, spastic paraparesis, behavioral problems, and schizophrenia. Early diagnosis and inception of a Phe-restricted diet after the newborn period prevents mental retardation and other neurological symptoms in PKU patients. With PKU, various mutations of the PAH gene have been identified along with their severity based on their enzyme activity [1]. One of the main motivations for measuring *brain* Phe levels is that new drugs may limit/reduce the transport of Phe into the brain. Thus, *plasma* Phe levels might be insufficient surrogate markers for *brain* Phe levels. However, the detection and quantitation of brain Phe with in vivo MR spectroscopy is uniquely challenging due to its low concentration and the position of Phe resonance (7.36 ppm) in a part of the spectrum that is generally not look at. Thus for measuring Phe accurately, a high level of expertise for acquiring high-quality data and advanced processing methods are required. It is for that reason, albeit phenylketonuria is a comparably frequently encountered metabolic disease, that only few groups have attempted to explore the value of MRS in PKU.

PKU was discovered in 1934 by Asbjörn Folling [2] after noticing excessive urinary excretion of phenylpyruvic acid. Subsequently, in 1953, Horst Bickel introduced a Phe-restricted diet that treated PKU patients but could not counter irreversible damage caused by the disease prior to treatment [3]. Ten years later, Robert Guthrie [4] described a simple technique to determine Phe concentrations in large populations using blood spot testing, a test currently routinely used for newborn screening in advanced societies. Blood Phe concentrations are considered normal within 40–80 μmol/l and are categorized as hyperphenylalaninemia (HPA) if higher than 240 μmol/l (>4 mg/dl). Severe HPA with concentrations greater than 1,200 μmol/l due to gene mutation for PAH enzyme is classified as classical PKU. A milder and less common form of HPA occurs when the PAH enzyme is normal but there is a deficiency in cofactor tetrahydrobiopterin (BH_4). In every case, the most effective treatment involves adherence to a severely Phe-restricted diet aiming at lowering plasma Phe concentrations thus brain Phe concentrations and preventing mental retardation. Additional Phe-free amino acid supplemental formulas are prescribed to provide other necessary amino acids and nutrients. In patients with BH_4 deficiency, BH_4 is orally administered to maintain plasma Phe concentrations within acceptable limits. It is preferable for women with PKU to maintain their plasma Phe levels between 120 and 240 μmol/l before and during pregnancy for the health of the fetus since higher blood Phe may lead to cardiac abnormalities, microcephaly, and mental retardation.

Numerous methodologies have been applied in the fields of radiology, electrophysiology, and cognitive neuroscience for evaluating impairments in PKU. Bone mineral density is decreased in children with PKU despite following dietary recommendations [5, 6]. Risk for Vitamin B-12 deficiency is elevated in PKU patients on relaxed diets [7]. The principal goal of imaging studies is the quantifying of brain Phe with respect to plasma Phe and clinical indicators such as Intelligence Quotient (IQ) in order to understand the impact of plasma Phe on neurological development. Transport of

Dr. Koch was a pioneer in providing medical services to the disabled and led the efforts that resulted in routine newborn screening for PKU and other inborn errors. We are grateful for his willingness to put together a chapter about MRS and PKU. Dr. Koch passed away on September 24th, 2011, at the age of 89.

A. Nagasunder, M.S. (✉)
Childrens Hospital Los Angeles, Los Angeles, CA 90027, USA

Rudi Schulte Research Institute, Santa Barbara, CA, USA
e-mail: anagasunder@chla.usc.edu

R. Koch, M.D.
Professor Emeritus, USC Keck School of Medicine, Los Angeles, CA, USA

S. Blüml and A. Panigrahy (eds.), *MR Spectroscopy of Pediatric Brain Disorders*,
DOI 10.1007/978-1-4419-5864-8_12, © Springer Science+Business Media, LLC 2013

a

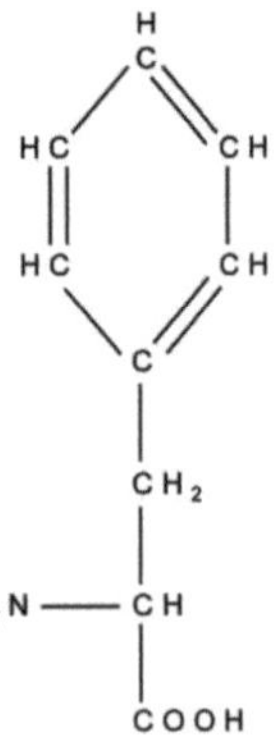

Molecule	Group	Chemical Shift ppm
Phenyl ring	CH	7.32
		7.42
		7.37
Non ring	CH_2	3.2
	CH	3.97

b
Lactate

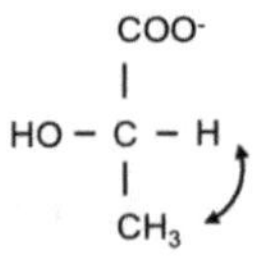

Fig. 12.1 (**a** and **b**) Molecular structure of Phe is shown. Resonances for ^{1}H MRS have been adapted from Govindaraju et al. [23]. Prominent chemical shift at 7.37 ppm is from the phenyl ring in the molecule. (Adapted from Govindaraju V, Young K, Maudsley AA. Proton NMR chemical shifts and coupling constants for brain metabolites. *NMR Biomed* 2000 May;13[3]:129–153, with permission.)

large neutral amino acids (LNAA), like Phe, from blood into the brain can probably be explained by selective absorption by the blood–brain barrier (BBB) whereas intraindividual variability indicates otherwise [8]. Transport mechanisms have been widely studied by various technologies [9–12]. Standard MR images as well as by diffusion tensor imaging (MR/DTI) showed that negligence in following a strict dietary regimen can lead to white matter abnormalities [13]. MR spectroscopy has been used for many years to noninvasively determine brain Phe levels [14]. The blood and brain Phe relationships have been studied widely but there are many inconsistencies reported with respect to the correlation between these concentrations [15–22]. Albeit the challenges of measuring brain Phe levels in individual patients accurately, MRS of the brain can still be used to measure average Phe levels in groups of subjects with PKU and might thus be a useful tool to research the impact of novel therapeutic interventions aiming to lower brain Phe levels.

MR Spectroscopy of PKU

Phenylalanine is an essential amino acid with the formula $HO_2CCH(NH_2)CH_2C_6H_5$ (Fig. 12.1) with a prominent resonance at ≈ 7.37 ppm in proton spectrum [23]. Normally, Phe is metabolized to tyrosine using the PAH enzyme along with the cofactor BH_4. In PKU patients, this reaction is absent and hence an accumulation of Phe leads to a deficiency of tyrosine. Excess Phe is converted to phenylacetate, phenyllactate, phenylpyruvate, and phenylethylamine detected in urine [24]. Although plasma Phe has been a primary marker in determining intellectual outcome of PKU patients, various studies [15–21] indicating inconsistencies in correlation between plasma and brain Phe as well as neurological abnormalities in PKU patients despite following diet control have driven researchers to devise new methodologies in measuring cerebral Phe effectively.

Cerebral Phe concentrations are closely related to clinical outcomes. Localized WM abnormalities associated with PKU have been shown on T2-weighted images as well as FLAIR (Fig. 12.2). Previous studies [14, 16, 20, 21] have used various quantitation methodologies in determining brain Phe using MRS (Table 12.1). Methodological approaches are summarized below:

1. Sequence Selection
   Selection of sequences is important in determining effective time as well as patient management in data acquisition.
   (a) Regular sequences (PRESS or STEAM)
   PRESS signals have better signal to noise ratio (SNR) than STEAM
   (b) Advanced sequences (CSI, COSY, etc.)
   Although the purpose of advanced spec sequences is to enhance understanding, they are not very effective in measuring Phe since it is a small signal concentration at higher-end of the ^{1}H spectrum. Independently, CSI requires a large voxel size. COSY or other advanced editing sequences increase acquisition time substantially and hence are impractical.
2. Parameter Determination
   Within an MRS sequence, it is important to choose appropriate protocol parameters, which would aid in Phe measurement. Important considerations include:
   (a) Echo time, TE = 20–35 ms
   (b) Repetition time, TR = 2,000–3,000 ms
   (c) Voxel Location and Placement (discussed below) (Figs. 12.3 and 12.4)
   (d) Volume within the voxel (discussed below)
   (e) Water Suppressed and Unsuppressed (water reference) signal acquisitions
3. Volume of Interest
   Many voxel locations have been investigated in prior PKU studies [14, 20, 21]. Large voxels with volumes of about 80 cm^3 placed in the supraventricular location (Fig. 12.3) encompassing mostly GM and surrounding

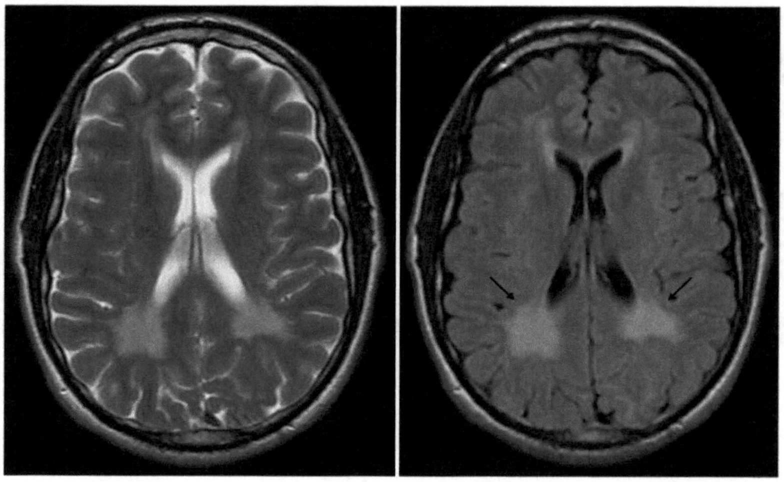

Fig. 12.2 WM abnormalities associated with PKU patients on T2-weighted and FLAIR sequences. *Black arrows* indicate extensive damage caused by high brain Phe levels. (Adapted from Leuzzi V, Tosetti M, Montanaro D, et al. The pathogenesis of the white matter abnormalities in phenylketonuria. A multimodal 3.0 tesla MRI and magnetic resonance spectroscopy (^{1}H MRS) study. *J Inherit Metab Dis*, 30: 209–216, 2007, with permission.)

Table 12.1 MRS studies of PKU

Study group	Reference	Method	Brain–blood Phe correlations	Location(s)	Notes
Leuzzi et al., Italy	*J Inherit Metab Dis* (2007) 30:209–216	Press TE=30 ms, TR=2 s ROI=8 cc, *N*=128	Linear ≤ 1,200 μmol; Intraindividual Variability > 1,200 μmol	1. Deep periventricular WM	Brain Phe not significantly different between normal and mentally retarded
Pietz et al., Rupp et al., Switzerland and Germany	*J Cereb. Blood Flow Metab* (2001) 3:276–284	PRESS TE=20 ms, TR=3 s ROI=84 cc, *N*=128	Linear ≤ 1,800 μmol; Intraindividual Variability > 1,800 μmol	1. Supraventricular and 2. Posterior-ventricular WM	
Möller et al. USA and Germany	*Brain Research* 778 (1997) 329–337	STEAM TE=20 ms, TR=1.6 s ROI=27–36 cc, *N*=512	Linear ≤ 1,500 μmol; Intraindividual Variability > 1,500 μmol	1. Posterior-ventricular brain 2. Frontal brain 3. Cerebellum	
Novotny et al. USA	*Pediatr. Res* (1995) 2:244–249.	ISIS TE=10–20 ms, TR=3–6 s ROI=15-32 cc, *N*=128	Intraindividual variability Weak correlation	1. Temporal lobe/parietal brain 2. Occipital cortex	
Moats et al., USA	*J Inherit Metab Dis*, 23: 7–14, 2000	STEAM TE=20 ms, TR=2 s ROI=72 cc, *N*=128–256	Intraindividual variability Weak correlation	1. Supraventricular mixed WM/GM	

PRESS point-resolved spectroscopy, *STEAM* stimulated echo acquisition mode, *ISIS* image-selected in vivo spectroscopy, *TE* echo time, *TR* repetition time, *ROI* region of interest, *N* number of signal averages, *WM* white matter, *GM* gray matter

peripheral WM tissue is effective in determining Phe concentrations. Presence of WM abnormalities in PKU patients has motivated researchers [14] to use a smaller voxel (20–30 cm^3) in the posterior periventricular WM region (Fig. 12.4). With either region, the popularly used upper part of the ^{1}H spectrum with resonances from Cr, Cho, mI and NAA is normal in PKU patients. Preference to any particular volume or MRS sequence depends on a compromise in SNR individuals are willing to take while aiming to understand the underlying pathology.

4. Postprocessing
   Standard quantitation procedures are inadequate in measuring Phe since they usually process chemical shifts until water signal, from 0 to 4.4 ppm. Consequently, investigators have their own custom-designed automatic processing approaches. For example, Kreis et al. [14] used the following methodology:

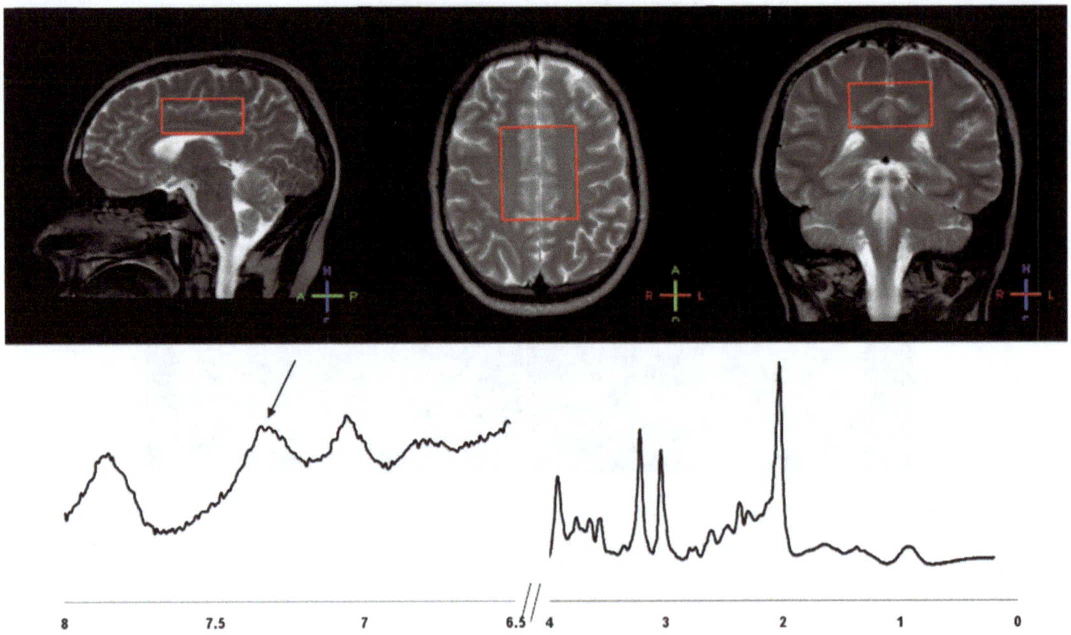

Fig. 12.3 Mixed GM/WM Location showing a large volume of interest used for Phe measurement using MRS. Upfield section as well as the lower part of ^{1}H MR spectrum is depicted. *Black arrow* indicated Phe peak. Signal with resonances from Cr, Cho, mI, and NAA are found normal in PKU patients

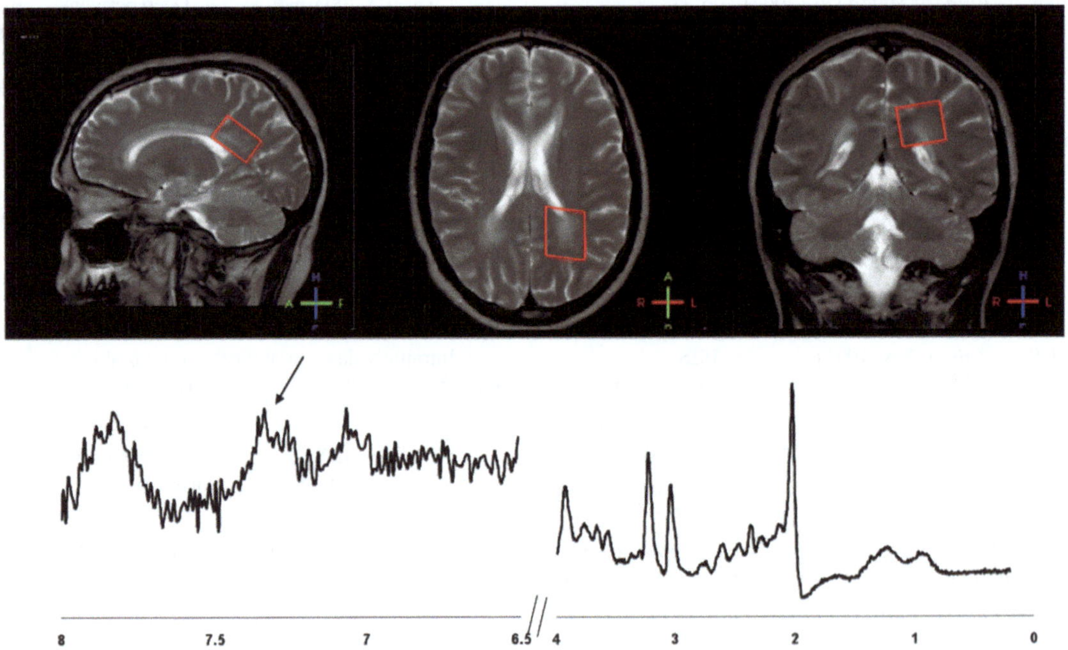

Fig. 12.4 Due to abnormalities on MRI, another region frequently studied in PKU patients is parietal WM

(a) Scaling
Spectra were divided by a fit to water signal decay. This aimed at eliminating contributions from metabolites other than Phe in brain tissue.

(b) Subtraction
Cr linewidths were matched using exponential line broadening on either the control or patient spectrum. Control spectrum was then subtracted from patient spectrum to determine residual Phe amplitude.

(c) Smoothing and Fitting
Lower-end of ^{1}H spectrum was smoothed. Signal with chemical shifts beyond the water signal was fitted to a Lorentzian line plus a quadratic baseline.

(d) Phe concentration
Total peak area was calculated as the ratio between total Phe signal from difference spectrum after all corrections and fit to water signal decay. Extensive calculations were performed to account for Phe contributions from CSF and blood within the volume of interest. Cerebral Phe for healthy patients determined to be 0.05 mM [25] was added to the final concentration.

Correlation of Brain and Blood Phenylalanine

Characteristics of Phe transport through BBB under various conditions were investigated [8]. Blood and brain Phe measurements were recorded simultaneously at specific times and a relationship curve of these results were obtained. Kreis et al. [8] showed a linear regression while likening Möller et al.'s [22] nonlinear relationship for blood–brain Phe to a selection of atypical PKU patients. Several inconsistencies have been reported in blood–brain ratios as well as the level of blood Phe which leads to a saturation of the brain. Possible explanation is the presence of intraindividual variability in Phe transport mechanism.

Clinical implications from various Phe transport mechanisms can be interpreted effectively by MRS along with IQ. Relationship between physiological factors and clinical outcome is still unclear. Recent advances in PKU treatment including LNAA therapy [10–12] are based on the rationalization that brain control and function is influenced by an imbalance in Phe transport through BBB. Not only do some amino acids block Phe through BBB, but they also block Phe at the gut from entering plasma. Modern alternative therapies also include treatment of specific causes of deficiency such as oral intake of biopterin, ammonia lyase therapy, and gene therapy. The overall purpose is to maintain moderate Phe levels to improve patient's quality of life.

A wide spectrum of severity of PKU leads to challenges in effective patient treatment strategies. Primary target of treatment is ensuring normal brain development. Although introducing dietary restrictions during the neonatal periods is carried out now universally, the duration of these restrictions or follow a diet for life is a topic of constant debate [26]. Previous arguments show that MRI changes may not be indicative of clinical parameters such as IQ or long-term dietary control but rather of the most recent event of dietary treatment [26]. Therefore, current goals of patient management include maintaining or improving the individual patient's quality of life by removing dietary restrictions. Particularly, pharmaceutical products that either prevent and reduce Phe uptake or accelerate Phe breakdown in the brain could be used. Periodic MRS is instrumental in measuring brain Phe decoupled from plasma Phe. It needs to be mentioned that most studies were carried out in adults or adolescents. It is possible that ratio of plasma to brain Phe is significantly different in newborns or small children. The newborn brain could be less protected by the blood-brain-barrier from excessive Phe than the mature brain.

References

1. Guldberg P, Rey F, Zschocke J, Romano V, Francois B, et al. A European multicenter study of phenylalanine hydroxylase deficiency: classification of 105 mutations and a general system for genotype-based prediction of metabolic phenotype. Am J Hum Genet. 1998;63:71–9.
2. Folling A. Ueber Ausscheidung von Phenylbrenztraubensaeure in den Harn als Stoffwechselanomalie in Verbindung mit Imbezillitaet. Ztschr Physiol Chem. 1934;227:169–76.
3. Bickel H, Gerrard J, Hickmans EM. The influence of phenylalanine intake on the chemistry and behaviour of a phenylketonuria child. Acta Ped. 1954;43(64–77):1954.
4. Guthriem R. A simple phenylalanine method for detecting phenylketonuria in large populations of newborn infants. Ada Susi. Pediatrics. 1963;32:338–43.
5. Zeman J, Bayer M, Stepán J. Bone mineral density in patients with phenylketonuria. Acta Paediatr. 1999;88(12):1348–51.
6. Allen J, Humphries I, Waters D, Roberts D, Lipson A, Howman-Giles R, Gaskin K. Decreased bone mineral density in children with phenylketonuria. Am J Clin Nutr. 1994;59(2):419–22.
7. Hvas AM, Nexo E, Nielsen JB. Vitamin B12 and vitamin B6 supplementation is needed among adults with phenylketonuria (PKU). J Inherit Metab Dis. 2006;29(1):47–53.
8. Rupp A, Kreis R, Zschocke J, Slotboom J, Boesch C, Rating D, Pietz J. Variability of blood–brain ratios of phenylalanine in typical patients with phenylketonuria. J Cereb Blood Flow Metab. 2001;21(3):276–84.
9. Hoeksma M, Reijngoud D, Pruim J, de Valk HW, Paans AM, van Spronsen FJ. Phenylketonuria: high plasma phenylalanine decreases cerebral protein synthesis. Mol Genet Metabol. 2009;96(4):177–82.
10. Matalon R, Surendran S, Matalon KM, Tyring S, Quast M, Jinga W, Ezell E, Szucs S. Future role of large neutral amino acids in transport of phenylalanine into the brain. Pediatrics. 2003;112(6):1570–4.
11. Pietz J, Kreis R, Rupp A, Mayatepek E, Rating D, Boesch C, Bremer HJ. Large neutral amino acids block phenylalanine transport into brain tissue in patients with phenylketonuria. J Clin Invest. 1999;103(8):1169–78.
12. Koch R, Moseley KD, Yano S, Nelson M, Moats RA. Large neutral amino acid therapy and phenylketonuria: a promising approach to treatment. Mol Genet Metabol. 2003;79(2):110–3.
13. Phillips MD, McGraw P, Lowe MJ, Mathews VP, Hainline BE. Diffusion-weighted imaging of white matter abnormalities in patients with phenylketonuria. AJNR Am J Neuroradiol. 2001;22(8):1583–6.
14. Kreis R, Pietz J, Penzien J, Herschkovitz N, Boesch C. Identification and quantitation of phenylalanine in the brain of patients with PKU by means of localized in vivo 1 H MRS. J Magn Reson B. 1995;107(3):242–51.
15. Rupp A, Kreis R, Zschocke J, Slotboom J, Boesch C, Rating D, Pietz J. Variability of blood–brain ratios of phenylalanine in typical patients with phenylketonuria. J Cereb Blood Flow Metab. 2001;21:276–84.
16. Leuzzi V, Tosetti M, Montanaro D, Carducci C, Artiola C, Antonozzi I, Burroni M, Carnevale F, Chiarotti F, Popolizio T, Giannatempo GM, D'Alesio V, Scarabino T. The pathogenesis of the white matter abnormalities in phenylketonuria. A multimodal 3.0 tesla MRI and magnetic resonance spectroscopy (1 H MRS) study. J Inherit Metab Dis. 2007;30:209–16.
17. Schindeler S, Ghosh-Jerath S, Thompson S, Rocca A, Joy P, Kemp A, Rae C, Green K, Wilcken B, Christodoulou J. The effects of large neutral amino acid supplements in PKU: an MRS and neuropsychological study. Mol Genet Metab. 2007;91:48–54.

18. Moats RA, Koch R, Moseley K, Guldberg P, Guttler F, Boles RG, Nelson Jr MD. Brain phenylalanine concentration in the management of adults with phenylketonuria. J Inherit Metab Dis. 2000; 23:7–14.
19. Koch R, Moats R, Guttler F, Guldberg P, Nelson Jr M. Blood–brain phenylalanine relationships in persons with phenylketonuria. Pediatrics. 2000;106:1093–6.
20. Möller HE, Vermathen P, Ullrich K, Weglage J, Koch H-G, Peters PE. In-vivo NMR spectroscopy in patients with phenylketonuria: changes of cerebral phenylalanine levels under dietary treatment. Neuropediatrics. 1995;26(4):199–202.
21. Novotny EJ, Avison MJ, Herschkowitz N, Petroff OA, Prichard JW, Seashore MR, Rothman DL. In vivo measurement of phenylalanine in human brain by proton nuclear magnetic resonance spectroscopy. Pediatr Res. 1995;37(2):244–9.
22. Möller HE, Weglage J, Wiedermann D, Vermathen P, Bick U, Ullrich K. Kinetics of phenylalanine transport at the human blood–brain barrier investigated in vivo. Brain Res. 1997;778(2): 329–37.
23. Govindaraju V, Young K, Maudsley AA. Proton NMR chemical shifts and coupling constants for brain metabolites. NMR Biomed. 2000;13(3):129–53.
24. Michals K, Matalon R. Phenylalanine metabolites, attention span and hyperactivity. Am J Clin Nutr. 1985;42(2):361–5.
25. Clarke DD, Lajtha AL, Maker HS. Intermediary metabolism. In: Siegel GJ et al., editors. Basic neurochemisty. 4th ed. New York: Raven; 1989. p. 541.
26. Moats RA, Scadeng M, Nelson MD. MR imaging and spectroscopy in PKU. Ment Retard Dev Disabil Res Rev. 1999;5(2):132–5.

13 Infection and Encephalitis

Kim M. Cecil and Diana M. Lindquist

Magnetic resonance spectroscopy (MRS) serves as a powerful tool in narrowing the differential diagnosis in pediatric brain disorders. Unfortunately, the literature provides only a limited number of case reports and larger patient series employing this technique in the diagnosis and monitoring of infectious and inflammatory conditions. For these conditions producing encephalitis, MRS often demonstrates a more benign spectral appearance, with minor changes in metabolite levels, which contrasts to the typically more dramatic and often aggressive spectral features recognized in neoplasms and metabolic disorders. One key exception is frank abscess, as this process depletes the metabolites found in normal brain parenchyma and replaces them with distinct amino acids. This chapter first describes some practical and technical concerns associated with conducting neurological MRS studies in the pediatric patients to confirm the diagnosis of an infectious and/or inflammatory process. A brief description of infectious disorders and inflammatory conditions with illustrative imaging and spectroscopy examples from our center and the literature will provide important information in diagnosing these conditions.

Practical and Technical Concerns

MRS performed in pediatric patients with suspected infectious encephalopathies requires the clinicians, radiologists, nurses, and technical staff to first recognize the effects of exogenous agents on the spectra. Exogenous agents used in the formulations of medications can contaminate the spectra, if present in relatively high concentrations. For example, 1,2-propane-diol (propylene glycol) is a vehicle used in the intravenous formulations of both pentobarbital (trade name, Nembutal) and phenobarbital to sedate, control seizures, and relieve anxiety, respectively. Propylene glycol may be confused with lactate, as it appears at 1.1 ppm on the spectrum, adjacent to where lactate resonates at 1.3 ppm. There is evidence that propylene glycol is metabolized via hepatic alcohol and aldehyde dehydrogenases to lactate [1]. Another agent, Lactated Ringer's solution is often used instead of saline in the administration of general anesthesia. Depending on the dosage in some patients, there is the potential to contaminate the proton MR spectrum with exogenous lactate. While it is necessary to sedate pediatric patients for imaging procedures and provide treatment for seizures, it is important to document exogenous agents which may contribute to the proton MRS spectrum and if possible, use alternative medications without propylene glycol, lactate, etc., when using MRS to diagnose and monitor therapy in pediatric patients.

Most imaging centers that perform MRS employ either single- or multivoxel (also referred to as spectroscopic imaging) acquisitions for proton MRS studies. No special sequences are necessary in the evaluation of patients for infectious or inflammatory disorders. However, it is always advisable to utilize at least two echo times to facilitate the detection and positive identification of metabolites, especially amino acids such lactate, alanine, glycine, etc.

Lactate is an important diagnostic feature provided by proton MRS. Many infectious processes have dramatically elevated concentrations of lactate, e.g., frank abscess. However, the elevated lactate levels for encephalitis are generally much lower than the levels detected for metabolic disorders or neoplasms. For the identification of lactate, proton MRS acquisition requires either sampling with a dedicated lactate editing sequence or using routine MRS localization techniques employing intermediate echo times on the order of 135–144 ms. This is necessary to separate macromolecule and lipid resonances found on short echo MRS. However, at higher fields such as 3 T, anomalous J-modulation can occur

K.M. Cecil, Ph.D. (✉)
Departments of Radiology, Pediatrics, Neuroscience and Environmental Health, Cincinnati Children's Hospital Medical Center, University of Cincinnati College of Medicine, Cincinnati, OH, USA
e-mail: kim.cecil@chmcc.org

D.M. Lindquist, Ph.D.
Departments of Radiology, Cincinnati Children's Hospital Medical Center, University of Cincinnati College of Medicine, Cincinnati, OH, USA

S. Blüml and A. Panigrahy (eds.), *MR Spectroscopy of Pediatric Brain Disorders*,
DOI 10.1007/978-1-4419-5864-8_13, © Springer Science+Business Media, LLC 2013

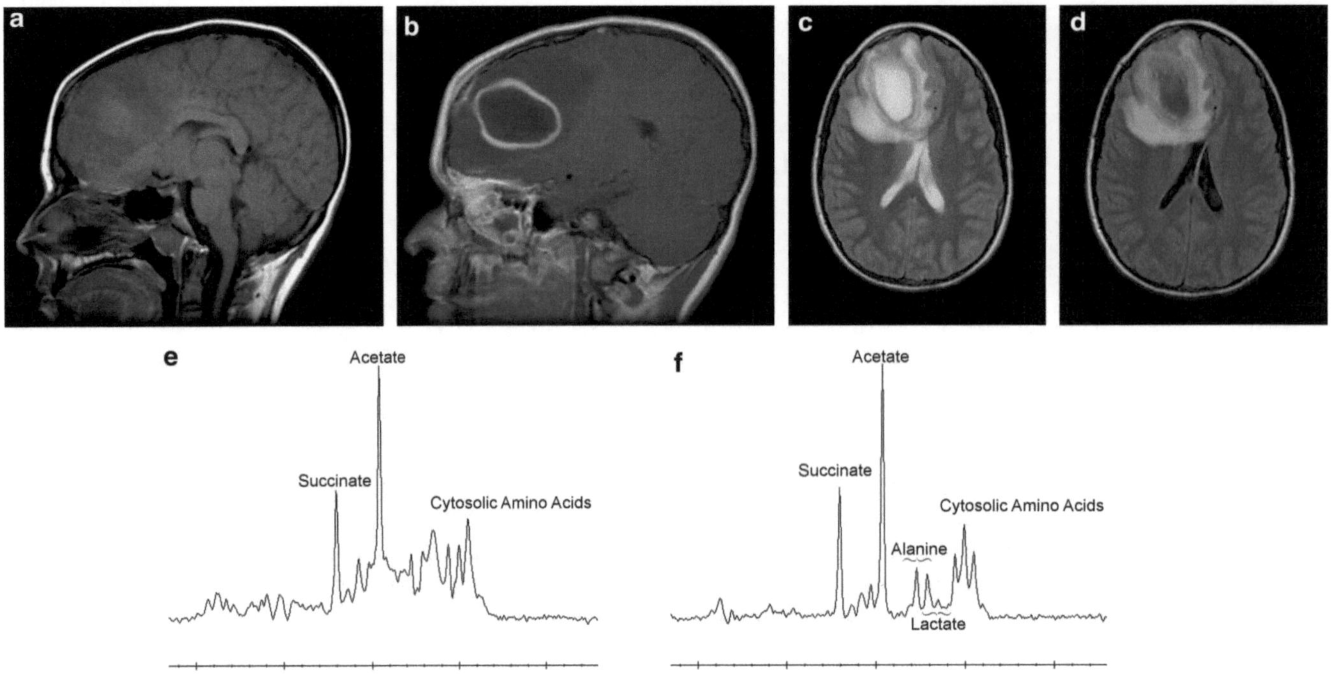

Fig. 13.1 MRI and MRS findings from a 13-year-old female patient diagnosed with a brain abscess. (**a**) T1-weighted pre-contrast image; (**b**) T1-weighted post-contrast image; (**c**) T2-weighted image; (**d**) FLAIR image; these sample images reveal the abscess core and wall accompanied with surrounding edema. (**e**) Short TE (35 ms) spectrum showing clear succinate and acetate peaks and a series of complicated peaks from alanine, lactate, and the cytosolic (leucine, isoleucine, valine) amino acids, which become clearer at long TE (288 ms, **f**). There is an absence of common brain metabolites (NAA, Cr, Cho) when sampling within the center of the abscess

which limits detection of lactate [2, 3]. Liu et al. have also shown that alanine (doublet appearing at 1.4 ppm) experiences greater effects of signal cancellation compared with other amino acids [4]. Combinations of short (35 ms or less), intermediate (135–144 ms), and long echo (270–288 ms) can be used to reliably delineate lactate and other amino acid elevations in the absence of a specialized editing sequence. Short echo acquisitions are important for other markers of infection such as glutamate, glutamine, and myo-inositol, besides the standard *N*-acetyl aspartate (NAA), creatine and phosphocreatine (Cr), and cholines (Cho).

Abscess

Brain abscesses form as an immune response to a bacterial or fungal infection or other foreign substance. Inflammation and swelling occur as a membrane forms around the infected brain cells, white blood cells, live and dead bacteria or fungi, collectively referred to as pus. Cytosolic amino acids are the end products of proteolysis by enzymes released from neutrophils in pus. The presence of cytosolic amino acids, such as isoleucine, leucine, and valine (0.9 ppm), with or without lactate (1.3 ppm), lipids (0.9–1.3 ppm), acetate (1.92), and succinate (2.4 ppm), represent a characteristic MRS profile for brain abscess (Fig. 13.1). Most of the spectroscopic literature of abscess is in adults; however, there are some large studies that include pediatric patients. Individual pediatric case reports have also been published. Age may influence the types of infections an individual may be vulnerable to in their life. The authors of this chapter know of no spectroscopic differences associated in abscess with age of the individual. The age of the abscess does influence the spectra as older, necrotic cores, and those patients treated with antibiotics usually demonstrate only a lactate resonance on proton MRS.

In a retrospective study of 194 patients (aged 3–60 years), Pal et al. evaluated pyogenic brain abscesses in vivo with proton MRS. After imaging and MRS were completed, pus aspirates were obtained for all patients to determine causative organisms [5]. For the majority (80%) of the abscesses, cytosolic amino acid resonances were detected on proton MRS. Obligate aerobes or facultative anaerobes demonstrated cytosolic amino acids and lactate with variable lipid content. Obligate anaerobes and some facultative anaerobes showed the presence of cytosolic amino acids, lactate, lipids, acetate with or without succinate. Acetate with or without succinate usually supports an anerobic bacterial origin, but not exclusively.

Fifty patients (aged 5–71 years) with intracranial cystic lesions ($N=21$ pyogenic abscesses, 23 tumor cysts, three epidermoid cysts and three arachnoid cysts) were evaluated with MRI and MRS [6]. The diagnostic accuracy of conventional MRI, DWI, and MRS, alone and in combinations, were determined to distinguish brain abscess or nonabscess cystic tumor. As in the previous study, the majority of abscesses demonstrated elevated lactate and cytosolic amino acids. DWI demonstrated high signal intensity, with low ADC values for abscesses indicating restricted diffusion. Combining the modalities, the diagnosis was accurately predicted in 96% of patients.

Luthra et al. retrospectively evaluated 110 patients (aged 3–55 years) for morphological features, ADC values, and metabolite features to discriminate surgically proven pyogenic, tubercular, and fungal brain abscesses [7]. Fungal abscesses demonstrated irregular walls with intra-cavitary projections. The wall and projections demonstrated low ADC, but the cavity high ADC. On MRS, the fungal abscess showed lipids (4/8), lactate (7/8), amino acids (4/8), and multiple peaks between 3.6 and 3.8 ppm assigned to trehalose (5/8). Pyogenic abscesses had smooth (55/91) and lobulated (36/91) walls, low ADC values in the wall and cavity, and elevated cytosolic amino acids (89/91), acetate (25/91), and succinate (18/91). Tubercular abscesses had smooth (4/11), lobulated (6/11), or crenated (1/11) walls with no intra-cavitary projections, low ADC values in the wall and cavity, and elevated lipids and lactate (11/11).

In an unusual presentation, Vajro et al. described the findings of an adolescent boy with a brain abscess due to *Klebsiella pneumoniae* 11 years postorthotopic liver transplantation [8]. The child was hospitalized for headache, weakness and mental confusion. Imaging (CT and MRI) revealed a cystic lesion with vasogenic edema. MRS revealed a very large lactate resonance suggestive of an inflammatory condition, which was confirmed poststereotactic drainage and antibiotic treatment. Chronic immunosuppression blunted the clinical and laboratory signs of inflammation.

Amoebic Mengioencephalitis

A previously healthy, 9-month-old female infant presented with acute onset of lethargy, fever, and development of seizure activity. MR imaging with diffusion-weighted imaging demonstrated a diffuse multifocal lesion pattern that revealed hypo-intense lesions on T1 weighted imaging predominately in cortical and deep gray matter, hyper-intense lesions on T2 weighted and diffusion weighted images (Fig. 13.2). The apparent diffusion coefficient map revealed hypo-intense lesions reflecting restricted diffusion. There was no appreciable contrast enhancement within the lesions. The proton MRS revealed elevated lactate and composite resonances for glutamate and glutamine. In the acute setting, the key metabolites,

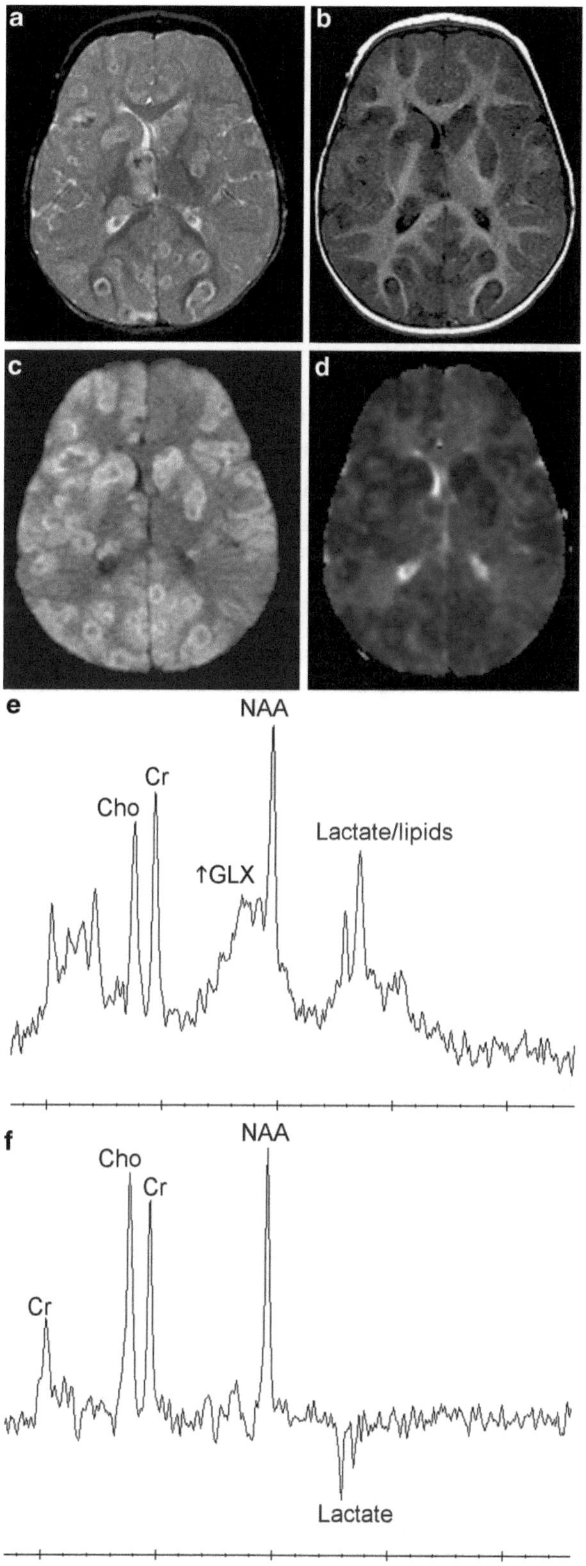

Fig. 13.2 MRI and MRS findings from a 9-month-old female with autopsy determined granulomatous amoebic encephalitis. (**a**) T1-weighted pre-contrast image; (**b**) T2-weighted image; (**c**) Diffusion-weighted image; (**d**) ADC map; these sample images demonstrate diffuse lesions throughout the brain, but primarily localized in cortical and deep gray matter. (**e**) Short TE (35 ms) spectrum showing normal levels

Fig. 13.2 (continued) of Cr, Cho, especially striking the preserved NAA levels, but elevated signal in the GLX region (*arrow*) as well as the presence of lactate, which was confirmed by its inversion at an intermediate TE (144 ms, **f**). The spectra were acquired within the left basal ganglia. (Patient imaging and information are courtesy of Charles M. Glasier, MD, and Arkansas Children's Hospital.)

NAA, Cr, and Cho were preserved. The lactate could arise from the immune response as well as the seizure activity, which is likely the source of the glutamate and glutamine elevation. Unfortunately, the child succumbed to the infection. An autopsy revealed the organism, *Balamuthia mandrillaris*. This deadly neurological condition is known as granulomatous amoebic encephalitis (GAE) (Courtesy of Charles M. Glasier, MD and Arkansas Children's Hospital).

Fungal Infections

Jain et al [9]. published a review of imaging features associated with CNS fungal infections. Their analyses indicated that fungal cranial infections (aspergillosis, cryptococcosis, mucomycosis, blastomyocosis, coccidioidomycosis, histoplasmosis, candidiasis) are known to produce a brain abscess secondary to the fungal infection. Fungal abscess show elevated lipids, lactate, alanine, acetate, succinate, choline, and a multiple resonances between 3.6 and 3.8 ppm thought to be unique for fungal origins. This resonance has been assigned to trehalose sugars.

Parasitic Infections

Neurocysticercosis

Cysticercosis is an infection caused by the pork tapeworm, *Taenia solium*. Infection occurs when the tapeworm larvae are ingested via contaminated food, water, or surfaces with contaminated feces. The larvae form cysticeri (cysts), which when found in the brain, are referred to as neurocysticercosis. Despite being the most common parasitic infection for children and young adults in developing nations, there are few MRS studies of patients with neurocysticercosis in the literature. As with many conditions, imaging features depend on the stage of infection and where the primary site of infection is located. For neurocysticercosis, four stages of cysts (vesicular, colloidal, nodular/granular, and calcified granulomas) within the brain parenchyma produce distinct imaging characteristics. The viable larval cyst represents a vesicular cyst with little to no host immune response and thus affords minimal signal change. The scolex can be distinguished as a nodule. As the cyst degenerates, fluid from the larval cyst leaks into the parenchyma, generating an inflammatory immune response recognized on imaging with contrast enhancement. Finally, the degenerating cyst produces a calcified granuloma. Cysts that lodge within or adjacent to the ventricles or cisterns may differ in their spectral appearance compared to the solitary parenchymal lesions. Detection of amino acids within large clusters of cysts is more easily afforded than in solitary cysts.

Kingsley reviewed MRS reports from adults with neurocysticercosis that describe spectral presentations with the elevation of Cho/Cr, pyruvate, alanine, lactate, and succinate [10]. The spectral variability may also arise from partial volume effects with adjacent brain parenchyma. For a patient who presented at the authors' institution, the lesion's cystic component is relatively small, so partial volume affects from adjacent parenchyma are observed. The ratios of NAA and Cho to Cr appear within normal limits (Fig. 13.3). However, lactate, lipids and possibly other amino acids appear elevated on the spectra.

Toxoplasmosis

Toxoplasmosis occurs after ingestion of a single-cell parasite known as *Toxoplasma gondii*. According to the US Centers for Disease Control, more than 60 million people in the USA may be infected with the parasite. For most healthy persons, the normal immune system prevents the parasite from causing illness. However, persons with compromised immune systems and pregnant women are more vulnerable to toxoplasmosis. In a retrospective review of MRS studies performed in pediatric and adult patients (aged 10–80 years), Ferraz-Filho et al [11]. found Cho/Cr and NAA/Cr levels were useful in discriminating toxoplasmosis ($N=42$) from WHO Grade III and IV glial neoplasms ($N=39$). The spectral pattern for glial neoplasms differs from toxoplasmosis by having greater elevations of Cho/Cr and lower levels of NAA/Cr. Upon analysis of the Receiver Operator Characteristics (ROC) curve, a discriminatory boundary for Cho/Cr alone was noted and used to detect neoplasms with 77% sensitivity and 79% specificity. Adding NAA/Cr to the model, specificity can be increased to nearly 98%.

Viral Processes

HIV and AIDS

The human immunodeficiency virus (HIV) is the virus that can lead to acquired immune deficiency syndrome (AIDS). HIV destroys the CD4+ T cells, which enable the body to fight disease. AIDS is the late stage of HIV infection. Proton MRS has been employed primarily in adult populations to differentiate tumor or progressive multifocal leukoencephalopathy from infectious processes in adults. Table 13.1 illustrates the utility of proton MRS in *adult* patients to distinguish multiple processes [12].

Outside of aiding differential diagnosis, other adult proton MRS studies monitor cognitive changes associated with HIV infection. However, few proton MRS studies examining cognitive or developmental changes in *pediatric* HIV and

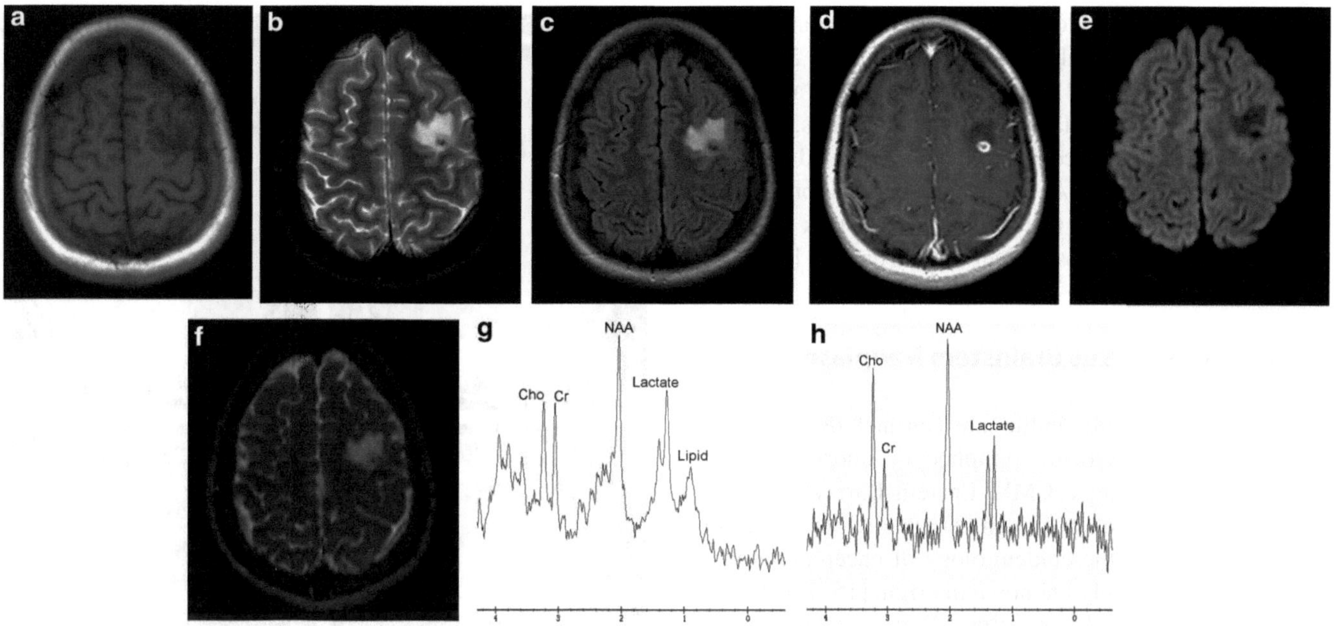

Fig. 13.3 MRI and MRS findings from a 16-year-old female diagnosed with neurocysticercosis. (**a**) Pre-contrast T1-weighted image; (**b**) T2-weighted image; (**c**) Post-contrast T1-weighted image; (**d**) FLAIR image; (**e**) Diffusion-weighted image; (**f**) ADC map; these representative images show the cyst formed from the tapeworm with associated edema. (**g**) Short TE (35 ms) spectrum shows apparently normal NAA/Cr and Cho/Cr from partial volume effects arising from sampling adjacent parenchyma; however, elevated lactate and lipids are appreciated as arising from the lesion. (**h**) Long TE (288 ms) spectrum clearly shows the lactate doublet

Table 13.1 Spectroscopy findings summarized for HIV and AIDS lesions in adult studies

Lesion in AIDS	NAA	Creatine	Choline	Myo-inositol	Lactate	Lipids
HIV WML	↓ in late stages	Mild elevation in early stages	↑	↑	May increase during acute encephalitis	–
PML	May decrease	–	↑	Variable	↑	↑
CMV	May decrease	–	↑	↑	May increase	–
Cryptococcoma	↓	↓	↓	↓	May increase	↑
Toxoplasmosis	↓	↓	↓	↓	↑	↑
Tuberculoma	Depleted	Depleted	Depleted	Depleted	–	↑
Lymphoma	↓	↓	↑	↓	↑	↑

AIDS acquired immunodeficiency syndrome, *NAA* N-acetyl aspartate, *HIV* human immunodeficiency virus, *WML* white matter lesions, *DEC* decreased, *INC* increased, *PML* progressive multifocal encephalopathy, *CMV* cytomegalovirus

AIDS have been reported. Keller and colleagues examined five brain regions including the frontal white matter, frontal gray matter and basal ganglia in HIV-infected children [13]. They found decreased choline in left frontal white matter of HIV-infected children compared with control subjects. For those children with higher viral loads (>5,000 HIV RNA copies/mL), decreased right basal ganglia Cr and Cho were found also compared to control subjects. Comparison within the HIV-infected children found higher Cho in frontal gray and lower mI in the right basal ganglia for children with higher viral loads. Correlating these metabolite findings with further analyses and with neuropsychological testing, Keller at al. suggested that normal brain development is affected in children with HIV at birth.

Cytomegalovirus

Cytomegalovirus (CMV) is a common viral infection, which is generally silent with no symptoms. However, in persons with weakened immune systems and babies prior to birth, CMV can cause serious injury. Congenital CMV infection causes birth defects, long-term brain, liver, lung, spleen problems, and even death. In the brain, congenital CMV infection and periventricular leukomalacia (PVL) affect the cerebral white matter in the same developmental period when immature oligodendrocytes are especially vulnerable to injury. In a study evaluating white matter lesions with diffusion tensor imaging, magnetization transfer imaging and proton MRS, pediatric patients with documented congenital cytomegalovirus infection were compared to patients with periventricular leukomalacia (mean group ages: 2.8 and 2.9 years, respectively) [14]. No differences were appreciated between the two populations. For both groups, increased ADC and myo-inositol concentrations were noted along with reduced FA, MTR, NAA, and Cho concentrations. van der Voorn et al. speculate that axonal losses, lack of myelin deposition and astrogliosis occur in both entities [14].

Encephalitis Versus Brainstem Neoplasm

Infectious encephalitis in humans can include herpes simplex viruses, arboviruses, lymphocytic choriomeningitis, measles virus, mumps, CMV, Epstein Barr virus (EBV), varicella-zoster virus 1, human herpes virus 6, and enteroviruses. However, the epidemiology of encephalitis in the USA is predominately unknown in origin [15, 16]. In a survey of pediatric brainstem lesions, Porto et al. reported the case of a 5-year-old male with left-sided horizontal and vertical nystagmus, double vision, and disequilibrium after coryzal illness [17]. The patient demonstrated isolated prolongation of T2 hyperintensity in the tegmentum of the pons and mesencephalon without contrast enhancement. Intermediate echo proton MRS at 1.5 T with PRESS localization revealed a normal spectrum. The child was treated with corticosteroids and showed clinical improvement. A repeat MRI 1 week later showed complete regression of the abnormal T2 signal. A presumptive diagnosis of encephalitis was made. After 4 years, there was no further clinical relapse reported.

Herpes Family of Viral Infections

Herpes encephalitis is the most common sporadic viral encephalitis. It favors manifestation in the temporal lobes. For adults, herpes simplex virus type 1 (HSV 1) is the primary source for fatal cases in adults. Sporadic cases of human herpes virus 6 (HHV6) have been described in those with lymphoproliferative disorders or immunocompromised patients. In neonates and children, herpes simplex virus type 2 (HSV 2) accounts for almost all congenital infections. Two historic case reports from the 1990s describe proton MRS features, specifically neuronal dysfunction, in pediatric herpes simplex encephalitis (HSE). Menon et al. reported the reduction of NAA/Cho in an 11-year-old boy that persisted at 8 and 16 weeks after the onset of symptoms [18]. Another HSE report described the restoration of NAA/Cr levels in an 11-year-old girl who fully recovered over the course of 1 year [19]. Patients with HSE from our institution demonstrate declines in NAA consistent with neuronal dysfunction, but also elevations of lactate, choline, and the composite neurotransmitters (glutamate, glutamine, etc.) (Figs. 13.4 and 13.5). Seizure activity alone may be associated in part with these additional findings.

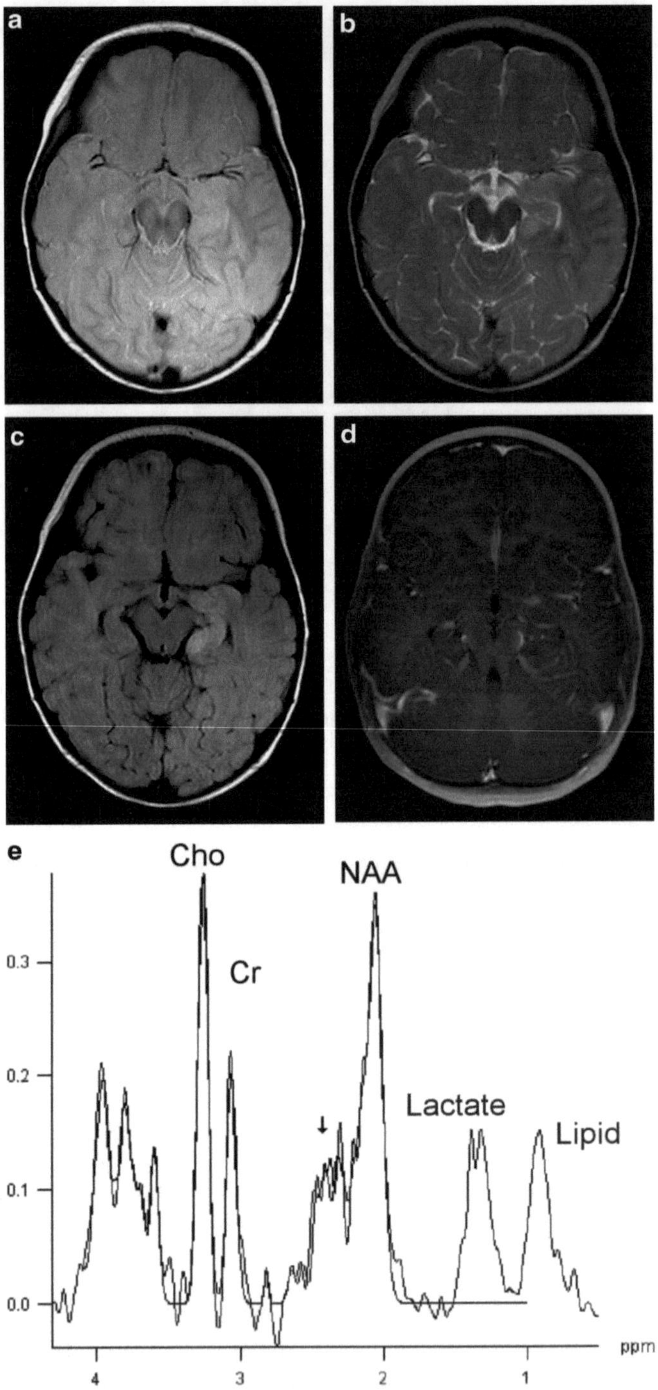

Fig. 13.4 MRI and MRS findings from a 12-month-old female diagnosed with herpes simplex encephalitis. (**a**) Proton density image; (**b**) T2-weighted image; (**c**) FLAIR image; (**d**) Post-contrast T1-weighted image; images feature abnormal signal within the left hippocampus and amygdala. (**e**) Short TE (35 ms) spectrum showing elevated signal in the GLX region (*arrow*), as well as elevated lipid and lactate. NAA/Cr appears slightly reduced on this spectrum acquired in the left hippocampus at 3 Tesla

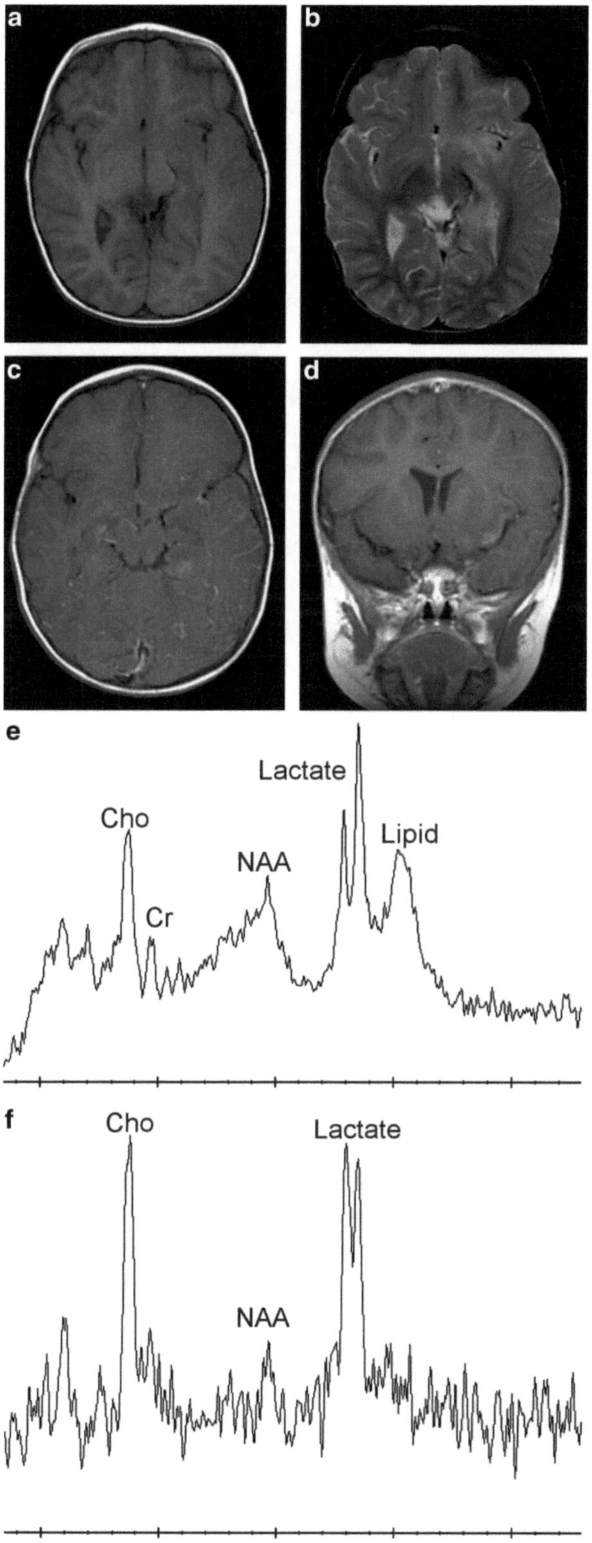

Fig. 13.5 MRI and MRS findings from a 20-month-old female diagnosed with herpes simplex encephalitis. (**a**) T1-weighted image; (**b**) T2-weighted image; (**c**) Post-contrast T1-weighted image; (**d**) Post-contrast T2-weighted image; these imaging examples show abnormal signal and leukomalacia within the left temporal lobe. (**e**) Short TE (35 ms) spectrum shows elevated lipid and lactate signals as well as elevated choline when sampled within the temporal lobe. (**f**) Long TE (288 ms) spectrum shows elevated lactate and severely reduced NAA and Cr

Epstein Barr Virus

EBV is among the most common human viruses and is also a member of the herpes virus family. Most persons become infected with EBV sometime in their life. In the USA, as much as 95% of adults between 35 and 40 years of age have been infected. In other developed countries, many persons are *not* infected with EBV in their childhood years. When infection with EBV occurs during adolescence or young adulthood, it causes infectious mononucleosis 35–50% of the time. Infants become susceptible to EBV as soon as maternal antibody protection (present at birth) disappears. Many children become infected with EBV, and these infections usually cause no symptoms or are indistinguishable from the other mild, brief illnesses of childhood. However, Cecil et al. reported imaging and proton MRS of a 12-month-old child with a 10-day history of fever and cough who presented with altered responsiveness, and opisthotonic posturing indicating seizure activity [20]. The child's CSF demonstrated no white cells, four red cells, 10 mg/dL protein; 75 mg/dL glucose and no culture growth. Serologic studies revealed acute EBV antibody titers and EBV IgM antinuclear antigen levels. Serum lactate and pyruvate were normal. Her CT images demonstrated symmetrically decreased attenuation in the basal ganglia. Subsequent MRI also demonstrated the bilateral signal abnormalities of the basal ganglia. The lesions revealed no contrast enhancement on either CT or MRI. The imaging appearance suggested many etiologies, such as hypoxic/ischemic injury, metabolic disorders, mitochondrial diseases, or toxin exposure as the primary considerations. Proton MRS was added to the imaging protocol, with the expectation that it would confirm a lactate resonance consistent with either the hypoxic-ischemic or metabolic etiologies. However, the resulting spectra from the basal ganglia indicated no evidence of lactate. Instead, minor declines in NAA with elevations of myo-inositol, lipid, macromolecules, and composite amino acids such as glutamate were found (Fig. 13.6). This more benign proton MRS pattern appeared to provide evidence supporting infection and inflammation in the acute setting.

Para- and Post-Infectious Encephalomyelitis

Acute Disseminated Encephalomyelitis

Acute disseminated encephalomyelitis (ADEM) is a post-infectious or post-immunization inflammatory disorder of the central nervous system (CNS) that is mediated by an immunologic response against myelin. By definition, ADEM is classified as a monophasic disease; however, reports of a remitting and relapsing course are referred to as multiphasic disseminated encephalomyelitis (MDEM). Children and

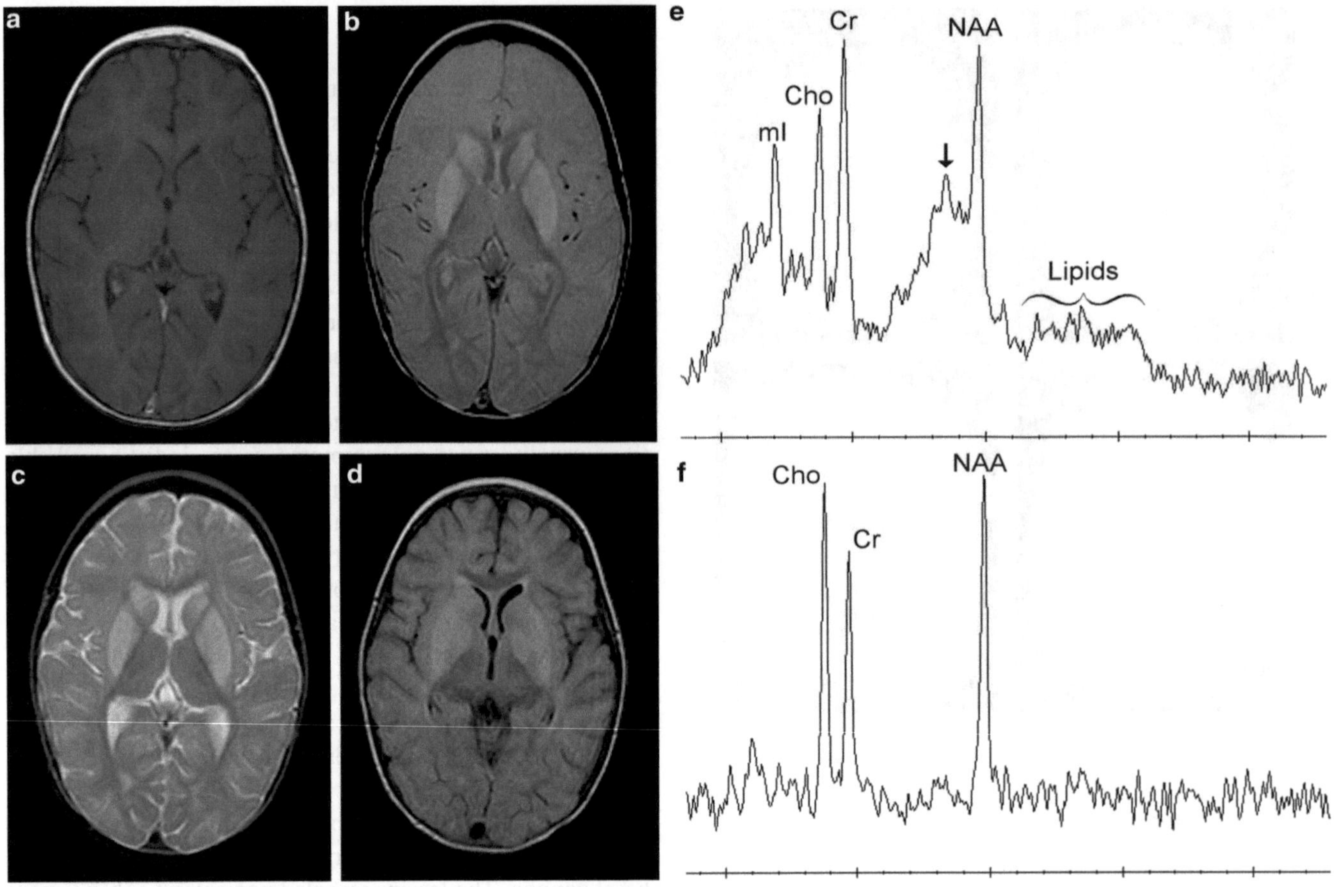

Fig. 13.6 MRI and MRS findings from a 12-month-old female diagnosed with Epstein Barr encephalitis. (**a**) T1-weighted image; (**b**) Proton density image; (**c**) T2 weighted image; (**d**) FLAIR image; abnormal signals are noted bilaterally in the caudate, globus pallidus and putamen. (**e**) Short TE (35 ms) spectrum showing elevated signal in the GLX region (*arrow*), with minimally elevated lipids and macromolecules. NAA/Cr appears slightly reduced on this spectrum acquired in the left basal ganglia. (**f**) Long TE (288 ms) spectrum shows no detectable elevation of lactate

adolescents are mainly affected with less frequent presentation in adults. The clinical and imaging features of ADEM are heterogeneous; however, the diagnosis relies on imaging and the analysis of cerebrospinal fluid. Most patients are previously healthy, with a history of a vaccination or minor infection occurring several days before the sudden onset of neurological symptoms that may include fever, altered mental state, headache, vomiting, ataxia, and seizures. Additional findings such as pyramidal and brainstem signs with cranial neuropathy, slurred speech, weakness, hemiplegia, and abnormal reflexes have also been described. Characteristic neuroimaging findings include multifocal regions of increased T2-weighted and FLAIR signal intensity with perifocal edema. Focal lesions usually demonstrate contrast enhancement. White matter lesions often appear in an asymmetric fashion adjacent to the ventricles and in subcortical regions. However, the cerebellum and deep gray matter regions such as the thalami, basal ganglia and brainstem may also be affected. Elevated CSF protein levels and pleocytosis are found in only half of suspected ADEM patients. With these variable patterns, proton MR spectroscopy can provide additional information to help distinguish ADEM from neoplasms.

Mader et al. described two distinct presentations of pediatric ADEM whose diagnosis was assisted using diffusion weighted imaging and proton MRS [21]. Their first described patient demonstrated a typical ADEM presentation. A 6-year-old girl with a history of an upper airway infection 10 days prior presented with fever, impaired consciousness, reduced motor movements, pyramidal signs, and aphasia. MRI studies revealed multiple hyperintense lesions in both hemispheres, in the thalami, pons, and the middle cerebellar peduncles, without contrast enhancement. Proton MRS of the lesions in the parietal lobe and pons demonstrated only a subtle elevation of lactate, as a sign of inflammation. Therapy with corticosteroids provided resolution of lesions and good clinical recovery. In another patient, Mader describes a more complicated picture of ADEM. In this case, a 13-year-old girl suffered minor head trauma followed by headaches, vomiting, adynamia, ataxia, paresthesia, and blurring of vision. CSF revealed elevated protein, but no pleocytosis, no oligoclonal banding and a normal IgG ratio with normal serological findings. An occipital lesion with hyperintense T2 signal with a peripheral rim of contrast enhancement without restricted diffusion was appreciated on MRI. Proton MRS revealed reduced NAA with increased levels of lactate, as well as macromolecules and lipids at 0.9, 1.2 and 1.4 ppm. The patient improved with corticosteroid therapy, but several relapses occurred with focal lesions appearing in the cerebellum and cerebral hemispheres, however, without localization in the periventricular white matter suggestive of multiple sclerosis.

At our institution, a 5-year-old girl presented with a 2-week history of headaches and emesis. The imaging revealed multifocal regions of abnormal signal with a large lesion within the right frontal lobe. The proton MRS revealed elevated lactate, glutatmate with glutamine, and choline with relatively good preservation of NAA and Cr. The preservation of NAA and Cr accompanied by low to normal mI suggested a demyelinating process over a neoplastic one. However, there were other features on imaging (i.e., mass effect, enhancement, edema) and clinical course that made a prospective diagnosis ADEM difficult. Ultimately, a biopsy was performed to provide a definitive diagnosis of ADEM (Fig. 13.7).

Acute Necrotizing Encephalopathy

Acute necrotizing encephalopathy is a rare neurological complication of viral infections such as influenza A and B, HHV6, varicella zoster, and mycoplasmal infection. This acute encephalopathy follows a viral febrile illness that manifests a rapid deterioration in the level of consciousness and produces seizures. On CT and MRI, symmetric focal brain lesions always involve the bilateral thalami, with lesions also commonly found in the cerebral periventricular white matter, internal capsule, putamen, upper brain stem tegmentum, and cerebellar medulla without other CNS involvement [22]. Due to the similarity of imaging presentation with mitochondrial disorders, it remains important to exclude mitochondrial and other metabolic diseases. Edema, perivascular hemorrhage, and necrosis are reported. The terminal branches of the intracerebral arteries generally supply the affected areas [22]. Histologic examinations of CNS lesions from patients with ANE demonstrate necrotic central neurons and glial cells [23, 24].

In a presumed diagnosis of ANE, a 16-month-old male child who presented with seizures, fever, and diarrhea at our institution had MR imaging with single voxel proton MRS acquired in the thalamus, basal ganglia, and white matter. The spectra obtained within the lesion located in the thalamus demonstrated a dramatically elevated lactate resonance with elevation of the glutamate and glutamine group of resonances, and choline coupled with a decline of NAA. MRS spectra acquired in lobar white matter and basal ganglia (caudate, putamen with internal capsule) revealed a similar pattern to that of the thalamus, but to a lesser extent (Fig. 13.8).

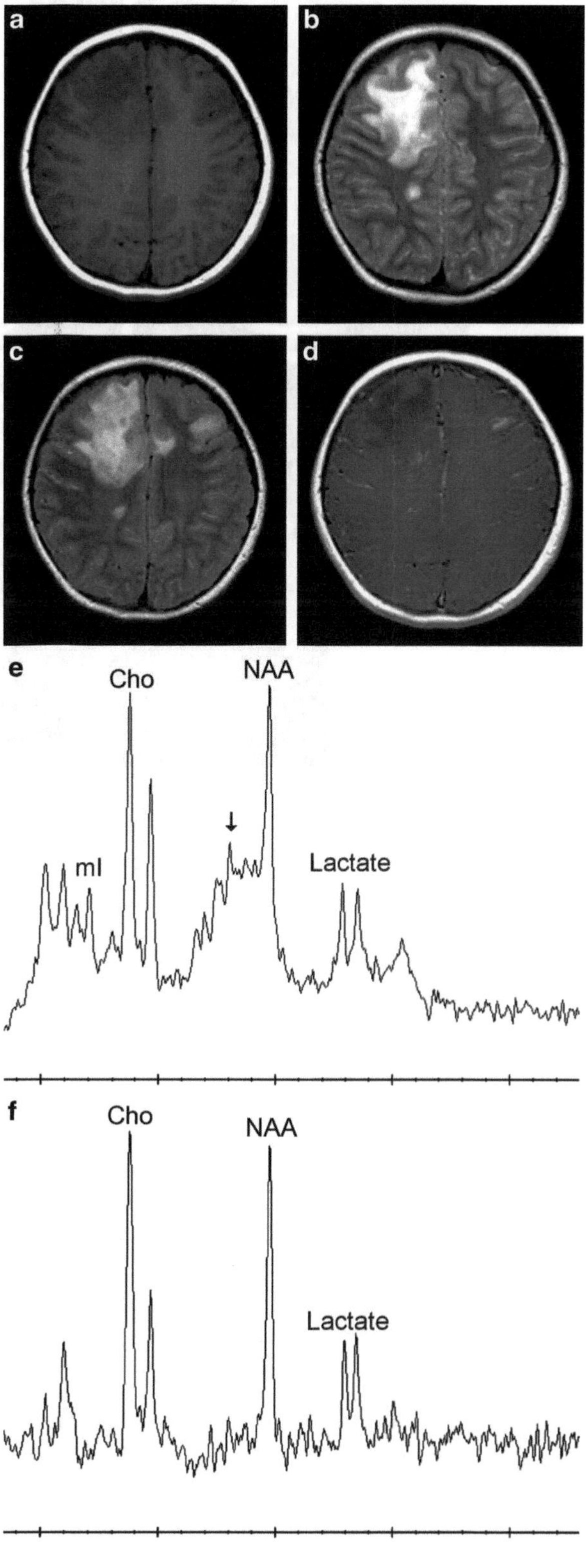

Fig. 13.7 MRI and MRS findings from a 5-year-old female with biopsy proven acute disseminated encephalitis (ADEM). (a) Precontrast T1-weighted image; (**b**) T2-weighted image; (**c**) FLAIR image; (**d**) Post-contrast T1-weighted image; abnormal heterogeneous signal primarily within a large lesion in the right frontal lobe is observed. (**e**) Short TE (35 ms) spectrum showing normal levels of Cr, and Cho, diminished NAA levels, elevated signal in the GLX region (*arrow*) as well as the presence of lactate and lipids; (**f**) Long TE (288 ms) spectrum reveals a highly significant elevation of lactate

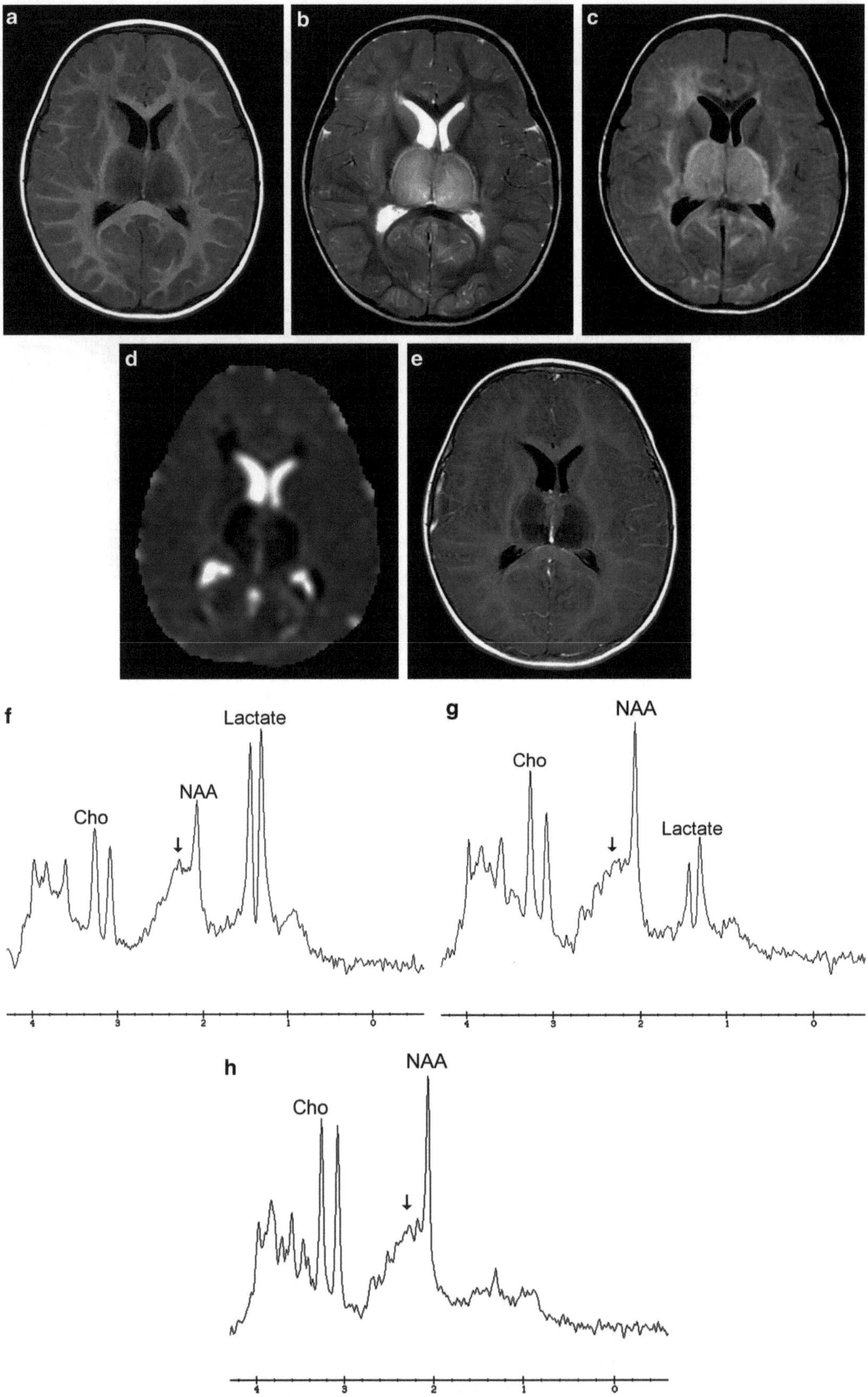

Fig. 13.8 MRI and MRS findings from a 16-month-old male diagnosed with acute necrotizing encephalopathy (ANE). (**a**) Pre-contrast T1-weighted image; (**b**) T2-weighted image; (**c**) FLAIR image; (**d**) ADC map; (**e**) Post-contrast T1-weighted image; abnormal signals are noted in the thalamus bilaterally, and within the white matter adjacent to the ventricles and external capsule. (**f**) Short TE (35 ms) spectrum of the thalamus; (**g**) Short TE (35 ms) spectrum of the left frontal lobe including cortical lesion (not seen on displayed level of images); (**h**) Short TE (35 ms) spectrum of the left basal ganglia. All spectra demonstrate elevated lactate, and GLX region (*arrow*) with amounts dependent upon lesion involvement

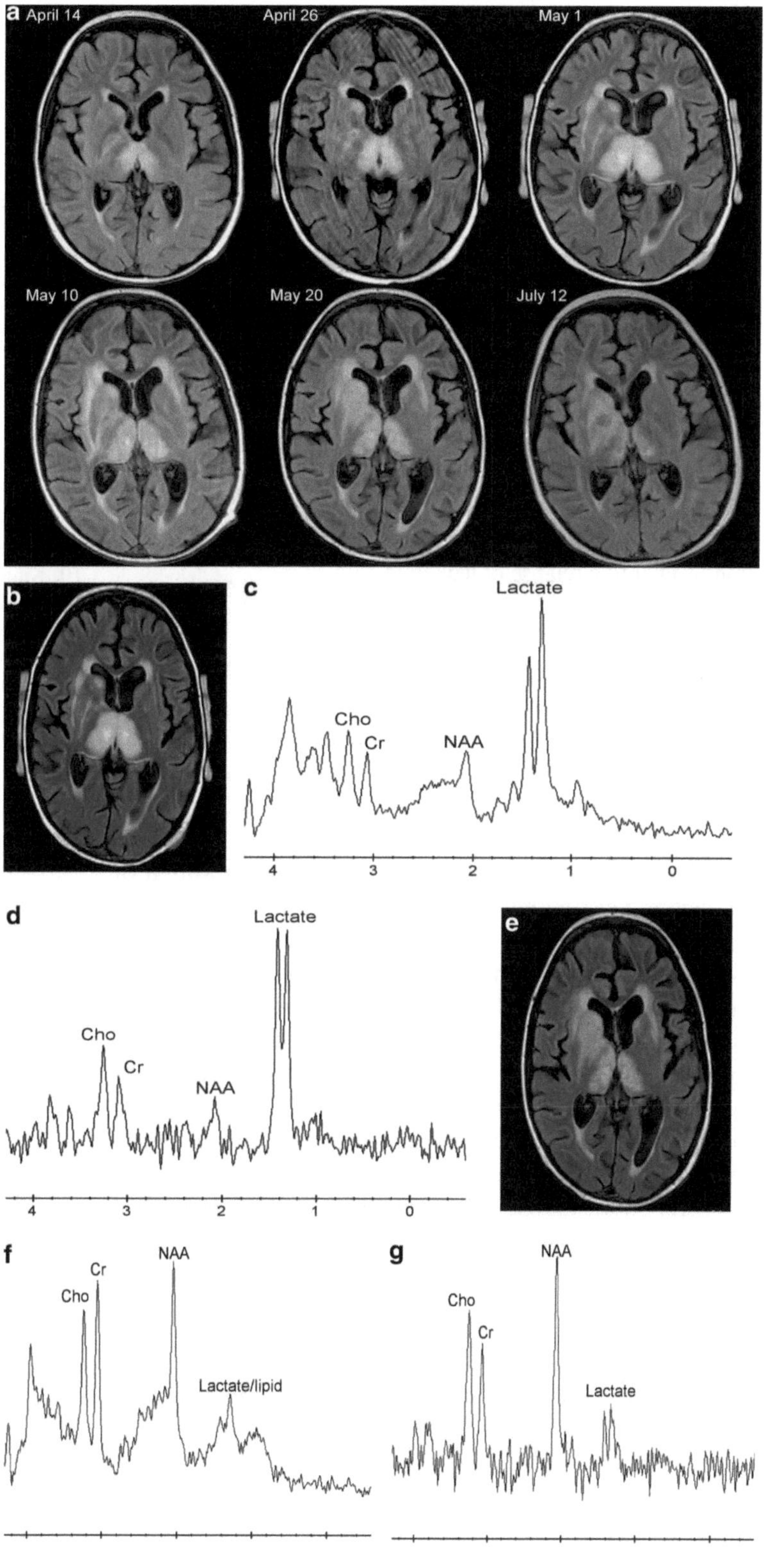

Fig. 13.9 MRI and MRS findings from a 13-year-old female who presented with respiratory alkalosis and mental status changes following a history of a bone marrow transplant for leukemia and subsequent fungal infections. Her relapse of acute lymphoblastic leukemia was treated with chemotherapy. (**a**) FLAIR images from April 14, April 26, May 1, May 10, May 20 and July 12 reveal an evolution of signal abnormalities beginning within the thalamus bilaterally and surrounding the lateral ventricles and expands to involve the caudate, internal and external capsule without significant volume loss. (**b–d**) FLAIR image from May 10 and short TE (35 ms) and long TE (288 ms) MRS obtained within the left thalamus demonstrate a dramatic elevation of lactate and glutamate with diminishment of NAA. (**e–g**) FLAIR image from May 20 indicates improvement of signal abnormalities, and there is significant clearance of lactate with restoration of NAA on short and long TE spectroscopic acquisitions. The evolving patterns on imaging and spectroscopy were most consistent with the diagnosis of acute disseminated encephalitis

Post-Treatment Infection

Patients with compromised immune systems or chronic medical histories following cancer treatment, or post-bone marrow transplants for genetic disorders are at risk for opportunistic infections and their complications. From a diagnostic standpoint, distinguishing recurrent illness from infection can be challenging with imaging alone. Proton MRS can often provide relevant information useful for narrowing the diagnostic differential.

A 10-year-old female was diagnosed with leukemia, underwent a bone marrow transplant 15 months post-diagnosis. She was subsequently followed for disseminated fungal infections and relapsed acute lymphoblastic leukemia (ALL) treated with chemotherapy (9-β-D-arabinofurnaosylguanine (Ara-G)) over the course of 2 years. During a period from April to July, the now 13-year-old female demonstrated on imaging multifocal areas of signal abnormality centered within the basal ganglia, thalami, and mid-brain (Fig. 13.9). The appearance of the lesions evolved over a short period of time. On spectroscopy, short and long echo voxels acquired within the left thalamus demonstrated dramatic elevation of lactate and diminution of NAA. Nineteen days later, the spectra demonstrated significant improvement with reduction of the lactate levels and improvement of NAA. This dramatic shift is most consistent with an infectious or para-infectious etiology. The patient was diagnosed during this period with ADEM. Unfortunately, the patient succumbed several months later to a relapse of leukemia.

Infections in the Masticator Space

Differentiating infection from malignant neoplasms can be very challenging with conventional imaging in the masticator space. In an exploratory study evaluating the utility of proton MRS to characterize lesions within the masticator space in pediatric and adult patients, there were a total of 24 lesions with pathologic outcomes defined [25]. From this group of 18 men and 6 women whose mean age was 40.6 years with ages ranging from 3 to 82 years, the pathologic analysis identified 7 chronic infections and 17 malignant neoplasms. Using criteria based on choline signal to noise levels, the mean value for chronic infections was 2.31 ± 0.19 compared to 5.76 ± 3.29 ($p < 0.01$) for malignant neoplasms. The chronic infections had absent or low choline levels; however, there was an overlap in low choline levels for some malignant neoplasms. For the two pediatric patients in the series, choline was detected in both infectious lesions.

Acknowledgments This work was supported by grants from the National Institutes of Health, NIEHS R01 ES015559, NCI R01 CA112182, and NIMH P50 MH077138. The authors have no competing financial or non-financial interests to declare.

References

1. Christopher MM, Eckfeldt JH, Eaton JW. Propylene glycol ingestion causes D-lactic acidosis. Lab Invest. 1990;62(1):114–8.
2. Lange T, Dydak U, Roberts TP, Rowley HA, Bjeljac M, Boesiger P. Pitfalls in lactate measurements at 3 T. AJNR Am J Neuroradiol. 2006;27(4):895–901.
3. Klomp DW, van der Graaf M, Willemsen MA, van der Meulen YM, Kentgens AP, Heerschap A. Transmit/receive headcoil for optimal 1 H MR spectroscopy of the brain in paediatric patients at 3 T. MAGMA. 2004;17(1):1–4.
4. Liu HS, Chung HW, Juan CJ, et al. Anomalous J-modulation effects on amino acids in clinical 3 T MR spectroscopy. AJNR Am J Neuroradiol. 2008;29(9):1644–8.
5. Pal D, Bhattacharyya A, Husain M, Prasad KN, Pandey CM, Gupta RK. In vivo proton MR spectroscopy evaluation of pyogenic brain abscesses: a report of 194 cases. AJNR Am J Neuroradiol. 2010;31(2):360–6.
6. Lai PH, Hsu SS, Ding SW, et al. Proton magnetic resonance spectroscopy and diffusion-weighted imaging in intracranial cystic mass lesions. Surg Neurol. 2007;68 Suppl 1:S25–36.
7. Luthra G, Parihar A, Nath K, et al. Comparative evaluation of fungal, tubercular, and pyogenic brain abscesses with conventional and diffusion MR imaging and proton MR spectroscopy. AJNR Am J Neuroradiol. 2007;28(7):1332–8.
8. Vajro P, Sokal EM, Maddaluno S, et al. Brain abscess due to Klebsiella pneumoniae in a liver-transplanted child. Transpl Infect Dis. 2009;11(4):341–5.
9. Jain KK, Mittal SK, Kumar S, Gupta RK. Imaging features of central nervous system fungal infections. Neurol India. 2007;55(3):241–50.
10. Kingsley PB, Shah TC, Woldenberg R. Identification of diffuse and focal brain lesions by clinical magnetic resonance spectroscopy. NMR Biomed. 2006;19(4):435–62.
11. Ferraz-Filho JR, Santana-Netto PV, Rocha-Filho JA, Sgnolf A, Mauad F, Sanches RA. Application of magnetic resonance spectroscopy in the differentiation of high-grade brain neoplasm and inflammatory brain lesions. Arq Neuropsiquiatr. 2009;67(2A):250–3.
12. Chang L, Miller BL, McBride D, et al. Brain lesions in patients with AIDS: H-1 MR spectroscopy. Radiology. 1995;197(2):525–31.
13. Keller MA, Venkatraman TN, Thomas A, et al. Altered neurometabolite development in HIV-infected children: correlation with neuropsychological tests. Neurology. 2004;62(10):1810–7.
14. van der Voorn JP, Pouwels PJ, Vermeulen RJ, Barkhof F, van der Knaap MS. Quantitative MR imaging and spectroscopy in congenital cytomegalovirus infection and periventricular leukomalacia suggests a comparable neuropathological substrate of the cerebral white matter lesions. Neuropediatrics. 2009;40(4):168–73.
15. Glaser CA, Gilliam S, Schnurr D, et al. In search of encephalitis etiologies: diagnostic challenges in the California Encephalitis Project, 1998–2000. Clin Infect Dis. 2003;36(6):731–42.
16. Whitley RJ. Viral encephalitis. N Engl J Med. 1990;323(4):242–50.
17. Porto L, Hattingen E, Pilatus U, et al. Proton magnetic resonance spectroscopy in childhood brainstem lesions. Childs Nerv Syst. 2007;23(3):305–14.
18. Menon DK, Sargentoni J, Peden CJ, et al. Proton MR spectroscopy in herpes simplex encephalitis: assessment of neuronal loss. J Comput Assist Tomogr. 1990;14(3):449–52.
19. Takanashi J, Sugita K, Ishii M, Aoyagi M, Niimi H. Longitudinal MR imaging and proton MR spectroscopy in herpes simplex encephalitis. J Neurol Sci. 1997;149(1):99–102.
20. Cecil KM, Jones BV, Williams S, Hedlund GL. CT, MRI and MRS of Epstein-Barr virus infection: case report. Neuroradiology. 2000;42(8):619–22.
21. Mader I, Wolff M, Nagele T, Niemann G, Grodd W, Kuker W. MRI and proton MR spectroscopy in acute disseminated encephalomyelitis. Childs Nerv Syst. 2005;21(7):566–72.
22. Seo HE, Hwang SK, Choe BH, Cho MH, Park SP, Kwon S. Clinical spectrum and prognostic factors of acute necrotizing encephalopathy in children. J Korean Med Sci. 2010;25(3):449–53.
23. Marco EJ, Anderson JE, Neilson DE, Strober JB. Acute necrotizing encephalopathy in 3 brothers. Pediatrics. 2010;125(3):e693–698.
24. Mastroyianni SD, Gionnis D, Voudris K, Skardoutsou A, Mizuguchi M. Acute necrotizing encephalopathy of childhood in non-Asian patients: report of three cases and literature review. J Child Neurol. 2006;21(10):872–9.
25. Yu Q, Yang J, Wang P. Malignant tumors and chronic infections in the masticator space: preliminary assessment with in vivo single-voxel 1 H-MR spectroscopy. AJNR Am J Neuroradiol. 2008;29(4):716–9.

Hepatic Encephalopathy in Children

14

Giulio Zuccoli and Gayathri Sreedher

Hepatic encephalopathy (HE) is a neurocognitive disorder associated with either acute or chronic liver disease (CLD). HE is also found in patients with either spontaneous or surgically created portosystemic shunts. The severity of HE spans from a mild neuropsychological impairment, detectable only at a psychometric evaluation, to coma. HE is a potentially reversible process. However, cirrhosis-associated neurological deficits may persist after liver transplant thus, supporting the hypothesis that HE may lead to irreversible neurological impairment [1].

Acute Liver Failure in Children

Acute liver failure (ALF) is characterized by a sudden and severe hepatic injury [2–4] followed by encephalopathy within 8 weeks of appearance of the symptoms [5]. However, in the pediatric population ALF is not always associated with HE, which may develop very late during the course of the disease [3]. Thus, ALF in children is considered a multisystem disorder with severe liver function impairment associated with significant coagulopathy with no sepsis or disseminated intravascular coagulation that is not correctable by the administration of parenteral vitamin K within 8 h. A detailed definition of ALF in children has been proposed in 2004 by the Working Group report of the second World Congress of Pediatric Gastroenterology. All definitions mentioned below imply the absence of previous liver disease [6].

G. Zuccoli, MD (✉) • G. Sreedher, MD
Department of Radiology, Children Hospital of Pittsburgh at the University of Pittsburgh Medical Center, Pittsburgh, PA 15224, USA
e-mail: giulio.zuccoli@gmail.com

Hyperacute

Coagulopathy due to acute liver dysfunction of 10 days or less of total duration by clinical criteria. In the hyperacute phase encephalopathy is variable.

Acute

Coagulopathy due to acute liver dysfunction of more than 10 days or less than 30 days of total duration by clinical criteria. Encephalopathy is absent or impossible to recognize, especially in younger patients. When present, encephalopathy tends to be preterminal.

Subacute

Coagulopathy due to acute liver dysfunction of more than 31 days but less than 6 months of total duration by clinical criteria. Jaundice is almost always present. Encephalopathy often marks preterminal deterioration. Subacute ALF is seen in association with autoimmune liver disease, Wilson disease, medications, and idiopathic causes. The idiopathic cases are characterized by poor prognosis.

Classification of HE of ALF in children differs from that of adults. In adults ALF is classified based on the severity of the encephalopathy in grades from 1 to 3 [7, 8]. In children, HE of ALF ranges from grade 1, characterized by confusion and mood changes, to grade 4A and B, the latter characterized by deep coma. HE patients with grades from 3 to 4B are likely candidates for liver transplantation [3, 9].

Etiology of ALF in Children

The cause of ALF varies according to patient's age, geographic distribution, medical, and social practices. Underlying metabolic condition represents the most frequent cause in

S. Blüml and A. Panigrahy (eds.), *MR Spectroscopy of Pediatric Brain Disorders*,
DOI 10.1007/978-1-4419-5864-8_14, © Springer Science+Business Media, LLC 2013

Europe and North America while the hepatitis A virus (HAV) is the commonest etiology in Asia and South America [3]. Cochran and Loseck [10] classified the etiology of ALF in children according to patient's age (Figs. 14.1 and 14.2).

Infective Etiology

Icterus and raised serum transaminase levels are usually found in children affected by ALF of viral origin. The most common virus associated with ALF is HAV. Association between underlying liver disease and HAV represents a predisposing factor to develop ALF in children. The hepatitis B virus (HBV) infection is less commonly seen in children than in adults with ALF. Infants born to mothers positive for the antibody to hepatitis B e antigen are a special group of patients that may present with ALF. The hepatitis C virus (HCV) infection and hepatitis D virus (HDV) are unlikely to be a cause of ALF in children. HCV and HDV infections are diagnosed by detecting anti-HCV antibody or HCV RNA in the serum and anti-HDV antibody in serum. The hepatitis E virus (HEV) infection is a common cause of ALF in chidren and the association between HAV and HEV infection has been reported in children affected by ALF in India, Pakistan, South Asia and Africa [2, 11]. Similar to HAV, HEV is transmitted via the fecal–oral route. Seronegative (Non-A-E) hepatitis may also be seen in ALF patients [11, 12]. Herpes simplex virus types 1 and 2, human herpes virus 6, varicella zoster virus, Epstein-Barr virus, cytomegalovirus, and parvovirus B19 may cause ALF in neonates and immunocompromised. Echovirus, Coxsackieviruses, and adenoviruses are other viruses that can cause ALF, particularly in newborns. Among bacteria, Salmonella, mycobacterium tuberculosis may cause ALF in the pediatric population. Zoonotic infections such as malaria, bartonella, and leptospirosis may be also responsible for ALF in children [2, 3].

Metabolic Etiology

The metabolic causes of ALF in children and infants comprise a special group. Timely diagnosis and prompt corrective treatment can be life saving. Urgent intervention with dietary manipulation for some cases is mandatory as liver transplantation may be contraindicated.

Neonatal hemochromatosis is associated with excess in iron deposition in the reticuloendothelial cells. Fetal liver injury, hepatic and extrahepatic siderosis occurs in NH. This can be fatal in >60 % of patients and future recurrence in siblings may be as high as 80 % [12, 13]. Neonatal hemochromatosis is the most common cause of ALF requiring liver transplantation in the perinatal period [14]. The severity of NH varies from asymptomatic to ALF. Prompt diagnosis and treatment are effective in prolonging survival. Serum Alfa Feto Protein and ferritin are the most sensitive tests for the diagnosis of NH. However, these tests are not specific [14]. Punch biopsy of the salivary glands and demonstration

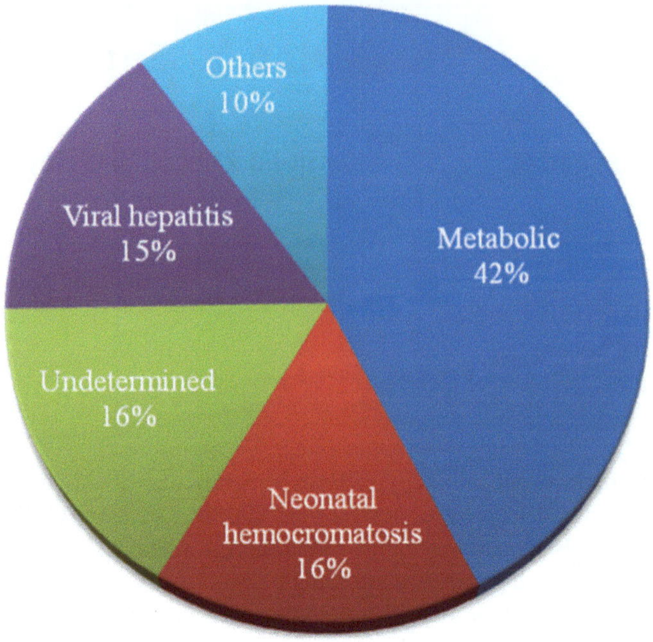

Fig. 14.1 Etiology of ALF in children younger than 1 year. (Modified from Cochran JB, Losek JD. Acute liver failure in children. Pediatr Emerg Care 2007; 23:129–35, with permission)

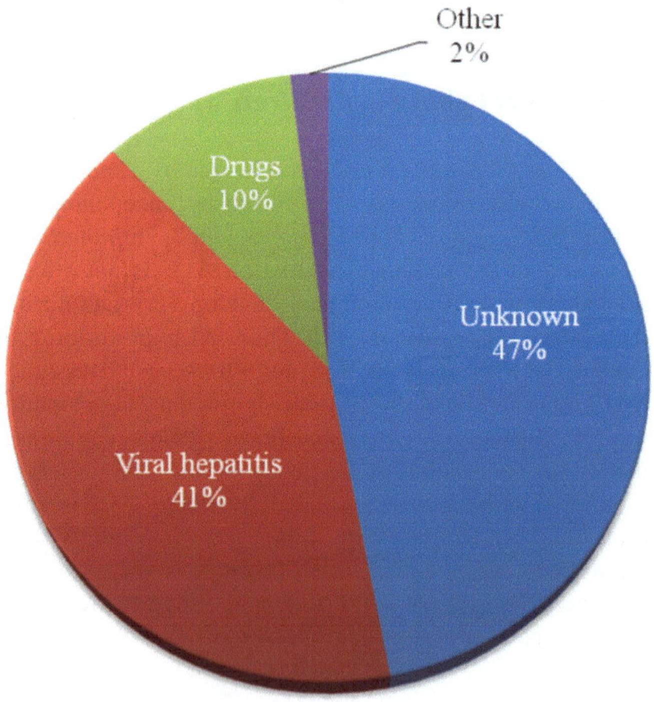

Fig. 14.2 Etiology of ALF in children 1 year and older (Modified from Cochran JB, Losek JD. Acute liver failure in children. Pediatr Emerg Care 2007; 23:129–35, with permission)

of iron is known to be useful for the diagnosis of NH [3]. Treatment includes administering iron chelating agents and antioxidants of debatable efficacy. Non-responders are candidates for early liver transplantation. Maternal treatment with immunoglobulins in subsequent pregnancies is known to decrease the incidence of NH in subsequent siblings [15].

Galactosemia is a disorder of galactose metabolism inherited in an autosomal-recessive pattern. Typical biochemical abnormalities include elevated galactitol, galactose-1-phosphate, and galactose in serum and urine analysis. Galactosemia is characterized by accumulation of these metabolic byproducts in the brain with development of mental retardation [16].

Tyrosinemia type I is a rare autosomal-recessive disorder affecting the liver, kidneys, and peripheral nerves. Symptomatology is varied and can range from ALF in infancy to CLD in later life. Regional predominance in areas like Quebec, Scandinavian countries, and the Indian subcontinent has been reported. When the disease manifests as ALF in infancy it is associated with bleeding diathesis and hepatomegaly. Increased association with hepatocellular carcinoma later in life has been reported. Biochemical markers include elevated serum and urine succinylacetone levels and decreased activity of fumarylacetoacetate hydrolase enzyme. Liver transplantation is curative. Treatment with NTBC 2-(2-nitro-4-trifluoromethylbenzoyl)-1, 3-cyclohexanedione) is also a clinical option and is known to diminish risk of ALF [17].

Wilson's disease is an autosomal-recessive disorder typically presenting in older kids in which copper accumulates in tissues. Biliary excretion of copper is reduced in Wilson disease, resulting in the accumulation of copper by the hepatocyte. Biochemical diagnosis includes a demonstration of low serum ceruloplasmin levels and increased serum copper levels, though the two may be normal in some patients. Opthalmological documentation of Kayser-Fleisher rings is helpful in diagnosis. Hemolytic anemia may be associated.

Other less common causes of ALF of metabolic origin in kids include enzyme disorders involving fatty chain oxidation, bile acid synthesis, mitochondrial respiratory chain disorders, and infantile fructose intolerance [3].

Chronic Liver Disease in Children

Numerous disorders are known to cause CLD in children. CLD is associated with a wide spectrum of diseases, including malformations, viruses, genetic metabolic, drug-induced, vascular and autoimmune hepatitis. CLD may present with hepatomegaly or splenomegaly, elevated liver enzymes, coaghulopathy, ascites, gastrointestinal bleeding or jaundice. They may also present with pulmonary arteriovenous shunting and pulmonary hypertension, bacterial

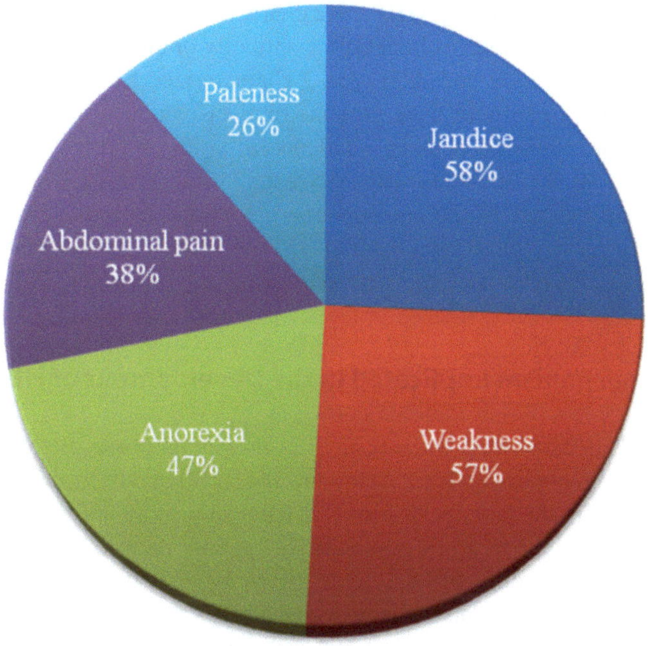

Fig. 14.3 Clinical findings in children with AIH (Modified from Oettinger R, Brunnberg A, Gerner P, et al. Clinical features and biochemical data of Caucasian children at diagnosis ofautoimmune hepatitis. J Autoimmun. 2005;24:79–84, with permission)

peritonitis or rarely with HE. Hepatitis B, hepatitis D virus, enteroviruses, cytomegalovirus, rubella virus, and herpes simplex are the predominant organisms implicated in CLD. Cirrhosis represents the end stage of any CLD. On histopathology, cirrhosis is characterized by regenerative nodules surrounded by fibrous bands [18]. Metabolic disorders associated with CLD in childhood are Alpha-1-antitrypsin deficiency, galactosemia, fructosemia, tyrosinosis, glycogen storage disease types III and IV, Niemann-Pick disease, Wolman disease, cystic fibrosis, and Wilson's disease [18]. More than 900 drugs, toxins, and herbal compounds have been described to cause acute and chronic liver damage. Apart from accidental exposure, drug-related hepatitis is rare in children. Drugs may directly affect the liver or mediate an autoimmune response. Autoimmune hepatitis (AIH) occurs in adults and children. The etiology of autoimmune hepatitis is unknown. Several factors, including viruses, drugs, and environment, may trigger autoimmunity. In the pediatric population AIH often presents acutely and has a more aggressive course than in adults. The peak of incidence of AIH in children is 10–20 years. Approximately one half of patients suffering from AH are younger than 20 years with a peak of incidence seen in premenstrual girls. Autoimmune hepatitis has also been reported in infants. Clinical findings in children with AIH are listed in Fig. 14.3 [19]. Three different types of autoimmune hepatitis have been described: AIH type-1 characterized by the presence of circulating anti smooth muscle antibodies and or antinuclear antibodies, AIH type-2 characterized by circulating liver-kidney microsomal type 1 antibody or anti-liver cytosol 1 antibody and AIH type-3 characterized by autoantibodies to soluble liver proteins or liver-pancreas antigen. AIH-2 shows a peak of incidence in younger patients. In fact 80 % of patients with AIH-2 are children. Type 2 AIH may be part of the autoimmune polyendocrinopathy-candidiasis-ectodermal dystrophy (APECED) syndrome, which is an autosomal-recessive monogenic disorder [19].

Mechanism Implicated in the Development of HE

HE is associated with ALF, CLD as well as portosystemic shunts bypassing liver. Many mechanisms have been implicated in the pathogenesis of HE. Clinically subtle HE which become apparent on psychometric testing alone is categorized into minimal HE. Acute HE is associated with acute hepatic insult. Episodic and persistent HEs are the other clinical presentation types of HE and are typically associated with persistent or long-standing liver insult. Mechanism and pathophysiology of neurocognitive impairment in HE can be better understood by sequentially considering the role of the major implicated toxins and their effects on brain neuronal function.

Role of Ammonia

Results of neuropathologic, spectroscopic, and neurochemical studies continue to support a major role for ammonia in the pathogenesis of the central nervous system injury of both acute and chronic liver failure. Ammonia remains central to the pathophysiology of HE since the late nineteenth century. Ammonia is normally detoxified in the liver. High ammonia levels in the arterial blood are related to increased risk of intracranial hypertension. The cause and effect relationship with ammonia is more definitive for acute liver insult. In cirrhosis the relationship between ammonia levels and HE severity are not as definitive.

Changes in Brain Astrocytes

Astrocytes are the most vulnerable glial cells to changes in blood ammonia levels. The reason for this is the presence of glutamine synthetase within astrocytes. This enzyme is absent in other neuronal cells. Glutamine synthetase takes up ammonia and converts it to glutamate and glutamine. Excessive glutamine can cause cell swelling, edema, and intracranial hypertension.

Damage to Blood–Brain Barrier

In liver failure the blood–brain barrier becomes more permeable. Ammonia levels may be partly related for this rather complex mechanism of increased permeability. The result of uncontrolled movement of plasma and water to extracellular space may lead to vasogenic edema in the brain. Several other factors may act synergistically and contribute to the clinical picture of HE.

Proinflammatory Markers

Systemic inflammation produces cytokines, which by brain capillary endothelial activation can increase the permeability of blood–brain barrier and may induce changes in brain-signaling mechanisms. The brain produces proinflammatory cytokines in ALF. This theory is also supported by the precipitation of ALF by sepsis, Systemic inflammatory response, and drug-induced ALF. Cirrhosis complicated by infective or systemic inflammation is a common precipitating factor for HE.

Oxidative Stress

Uptake of ammonia and excess glutamine production elevates mitochondrial glutamine levels and stimulates production of reactive oxygen species (ROS). This is implicated in the increase of oxygen free radicals which can compromise membrane integrity of neighboring neurons as well [4]. A single mechanism has not been postulated for HE changes. In varied clinical scenarios, simultaneous presence of one or more of the above implicating factors may act in a synergistic manner in the pathogenesis of HE.

Neuroimaging Findings of HE

Pathogenic mechanisms responsible for HE are thought to be related to accumulation in the blood of several compounds that are efficiently metabolized by the liver under normal circumstances. These substances include manganese and ammonia, which can modify astrocyte and neuron function [20–23]. The hypermanganesemia exerts a neurotoxic effect, thus inducing reactive gliosis and selective neuronal loss in the basal ganglia and the midbrain structures [24]. Ammonia is the most important toxin implicated in the pathogenesis of hepatic encephalopathy causing disturbance in the glutaminergic, GABAergic and benzodiazepine transmission. In HE there is proliferation of Alzheimer type-II cells in the gray matter [20]. Neuropathological changes in children affected by acquired hepato-cerebral degeneration may also show focal areas of spongiosis and neuronal loss, diffuse gliosis, and Alzheimer type II cells. Patients affected by acquired hepato-cerebral degeneration clinically may resemble valproate-associated hepatotoxicity [25]. Changes in MR imaging of the brain parenchyma in children and adults with HE include increased T1-weighted signal intensity in the basal ganglia, particularly in the globus pallidus atrophy, normal T2-weighted signal intensity [26, 27]. The paramagnetic properties of manganese are felt to be responsible for the increase in the signal intensity in T1-weighted images extending from the globus pallidus, putamen, internal capsule, pituitary gland, midbrain surrounding the red nucleus,

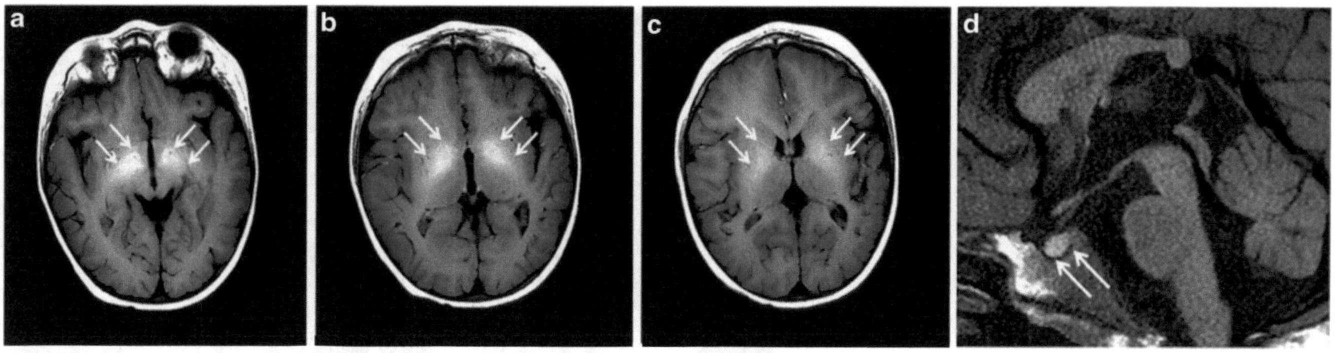

Fig. 14.4 (**a–c**) A 3-year-old boy suffering from hepatic encephalopathy. Increased signal intensity alteration is noted in the bilateral cerebral peduncle (**a**) and globus pallidus (**b, c**) on T1-weighted images (*arrows*). (**d**) Diffuse increased T1 signal involves the pituitary gland (*arrows*) in a 3-year-old child suffering from hepatic encephalopathy

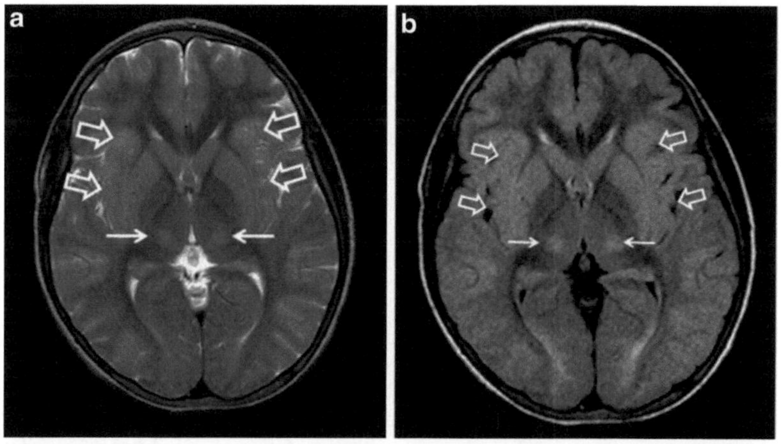

Fig. 14.5 (**a–b**) Increased T2-FLAIR signal is noted in the thalami (*arrows*) and cortex (*empty arrows*) in a 12-year-old female affected by hepatic encephalopathy

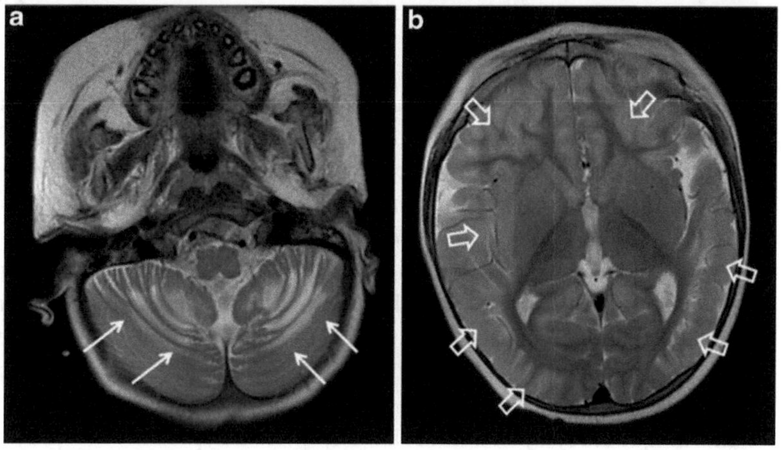

Fig. 14.6 (**a–b**) Bilaterally increased signal on T2-weighted images is noted in the cerebellum (**a**, *arrows*) and in the cortex, supratentorially (**b**, *empty arrows*)

and the white matter (Fig. 14.4) [26, 27]. However, normal T2-weighted decreased intensity caused by iron accumulation does not allow identifying manganese accumulation on T2-weighted images. In acute HE increased T2-weighted signal intensity in the cerebral cortex may be observed in children (Fig. 14.5) [28].

Diffusion properties of the brain in hepatic encephalopathy in children have not been evaluated. Few studies have been performed in adult patients. Patients with acute hepatic encephalopathy may exhibit characteristic regions of involvement on T2-wehighted images with DWI\ADC findings that can be reversible [29]. Extent of the signal intensity alteration seen on T2-weighted images and on DWI\ADC images correlates with the plasma ammonia levels. In acute hyper-ammoniemic encephalopathy typical symmetric increased T2 signal and restricted diffusion may be observed in the posterior limb of the internal capsule, periventricular white matter, thalamus, dorsal brainstem, cerebellar white matter, basal ganglia, and cerebellum (Figs. 14.6 and 14.7) [29].

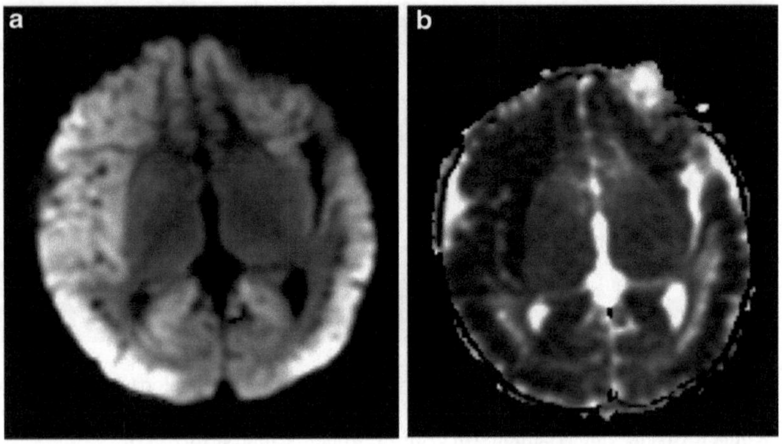

Fig. 14.7 (**a–b**) Bilaterally increased signal on DWI (**a**) and decreased signal on ADC map (**b**) consistent with cytotoxic edema is noted in the brain cortex

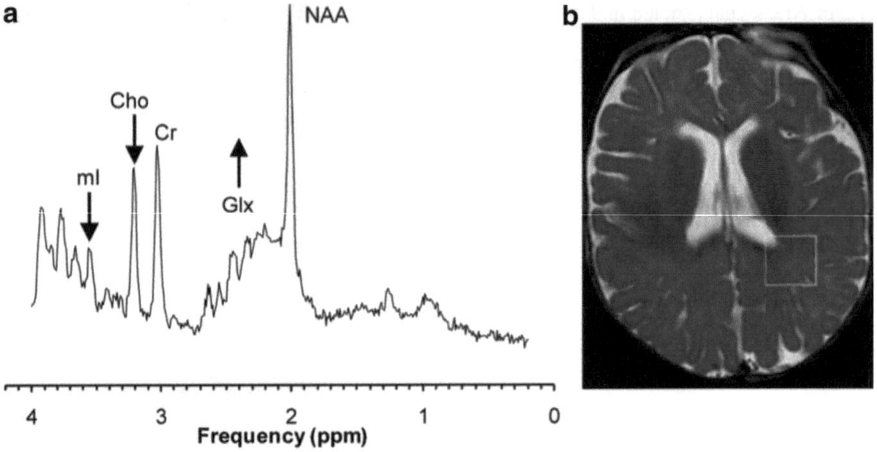

Fig. 14.8 MR Spectroscopy (MRS) shows different findings in patients with minimal hepatic encephalopathy, acute encephalopathy, and chronic liver disease

In chronic liver disease and minimal hepatic encephalopathy as well as ALF, the apparent diffusion coefficient (ADC) is increased in frontal and parietal white matter, dorsal brain stem, internal capsule, thalamus, and cerebral cortex [29–31]. Fractional anisometry is reduced in the periventricular white matter [30, 31]. High mean diffusivity in cortical gray matter as well as subcortical white matter is seen in minimal hepatic encephalopathy [31–33]. These findings support the hypothesis that in HE interstitial cerebral edema plays an important role.

In a unique study by Mardini et al. [34] where a hyperammonemic state was induced in patients with cirrhosis, interesting findings were revealed. The study used diffusion tensor images to generate ADC maps. They found an increase in ADC values, which correlated with increase in blood ammonia levels. These findings confirm the theory of ammonia leading to brain edema and subsequent changes in brain diffusion properties. Following treatment of hepatic encephalopathy reversal of these changes may be observed [35].

MR Spectroscopy (MRS) shows different findings in patients with minimal hepatic encephalopathy, acute encephalopathy, and chronic liver disease (Figs. 14.8 and 14.9). In MRS total creatine, which is composed of resonances from creatine and phosphocreatine, is used as an internal reference. Changes in metabolite ratios are often measured as ratios with creatine as the denominator. This is because total creatine (Cr) remains stable in size despite bioenergetic abnormalities. Glutamine (Gln) is a precursor of glutamate (Glu) in the brain. Glutamine is located in astrocytes. The two are structurally similar and their sum resonance in MRS is commonly denoted as Glx [36]. In patients with HE there is an increase in Glutamine content of gray and white matter with a decrease in choline and myoinositol levels. Myo-inositol, which is seen at short TE MRS, is believed to be essential for cell growth [36]. The increased glutamine in white matter correlates with increased plasma ammonia levels [37]. In ALF with HE in children there is an increase in glutamine and lactate in white matter [38]. Lactate is produced by anaerobic metabolism, and it measures glucose utilization [36].

In children with MHE there is a decrease in myo-inositol levels in gray and white matter. The decrease in myo-inositol correlates with plasma branched chain and aromatic amino acid ratios [37]. This ratio of amino acids is raised in patients

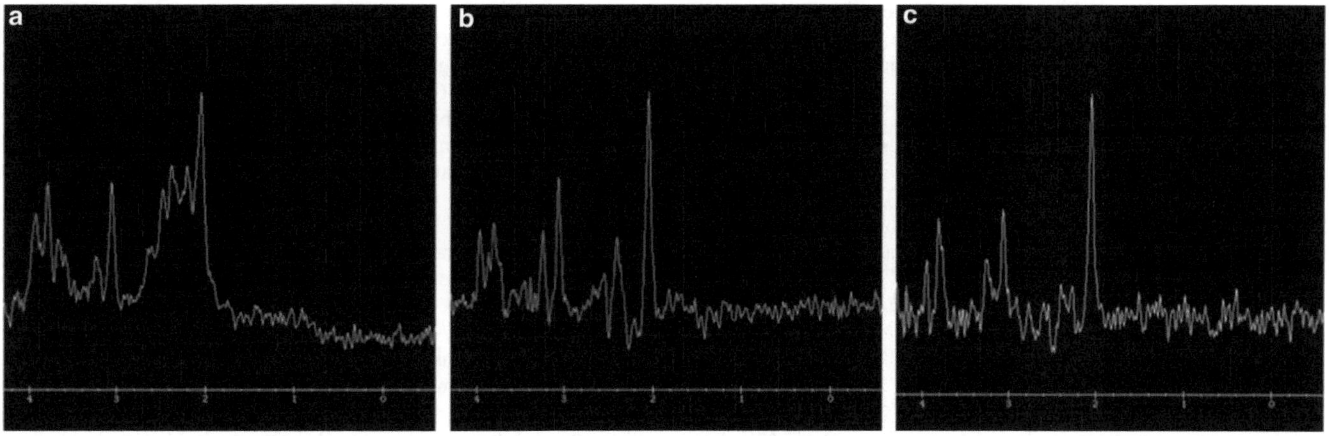

Fig. 14.9 Acute hepatic encephalopathy. (**a**) Thalamus 35TE. (**b**) Thalamus 144TE. (**c**) Thalamus 288TE

with impaired liver function. Increased glutamine/creatine ratios and decreased myo-inositol/creatine are also seen in adults with ALF and HE [39]. *N*-acetylaspartate (NAA)/creatine ratios are also decreased in patients with chronic liver disease and HE (Verma A et al. 2008). NAA is found in neurons and serves as a marker of neuronal density [36].

Reversal of these changes may be demonstrated by MRS after treatment of hepatic encephalopathy. Usually, clinical improvement precedes MRS changes. Reversal of the elevated glutamine/creatine to baseline and reversal of decreased choline/creatine to normal levels are seen following clinical improvement in patients with ALF. Persistent decrease in choline/creatine points toward poor prognosis [40].

Following liver transplantation the sequence of reversal of MRS changes was studied by Cordoba and colleagues [41–43]. The first peak to normalize is choline/creatine, within 6–8 weeks. Glutamine/creatine normalizes next after 8–9 weeks. Myo-inositol/creatine reverses last, taking up to 3–7 months.

References

1. Mechtcheriakov S, Graziadei IW, Mattedi M, Bodner T, Kugener A, Hinterhuber HH, Marksteiner J, Vogel W. Incomplete improvement of visuo-motor deficits in patients with minimal hepatic encephalopathy after liver transplantation. Liver Transplant. 2004;10:77–83.
2. Bernal W, Auzinger G, Dhawan A, Wendon J. Acute liver failure. Lancet. 2010;376:190–201.
3. Dhawan A. Etiology and prognosis of acute liver failure in children. Liver Transpl. 2008;14 Suppl 2:S80–4.
4. Seyan AS, Hughes RD, Shawcross DL. Changing face of hepatic encephalopathy: role of inflammation and oxidative stress. World J Gastroenterol. 2010;16:3347–57.
5. Trey C, Davidson C. The management of fulminant hepatic failure. In: Popper H, Schaffner F, editors. Progress in liver diseases, vol. 111. New York, NY: Grun and Stratten; 1970. p. 282–98.
6. Baker A, Alonso ME, Aw MM, Ciocca M, Porta G, Rosenthal P. Hepatic failure and liver transplant: Working Group report of the second World Congress of Pediatric Gastroenterology, Hepatology, and Nutrition. J Pediatr Gastroenterol Nutr. 2004;39 Suppl 2:S632–9.
7. O'Grady JG, Schalm SW, Williams R. Acute liver failure: redefining the syndromes. Lancet. 1993;342:273–5.
8. Ichai P, Samuel D. Etiology and prognosis of fulminant hepatitis in adults. Liver Transpl. 2008;14 suppl 2:S67–79.
9. Aw MM, Dhawan A. Acute liver failure. Indian J Pediatr. 2002;69:87–91.
10. Cochran JB, Losek JD. Acute liver failure in children. Pediatr Emerg Care. 2007;23:129–35.
11. Arora NK, Nanda SK, Gulati S, Ansari IH, Chawla MK, Gupta SD, Panda SK. Acute viral hepatitis types E, A, and B singly and in combination in acute liver failure in children in north India. J Med Virol. 1996;48:215–21.
12. Whittington PF. Fulminant hepatic failure in children. In: Suchy FJ, editor. Liver disease in children. Philadelphia, PA: Lippincott Williams & Wilkins; 2001. p. 63–88.
13. Flynn DM, Mohan N, McKiernan P, Beath S, Buckels J, Mayer D, Kelly DA. Progress in treatment and outcome for children with neonatal haemochromatosis. Arch Dis Child Fetal Neonatol Ed. 2003;88:F124–7.
14. Ekong Udeme D, Kelly S, Whitington PF. Disparate clinical presentation of neonatal hemochromatosis in twins. Pediatrics. 2005;116:880–4.
15. Whitington PF, Hibbard JU. High-dose immunoglobulin during pregnancy for recurrent neonatal haemochromatosis. Lancet. 2004;364:1690–8.
16. Wang ZJ, Berry GT, Dreha SF, Segal S, Zimmerman RA. In vivo proton brain MRS of galactosemia. Ann Neurol. 2001;50:266–9.
17. Bijarnia S, Puri RD, Ruel J, Gray GF, Jenkinson L, Verma IC. Tyrosinemia Type I—diagnostic issues and prenatal diagnosis. Indian J Pediatr. 2006;73:63–165.
18. Mews C, Sinatra F. Chronic liver disease in children. Pediatr Rev. 1993;14:436–43.
19. Mieli-Vergani G, Vergani D. Autoimmune hepatitis in children: what is different from adult AIH? Semin Liver Dis. 2009;29:297–306.
20. Butterworth RF. Pathophysiology of hepatic encephalopathy: a new look at ammonia. Metab Brain Dis. 2002;17:221–7.
21. Rao KV, Norenberg MD. Cerebral energy metabolism in hepatic encephalopathy and hyperammonemia. Metab Brain Dis. 2001;16:67–78.

22. Normandin L, Hazell AS. Manganese neurotoxicity: an update of pathophysiologic mechanisms. Metab Brain Dis. 2002;17:375–87.
23. Hazell AS. Astrocytes and manganese neurotoxicity. Neurochem Int. 2002;41:271–7.
24. Rose C, Butterworth RF, Zayed J, Todd K, Michalak A, Spahr L, Huet PM, Pomier-Layrargues G. Manganese deposition in basal ganglia structures results from both portal-systemic shunting and liver dysfunction. Gastroenterology. 1999;117:640–4.
25. Bicknese AR, May W, Hickey WF, Dodson WE. Early childhood hepatocerebral degeneration misdiagnosed as valproate hepatotoxicity. Ann Neurol. 1992;32:767–75.
26. Genovese E, Maghnie M, Maggiore G, Tinelli C, Lizzoli F, De Giacomo C, Pozza S, Campani R. MR Imaging of CNS involvement in children affected by chronic liver disease. AJNR Am J Neuroradiol. 2000;21:845–51.
27. Zuccoli G, Siddiqui N, Cravo I, Bailey A, Gallucci M, Harper C. Neuroimaging findings in alcoholic encephalopathies. AJR Am J Roentenol. 2010;195:1378–84.
28. Bindu PS, Sinha S, Taly AB, Christopher R, Kovoor JME. Cranial MRI in acute hyperammonemic encephalopathy. Pediatr Neurol. 2009;41:139–42.
29. McKinney AM, Lohman BD, Sarikaya B, Uhlmann E, Spanbauer J, Singewald T, Brace JR. Acute hepatic encephalopathy: diffusion-weighted and fluid-attenuated inversion recovery findings, and correlation with plasma ammonia level and clinical outcome. Am J Neuroradiol. 2010;31:1471–9.
30. Sugimoto R, Iwasa M, Maeda M, Urawa N, Tanaka H, Fujita N, Kobayashi Y, Takeda K, Kaito M, Takei Y. Value of the apparent diffusion coefficient for quantification of low-grade hepatic encephalopathy. Am J Gastroenterol. 2008;103:1413–20.
31. Kumar R, Gupta RK, Elderkin-Thompson V, Huda A, Sayre J, Kirsch C, Guze B, Han S, Thomas MA. Voxel-based diffusion tensor magnetic resonance imaging evaluation of low-grade hepatic encephalopathy. J Magn Reson Imaging. 2008;27(5):1061–8.
32. Goel A, Yadav S, Saraswat V, Srivastava A, Thomas MA, Pandey CM, Rathore R, Gupta R. Cerebral oedema in minimal hepaticencephalopathy due to extrahepatic portalvenous obstruction. Liver Int. 2010;30(8):1143–51.
33. Rai V, Nath K, Saraswat VA, Purwar A, Rathore RK, Gupta RK. Measurement of cytotoxic and interstitial components of cerebral edema in acute hepatic failure by diffusion tensor imaging. J Magn Reson Imaging. 2008;28:334–41.
34. Mardini H, Smith FE, Record CO, Blamire AM. Magnetic resonance quantification of water and metabolites in the brain of cirrhotics following induced hyperammonaemia. J Hepatol. 2011;54(6):1154–60.
35. Rovira A, Córdoba J, Raguer N, Alonso J. Magnetic resonance imaging measurement of brain edema in patients with liver disease: resolution after transplantation. Curr Opin Neurol. 2002; 15:731–7.
36. Atlas SW (2009) Magnetic resonance spectroscopy and the biochemical basis of neurologic disease. In Eva MR, Gilberto González R (Eds.) Magnetic resonance imaging of the brain and spine, 4th Edn (1844–1845). Philadelphia: Lippincott Williams & Wilkins; 2009
37. Foerster BR, Conklin LS, Petrou M, Barker PB, Schwarz KB. Minimal hepatic encephalopathy in children: evaluation with proton MR spectroscopy. AJNR Am J Neuroradiol. 2009;30:1610–13.
38. Sijens P, Alkefaji H, Lunsing R, Spronsen F, Meiners L, Oudkerk M, Verkade M. Quantitative multivoxel ^{1}H MR spectroscopy of the brain in children with acute liver failure. Eur Radiol. 2008;18:2601–9.
39. Verma A, Saraswat VA, Radha Krishna Y, Nath K, Thomas MA, Gupta RK. In vivo 1H magnetic resonance spectroscopy-derived metabolite variations between acute-on-chronic liver failure and acute liver failure. Liver Int. 2008;28(8):1095–103.
40. Saksena S, Rai V, Saraswat VA, Rathore RS, Purwar A, Kumar M, Thomas MA, Gupta RK. Cerebral diffusion tensor imaging and in vivo proton magnetic resonance spectroscopy in patients with fulminant hepatic failure. J Gastroenterol Hepatol. 2008;23: e111–9.
41. Cordoba J, Olive G, Alonso J, Rovira A, Segarra A, Perez M, Jacas C, Vargas V. Improvement of magnetic resonance spectroscopic abnormalities but not pallidal hyperintensity followed amelioration of hepatic encephalopathy after occlusion of a large spleno-renal shunt. J Hepatol. 2001;34:176–8.
42. Naegele T, Grodd W, Viebahn R, Seeger U, Klose U, Seitz D, Kaiser S, Mader I, et al. MR imaging and (1)H spectroscopy of brain metabolites in hepatic encephalopathy: time-course of renormalization after liver transplantation. Radiology. 2000;216:683–91.
43. Cordoba J, Alonso J, Rovira A, Jacas C, Sanpedro F, Castells L, et al. The development of low-grade cerebral edema in cirrhosis is supported by the evolution of (1)H- magnetic resonance abnormalities after liver transplantation. J Hepatol. 2001;35:598–604.

Magnetic Resonance Spectroscopy in Epilepsy

15

Elka Miller and Elysa Widjaja

Magnetic Resonance Spectroscopy (MRS) enables us to assess the metabolic changes in the brain of patients with epilepsy. Therefore it can provide complementary information to structural imaging. Structural MRI plays an important role in identifying the underlying epileptogenic substrate responsible for epilepsy. MRS identifies metabolic changes in the epileptogenic brain, which could be used to lateralize seizure focus, detect bilateral brain abnormalities such as bilateral temporal lobe epilepsy, identify the metabolic abnormalities in the epileptic brain, assess metabolic abnormalities in the epileptogenic zone that appears normal on structural MRI, predict surgical outcome, and improve our understanding of the pathophysiology of epileptogenic substrate.

The neuronal marker *N*-acetylaspartate (NAA) has been shown to be reduced in epilepsy [1] (Fig. 15.1), and this could be related to neuronal metabolite dysfunction or neuronal loss. Experimental and clinical studies have suggested that reduced NAA values can return to normal baseline levels if the patients became seizure free [2, 3]. This reduction could be explained by the fact that NAA reflects the function of neuronal mitochondria, which may be altered in the epileptic brain [4]. In animal studies, NAA/Cr ratios have been shown to increase during the ictal phase, return to pretreatment levels 5 h after the ictal event, and then decrease to subnormal levels 24 h postictally [2]. This reduction in NAA level was related to neuronal loss, which was confirmed by histopathology [2, 5, 6]. Seizures may result in an abnormal elevation of lactate peak secondary to anaerobic metabolism from hypoxia or increased metabolic demand that exceeds tissue perfusion. Animal models of epilepsy have demonstrated ictal and persistent postictal lactate peak after kainic acid injection is reliant on the expression of seizure-induced damage rather than non-damaging electroclinical seizures [7]. Therefore, lactate can be used as a marker for seizure-induced neuronal damage. Glutamate is the principal excitatory neurotransmitter in the mammalian brain and γ-amino butyric acid (GABA) is the major inhibitor neurotransmitter in the human brain. Disorders with GABA and glutamate are closely linked with seizure disorders [8, 9]. Elevated in vitro glutamate concentrations have been identified in epileptic tissue [10, 11]. Ictal studies in adults have shown increased glutamine/glutamate concentrations ipsilateral to the epileptogenic focus [12]. Interictally, both increase [8] and decrease [12] of glutamine/glutamate have been reported.

Two different types of MR spectroscopic acquisition can be performed, a localized single-voxel spectroscopy or chemical shift imaging (CSI), also termed MR spectroscopic imaging (MRSI) or spectroscopic imaging. Single-voxel MRS measures the MR signal of a single selected region of interest whereas signal outside this area is suppressed. On the other hand, in 2-D or 3-D CSI multiple spatially arrayed spectra (typically more than 100 spectra per slice) from slices or volumes are acquired simultaneously, which is helpful to obtain information from different parts of the brain and allows retrospective assessment of regions of interest. Advantages of a single voxel spectroscopy include shorter acquisitions (about 5 min), more explicit spatial localization, more homogeneous shimming, and better water suppression. Single voxel spectroscopy is easy to interpret, can provide higher quality spectra, and avoid the need for time-consuming post-processing. However, only one spectrum can be obtained from one data acquisition of single voxel spectroscopy. On the other hand, CSI has the advantage of obtaining multiple spectra simultaneously during one measurement. However, with CSI the acquisition time can be longer, 10–15 min depending on the area of acquisition, and the data processing is more complex and time consuming. The longer

E. Miller, M.D. (✉)
Department of Diagnostic Imaging, Children's Hospital of Eastern Ontario, Ottawa, ON, Canada
e-mail: emiller@cheo.on.ca

E. Widjaja, M.B.B.S., M.R.C.P., F.R.C.R., M.D.
Department of Diagnostic Imaging, Hospital for Sick Children, University of Toronto, Toronto, ON, Canada

S. Blüml and A. Panigrahy (eds.), *MR Spectroscopy of Pediatric Brain Disorders*,
DOI 10.1007/978-1-4419-5864-8_15, © Springer Science+Business Media, LLC 2013

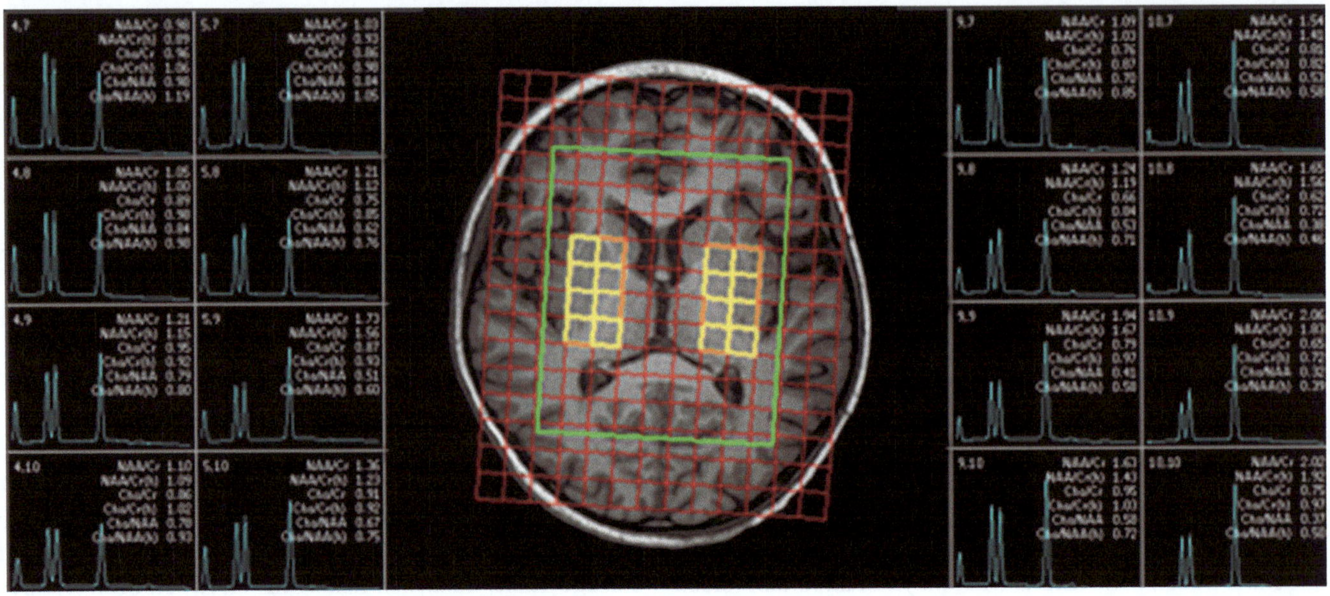

Fig. 15.1 Eight-year old with status epilepticus with no underlying etiology identified. Multivoxel spectroscopy at the level of the basal ganglia demonstrates reduced *N*-acetyl aspartate relative to creatine bilaterally

scan times are of a greater disadvantage in children, especially in the non-sedated children undergoing MRI. With rapid improvement of MR techniques and data processing, the use of CSI technique in seizure evaluation in children will undoubtedly increase. In pediatric epilepsy, it is easier to obtain single voxel spectroscopy in cases where a lesion is visible on structural imaging or in dedicated studies of the hippocampus. However, in *non-lesional* epilepsy, CSI acquisition needs to be considered as it has the advantage of comparing spectra from multiple brain regions simultaneously as CSI covers a larger brain area.

In this chapter, we will describe the MRS patterns of different epileptic syndromes, as defined using the International League Against Epilepsy (ILAE) classification of epileptic syndromes [6], and also the MRI and MRS pattern of specific epileptogenic substrates encountered in children with partial epilepsy.

MR Spectroscopy in Epilepsy Syndromes

Neonate

Early Myoclonic Encephalopathy

Early myoclonic encephalopathy is an epileptic syndrome of early onset, either in the neonatal period or first months of life, and is characterized by erratic, fragmentary, or massive myoclonus, partial seizures, and late tonic spasms. The prognosis is poor and multiple etiologies have been related to the syndrome. Inborn errors of metabolism are one of the most common causes, including nonketotic hyperglycinemia, and amino-acid and organic acidopathies such as propionic aciduria and D-glyceric acidemia can be of concern. EEG consistently reveals a suppression–burst pattern [13]. MR imaging including MRS shows changes related to the underlying etiology. For instance, in nonketotic hyperglycinemia, abnormalities of corpus callosum, delayed myelination, and volume loss can be seen; MRS detects glycine peak on the intermediate or long TE sequence (Fig. 15.2). With disease progression, cortical and periventricular atrophy develops in many cases.

Ohtahara Syndrome

Ohtahara syndrome or early infantile epileptic encephalopathy with burst–suppression (EIEE) is a rare progressive epileptic encephalopathy. The syndrome is characterized by tonic spasms and partial seizures with onset in the neonatal and early infantile period. The more elaborate name comes from the pattern of burst activity on EEG. It is an extremely debilitating progressive neurological disorder, involving intractable seizures and severe mental retardation. No single cause has been identified, although in many cases structural brain damage is present. The etiology of OS has been related to many different structural brain malformations such as hemimegalencephaly, porencephaly, Aicardi syndrome, destructive encephalopathy following hypoxic ischemic encephalopathy, and migrational disorders. Occasionally, MRI reveals no structure abnormality but the syndrome might be related to a metabolic disorder. Seo et al [14]. reported a case of a 36-week female with OS and NADH dehydrogenase deficiency; the first brain MRI at 3 months of age showed no structural abnormality, but

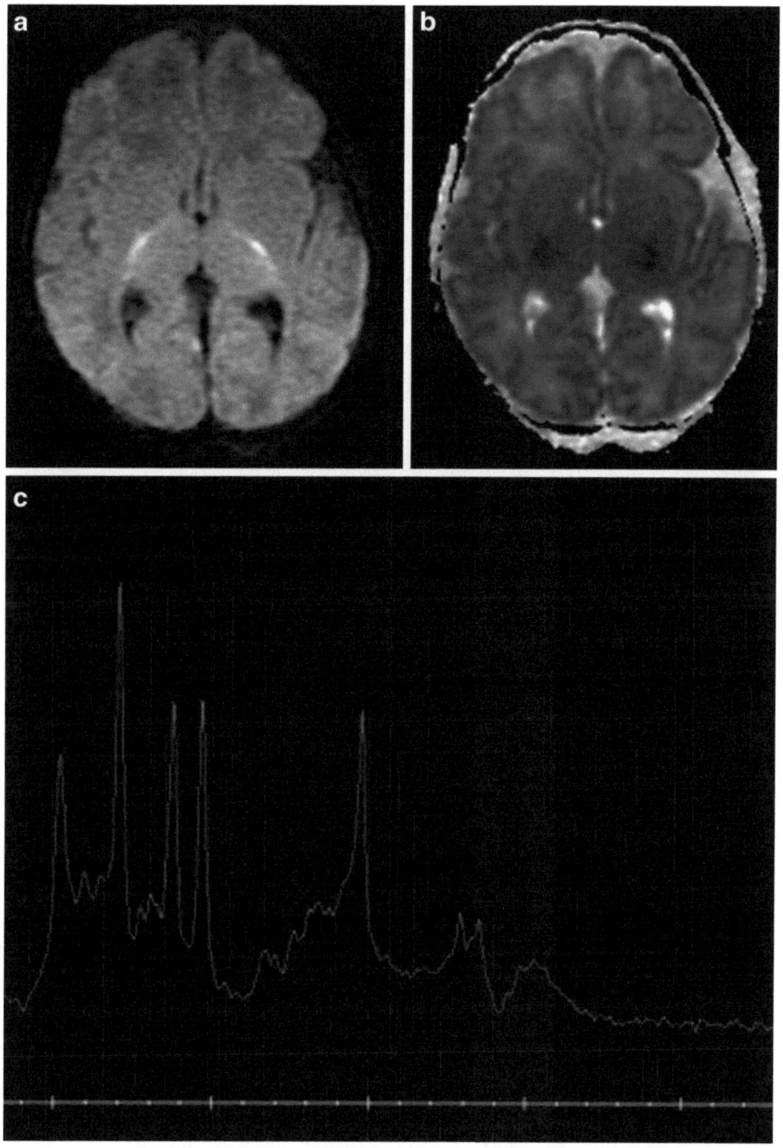

Fig. 15.2 Neonate presenting with seizures. Axial (**a**) diffusion and (**b**) ADC map show diffusion restriction in the posterior limb of internal capsules. (**b**) Single voxel MR spectroscopy with TE = 144 ms shows the presence of glycine at 3.5 ppm, in keeping with nonketotic hyperglycinemia

the MRS demonstrated a large peak of lactate in the right basal ganglia and right frontal white matter. The lactate peak may provide a clue of an underlying metabolic disorder, such as mitochondrial disorder. Interestingly enough, lactate peak tends to resolve following treatment and/or partial or complete resolution of the seizures.

Infancy

West Syndrome

West syndrome is defined by a triad of spasms in clusters, mental retardation, and diffuse and profound paroxysmal EEG abnormalities called hypsarrhythmias. This is an age-dependent epilepsy syndrome that usually begins in infancy between 4 and 6 months and before 12 months in over 90% of the cases [15], but can occur later up to 4 years of age. West syndrome can be caused by various brain disorders. MRI is helpful for detecting underlying conditions such as focal cortical dysplasia, tumor, hypoxic ischemic injury, post-infection, metabolic, and other unknown causes. The role of MRS is related to the diagnosis of the underlying condition responsible for West syndrome.

West syndrome is resistant to many conventional antiepileptic drugs, and only valproic acid, benzodiazepines, adrenocorticotropic hormone (ACTH), corticosteroids, and vigabatrin have been found efficacious. ACTH is the treatment of choice for infantile spasms, but frequent and sometimes serious side effects such as infections and hypertension have occurred during ACTH therapy. Imaging of the brain during treatment usually demonstrate atrophy that could be related to a variety of causes, including the catabolic effect of

ACTH, mineralocorticoid effect resulting in loss of water and/or an increase in cerebrospinal fluid (CSF) pressure compressing the brain. MRS in these cases can demonstrate a decrease in NAA, which could be related to a reduction in NAA synthesis in mitochondria and leakage of NAA from cell membrane [16]. The changes in NAA may be related to the underlying infantile spasm or to the effect of treatment. Maeda et al. [16] have obtained MRS from the left centrum semiovale of patients with infantile spasm before ACTH treatment, immediately at the initiation of ACTH treatment and several months after treatment [16]. They demonstrated a significant decrease in NAA concentration immediately after initiation of treatment, which suggested that the changes were more likely related to ACTH treatment. These changes also appear to be reversible as there was some improvement of the NAA concentrations following cessation of ACTH treatment. Therefore, alterations in NAA could be secondary to ACTH-related brain volume loss.

Epilepsy of Infancy with Migrating Focal Seizures

Malignant migrating partial seizure in infancy (MMPSI) is an epileptic encephalopathy characterized by seizure onset in the first 6 months of life, and of rapidly progressive partial seizures that become continuous [17]. The EEG discharges are random and involve multiple independent sites and seizures migrate from one area of the cortex to another. The seizures last several minutes longer than the usual partial seizures in infancy. It is associated with major deterioration in psychomotor abilities. Microcephaly is a common feature. With time, the seizures tend to be more frequently generalized and myoclonus is rare. By the end of the first year of life, seizures become almost continuous and occur in clusters with clinical deterioration. The etiology of these seizures is unknown. MRI is frequently negative [18], but hippocampal gliosis and atrophy resembling hippocampal sclerosis can be found [19]. MRS has been reported in one subject and revealed reduction of NAA in the basal ganglia and frontal cortex [20]. However, this patient also had cortical and subcortical atrophy. The decrease in NAA could be secondary to the loss of neuron related to atrophy and not necessarily attributed to excessive excitatory neurotransmitter activity.

Dravet Syndrome

Dravet syndrome or severe myoclonic epilepsy in infancy (SMEI) is a malignant epilepsy syndrome characterized by early prolonged febrile and afebrile seizures followed by intractable seizures of different types and secondary psychomotor delay [21, 22]. Abnormal neurologic signs include ataxia and pyramidal tract damage. EEGs are usually normal in the early course of the disease; however, generalized interictal epileptiform discharges appear in the second year of life. The main clinical distinction is with febrile convulsion but febrile convulsion usually occurs later between 18 and 22 months.

In some studies, there were no MRI abnormalities related to SMEI [21, 23], but in other studies, brain abnormalities including focal cortical dysplasia and mesial temporal sclerosis were reported in infants with SMEI [24, 25]. Mesial temporal sclerosis has been reported several months or years after the initial presentation of SMEI. There is no study reporting the MRS features of SMEI. The MRS features related to the underlying brain abnormalities such as focal cortical dysplasia or mesial temporal sclerosis will be discussed later.

Myoclonic Encephalopathy

Myoclonic encephalophaty is a syndrome characterized by severe recurrent seizures, principally massive myoclonic jerks at the onset of the disorder and a striking burst–suppression pattern on EEG. It begins in the neonatal and early infantile periods. Seizures in this syndrome are difficult to treat, and the patients are rarely seizure free. Nonketotic hyperglycinemia is one of the most common causes of early myoclonic encephalopathy. The MRI features of this metabolic abnormality include hypomyelination, hypoplastic corpus callosum, and myelin vacuolation resulting in diffusion restriction within the pyramidal tracts, middle cerebellar peduncles, and dentate nuclei. Proton MRS can identify elevated glycine. At short echo time (e.g., TE = 30 ms), the spectral peak generated by glycine may overlap with myo-Inositol (MI) signal, as both glycine and MI resonate approximately at 3.56 ppm. However, MI has much shorter T_2 relaxation time than glycine, and hence its signal significantly reduces at longer echo times (such as TE = 144 ms). In patients with nonketotic hyperglycinemia, an abnormal peak at 3.56 ppm (glycine) remains conspicuous at longer echo times (Fig. 15.2). MRS findings should be confirmed with plasma or CSF glycine levels.

Childhood

Febrile Seizures

Febrile seizures (FS) occur in 2–5% of children. FS are classified as simple or complex. The "simple FS" are generalized tonic–clonic seizures that last for less than 15 min without recurrence within the next 24 hours while "complex FS" are focal, prolonged for more than 15 min, or occurring in a cluster of two or more convulsions within 24 hours. These seizures are known to be benign but 2–3% of children will later develop epilepsy, most likely of temporal lobe origin [26].

Studies in adult patients with antecedent prolonged febrile convulsions in early childhood had demonstrated volume loss of the hippocampus and amygdala [27, 28]. Nevertheless, it is still not clear whether complex febrile seizures are an epiphenomenon or a causative factor. MRI studies in familial mesial temporal lobe epilepsy (MTLE) have suggested that a genetically determined mechanism might play an important role in the hippocampal damage [29, 30].

Children with TLE and history of FS in early childhood are inclined to have lower NAA/ (Cr _Cho) ratios ipsilateral to seizure focus, indicating an element of neuronal loss. Decreased NAA/Cr ratio can also be observed in the contralateral side in children with FS, but to a lesser extent than the affected side [31]. The reason for these metabolites changes contralateral to seizure focus is not well understood. MRS is able to demonstrate alterations in the hippocampus in children with FS [32]. These changes are, however, nonspecific and do not determine the seizure type, as similar changes can be seen in non-complex febrile seizures [31].

Epilepsy with Myoclonic Atonic (Previously Astatic) Seizures

Myoclonic–astatic epilepsy is a syndrome that begins between 2 and 5 years of age. It begins with generalized tonic–clonic seizures with generalized spike waves in a previously normal child. Most patients recover within 1 to 3 years, but others develop myoclonic status and major cognitive decline. No etiology or gene has been identified. Parker et al. [33] reported one case of a 5-year-old male with myoclonic astatic epilepsy. The FDG/PET study demonstrated hypometabolism in the left temporo-parietal lobe, but interestingly the MRS spectra acquired from the region of hypometabolism demonstrated elevated NAA/Cho ratios (2.13 in the left and 1.61 in the contralateral side). The reason for the elevated NAA/Cho ratio is not known.

Benign Childhood Epilepsy with Centrotemporal Spikes (Rolandic Epilepsy)

Benign childhood epilepsy (BCE) or Rolandic epilepsy is considered the most common epilepsy syndromes in childhood. In studies conducted in North America and Europe, the incidence ranges from 5 to 15% of childhood epilepsy syndromes. The onset is usually between 2 and 13 years of age in children without neurological or intellectual deficits. Patients usually are seizure free before age 16. Benign Rolandic epilepsy are characterized by brief, usually simple partial, hemifacial motor seizures, often preceded or accompanied by somatosensory symptoms, with a tendency to evolve into generalized tonic–clonic seizures. The EEG reflects characteristic features with discharges in the precentral and postcentral gyri in the suprasylvian region, with motor, sensory, and autonomic manifestations in the face, mouth, and throat. In recent years, there has been some evidence that BCE is less than benign for certain patients, who have demonstrated cognitive and/or motor difficulties [34]. Some of these patients may have focal cortical dysplasia responsible for the Rolandic epilepsy.

Single voxel MRS of 13 children with BCE [35] demonstrated a significantly higher asymmetry of the NAA/Cr ratios in the hippocampal region when compared with controls. Lateralization of the EEG discharge interictally corresponded with the lower NAA/Cr ratios in the hippocampal region. The lower NAA/Cr could be interpreted as an indicator of neuronal dysfunction. The abnormal metabolites in the hippocampal region may be related to spreading of seizure focus from the Rolandic to the hippocampal region via white matter pathways [36].

Lennox-Gastaut Syndrome

Lennox-Gastaut syndrome (LGS) is one of the most intractable catastrophic epilepsies in children. It is characterized by a combination of multiple seizures types including tonic and atonic seizures, atypical absences, myoclonic seizures, and spasm, as well as generalized slow spike waves and/or generalized paroxysmal fast activity on EEG and progressive cognitive impairment. The majority of patients with LGS have bilateral diffuse encephalopathy and normal MRI. However, a variety of multifocal or diffuse abnormalities can be found on MRI in the symptomatic cases, including microdysgenesis, pachygyria, neuronal necrosis, and hypoxic lesion in the neocortex. Consequently, the role of MRI is to clarify the etiology rather than establish the diagnosis of epilepsy syndrome. Lee et al. [37] evaluated 27 children and adolescents who had LGS and found cerebral lesions in 23 patients, with the most common pathology being malformations of cortical development (20/23). Reduction of NAA/Cho or NAA/Cr has been found in the region of focal cortical dysplasia in three patients. The NAA/Cho or NAA/Cr ratios were not lateralized in four patients, including two patients without abnormalities on MRI.

Childhood Absence Epilepsy

Absences are generalized non-convulsive seizures. The ILAE proposed the classification of three syndromes of idiopathic generalized epilepsy (IGE) with absence seizures: childhood absence epilepsy, juvenile absence epilepsy, and juvenile myoclonic epilepsy [38]. Typical absence seizures present with bilateral synchronous, symmetric 3 Hz generalized spike, and slow wave discharge on EEG [39].

Childhood absence epilepsy is a relatively common epilepsy syndrome presenting in school age children. The main mechanism of this type of seizures, as well as juvenile absence epilepsy and juvenile myoclonic epilepsy, is unknown. Two main hypotheses have been proposed to explain the pathogenesis of absence seizures in animal models (1) excessive thalamic oscillation due to hypersynchronization and/or (2) cortical hyperexcitability, which may amplify physiological rhythmic oscillations originating in the thalamus. Such dysfunctions may result from alterations affecting: (1) synaptic communications within the thalamo-cortical network; (2) intrinsic properties in cortical and/or thalamic neurons; or (3) morphological abnormalities within the thalamo-cortical circuit [40–42]. MR spectroscopy in patients with absence epilepsy has demonstrated reduced NAA/Cr ratio in both thalami [43, 44], indicating the presence of neuronal dysfunction in the thalami of patients with absence epilepsy. Neither the cortex nor the thalamus alone can sustain these discharges, suggesting that both structures are involved in the generation of discharges. By co-registering MRI to subtraction ictal–interictal single photon emission computed tomography (SPECT), Nehling et al. [45] found diffuse nonspecific decreased blood flow during the ictal phase and generalized increased blood flow during the postictal phase in typical childhood absence seizures. These data suggest that seizures are not limited to the thalamo-cortical circuit in which absence seizures originate. However, which particular structure initiates the seizure onset remains uncertain.

Adolescence

Juvenile Absence Epilepsy

Juvenile absence epilepsy (JAE) is the only syndrome in which the ictal manifestations of absence seizures show clinical and EEG similarities to those of childhood absence epilepsy. However, in JAE the frequency of the absences is low and the symptoms are milder. Furthermore, the diagnosis can be disregarded until generalized tonic–clonic seizures appear. Age at seizure onset is usually between 10 and 17 years, with a peak between 10 and 12 years. Severe impairment of consciousness is the essential feature of the absence seizure in JAE but a crucial characteristic is that neurologic examination and neuroimaging results are normal.

Although the mechanism is unknown, the occurrence of abnormalities in corticothalamic network has been shown to be the functional basis of absence seizure generation [41]. Using EEG-correlated functional MRI, Salek-Haddadi et al. [46] found marked bilateral thalamic activation and cortical deactivation during prolonged absences, suggestive of a reduction in cortical blood flow in a patient with intractable juvenile absence epilepsy. Reduced NAA levels and NAA/Cr ratios in both thalami have been reported in the early stage of JAE [44]. This has been attributed to neuronal dysfunction and/or subtle changes in neuronal density.

Juvenile Myoclonic Epilepsy

Juvenile myoclonic epilepsy (JME) is a common hereditary epileptic syndrome that comprises 5–11% of patients with epilepsy [47]. The onset of JME occurs from 6 to 22 years of age. It is characterized by myoclonic jerks, generalized tonic–clonic seizures, and absence seizures. JME is non-progressive, and there are no abnormalities on clinical examination and no intellectual deficits. Psychiatric disorders may coexist. Generalized polyspike-and-waves are the most characteristic EEG pattern. Dense array EEG demonstrated epileptiform discharges that localized to sources that included orbitofrontal/medial frontopolar cortex, and also frequently included basal medial temporal lobe structures as the dominant contributors to the discharges [48]. The exact mechanism of the generalized seizures remains unclear but the pathophysiology of JME and other epilepsies has been linked to the thalamic and cortico-thalamic tracts generating spike and wave discharges and creating an abnormal thalamocortical circuitry, respectively. MRS studies of those with JME demonstrated low NAA/Cr values and low absolute NAA levels in the thalamus [49, 50]. The decreased NAA/Cr ratio supports the hypothesis of thalamic dysfunction as part of the underlying mechanism in this generalized epilepsy. Decrease in NAA/Cr and glutamate–glutamine/Cr ratios in primary motor cortex and medial prefrontal cortex showed the strongest correlation between thalamus and cortex [51].

Progressive Myoclonus Epilepsy

Lafora disease (LD) is a progressive myoclonus epilepsy syndrome, inherited as an autosomal recessive trait, with onset in late childhood or adolescence. This disorder is characterized by sporadic myoclonus, occipital lobe seizures and/or generalized seizures, behavioral changes, and cognitive decline. Prognosis is poor, with death occurring less than a decade from diagnosis. Pathological studies demonstrate Lafora bodies or acid Schiff positive cytoplasmic inclusions. Lafora bodies are predominantly located in neurons but can be found in other organs such as the liver, skin, mucosa, muscle, and myocardium. Diagnosis is made with biopsy and demonstration of EPM2A gene in 6q23–25 mutation, which occurs in 70–80% of the cases, or EPM2B gene in 6P22.3 mutation [52].

Proton MRS has been performed in ten patients with LD, demonstrating a reduction in NAA/Cr ratio in the cortex, especially frontal cortex, basal ganglia, and cerebellum [53]. Another study correlated MRS metabolic changes in the gray and white matter with cognitive impairment in five patients with LD and found significant reduction in NAA/MI and NAA/Cr in the gray matter and white matter of patients compared to controls, more significant in the frontal regions [54]. They have also found that NAA/MI was the most statistically significant altered parameter in the frontal lobe and the only significant altered ratio that demonstrated strong correlation with intellectual and executive impairments.

Distinctive Constellations of Epilepsy

Mesial Temporal Lobe Epilepsy

Mesial temporal lobe epilepsy (TLE) is less frequently encountered in children compared to adults. In MRI studies of pediatric patients with TLE, hippocampal sclerosis (HS) was noted in 21% of patients 15 years of age or younger with new-onset TLE [55] and 57% of patients 2–17 years of age with refractory temporal lobe epilepsy [56–58]. The etiology of hippocampal sclerosis is unknown, but a link with febrile seizures has been suggested [27]. MRI enables detection of structural abnormalities, most commonly signal abnormalities and atrophy of the hippocampus and amygdala. However, a proportion of patients remain with intractable TLE in whom no MRI changes can be detected. In mesial TLE, MRS can be helpful in lateralizing the seizure focus, detecting bilateral abnormalities, and identifying metabolic abnormalities in the epileptogenic brain. The abnormalities typically consist of a decrease in NAA/Cr, NAA/Cho, NAA/[Cr + Cho] in the epileptogenic zone within the temporal lobe [59, 60 61, 62]. Asymmetry in NAA/Cr between right and left sides lateralized 92.5% of TLE patients who had lateralization by ictal EEG [59]. Increased myoinositol (MI) has been reported as a consequence of induction of Na+/MI cotransporter following seizure activity [63]. The reduction in NAA has been correlated with neuronal cell loss and reactive astrogliosis in HS [64, 65]. Changes in NAA are not limited to chronic seizures. Reduced NAA has also been observed in newly diagnosed TLE, implying that neuronal abnormalities can be detected before the typical structural MRI abnormalities develop [66].

Abnormal NAA has been detected both ipsilateral and contralateral to the site of seizure onset and the abnormal NAA reversed in patients who become seizure free after surgery [67, 68]. This suggests that the contralateral NAA abnormalities could represent transient neuronal dysfunction related to spread of seizures. However, bilateral metabolic changes may be associated with poor postoperative seizure outcome [69], particularly when the metabolic dysfunction is worse in the area contralateral to resection. MRS abnormalities have also been identified in the extratemporal lobe in TLE. Reduction in MI has been identified in the frontal lobe of patients with TLE, which may be a temporary effect following recent seizure activity or the cumulative effect of chronic seizures [70]. CSI or multislice proton MRS imaging has demonstrated decreased NAA concentration in the frontal, parietal, and occipital lobes both in the ipsilateral and contralateral hemispheres in TLE [71]. The cause for this extensive NAA abnormality is not well understood, but may be related to widespread epileptogenic process that extends outside the primary epileptogenic zone. The excitotoxic process that leads to a reduction in NAA in the hippocampus can induce NAA reduction in regions involved in the seizure spread. The loss of efferent neurons in the hippocampus may lead to differentiation and alteration in the function of neurons in other brain regions. Another potential cause of the widespread reduction in NAA may be related to treatment effects from antiepileptic drugs.

Extratemporal Lobe Epilepsy

There are fewer studies on MRS in extratemporal lobe epilepsy compared to TLE. The potential for seizure lateralization is lower in patients with extratemporal lobe epilepsy compared with TLE. Seizure lateralization was achieved in approximately 50% of patients with frontal lobe epilepsy [72, 73]. Furthermore, due to widespread NAA reduction in extratemporal lobe epilepsy, MRS abnormalities may not be adequately localized to identify the seizure focus in extratemporal lobe epilepsy [73].

Hemiconvulsion–Hemiplegia–Epilepsy Syndrome

Hemiconvulsion–hemiplegia–epilepsy syndrome (HHE) is an uncommon consequence of prolonged febrile convulsion that occurs in children without antecedents, between 5 months and 4 years old, with a peak incidence during the first 2 years of life. The mechanism underlying the syndrome is unknown. The differential diagnosis of HHE in the acute phase remains a challenge, and requires exclusion of infective, vascular, and metabolic causes. MR imaging demonstrates unilateral edematous swelling of the affected hemispheres in the acute phase, with diffusion restriction secondary to cytotoxic edema [74]. In the chronic stage, global volume loss develops, which is independent of a vascular territory. Freeman et al. [75] reported decrease in NAA peak in the affected hemispheres in comparison to the contralateral side in one of the three patients. Decreased level of NAA in the affected hemisphere is likely related to the diffuse edema and/or neuronal loss.

MRS of Epileptogenic Substrates

Malformations of Cortical Development

Malformations of cortical development (MCD) are congenital anomalies of the cortex that occur as a result of insult occurring during proliferation, migration, and/or organization of neuronal cells. In a series of autopsied brains from patients with epilepsy, 14% had congenital malformations, and of those 46.5% had MCD [76]. These lesions are widely recognized as an important cause of refractory epilepsy and their identification with MRI remains one of the most important factors in determining surgical outcomes. The MRS abnormality most frequently found in MCD is decreased NAA or NAA/Cr ratio in the lesion compared to controls [1], but the findings can be heterogeneous and increase in NAA [77] or no abnormalities [78] has been reported in studies evaluating MCD. A decrease or an increase in Cr/phosphocreatine and an increase in Cho compounds [79] have been reported. In adults, large MCD had abnormal levels of

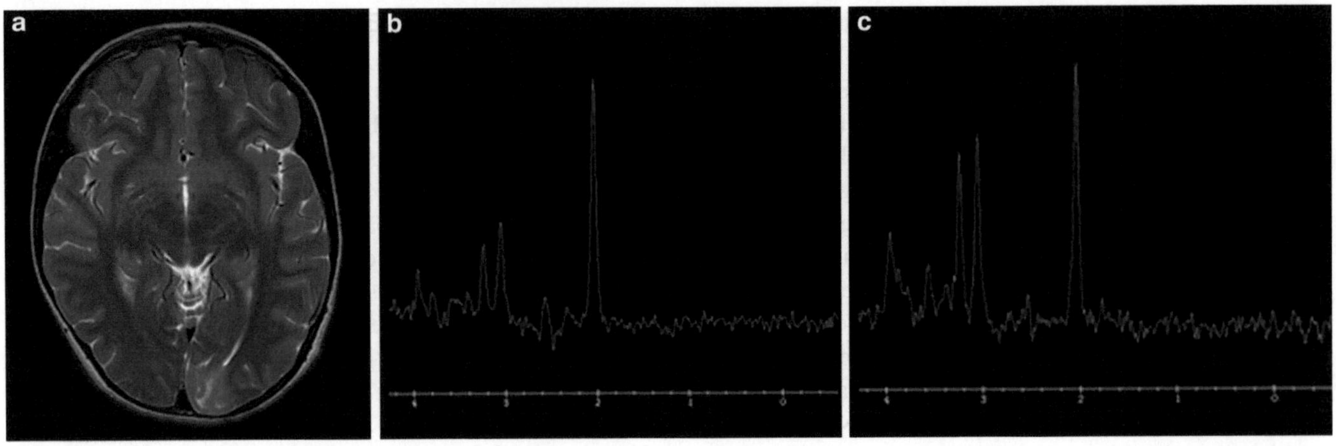

Fig. 15.3 Thirteen-year old with seizures. Axial (**a**) T2 shows increased signal in the left occipital lobe cortex and subcortical white matter, in keeping with focal cortical dysplasia. Single voxel MR spectroscopy acquired from the (**b**) right and (**c**) left occipital lobes relative reduction in NAA in the left occipital lobe compared to the right occipital lobe

glutamine and GABA plus homocarnosine (GABA+)/Cr [80]. Studies in adults with MCD [77, 79] described normal-appearing perilesional zone that demonstrated metabolic abnormalities similar to that in MCD. Therefore, the MRI-visible lesion is likely to be only the "tip of the iceberg" and could explain why surgical resection does not yield good results with respect to epilepsy control in some patients with focal MCD. Abnormal metabolites have been found not only adjacent to MCD, but also contralateral to MCD [81].

Hemimegalencephaly is a malformation due to abnormal neuronal proliferation. In a report of two cases of hemimegaencephaly [82], single voxel MRS demonstrated metabolic disturbances such as marked reduction of glutamate and NAA in the white matter, with less severe or no alterations in cortical gray matter, basal ganglia, and cerebellum. Both these cases also had mildly decreased NAA level in the white matter of the contralateral hemisphere. The spectroscopic findings indicate loss of neuronal tissue and glial cell proliferation, which affect not only the abnormal hemisphere, but also the normal appearing contralateral hemisphere to a lesser extent.

Focal cortical dysplasia (FCD), as initially defined by Taylor and co-workers [83], closely mimics the histopathologic appearance of cortical tubers in tuberous sclerosis but fails to demonstrate the additional pathologic stigmata, family history, or clinical presentation. FCD is one of the most common epileptogenic substrate responsible for intractable epilepsy in children. MRI appearance of FCD includes thickening of the cortex, increased signal on T2- and FLAIR images in the subcortical white matter and cortex, loss of gray/white demarcation, and abnormal sulci. MRS of FCD has shown reduced NAA/Cr within the lesion compared to the contralateral side [84] (Fig. 15.3).

Gray matter heterotopias are collections of neurons and glia in abnormal location secondary to the arrest of neuronal migration. Arrest of neuronal migration can occur at different stages of maturation. Therefore, some neurons might be less mature and improperly connected, while other neurons are more mature. Histology has shown the presence of normal appearing neurons in heterotopia [85]. This variability in neuronal maturation within gray matter heterotopia may account for the variability in NAA metabolite observed on in vivo MRS. Some studies have shown no significant differences of NAA/Cr ratios in areas of gray matter heterotopia compared with normal brain or controls [86, 87]; others have found a reduction in NAA level [88–91]; and in one study, MRS of a large gray matter heterotopia showed increased NAA level [92].

Band heterotopia is a MCD characterized by disruption of neuronal migration, demonstrating extensive bilateral symmetric plates of heterotopic gray matter, usually in the centrum semiovale below the normal cortex. Individuals with this abnormality may present clinically with mental retardation and intractable epilepsy. Band heterotopia may be caused by mutations in the doublecortin gene Xq22.3 or LISI gene on chromosome 17 [93]. On histology, the external cortex appears close to normal with the usual six layers and relatively well differentiated neurons; that may account for the normal NAA/Cr [94] reported in band heterotopia. However, decrease in NAA/Cr ratio has also been demonstrated within band heterotopia [89], which could be related to dysfunctional neurons. Differences in NAA/Cr ratios reported in the literature may be related to slight differences in neuronal maturation or neuronal dysfunction or differences in MRI acquisition techniques.

Polymicrogyria is a malformation due to abnormal late neuronal migration and cortical organization. This abnormality

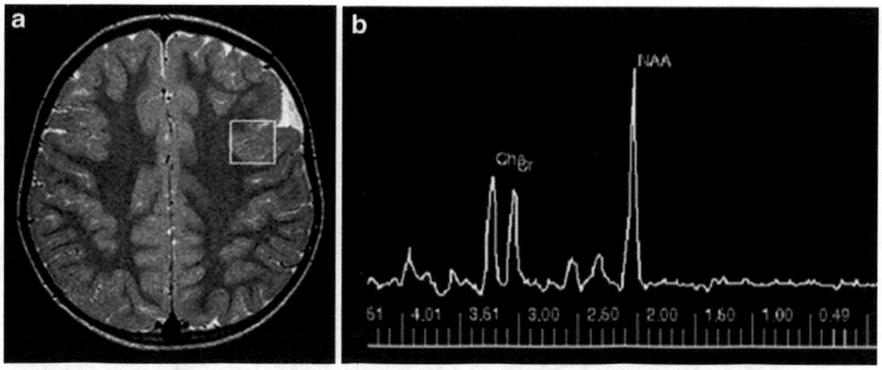

Fig. 15.4 (**a**) Axial T2 demonstrates cortical thickening and irregular gray–white matter junction in the left frontal lobe, features in keeping with polymicrogyria. (**b**) Single voxel MR spectroscopy with TE = 144 ms acquired from the polymicrogyria shows relatively normal *N*-acetyl aspartate (NAA) relative to creatine

appears on MRI as an area of thickened cortex with an undulating gray–white matter interface and often with abnormal adjacent white matter. On histology, polymicrogyria has a common derangement of the typical six-layered lamination of the cortex. The insult leading to the development of polymicrogyria occurs when the neurons are more mature and have normal cellular structure. Variable MRS abnormalities have been demonstrated in the literature. Widjaja et al. [86] studied 22 children (mean age 16 years) with polymicrogyria and showed no significant reduction in NAA/Cr ratio in polymicrogyria compared with the normal brain (Fig. 15.4). Simone et al. [90] applied MRS in five patients with polymicrogyria (mean age 32 years) and reported reduced NAA/Cr and NAA/Cho ratios in areas affected by polymicrogyria. The differences in the results were postulated to be due to differences in age groups, as metabolites levels change with growth, or due to acquisition limitations as MRS were acquired from different regions of the brain and therefore ratios can vary significantly depending on their locations in the brain parenchyma.

Neurocutaneous Syndromes

Tuberous Sclerosis Complex

Tuberous sclerosis complex (TSC) is an autosomal dominant disorder that affects multiple systems including brain, eyes, heart, kidney, skin, and lungs. Two genetic abnormalities have been described related to TSC (TSC 1 on chromosome 9q34 and TSC 2 on chromosome 16pI3). Intracranial manifestations of TSC include cortical tubers, subependymal nodules, and giant cell astrocytomas, and these patients present with epilepsy and mental retardation. Cortical tubers demonstrate a low NAA/Cr (Fig. 15.5), increased Cho/Cr, and a lactate peak. The presence of a lactate peak that correlates with EEG or MEG could add valuable information if surgery is considered [95], but does not identify the epileptogenic tuber. Yapici et al. [95] reported four of the six patients who showed lactate peak had seizures within 2 days of the spectroscopy study, and lactate peak was also detected in four tubers not associated with an epileptogenic focus, as well as in two individuals with good seizure control and no interictal spiking on EEG. Therefore, a lactate peak is not a specific marker of an epileptogenic focus, but may reflect changes related to refractory seizures. Myoinositol/creatine ratio has a propensity to be increased in cortical tubers [95, 96]. An increase in MI level is expected when there is an increase in membrane turnover due to myelin sheath repair. Therefore, MI in cortical tubers suggests the presence of gliosis and demyelination within cortical tubers. MRS of subependymal giant cell astrocytoma has demonstrated a decrease in NAA/Cr and an increase in Cho/Cr compared to the contralateral non-affected side [97].

Sturge-Weber Syndrome

Sturge-Weber syndrome or encephalotrigeminal angiomatosis is characterized by facial port-wine stain, epilepsy, and mental retardation. MRI shows leptomeningeal angiomatosis, enlargement of the choroid plexus, parenchymal atrophy, calvarial changes, and calcifications. MRS could be valuable for early characterization and monitoring of neuronal dysfunction or neuronal loss in infants and children with Sturge-Weber syndrome. NAA peak has been shown to decrease (Fig. 15.6), and choline peak increased on the affected side. Reduced NAA has been attributed to neuronal loss, as a consequence of the leptomeningeal angiomatosis, and associated cerebral volume loss and calcification. Others have postulated that the decrease in NAA is related to neuronal dysfunction secondary to seizures [98, 99].

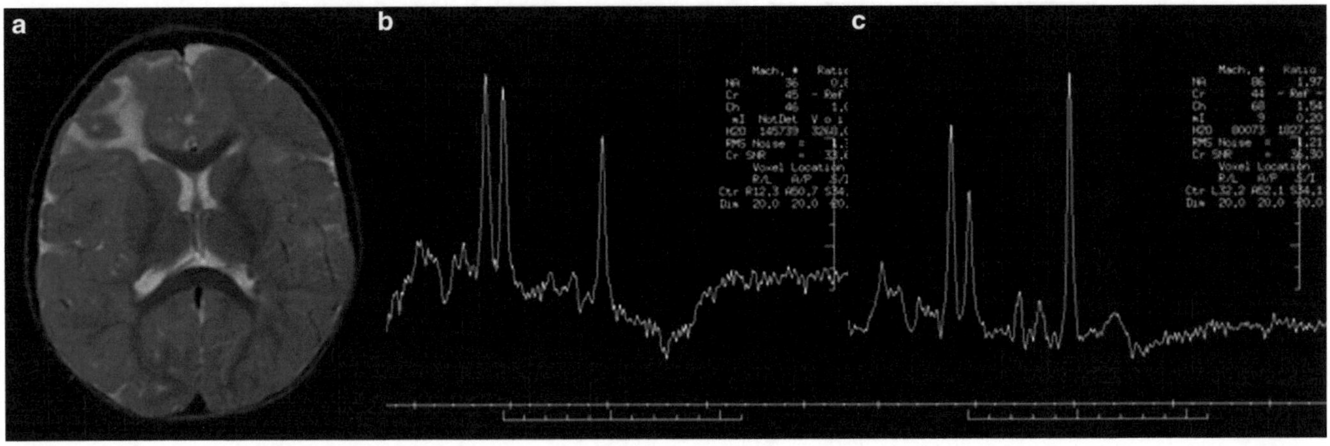

Fig. 15.5 Eighteen-month-old girl with tuberous sclerosis complex. (**a**) Axial T2 demonstrating a right frontal cortical tuber. Single voxel MR spectroscopy from (**b**) the right frontal cortical tuber shows reduced N-acetyl aspartate compared to (**c**) the normal appearing left frontal lobe

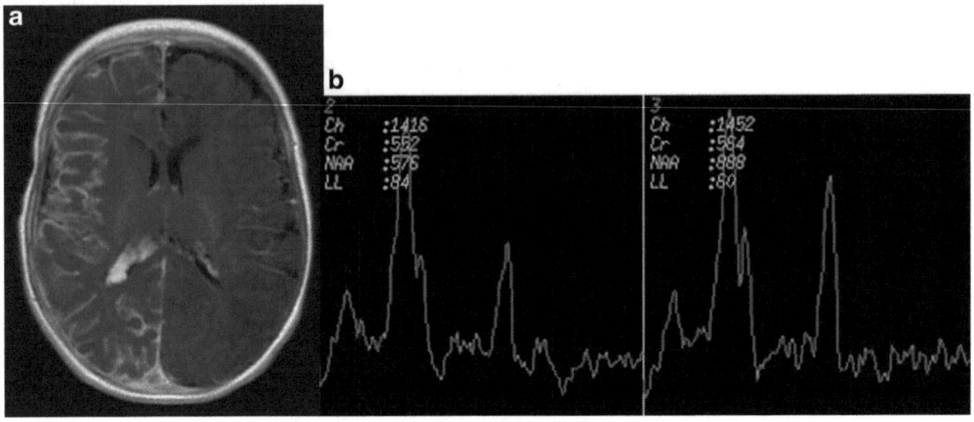

Fig. 15.6 Three-month old with Sturge Weber syndrome. (**a**) Axial T1 post-contrast shows leptomeningeal enhancement in the right hemisphere and enlarged right choroid plexus. (**b**) On chemical shift imaging, there is reduced N-acetyl aspartate in the right frontal lobe compared to the left frontal lobe

Tumor

Epilepsy-associated developmental tumor may account for up to two-thirds of the surgical pathologic substrate [100–103] in epilepsy surgery. These tumors originate in and develop from the cortex and therefore clinically present with seizures. They are slow growing tumor with well-defined margins, without associated edema or necrosis. Complete removal results in good seizure control or render the patients seizure free. The epilepsy-associated tumor includes ganglioglioma and dysembryoplastic neuro-epithelial tumor (DNET).

Ganglioglioma are slightly more common in males and are ten times more common in children than in adults [104]. They are associated with chronic epilepsy in 85% of cases, and are located mostly in the temporo-mesial (50%) or temporo-lateral (29%) location [105]. Ganglioglioma may present as a solid mass in 43%, a cyst in 5%, and a mixed lesion in 52% [106]. They involve the cortex, usually broaden the gyri, and may cause remodeling of the adjacent bone. On CT, ganglioglioma may present as hypo- (38%), iso- (15%), hyper-attenuating (15%), or mixed attenuation mass (32%). Calcification may be seen in about 30–50% of cases. On MR, the tumor may appear hypo- or iso-intense to gray matter on T1WI and hyper-intense on T2WI. Some may demonstrate intrinsic high T1 signal [106]. Enhancement following gadolinium administration is common in up to 60% of cases. It can be nodular, ring-like, or solid. On MRS, ganglioglioma showed reduced Cho/Cr and NAA/Cr and increased Cho/NAA ratio compared to contralateral side [107] (Fig. 15.7). Patients with ganglioglioma had the best outcome compared

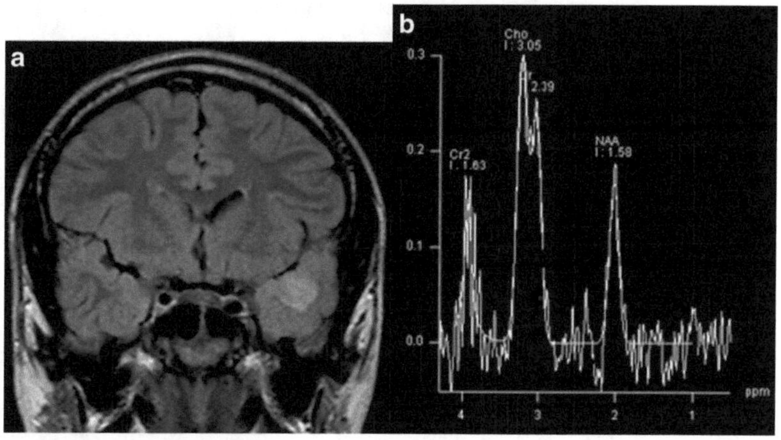

Fig. 15.7 Sixteen-year-old boy with ganglioglioma. (**a**) Coronal FLAIR shows the well-defined tumor in the left anterior temporal lobe. (**b**) Single voxel MR spectroscopy acquired from the tumor shows reduced N-acetyl aspartate relative to creatine and elevated choline

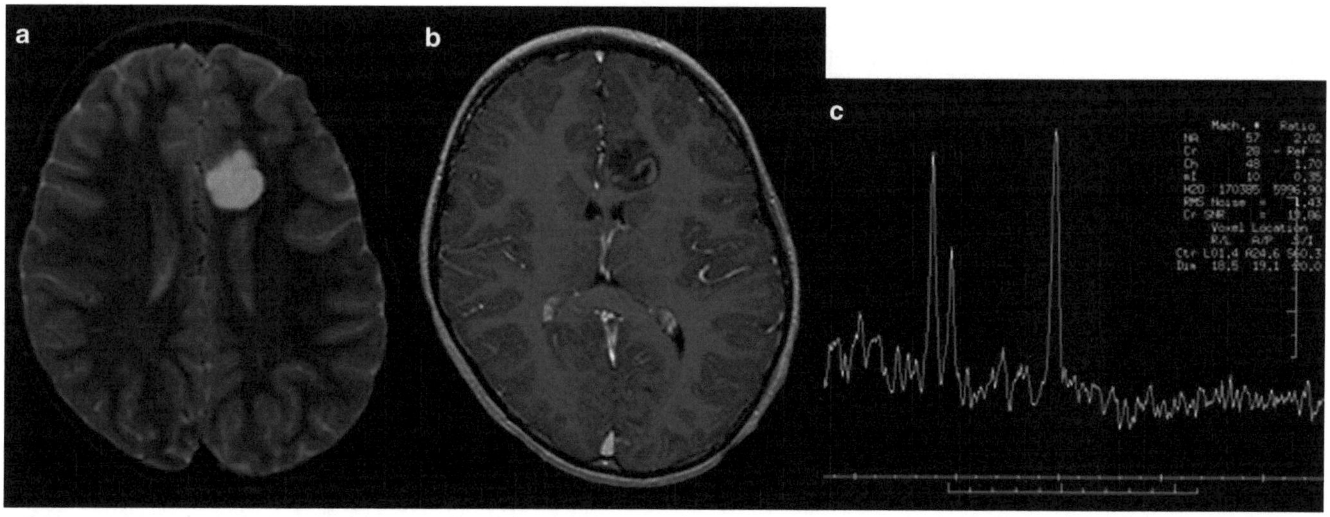

Fig. 15.8 Seven-year-old girl with dysembryoplastic neuro-epithelial tumor. (**a**) Axial T2 shows hyperintense lesion in the left mesial frontal lobe, (**b**) with minimal enhancement on the post-contrast scan. (**c**) Single voxel MR spectroscopy acquired from the tumor shows normal *N*-acetyl aspartate relative to creatine and slightly elevated choline

to other types of epilepsy-associated tumors (92% Engel class I and II) [100, 102, 105].

DNET affects the temporal and frontal lobes predominantly. DNET (14%) is less common in children compared to ganglioglioma (43%) [102]. The lesion may have a well-demarcated margin (50%) or the margins may be slightly blurred [108]. The tumor may cause broadening of the gyri, effacement of the sulci, and distortion of the ventricles [108]. The tumor may also result in remodeling of the overlying skull vault in 44% of cases [109]. On MR imaging, the tumor is of low T1/high T2 signal, often with multi-cystic, multinodular changes, and "bubbly" appearance [108], and may have a thin rim of high signal on FLAIR sequence. The tumor appears wedge-shaped and extends to the ventricle in 30% of cases. One-third of the cases show faint punctate or ring enhancement. DNET can demonstrate slightly reduced or similar NAA signal when compared to the contralateral normal side; the choline peak can be slightly elevated but usually are lower than in higher grade tumor, indicative of minor or non-active membrane turnover (Fig. 15.8). This supports the benign biologic behavior of this indolent tumor. [110, 111]

Differentiating low-grade tumor from focal cortical dysplasia (FCD) based on imaging can be challenging but important for treatment planning. Studies have been performed to differentiate low-grade tumor from FCD [110, 112]. Vouri et al. [110] suggested that changes in NAA and Choline could help differentiate low-grade tumor from FCD. The main difference was low levels of NAA in gliomas ($n=10$) compared to nearly normal levels of NAA in FCD ($n=5$) and DNET ($n=3$). In contrast, there were increased Cho levels in low-grade glioma compared to FCD. Changes in Cho and Cr can help differentiate astrocytoma from oligodendroglioma and oligoastrocytoma. In oligoastrocytoma both Cho and Cr were elevated, whereas in astrocytoma Cho was modestly increased and Cr was decreased. The higher cell density in

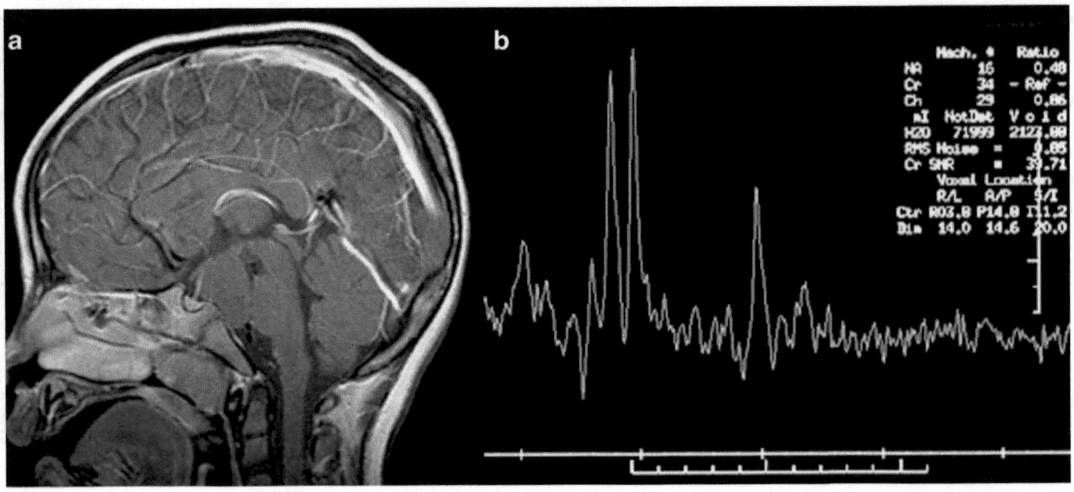

Fig. 15.9 Four-year-old girl with hypothalamic hamartoma. (**a**) Sagittal T1 post-contrast demonstrates a non-enhancing mass in the hypothalamus, in keeping with hypothalamic hamartoma. (**b**) Single voxel MR spectroscopy acquired from the tumor with TE = 144 ms shows reduced *N*-acetyl aspartate relative to creatine

oligodendroglioma may account for the elevated level of Cho in the tumor. However, transient seizures can elevate choline levels [113], therefore caution should be exercised when interpreting MRS in the setting of acute seizures.

Hypothalamic Hamartoma

Hypothalamic hamartoma are developmental malformations associated with central precocious puberty and gelastic (laughing) seizures. Seizures usually begin in infancy and childhood and later may be accompanied by cognitive decline. The relation between seizures and hamartoma has been documented using stereotactic depth recording, and with ictal single photon emission computed tomography studies showing hyperperfusion in hypothalamic hamartoma [114]. MR appearance of this lesion is isointense to increase signal on T2-weighted images relative to cortical and deep gray matter, slightly decreased signal on T1-weighted images, and higher signal intensity compared with gray matter on fluid attenuated inversion recovery imaging. Proton MRS demonstrated lower NAA content and higher MI concentration than either normal thalamic gray matter or frontal lobe gray and white matter [115, 116] (Fig. 15.9). The decrease in NAA suggested reduced neuronal density in the hypothalamic hamartoma and the increase in MI likely reflects gliosis.

Rasmussen Syndrome

Rasmussen encephalitis is a rare, progressive disease beginning in the first decade in previously healthy children [117]. It is characterized by acute presentation with refractory partial seizures, often with epilepsia partialis continua, which presents as clonic twitching of one group of muscles, repeated every few seconds, and persisting for hours, days, or longer. The disease usually follows a progressive neurological and cognitive deterioration with the development of hemiplegia. In the acute stages, MRI demonstrates cortical hyper-intensity on T2-weighted images that progress to volume loss in the chronic stages, with loss of the acute increased signal on T2-weighted MRI. MRS studies had focused predominantly on NAA level, which is usually decreased in the affected hemisphere [118–121], suggestive of neuronal loss and correspond to the volume loss seen with conventional MR sequences. Abnormally high concentration of Cho was reported in one study [120] but not in others [118, 119], suggestive of variable changes in membrane turnover. Increased lactate has been observed in Rasmussen encephalitis patients imaged during complex partial status epilepticus, indicative of the occurrence of anaerobic metabolism. However, the abnormalities on MRS tend to resolve completely on subsequent scans when seizures are under better control [122]. Consequently, care should be taken when interpreting the MRS in these patients on the basis of a single spectroscopy study. Increase in MI has also been reported in the late stages of the disease [118], which suggests prominent gliotic activity or scar.

Treatment and MRS

Vigabatrin is an irreversible inhibitor of GABA transaminase, the enzyme that catalyzes the metabolism of GABA in the brain. Vigabatrin has been shown to have an anticonvulsant

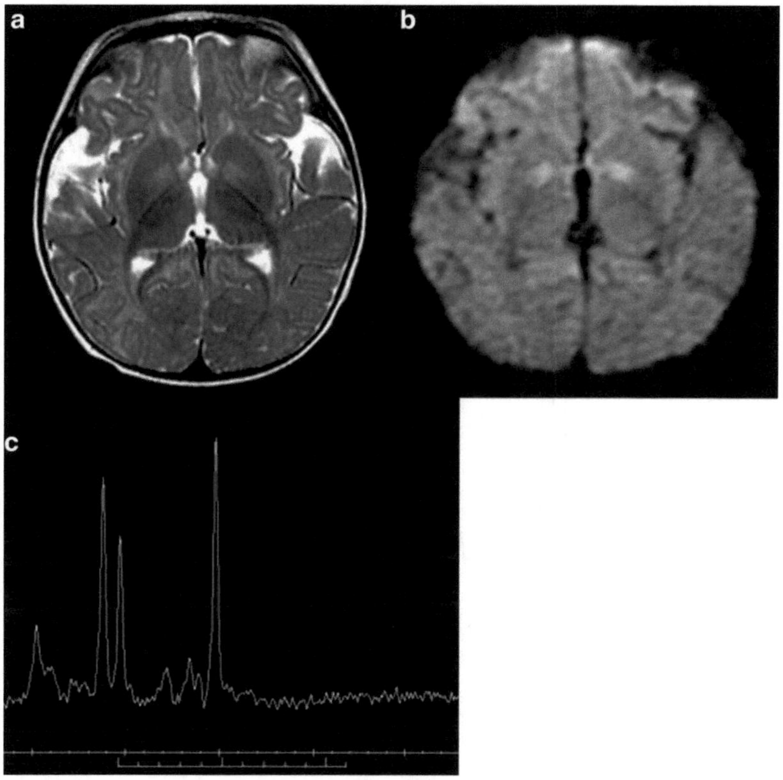

Fig. 15.10 Six-month old with infantile spasm treated with vigabatrin. Axial (**a**) T2 and (**b**) diffusion weighted imaging shows increased signal in the globi pallidi. (**c**) Single voxel MR spectroscopy acquired with TE = 144 ms shows normal spectra for age

effect in animal models of epilepsy and in human epileptic patients. Patients with infantile spasm treated with Vigabatrin may exhibit a transient MRI hyperintensity on T2 and diffusion-weighted sequences in the dentate nuclei, globi pallidi, posterior brainstem, and thalami. The signal changes have been observed in approximately 20–30% of infantile spasm treated with Vigabatrin and can be observed 1–12 months after commencing Vigabatrin [123]. These transient hyperintensities do not demonstrate a lactate peak or significant metabolite abnormality on MRS (Fig. 15.10). The exact significance of these alterations is not well understood [124].

Ketogenic diet, a diet high in fat and low in carbohydrate, is a highly effective treatment in controlling seizures in children. The mechanism by which ketogenic diet achieves seizure control is poorly understood but it is believed that the diet affects intermediary metabolism that influences the dynamics of the major inhibitory and excitatory neurotransmitter system in the brain. Three water-soluble compounds, *β-hydroxybutyrate, acetoacetate, and acetone* (known collectively as *ketone bodies*), are produced by the liver in otherwise healthy people when they fast or are under a ketogenic diet. The level of ketosis in patients is monitored by measuring urine ketone level; however, MRS can also detect these metabolites. Ketone has a single resonance at 2.2 ppm, while acetoacetate has two peaks at 2.26 and 3.46 ppm. Ketone is a metabolite that has been identified in epileptic patients treated with ketogenic diet, which is an indicator of excess acetone (Fig. 15.11). The other two metabolites are not detected in the spectra, likely due to lower concentrations. MRS in patients on ketogenic diet may additionally show a reduction in NAA and Cr while on the diet [125].

Conclusion

MRS is a non-invasive tool that allows in vivo assessment of brain metabolism, and therefore could potentially be used to lateralize seizure focus in TLE and to assist in the understanding of the pathophysiology of epilepsy syndromes and brain malformations. The ability of MRS to lateralize and localize seizure focus is still limited in extratemporal lobe epilepsy, which is more common than TLE in children with intractable epilepsy. Whole-brain CSI may assist in seizure localization in those with cryptogenic focal epilepsy. However, due to the longer acquisition time and more complex processing, CSI is not commonly used in the pediatric population. Further technical developments in CSI and post-processing may allow whole-brain MRS to be performed within an acceptable time, thereby allowing more widespread use of CSI in clinical practice.

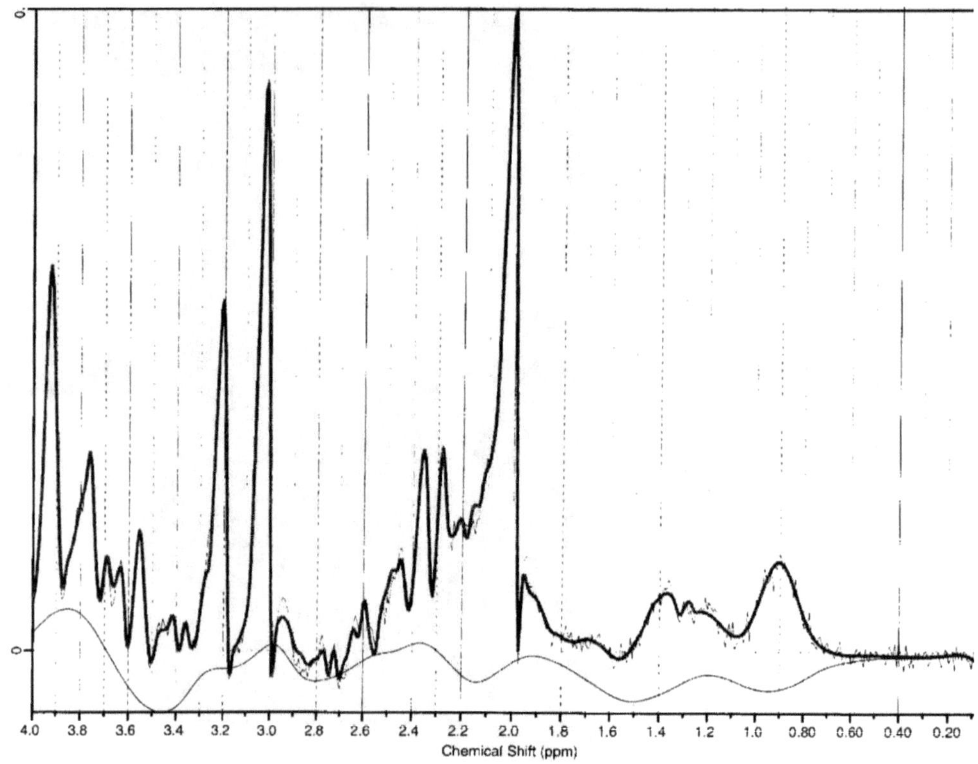

Fig. 15.11 Twenty-two-month old with spasm and tonic seizures on ketogenic diet. Single voxel MR spectroscopy with TE=35 ms shows the presence of ketones at 2.2 ppm, which is an indicator of excess acetone in patients on ketogenic diet

References

1. Urenjak J, Williams SR, Gadian DG, Noble M. Specific expression of N-acetylaspartate in neurons, oligodendrocyte-type-2 astrocyte progenitors, and immature oligodendrocytes in vitro. J Neurochem. 1992;59(1):55–61.
2. Najm IM, Wang Y, Hong SC, Luders HO, Ng TC, Comair YG. Temporal changes in proton MRS metabolites after kainic acid-induced seizures in rat brain. Epilepsia. 1997;38(1):87–94.
3. Baslow MH. Evidence supporting a role for N-acetyl-L-aspartate as a molecular water pump in myelinated neurons in the central nervous system. An analytical review. Neurochem Int. 2002;40(4):295–300.
4. Varho T, Komu M, Sonninen P, Lahdetie J, Holopainen IE. Quantitative HMRS and MRI volumetry indicate neuronal damage in the hippocampus of children with focal epilepsy and infrequent seizures. Epilepsia. 2005;46(5):696–703.
5. Hiremath GK, Najm IM. Magnetic resonance spectroscopy in animal models of epilepsy. Epilepsia. 2007;48 Suppl 4:47–55.
6. Berg AT, Berkovic SF, Brodie MJ, et al. Revised terminology and concepts for organization of seizures and epilepsies: report of the ILAE Commission on Classification and Terminology, 2005–2009. Epilepsia. 2010;51(4):676–85.
7. Najm IM, Wang Y, Shedid D, Luders HO, Ng TC, Comair YG. MRS metabolic markers of seizures and seizure-induced neuronal damage. Epilepsia. 1998;39(3):244–50.
8. Woermann FG, McLean MA, Bartlett PA, Parker GJ, Barker GJ, Duncan JS. Short echo time single-voxel 1 H magnetic resonance spectroscopy in magnetic resonance imaging-negative temporal lobe epilepsy: different biochemical profile compared with hippocampal sclerosis. Ann Neurol. 1999;45(3):369–76.
9. Simister RJ, McLean MA, Barker GJ, Duncan JS. A proton magnetic resonance spectroscopy study of metabolites in the occipital lobes in epilepsy. Epilepsia. 2003;44(4):550–8.
10. Sherwin A, Robitaille Y, Quesney F, et al. Excitatory amino acids are elevated in human epileptic cerebral cortex. Neurology. 1988;38(6):920–3.
11. Petroff OA, Pleban LA, Spencer DD. Symbiosis between in vivo and in vitro NMR spectroscopy: the creatine, N-acetylaspartate, glutamate, and GABA content of the epileptic human brain. Magn Reson Imaging. 1995;13(8):1197–211.
12. Pfund Z, Chugani DC, Juhasz C, et al. Evidence for coupling between glucose metabolism and glutamate cycling using FDG PET and 1 H magnetic resonance spectroscopy in patients with epilepsy. J Cereb Blood Flow Metab. 2000;20(5):871–8.
13. Ohtahara S, Yamatogi Y. Epileptic encephalopathies in early infancy with suppression-burst. J Clin Neurophysiol. 2003;20(6):398–407.
14. Seo JH, Lee YM, Lee JS, Kim SH, Kim HD. A case of Ohtahara syndrome with mitochondrial respiratory chain complex I deficiency. Brain Dev. 2010;32(3):253–7.
15. Kellaway P, Hrachovy RA, Frost Jr JD, Zion T. Precise characterization and quantification of infantile spasms. Ann Neurol. 1979;6(3):214–8.
16. Maeda H, Furune S, Nomura K, et al. Decrease of N-acetylaspartate after ACTH therapy in patients with infantile spasms. Neuropediatrics. 1997;28(5):262–7.
17. Coppola G, Plouin P, Chiron C, Robain O, Dulac O. Migrating partial seizures in infancy: a malignant disorder with developmental arrest. Epilepsia. 1995;36(10):1017–24.

18. Wilmshurst JM, Appleton DB, Grattan-Smith PJ. Migrating partial seizures in infancy: two new cases. J Child Neurol. 2000;15(11):717–22.
19. Coppola G, Dulac O. Malignant migrating partial seizures in infancy. In: Roger J, Bureau M, Dravet C, Genton P, Tassinari C, Wolf P, editors. Epileptic syndromes in infancy, childhood and adolescence. 3rd ed. London: John Libbey & Company Ltd; 1995. p. 65–8.
20. Gross-Tsur V, Ben-Zeev B, Shalev RS. Malignant migrating partial seizures in infancy. Pediatr Neurol. 2004;31(4):287–90.
21. Guerrini R, Dravet C. Severe epileptic encephalopathies of infancy, other than West syndrome. In: Engel Jr J, Pedley A, editors. Epilepsy: a comprehensive textbook. Philadelphia: Lippincott-Raven; 1997. p. 2285–302.
22. Dravet C, Bureau M, Oguni H, Fukuyama Y, Cokar O. Severe myoclonic epilepsy in infancy: Dravet syndrome. In: Delgado-Escueta AV GR, Medina MT, Genton P, Bureau M, Dravet C. , ed. *Advance in Neurology*. Philadelphia: Lippincott Williams and Wilkins; 2005:71–102.
23. Nabbout R, Gennaro E, Dalla Bernardina B, et al. Spectrum of SCN1A mutations in severe myoclonic epilepsy of infancy. Neurology. 2003;60(12):1961–7.
24. Siegler Z, Barsi P, Neuwirth M, et al. Hippocampal sclerosis in severe myoclonic epilepsy in infancy: a retrospective MRI study. Epilepsia. 2005;46(5):704–8.
25. Striano P, Mancardi MM, Biancheri R, et al. Brain MRI findings in severe myoclonic epilepsy in infancy and genotype-phenotype correlations. Epilepsia. 2007;48(6):1092–6.
26. Berg AT, Shinnar S, Darefsky AS, et al. Predictors of recurrent febrile seizures. A prospective cohort study. Arch Pediatr Adolesc Med. 1997;151(4):371–8.
27. Cendes F. Febrile seizures and mesial temporal sclerosis. Curr Opin Neurol. 2004;17(2):161–4.
28. Davies KG, Hermann BP, Dohan Jr FC, Foley KT, Bush AJ, Wyler AR. Relationship of hippocampal sclerosis to duration and age of onset of epilepsy, and childhood febrile seizures in temporal lobectomy patients. Epilepsy Res. 1996;24(2):119–26.
29. Kobayashi E, Facchin D, Steiner CE, et al. Mesial temporal lobe abnormalities in a family with 15q26qter trisomy. Arch Neurol. 2002;59(9):1476–9.
30. Berkovic SF, Scheffer IE. Febrile seizures: genetics and relationship to other epilepsy syndromes. Curr Opin Neurol. 1998;11(2):129–34.
31. Holopainen IE, Valtonen ME, Komu ME, et al. Proton spectroscopy in children with epilepsy and febrile convulsions. Pediatr Neurol. 1998;19(2):93–9.
32. Wu WC, Huang CC, Chung HW, et al. Hippocampal alterations in children with temporal lobe epilepsy with or without a history of febrile convulsions: evaluations with MR volumetry and proton MR spectroscopy. AJNR Am J Neuroradiol. 2005;26(5):1270–5.
33. Parker AP, Ferrie CD, Keevil S, et al. Neuroimaging and spectroscopy in children with epileptic encephalopathies. Arch Dis Child. 1998;79(1):39–43.
34. Otsubo H, Chitoku S, Ochi A, et al. Malignant rolandic-sylvian epilepsy in children: diagnosis, treatment, and outcomes. Neurology. 2001;57(4):590–6.
35. Lundberg S, Weis J, Eeg-Olofsson O, Raininko R. Hippocampal region asymmetry assessed by 1 H-MRS in rolandic epilepsy. Epilepsia. 2003;44(2):205–10.
36. Bhardwaj RD, Mahmoodabadi SZ, Otsubo H, Snead 3rd OC, Rutka JT, Widjaja E. Diffusion tensor tractography detection of functional pathway for the spread of epileptiform activity between temporal lobe and Rolandic region. Childs Nerv Syst. 2010;26(2):185–90.
37. Lee YJ, Kang HC, Lee JS, et al. Resective pediatric epilepsy surgery in Lennox-Gastaut syndrome. Pediatrics. 2010;125(1):e58–66.
38. Proposal for revised classification of epilepsies and epileptic syndromes. Commission on Classification and Terminology of the International League Against Epilepsy. Epilepsia. Jul–Aug 1989;30(4):389–399.
39. Porter RJ. The absence epilepsies. Epilepsia. 1993;34 Suppl 3:S42–48.
40. Futatsugi Y, Riviello Jr JJ. Mechanisms of generalized absence epilepsy. Brain Dev. 1998;20(2):75–9.
41. Chan CH, Briellmann RS, Pell GS, Scheffer IE, Abbott DF, Jackson GD. Thalamic atrophy in childhood absence epilepsy. Epilepsia. 2006;47(2):399–405.
42. Gloor P, Fariello RG. Generalized epilepsy: some of its cellular mechanisms differ from those of focal epilepsy. Trends Neurosci. 1988;11(2):63–8.
43. Fojtikova D, Brazdil M, Horky J, et al. Magnetic resonance spectroscopy of the thalamus in patients with typical absence epilepsy. Seizure. 2006;15(7):533–40.
44. Kabay SC, Gumustas OG, Karaman HO, Ozden H, Erdinc O. A proton magnetic resonance spectroscopic study in juvenile absence epilepsy in early stages. Eur J Paediatr Neurol. 2010;14(3):224–8.
45. Nehlig A, Valenti MP, Thiriaux A, Hirsch E, Marescaux C, Namer IJ. Ictal and interictal perfusion variations measured by SISCOM analysis in typical childhood absence seizures. Epileptic Disord. 2004;6(4):247–53.
46. Salek-Haddadi A, Lemieux L, Merschhemke M, Friston KJ, Duncan JS, Fish DR. Functional magnetic resonance imaging of human absence seizures. Ann Neurol. 2003;53(5):663–7.
47. Dreifuss FE. Juvenile myoclonic epilepsy: characteristics of a primary generalized epilepsy. Epilepsia. 1989;30 Suppl 4:S1–7. discussion S24–27.
48. Holmes MD, Quiring J, Tucker DM. Evidence that juvenile myoclonic epilepsy is a disorder of frontotemporal corticothalamic networks. Neuroimage. 2010;49(1):80–93.
49. Mory SB, Li LM, Guerreiro CA, Cendes F. Thalamic dysfunction in juvenile myoclonic epilepsy: a proton MRS study. Epilepsia. 2003;44(11):1402–5.
50. Haki C, Gumustas OG, Bora I, Gumustas AU, Parlak M. Proton magnetic resonance spectroscopy study of bilateral thalamus in juvenile myoclonic epilepsy. Seizure. 2007;16(4):287–95.
51. Lin K, Carrete Jr H, Lin J, et al. Magnetic resonance spectroscopy reveals an epileptic network in juvenile myoclonic epilepsy. Epilepsia. 2009;50(5):1191–200.
52. Baykan B, Striano P, Gianotti S, et al. Late-onset and slow-progressing Lafora disease in four siblings with EPM2B mutation. Epilepsia. 2005;46(10):1695–7.
53. Villanueva V, Alvarez-Linera J, Gomez-Garre P, Gutierrez J, Serratosa JM. MRI volumetry and proton MR spectroscopy of the brain in Lafora disease. Epilepsia. 2006;47(4):788–92.
54. Pichiecchio A, Veggiotti P, Cardinali S, Longaretti F, Poloni GU, Uggetti C. Lafora disease: spectroscopy study correlated with neuropsychological findings. Eur J Paediatr Neurol. 2008;12(4):342–7.
55. Harvey AS, Berkovic SF, Wrennall JA, Hopkins IJ. Temporal lobe epilepsy in childhood: clinical, EEG, and neuroimaging findings and syndrome classification in a cohort with new-onset seizures. Neurology. 1997;49(4):960–8.
56. Harvey AS, Grattan-Smith JD, Desmond PM, Chow CW, Berkovic SF. Febrile seizures and hippocampal sclerosis: frequent and related findings in intractable temporal lobe epilepsy of childhood. Pediatr Neurol. 1995;12(3):201–6.
57. Grattan-Smith JD, Harvey AS, Desmond PM, Chow CW. Hippocampal sclerosis in children with intractable temporal lobe epilepsy: detection with MR imaging. AJR Am J Roentgenol. 1993;161(5):1045–8.
58. Mohamed A, Wyllie E, Ruggieri P, et al. Temporal lobe epilepsy due to hippocampal sclerosis in pediatric candidates for epilepsy surgery. Neurology. 2001;56(12):1643–9.
59. Cendes F, Caramanos Z, Andermann F, Dubeau F, Arnold DL. Proton magnetic resonance spectroscopic imaging and magnetic

resonance imaging volumetry in the lateralization of temporal lobe epilepsy: a series of 100 patients. Ann Neurol. 1997;42(5):737–46.
60. Simister RJ, Woermann FG, McLean MA, Bartlett PA, Barker GJ, Duncan JS. A short-echo-time proton magnetic resonance spectroscopic imaging study of temporal lobe epilepsy. Epilepsia. 2002;43(9):1021–31.
61. Riederer F, Bittsansky M, Schmidt C, et al. 1 H magnetic resonance spectroscopy at 3 T in cryptogenic and mesial temporal lobe epilepsy. NMR Biomed. 2006;19(5):544–53.
62. Ng TC, Comair YG, Xue M, et al. Temporal lobe epilepsy: presurgical localization with proton chemical shift imaging. Radiology. 1994;193(2):465–72.
63. Novotny E, Ashwal S, Shevell M. Proton magnetic resonance spectroscopy: an emerging technology in pediatric neurology research. Pediatr Res. 1998;44(1):1–10.
64. Blumcke I, Pauli E, Clusmann H, et al. A new clinico-pathological classification system for mesial temporal sclerosis. Acta Neuropathol. 2007;113(3):235–44.
65. Hammen T, Hildebrandt M, Stadlbauer A, et al. Non-invasive detection of hippocampal sclerosis: correlation between metabolite alterations detected by (1)H-MRS and neuropathology. NMR Biomed. 2008;21(6):545–52.
66. Miller SP, Li LM, Cendes F, et al. Neuronal dysfunction in children with newly diagnosed temporal lobe epilepsy. Pediatr Neurol. 2000;22(4):281–6.
67. Hugg JW, Kuzniecky RI, Gilliam FG, Morawetz RB, Fraught RE, Hetherington HP. Normalization of contralateral metabolic function following temporal lobectomy demonstrated by 1 H magnetic resonance spectroscopic imaging. Ann Neurol. 1996;40(2):236–9.
68. Serles W, Li LM, Antel SB, et al. Time course of postoperative recovery of N-acetyl-aspartate in temporal lobe epilepsy. Epilepsia. 2001;42(2):190–7.
69. Kuzniecky R, Hugg J, Hetherington H, et al. Predictive value of 1 H MRSI for outcome in temporal lobectomy. Neurology. 1999;53(4):694–8.
70. Mueller SG, Suhy J, Laxer KD, et al. Reduced extrahippocampal NAA in mesial temporal lobe epilepsy. Epilepsia. 2002;43(10): 1210–6.
71. Capizzano AA, Vermathen P, Laxer KD, et al. Multisection proton MR spectroscopy for mesial temporal lobe epilepsy. AJNR Am J Neuroradiol. 2002;23(8):1359–68.
72. Garcia PA, Laxer KD, van der Grond J, Hugg JW, Matson GB, Weiner MW. Proton magnetic resonance spectroscopic imaging in patients with frontal lobe epilepsy. Ann Neurol. 1995;37(2):279–81.
73. Stanley JA, Cendes F, Dubeau F, Andermann F, Arnold DL. Proton magnetic resonance spectroscopic imaging in patients with extratemporal epilepsy. Epilepsia. 1998;39(3):267–73.
74. Auvin S, Devisme L, Maurage CA, et al. Neuropathological and MRI findings in an acute presentation of hemiconvulsion-hemiplegia: a report with pathophysiological implications. Seizure. 2007;16(4):371–6.
75. Freeman JL, Coleman LT, Smith LJ, Shield LK. Hemiconvulsion-hemiplegia-epilepsy syndrome: characteristic early magnetic resonance imaging findings. J Child Neurol. 2002;17(1):10–6.
76. Meencke HJ, Veith G. Migration disturbances in epilepsy. In: Engel Jr J, Wasterlain C, Cavalheiro EA, editors. Molecular neurobiology of epilepsy. New York: Elsevier; 1992. p. 31–40.
77. Woermann FG, McLean MA, Bartlett PA, Barker GJ, Duncan JS. Quantitative short echo time proton magnetic resonance spectroscopic imaging study of malformations of cortical development causing epilepsy. Brain. 2001;124(Pt 2):427–36.
78. Lee BC, Schmidt RE, Hatfield GA, Bourgeois B, Park TS. MRI of focal cortical dysplasia. Neuroradiology. 1998;40(10):675–83.
79. Mueller SG, Laxer KD, Barakos JA, et al. Metabolic characteristics of cortical malformations causing epilepsy. J Neurol. 2005;252(9):1082–92.
80. Simister RJ, McLean MA, Barker GJ, Duncan JS. Proton magnetic resonance spectroscopy of malformations of cortical development causing epilepsy. Epilepsy Res. 2007;74(2–3):107–15.
81. Leite CC, Lucato LT, Sato JR, Valente KD, Otaduy MC. Multivoxel proton MR spectroscopy in malformations of cortical development. AJNR Am J Neuroradiol. 2007;28(6):1071–5. discussion 1076–1077.
82. Hanefeld F, Kruse B, Holzbach U, et al. Hemimegalencephaly: localized proton magnetic resonance spectroscopy in vivo. Epilepsia. 1995;36(12):1215–24.
83. Taylor DC, Falconer MA, Bruton CJ, Corsellis JA. Focal dysplasia of the cerebral cortex in epilepsy. J Neurol Neurosurg Psychiatry. 1971;34(4):369–87.
84. Colon AJ, Hofman P, Ossenblok PP, et al. MRS-lateralisation index in patients with epilepsy and focal cortical dysplasia or a MEG-focus using bilateral single voxels. Epilepsy Res. 2010;89(1):148–53.
85. Battaglia G, Arcelli P, Granata T, et al. Neuronal migration disorders and epilepsy: a morphological analysis of three surgically treated patients. Epilepsy Res. 1996;26(1):49–58.
86. Widjaja E, Griffiths PD, Wilkinson ID. Proton MR spectroscopy of polymicrogyria and heterotopia. AJNR Am J Neuroradiol. 2003;24(10):2077–81.
87. Kuzniecky R, Hetherington H, Pan J, et al. Proton spectroscopic imaging at 4.1 tesla in patients with malformations of cortical development and epilepsy. Neurology. 1997;48(4):1018–24.
88. Kaminaga T, Kobayashi M, Abe T. Proton magnetic resonance spectroscopy in disturbances of cortical development. Neuroradiology. 2001;43(7):575–80.
89. Li LM, Cendes F, Bastos AC, Andermann F, Dubeau F, Arnold DL. Neuronal metabolic dysfunction in patients with cortical developmental malformations: a proton magnetic resonance spectroscopic imaging study. Neurology. 1998;50(3):755–9.
90. Simone IL, Federico F, Tortorella C, et al. Metabolic changes in neuronal migration disorders: evaluation by combined MRI and proton MR spectroscopy. Epilepsia. 1999;40(7):872–9.
91. Preul MC, Leblanc R, Cendes F, et al. Function and organization in dysgenic cortex. Case report. J Neurosurg. 1997;87(1):113–21.
92. Castillo M, Kwock L, Mukherji SK. Clinical applications of proton MR spectroscopy. AJNR Am J Neuroradiol. 1996;17(1):1–15.
93. des Portes V, Francis F, Pinard JM, et al. Doublecortin is the major gene causing X-linked subcortical laminar heterotopia (SCLH). Hum Mol Genet. 1998;7(7):1063–70.
94. Munakata M, Haginoya K, Soga T, et al. Metabolic properties of band heterotopia differ from those of other cortical dysplasias: a proton magnetic resonance spectroscopy study. Epilepsia. 2003;44(3):366–71.
95. Yapici Z, Dincer A, Eraksoy M. Proton spectroscopic findings in children with epilepsy owing to tuberous sclerosis complex. J Child Neurol. 2005;20(6):517–22.
96. Mizuno S, Takahashi Y, Kato Z, Goto H, Kondo N, Hoshi H. Magnetic resonance spectroscopy of tubers in patients with tuberous sclerosis. Acta Neurol Scand. 2000;102(3):175–8.
97. de Carvalho Neto A, Gasparetto EL, Bruck I. Subependymal giant cell astrocytoma with high choline/creatine ratio on proton MR spectroscopy. Arq Neuropsiquiatr. 2006;64(3B):877–80.
98. Moore GJ, Slovis TL, Chugani HT. Proton magnetic resonance spectroscopy in children with Sturge-Weber syndrome. J Child Neurol. 1998;13(7):332–5.
99. Sijens PE, Gieteling EW, Meiners LC, et al. Diffusion tensor imaging and magnetic resonance spectroscopy of the brain in a patient with Sturge-Weber syndrome. Acta Radiol. 2006;47(9):972–6.
100. Benifla M, Otsubo H, Ochi A, et al. Temporal lobe surgery for intractable epilepsy in children: an analysis of outcomes in 126 children. Neurosurgery. 2006;59(6):1203–13. discussion 1213–1204.

101. Mittal S, Montes JL, Farmer JP, et al. Long-term outcome after surgical treatment of temporal lobe epilepsy in children. J Neurosurg. 2005;103(5 Suppl):401–12.
102. Luyken C, Blumcke I, Fimmers R, et al. The spectrum of long-term epilepsy-associated tumors: long-term seizure and tumor outcome and neurosurgical aspects. Epilepsia. 2003;44(6):822–30.
103. Clusmann H, Kral T, Gleissner U, et al. Analysis of different types of resection for pediatric patients with temporal lobe epilepsy. Neurosurgery. 2004;54(4):847–59. discussion 859–860.
104. Blumcke I, Lobach M, Wolf HK, Wiestler OD. Evidence for developmental precursor lesions in epilepsy-associated glioneuronal tumors. Microsc Res Tech. 1999;46(1):53–8.
105. Luyken C, Blumcke I, Fimmers R, Urbach H, Wiestler OD, Schramm J. Supratentorial gangliogliomas: histopathologic grading and tumor recurrence in 184 patients with a median follow-up of 8 years. Cancer. 2004;101(1):146–55.
106. Koeller KK, Henry JM. From the archives of the AFIP: superficial gliomas: radiologic-pathologic correlation. Armed Forces Institute of Pathology. Radiographics. 2001;21(6):1533–56.
107. Im SH, Chung CK, Cho BK, Lee SK. Supratentorial ganglioglioma and epilepsy: postoperative seizure outcome. J Neurooncol. 2002;57(1):59–66.
108. Ostertun B, Wolf HK, Campos MG, et al. Dysembryoplastic neuroepithelial tumors: MR and CT evaluation. AJNR Am J Neuroradiol. 1996;17(3):419–30.
109. Stanescu Cosson R, Varlet P, Beuvon F, et al. Dysembryoplastic neuroepithelial tumors: CT, MR findings and imaging follow-up: a study of 53 cases. J Neuroradiol. 2001;28(4):230–40.
110. Vuori K, Kankaanranta L, Hakkinen AM, et al. Low-grade gliomas and focal cortical developmental malformations: differentiation with proton MR spectroscopy. Radiology. 2004;230(3):703–8.
111. Lee DY, Chung CK, Hwang YS, et al. Dysembryoplastic neuroepithelial tumor: radiological findings (including PET, SPECT, and MRS) and surgical strategy. J Neurooncol. 2000;47(2):167–74.
112. Pillai JJ, Hessler RB, Allison JD, Park YD, Lee MR, Lavin T. Advanced MR imaging of cortical dysplasia with or without neoplasm: a report of two cases. AJNR Am J Neuroradiol. 2002;23(10):1686–91.
113. Ende G, Braus DF, Walter S, Weber-Fahr W, Henn FA. The hippocampus in patients treated with electroconvulsive therapy: a proton magnetic resonance spectroscopic imaging study. Arch Gen Psychiatry. 2000;57(10):937–43.
114. Wakai S, Nikaido K, Nihira H, Kawamoto Y, Hayasaka H. Gelastic seizure with hypothalamic hamartoma: proton magnetic resonance spectrometry and ictal electroencephalographic findings in a 4-year-old girl. J Child Neurol. 2002;17(1):44–6.
115. Freeman JL, Coleman LT, Wellard RM, et al. MR imaging and spectroscopic study of epileptogenic hypothalamic hamartomas: analysis of 72 cases. AJNR Am J Neuroradiol. 2004;25(3):450–62.
116. Tasch E, Cendes F, Li LM, et al. Hypothalamic hamartomas and gelastic epilepsy: a spectroscopic study. Neurology. 1998;51(4): 1046–50.
117. Rasmussen T, Olszewski J, Lloydsmith D. Focal seizures due to chronic localized encephalitis. Neurology. 1958;8(6):435–45.
118. Matthews PM, Andermann F, Arnold DL. A proton magnetic resonance spectroscopy study of focal epilepsy in humans. Neurology. 1990;40(6):985–9.
119. Cendes F, Andermann F, Silver K, Arnold DL. Imaging of axonal damage in vivo in Rasmussen's syndrome. Brain. 1995;118(Pt 3):753–8.
120. Turkdogan-Sozuer D, Ozek MM, Sav A, Dincer A, Pamir MN. Serial MRI and MRS studies with unusual findings in Rasmussen's encephalitis. Eur Radiol. 2000;10(6):962–6.
121. Park YD, Allison JD, Weiss KL, Smith JR, Lee MR, King DW. Proton magnetic resonance spectroscopic observations of epilepsia partialis continua in children. J Child Neurol. 2000;15(11):729–33.
122. Wellard RM, Briellmann RS, Wilson JC, et al. Longitudinal study of MRS metabolites in Rasmussen encephalitis. Brain. 2004;127(Pt 6):1302–12.
123. Dracopoulos A, Widjaja E, Raybaud C, Westall CA, Snead 3rd OC. Vigabatrin-associated reversible MRI signal changes in patients with infantile spasms. Epilepsia. 2010;51(7):1297–304.
124. Milh M, Villeneuve N, Chapon F, et al. Transient brain magnetic resonance imaging hyperintensity in basal ganglia and brain stem of epileptic infants treated with vigabatrin. J Child Neurol. 2009;24(3):305–15.
125. Seymour KJ, Bluml S, Sutherling J, Sutherling W, Ross BD. Identification of cerebral acetone by 1 H-MRS in patients with epilepsy controlled by ketogenic diet. MAGMA. 1999;8(1): 33–42.

^{1}H Magnetic Resonance Spectroscopy of the Brain During Adolescence: Normal Brain Development and Neuropsychiatric Disorders

16

Alena Horská and E. Mark Mahone

Adolescence, a transitional period between childhood and adulthood (12–18 years of age), is characterized by maturation of cognitive and behavioral abilities [156]. Compared to brain development in perinatal and early childhood, neurobiological changes occurring during later childhood and adolescence are less dramatic but have critical importance for development of normal brain functions [47]. The combinations of genetic vulnerability, endocrine changes during puberty, and environmental factors render adolescents at risk for developing psychiatric disorders [110, 172]. In the developed world, mental and addictive disorders can be considered the primary chronic diseases of childhood and adolescence. Attention Deficit/Hyperactivity Disorder (ADHD) and Autism Spectrum Disorders (ASD) are associated with childhood. The onset of mood and anxiety disorders generally occurs in adolescence, although the diagnoses may be delayed until adulthood. Many psychiatric disorders that emerge in childhood and adolescence can be understood as dysfunctions within established brain circuits [75, 160]. Therefore, an understanding of normal development of the brain and its circuitry is important for both identifying the causes of psychiatric disorders and for development of effective treatments [160].

Advanced techniques of neuroimaging make possible studies of brain structure, physiology, function, and metabolism in the critical periods of childhood and adolescence [45]. MRI was the first neuroimaging technique that enabled noninvasive studies of neuroanatomical correlates of cognition, behavior, and emotions and permitted serial observations in individual subjects [100]. This chapter is an overview of the applications of ^{1}H Magnetic Resonance Spectroscopy (MRS) to brain development during adolescence, and to major neuropsychiatric disorders, except ADHD and ASD, which are subjects of separate chapters in this volume. ^{1}H MRS allows for testing of novel hypotheses on specific regional metabolic patterns and their changes over time in psychiatric disorders associated with childhood and adolescence, in populations not affected by a chronic disease or long-term medications.

A. Horská, Ph.D (✉)
The Russell H. Morgan Department of Radiology and Radiological Science, Johns Hopkins University,
600 N Wolfe St, Park Bldg, 3rd Floor, Rm 367 H, Baltimore, MD 21287, USA
e-mail: ahorska@jhmi.edu

E.M. Mahone, Ph.D.
Department of Neuropsychology, Kennedy Krieger Institute, Baltimore, MD, USA

Normal Brain Development

Imaging of Brain Development During Adolescence

MRI studies revealed regional and sex-related heterogeneity of rates of maturation of gray and white matter. Considering the differences between males and females in prevalence, age of onset and presentation of symptoms of neuropsychiatric disorders, sex-related differences in developmental brain trajectories are of high relevance for studies of pathology [55]. However, the differences in morphology may not reflect sexually dimorphic differences in functionally relevant factors such as neuronal connectivity and receptor density [100].

Earlier cross-sectional and later longitudinal quantitative MRI studies in typically developing children and adolescents examined age-related changes in total brain volumes and volumes of gray matter, white matter, and subcortical structures between the ages of 4 and 20 years [56–58, 79, 129]. Total cerebral volume peaks at the age or 14.5 years in boys and at 10.5 years in girls, with the male brain having an approximately 9% larger mean volume (Fig. 16.1a).

Cortical gray matter volumes follow a nonlinear developmental course, with an increase during preadolescence and decrease in the postadolescence period. The maximum gray matter volumes are detected around the age of 12 years in the frontal and parietal lobes, and around the age of 16 years in the

S. Blüml and A. Panigrahy (eds.), *MR Spectroscopy of Pediatric Brain Disorders*,
DOI 10.1007/978-1-4419-5864-8_16, © Springer Science+Business Media, LLC 2013

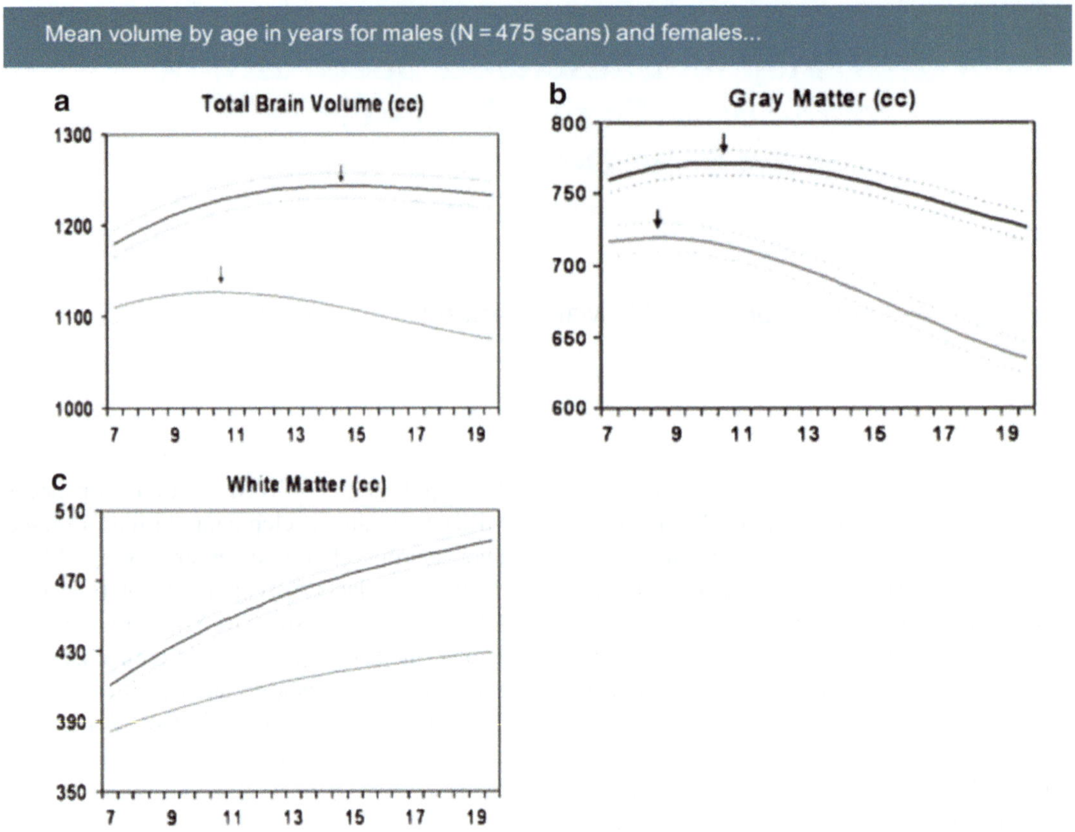

Fig. 16.1 Mean volume by age in years is shown for males (upper trace; $N=475$ scans) and females (lower trace; $N=354$ scans). Middle lines in each set represent mean values, and upper and lower lines represent upper and lower 95% confidence intervals. (**a**) Total brain volume, (**b**) gray matter volume, (**c**) white matter volume. Brain volume follows an inverted U shape trajectory, which peaks at approximately age 10.5 in girls and 14.5 in boys. Cortical gray matter follows an inverted U shape developmental trajectory, with peak sizes occurring at different times in different regions. White matter volumes increase throughout childhood and adolescence. (From Giedd JN, et al. *Anatomic Magnetic Resonance Imaging of the Developing Child and Adolescent Brain and Effects of Genetic Variation. Neuropsychol Rev 2010 11–19, with permission.*)

temporal lobe; the volumes of occipital gray matter continue to increase through the age of 20 years (Fig. 16.1b). A similar pattern of nonlinear developmental changes has also been described for the number of synapses, glucose utilization rate, EEG power, and neurotransmitter receptor densities [55]. For example, one PET study showed that at birth, the regional cerebral metabolic rates of glucose utilization are about 30% lower than the rates measured in adults. Between the ages of 4 years and 9–10 years, a high plateau of glucose utilization rate twice as high as in the adult brain is reached, followed by a decline until 16–18 years when the glucose utilization rates stabilize [28]. It was noted that the ascending rate of glucose utilization until 4 years of age corresponds to the period of synaptic proliferation, and the high plateau during childhood represents the period of synaptic stabilization and the decline during adolescence is associated with the period of synaptic elimination and diminishing energy requirement [28].

The volumes of white matter tend to increase linearly throughout childhood and adolescence, with smaller variability among regions [56, 57, 59] (Fig. 16.1c). Age-related differences in structural integrity and organization of white matter can be assessed with diffusion tensor imaging (DTI), by measuring water diffusion properties along white matter tracts. After prominent changes in DTI parameters (e.g., mean diffusivity (MD)) or fractional anisotropy (FA)) observed during infancy and early childhood, continuing but more subtle age-related decreases in MD and increases in FA were detected in several white matter tracts [14, 63, 98]. Increases in white matter FA, as detected by DTI, and white matter volumes, as reported by morphometric MRI, may be attributed to continuing myelination and other factors, including increase in the fiber diameter [62]. Maturation of white matter is associated with development of specific cognitive functions [118]. For example, one DTI study of adolescent boys reported a relationship between language and semantic memory and FA in the arcuate fasciculus [4]. In planning of future studies of neuropsychiatric disorders, it should be considered that impairment of white matter is involved in a wide range of psychiatric disorders and neurodevelopmental cognitive and emotional disorders [47, 48].

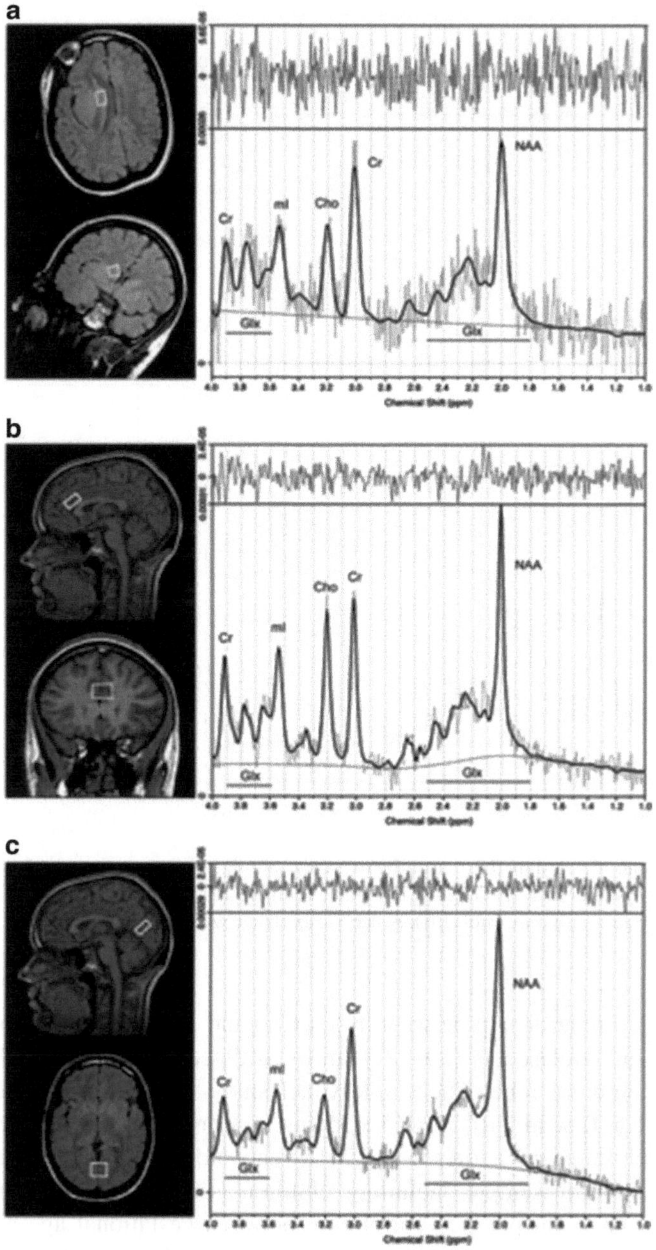

Fig. 16.2 Localizer images and ¹H MR spectra of (**a**) right caudate nucleus, (**b**) anterior cingulate gyrus, and (**c**) occipital cortex, brain regions frequently examined in patients with neuropsychiatric disorders. The spectra show signals of choline (Cho), creatine (Cr), myo-inositol (mI), *N*-acetylaspartate (NAA), and complex unresolved signals of glutamate and glutamine (Glx). The spectra were acquired at 1.5 T with 2 s repetition time and 30 ms echo time. (From Starck, Goran, et al.: *A ¹H magnetic resonance spectroscopy study in adults with obsessive compulsive disorder: relationship between metabolite concentrations and symptom severity. J Neural Transmission 2008, 7–2, with permission*

¹H MRS of Brain Development During Adolescence

Psychiatric disorders may be a result of impairment in complex biological and psychological processes [75]. If aberrations in biological substrates precede the emerging of symptoms, noninvasive neuroimaging techniques such as ¹H MRS may have an invaluable role in identifying potential biomarkers of specific diseases. Knowledge of age-related changes in concentrations of these biomarkers would be important for detection and understanding of pathological findings in neuropsychiatric diseases associated with abnormal brain development during childhood and adolescence.

¹H MRS can detect differences in metabolic patterns between gray and white matter [8, 10, 34, 77, 132] and within specific gray and white matter regions [3, 81]. Figure 16.2 shows examples of spectroscopic patterns in three gray matter regions of interest often examined in patients with neuropsychiatric disorders—caudate nucleus, anterior cingulate, and occipital cortex. The spectra show signals of *N*-acetylaspartate (NAA), choline (Cho), creatine (Cr), myo-inositol (Ins), and complex resonances of overlapping signals of glutamate (Glu) and glutamine (Gln), denoted Glx. A short TE spectrum collected at 7 T in a 5.5-year-old healthy boy (Fig. 16.3) demonstrates a superior signal resolution compared with 1.5 T. The major advantage of ultra-high field MRS for studying neuropsychiatric disorders is improved reliability of quantitative assessment, in particular of metabolites at low concentrations or with a complex signal pattern [166]. NAA, located both in neuronal cell bodies and axons, is considered a marker of neuronal integrity and function. Signals of N-acetylaspartate and N-acetylaspartyl glutamate contribute to the “NAA” resonance. The Cho signal represents compounds associated with cell membrane turnover (mainly glycerophosphocholine, phosphocholine, and free choline). The Cr resonance includes creatine and phosphocreatine, compounds involved in high-energy cell metabolism. Myo-inositol, located primarily in glial cells, is considered a glial marker [16]. The metabolism of Glu (an excitatory neurotransmitter), GABA (an inhibitory neurotransmitter), and Gln are linked via the Glu/GABA-Gln cycle, involving neurons and astrocytes [7]. Recent publications cover technical aspects and clinical applications of ¹H MRS [9] and present lists of chemical shifts of MRS-detected compounds [33, 67].

The knowledge of age-related differences during brain development, maturation, and aging is important for interpretation of data in patients with neuropathologies [69, 74, 81, 95, 123]. Age-related metabolic differences are most prominent within the first 2–3 years of life [95, 123] compared with changes observed during childhood, adolescence, or aging.

In the *gray matter*, a single voxel MRS study of a mid-parietal region reported a gradual increase in the total NAA concentration and a decrease in taurine (Tau) from infancy to adulthood [132]. No age-related differences in Cho, Cr, Ins, Glu, and Gln were detected after the age of 1 year. Spectra were obtained at 2.0 T using the STEAM technique,

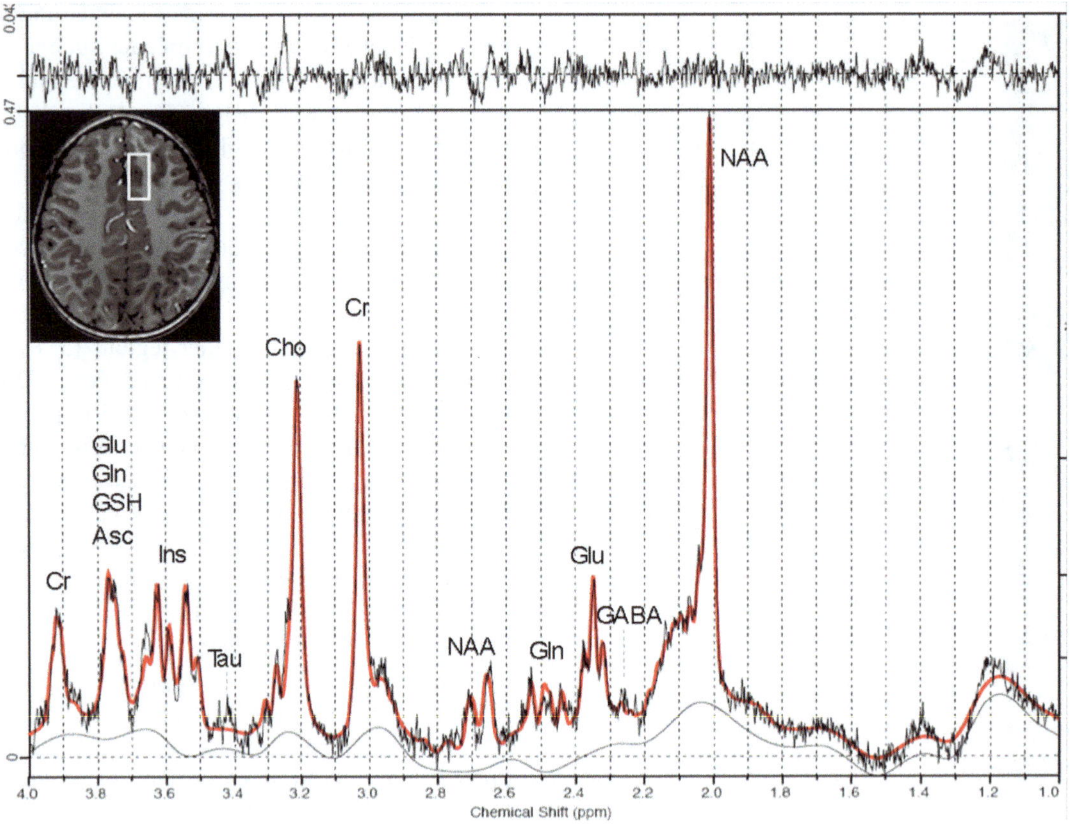

Fig. 16.3 Localizer image and ^{1}H MR spectrum collected at 7 T with repetition time of 3 s, echo time of 14 ms, and 96 acquisitions, in the anterior medial frontal region in a 5.5-year-old healthy boy. The signals can be assigned to ascorbate (Asc), choline (Cho), creatine (Cr), γ-aminobutyrate (GABA), glutamate (Glu), glutamine (Gln), glutathione (GSH), myo-inositol (Ins), *N*-acetylaspartate (NAA), and taurine (Tau)

with repetition time (TR)/mixing time (TM)/echo time (TE) = 6 s/10 or 30 ms/20 ms. The study included 17 children aged 5–10 years and 26 children aged 10–18 years, in addition to younger children and a group of adults [132]. No age-related differences in Cho, Cr, and NAA concentrations were detected in cortical gray matter (frontal, parietal, medial premotor, and motor cortices) in a MRSI study performed at a long TE of 272 ms [74]; the study included 15 children 3–18 years old. The only significant finding was a slight decline in mean gray matter NAA/Cho ratio after the age of 10 years [74]. This is in agreement with a study by Kadota et al., reporting a gradual linear decrease in the NAA/Cho ratio from childhood to old age in the midline gray matter at the level of the centrum semiovale [81]. Their MRSI study was carried out at 1.5 T with TR/TE = 1.5 s/270 ms in 90 healthy volunteers aged 4–88 years [81]. A nonlinear relationship between cortical gray matter NAA concentrations and age was reported in a ^{1}H and ^{31}P MRSI study (1.5 T, TR/TE = 1.5 s/30 ms) including 105 healthy children 6–18 years old; no difference in NAA concentration between the youngest and oldest children was detected [65]. The concentration of phosphocreatine (detected with ^{31}P MRS) was increasing with age [65]. No relationship between NAA/Cho and age in 21 children and adolescents (10–18 years) was detected in the medial temporal lobe. The single-voxel study was performed at 1.5 T, with TR/TE = 1.5 s/35 ms in a group of 21 healthy children and adolescents 10–18 years old [60]. However, in a larger sample including children born prematurely, a significant positive correlation between gestational age at birth and NAA and Cr concentrations was detected [61].

In the *white matter*, a gradual increase in NAA concentration; a slow decrease in Cho concentration; and reductions in Gln, taurine, and GABA with increasing age were noted in the parieto-occipital region [132]. A small linear increase in the ratio NAA/Cho averaged from the frontal and the parietal white matter between the ages 6 and 18 years was reported in another study [74]. In the study by Kadota et al., the white matter NAA/Cho ratio measured in the centrum semiovale increased during childhood, and after reaching a maximum around 15.9 years in the posterior regions, around 17.6 years in the central regions, and around 21.9 years in the anterior regions, a steady decline was observed [81]. Figure 16.4 shows age-related differences in Cho/Cr and NAA/Cr ratios obtained in healthy children and adolescents in two white matter regions. A relatively small but significant age-related decrease in the Cho/Cr ratio and a

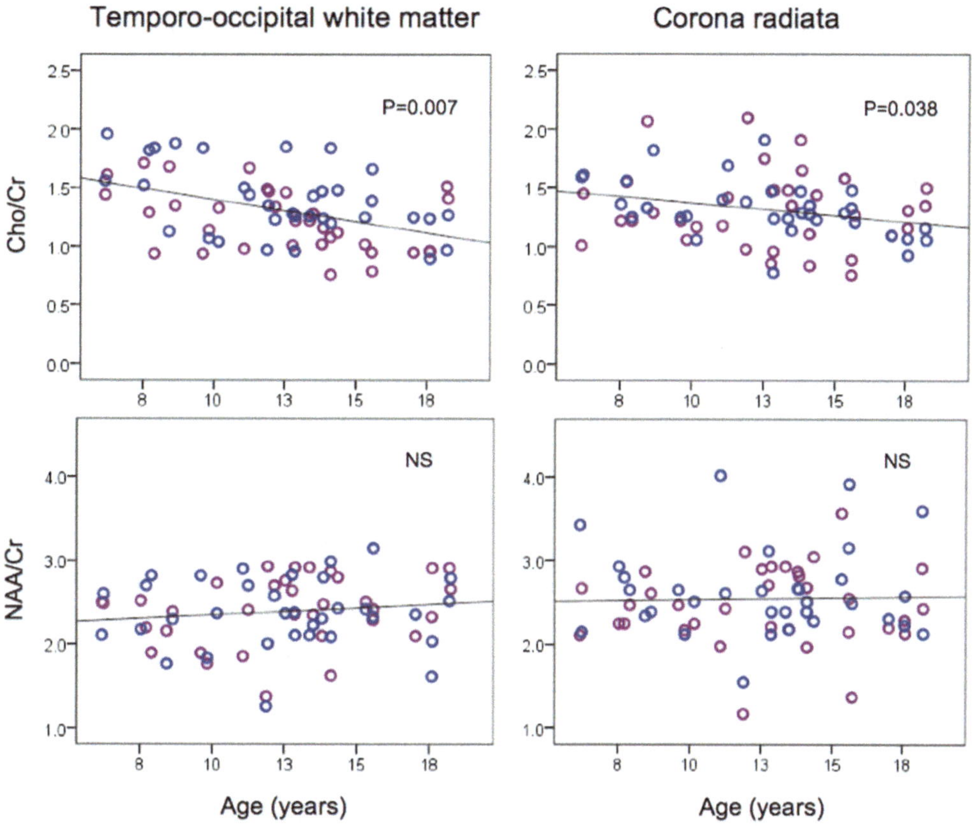

Fig. 16.4 Age-related decrease of the Cho/Cr ratio and stable NAA/Cr ratio in the temporo-occipital white matter and the corona radiata. The ¹H MRSI data were collected in a group of 37 healthy children and adolescents at 1.5 T, with repetition time of 2 s and echo time of 140 ms

nonsignificant relationship between the NAA/Cr ratio and age were detected in the temporo-occipital white matter and the corona radiata (Horska et al. unpublished results).

In the *basal ganglia*, the concentrations of Cho, Cr, NAA, Ins, Glu, and Gln were stable from infancy to adulthood [132]. In the *thalamus*, a slight increase in total NAA concentration during childhood and adolescence was observed at a short TE [132] while no effect of age on metabolite concentrations or the NAA/Cho ratio was detected in a long TE study including a smaller number of subjects [74].

In the *cerebellum*, mean NAA levels were slightly higher in older children and adolescents compared to infants and younger children [132]. A decrease in mean Ins concentration from infancy to adulthood was also detected [132].

While morphologic MRI studies reported differences in brain sizes and developmental trajectories between boys and girls, no sex-related differences in metabolite levels were detected in most of the MRS studies discussed above, likely due to both limited sample sizes and cross-sectional design. However, the study by Kadota et al. found a faster increase in white matter NAA/Cho ratio with age in boys than in girls [81]. Regarding left–right differences, the same study also reported a higher white matter NAA/Cho ratio in the right hemisphere compared with the left hemisphere in children and adolescents [81]. In an older age group of healthy controls (mean age 29.6±5.3 years), ¹H MRSI performed at 1.5 T did not detect any differences between male and female subjects in Cho, Cr, and NAA concentrations and metabolite ratios in functionally lateralized cortical regions—the hippocampal and parahippocampal gyri, thalamus, insula, Broca's and Wernicke's areas, primary and secondary visual areas, temporal, inferior, parietal, cingulate, supplemental motor, dorsolateral prefrontal, and sensorimotor areas [117]. NAA concentration was 21.9% higher in the left thalamus and 13% higher in the region contralateral to the Wernicke's area [117]. However, the study was limited to 20 controls and a younger age group was not available to determine if these left–right differences can also be detected in children and adolescents.

Studies of normal brain development demonstrated that ¹H MRS is a sensitive technique that can detect age-related differences in brain metabolism, consistent with continuing brain maturation during childhood and adolescence. Considering the importance of early detection of abnormalities in brain development that may contribute to early onset neuropsychiatric disorders, more detailed longitudinal studies of normal brain development are needed to better understand and interpret developmental metabolic trajectories in patient populations. The focus of future studies may also be on regional age-related changes in concentrations of neurotransmitters implied in psychiatric disorders, such as Glu and GABA.

Metabolic Correlates of Neuropsychological Performance in Healthy Children and Adolescents

^{1}H MRS has been used to study cognitive processes in neurological and neuropsychiatric disorders [140]. Studies in typically developing children and adolescents can improve our understanding of localization of specific cognitive functions.

In the *frontal lobe*, a ^{1}H MRSI study (1.5 T, TR/TE=2 s/140 ms) in 51 healthy boys and girls 6–18 years old identified a positive relationship between frontal white matter NAA/Cr ratio and performance on two neuropsychological tests associated with frontal lobe function [122]. Positive correlations between the NAA/Cr ratio in the left frontal white matter and the performance on the Purdue Pegboard right hand scores (a test of manual dexterity and speed) and between the NAA/Cr ratio in the right frontal white matter and Stanford-Binet-IV Bead Memory scores (a test of visual working memory) were detected. No significant relationship between the test scores and frontal gray matter NAA/Cr ratios was observed [122]. In a group of 20 normal developing 24 boys 7–12 years old [176], NAA and Cr concentrations in right frontal white matter positively correlated with working memory skills assessed by the Visual Two-Back Memory Test. Since no significant correlations between the MRS measures and the Visual Temporal Order Memory Test and estimated full-scale IQ were detected, it was concluded that the results may be specific to visual working memory. The ^{1}H MRS study was performed at 1.5 T with TR/TE=1.5 s/30 ms [176].

In the *medial temporal lobe,* NAA/Cho ratio was positively correlated with performance on several memory variables (learning, immediate recall, face–name recognition) and negatively correlated with long-term memory loss; modified version of the Auditory Verbal Learning test and a face–name memory task were used in the experiments. No significant relationship between NAA/Cho ratio and global intelligence assessed by Wechsler intelligence scales was detected [60].

In the $^{31}P/^{1}H$ MRSI study evaluating gray matter, white matter, and deep brain nuclei in one slice at the *level of the basal ganglia* [65], mean NAA concentration was correlated only with the visual–spatial construction domain, while mean phosphocreatine levels (and also gray matter volumes) showed significant correlations with language, visual–spatial construction, and memory domains. Composite scores were used in the correlation analyses; for the Visual Spatial cognitive domain, Wechsler Block Design, Visual Motor Integration Test, and Test of Visual Perception were used. The results of this study suggest that, in some instances, phosphocreatine concentration (measured by ^{31}P MRS) may be a more sensitive biomarker of neurocognitive development than NAA.

Neuropsychiatric Disorders of Childhood and Adolescence

A critical skill underlying multiple childhood psychopathologies is the ability to control behaviors that conflict with societal norms [108]. This "self-regulatory control" is crucial for a child's progressive ability to organize behaviors, thoughts, and emotions in order to attain goals [11, 131]. Early disturbance to the maturation of self-regulatory control skills can contribute to the development of a variety of childhood psychiatric disorders—especially those involving atypical behavioral, emotional, and cognitive regulation [154]. There is evidence suggesting that the neural substrate underlying these skills is supported by a disturbed neural network with cortical and subcortical components including the frontal cortex and its striatal-thalamic-cerebellar connections [42].

Anomalous early development of fronto-striatal-cerebellar circuitry in children is associated with onset of atypical behaviors, including those involving insufficient self-regulation (e.g., *Attention Deficit/Hyperactivity Disorder (ADHD), Tourette syndrome, Bipolar Disorder*) [141], excessive self-regulation (e.g., *Anorexia Nervosa, Autism Spectrum Disorders*), or both (e.g., *Obsessive Compulsive Disorder, Childhood Schizophrenia, Bulimia Nervosa*) [108].

Current neurological models of frontal system structure and function have their basis in a well-described series of at least five parallel frontal-subcortical circuits [42], of which two are related to motor function, originating in supplementary motor area (skeletomotor) and frontal eye fields (oculomotor) regions of the cortex; the other three, originating in dorsolateral prefrontal, anterior cingulate, and lateral orbitofrontal cortices, are thought to be crucial in cognitive ("executive") and socioemotional self-regulation. Frontal projections to the basal ganglia and cerebellum form a series of frontal-striatal-thalamo-frontal (Fig. 16.5) and frontal-cerebello-frontal circuits (Fig. 16.6) [94]. These circuits link specific regions of the frontal lobes to subcortical structures, supply modality-specific mechanisms for interaction with the environment, and provide the framework for understanding the neurobiological relationship among different childhood psychiatric disorders [108]. There are major periods of gain in self-regulatory skills that are thought to correspond to periods of myelination and maturation of the prefrontal cortex and frontal-striatal brain systems [17]. The frontal systems that support executive function have a protracted period of development [162] and are vulnerable to disruption via a variety of etiologies. This is likely why so many children who develop childhood psychiatric disorders present behavioral difficulties involving insufficient or excessive self-regulation.

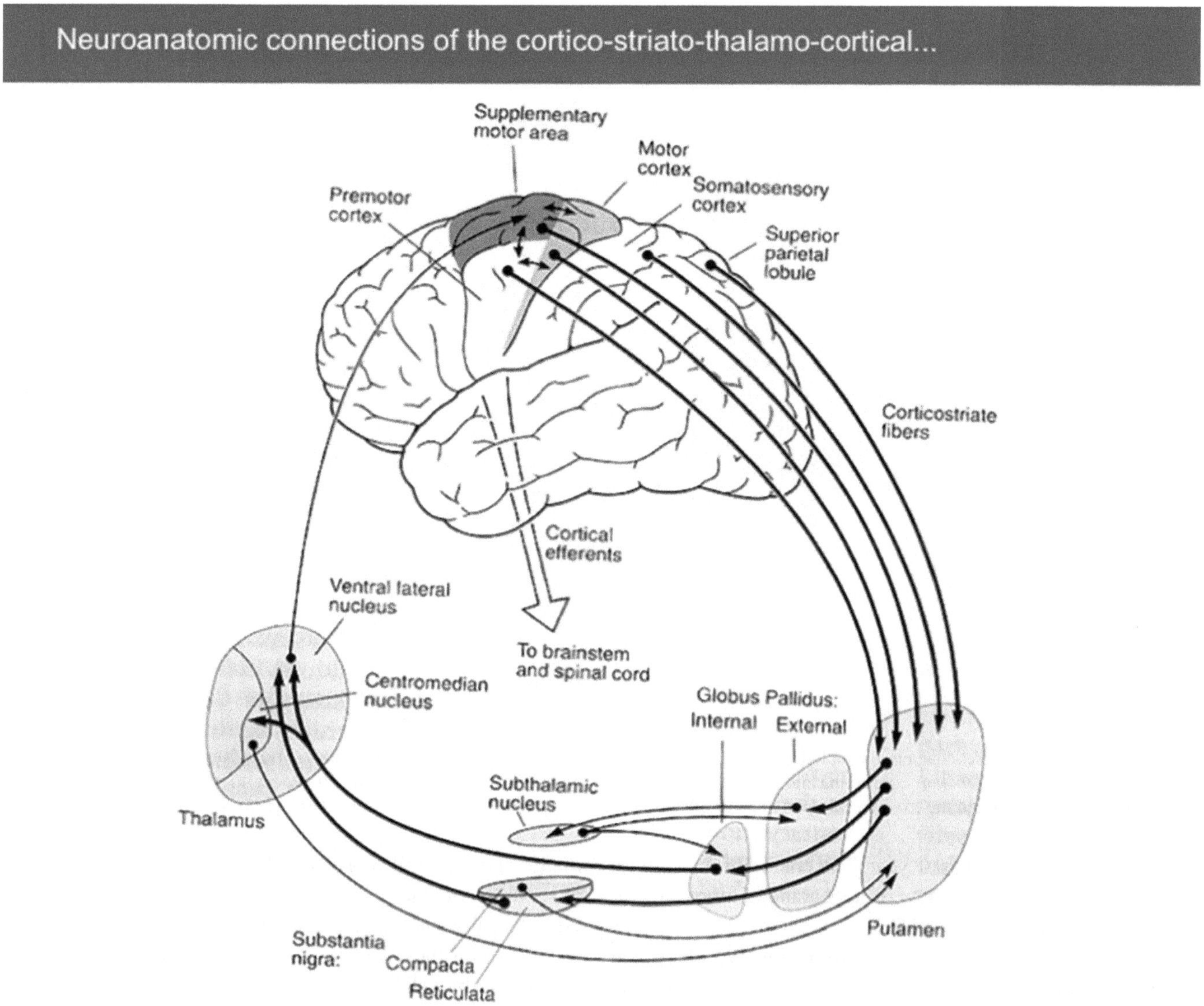

Fig. 16.5 The prefrontal portions of cortico–striato–thalamo–cortical circuits project to specific regions of the striatum, which, in turn, project directly or indirectly to specific regions of the internal segment of the globus pallidus and the substantia nigra pars reticulata. These nuclei then project to the thalamus, which closes the loop by projecting back to the cortex. In each circuit, information flows predominantly through either a direct or an indirect pathway, both of which are modulated by dopamine. (From Rostain AL, *Frontal Lobe Disorders in Pediatric Neuropsychology: Attention-Deficit Hyperactivity Disorder and Tourette Disorder. Handbook of Medical Neuropsychology, springer 2010, with permission*

Tourette syndrome

Tourette syndrome is a childhood-onset neuropsychiatric disorder characterized by the presence of multiple chronic motor and vocal tics, commonly associated with obsessive compulsive symptoms and disturbances of attention [97, 141]. A tic is considered a sudden, rapid, involuntary, non-rhythmic repetitive movement, gesture, or vocalization that typically mimics some fragments of normal behavior. Patients with Tourette syndrome typically start presenting symptoms around the age of 4–6 years, with simple motor tics manifesting at 6–8 years of age and complex motor tics at the age of 8–10 years [141].

The formal diagnostic criteria for Tourette syndrome, as defined by the *Tourette Syndrome Classification Group* (1993) includes the following (1) onset of symptoms before age 21 years; (2) presence of multiple motor and at least one vocal tic (not necessarily concurrently); (3) waxing and waning course; (4) presence of tic symptoms for at least 1 year; (5) absence of a precipitating illness; and (6) observation of the tics by a knowledgeable individual. The *DSM-IV-TR* [1] recognizes three types of tic disorders. *Transient tic disorders* involve multiple motor and/or vocal tics, many times a day, often in bouts, lasting at least 1 month, but not more than 1 year. *Chronic motor/vocal tic disorders* are identical to transient tic disorders, except that motor *or* vocal tics (but

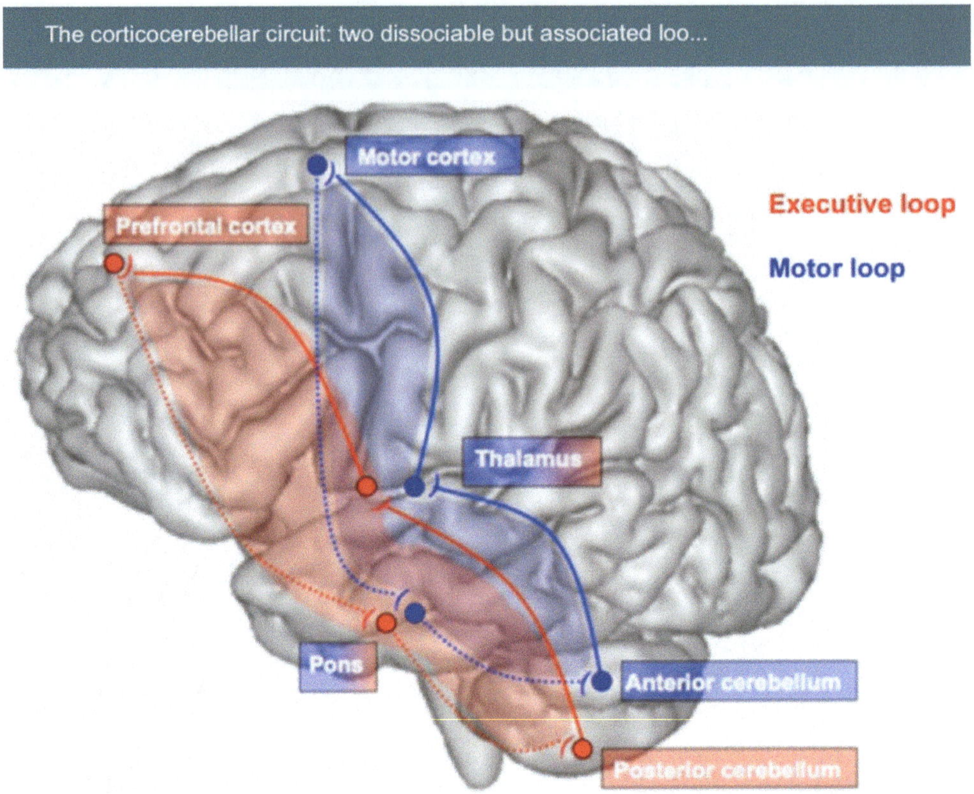

Fig. 16.6 The corticocerebellar circuit includes two dissociable but associated loops, the *motor loop* connecting motor cortex, thalamus, and anterior cerebellum and the *executive loop* connecting prefrontal-pontine-posterior cerebellar sites. (From Zahr NM, et al. *Contributions of Studies on Alcohol Use Disorders to Understanding Cerebellar Function. Neuropsychol Rev 2010 9–13, with permission*)

not both) occur for at least 1 year. The course of the disease is variable; patients may show disappearance, improvement, or worsening of symptoms [150].

Pathophysiology of Tourette syndrome involves disrupted neuronal circuits and neurotransmitter abnormalities involving the frontostriatal circuits [108, 141], limbic, and associative circuits [99]. A strong evidence supporting abnormalities of the dopaminergic and noradrenergic neurotransmission is present, although the specific mechanisms remain to be elucidated [99].

Neuroimaging techniques were applied in Tourette syndrome to assess anatomical, functional, and neurochemical aspects of this disorder. A recent comprehensive review summarized different methodologies and major findings obtained in functional neuroimaging studies (SPECT, PET, fMRI) [136]. Anatomical findings in children and adolescents with Tourette syndrome include reduced thickness of frontal and parietal cortical gray matter, most prominent in ventral portions of the sensory and motor regions. In the sensorimotor regions, cortical thickness was negatively correlated with tic severity [155]. Lower caudate and thalamic volumes were also detected [105]. Volumetric studies of Tourette syndrome are complicated, however, by the comorbidities with ADHD. For example, in children with "pure" Tourette syndrome (TS), for whom disproportionate *increases* in frontal white matter and rostral corpus callosum volume have been observed (compared to controls)—a pattern that contrasts with that observed in children with "pure" ADHD, in whom *reductions* in these regions were observed, and in children with comorbid TS and ADHD, in whom no differences with controls were observed in these regions [52]. DTI studies also revealed white matter impairment in Tourette syndrome. For example, a DTI study in 15 children with Tourette syndrome (mean age 11.6 ± 2.5 years) revealed increased ADC in the gray matter (orbitofrontal cortex bilaterally, left putamen, and left insular cortex) and white matter (corticostriatal projection pathways) compared with healthy controls [66]. Microstructural DTI-assessed abnormalities in several regions were related to tic severity and neurobehavioral scores [66, 76]. DTI also demonstrated reduced connectivity in the corpus callosum [130] and within the frontostriatothalamic circuit [105, 106].

A multislice ^{1}H MRSI study (TI/TE/TR = 230 ms/135 ms/1.8 s) performed at a head-only 3 T MRI scanner evaluated data collected in the premotor cortex, caudate head, putamen, and thalamus of 25 boys (age range 7–17 years) with Tourette syndrome and 36 age-matched healthy controls [38]. In the putamen, Cho and NAA concentrations (expressed in institutional units) were reduced in the left hemisphere and Cr levels were reduced bilaterally in the patient group. In the frontal cortex, patients had reduced NAA bilaterally, reduced Cr in the right hemisphere, and reduced Ins in the left hemisphere. No group differences in Glx were detected. Exploratory analyses also suggested lower Cr in the caudate head and in the thalamus and lower NAA in the thalamus, bilaterally. Of the examined brain regions and metabolites, the only significant relationship between metabolite levels and clinical parameters was a negative correlation between left frontal cortex Ins and duration of tic symptoms. The study results—lower cortical and subcortical NAA concentrations—are suggestive of impairment neuronal integrity or neuronal function in brain regions involved in Tourette syndrome neuropathology. Future ^{1}H MRS studies, in particular those performed at high fields may be able to assess concentrations of relevant synaptic neurotransmitters, including glutamate and GABA.

Pediatric Bipolar Disorder

Pediatric bipolar disorder is a severe and persistent, cycling mood disorder, with lifetime prevalence estimates around 1% [78, 101]. The *Diagnostic and Statistical Manual of Mental Disorders* (DSM-IV) differentiates between bipolar I disorder (patients may experience additional psychotic symptoms, such as delusions or hallucinations) while patients with bipolar II disorder have hypomanic (but not manic) episodes in addition to having one or more major depressive episodes. The course is often chronic, involving mixed symptoms and rapid changes [177]. While many of the symptoms of pediatric bipolar disorder overlap with those of childhood ADHD, the presence of mixed symptoms, severe irritability, elated mood and grandiosity, and reduced need for sleep without fatigue, more commonly associate with bipolar disorder [111]. Children with bipolar disorder also appear to display different patterns of motor dysfunction, compared to children with ADHD—the latter group showing greater impairment on basic motor speed, and children with bipolar disorder group showing dysfunction only on complex (sequenced) movements [40]. Severe irritability is a prominent mood feature in pediatric bipolar disorder than grandiosity [175], and the irritability associated with pediatric bipolar disorder has been found to be more functionally impairing than that observed in ADHD or Oppositional Defiant Disorder (ODD) [112]. Bipolar disorder in children and adolescents has unique symptoms not commonly seen in adults (ultra-rapid mood cycling or extreme irritability) and the form of the illness is usually more severe than in adult-onset bipolar disorder [170].

The neurobiological substrate of pediatric bipolar disorder occurs at the interface between affect and cognition [124], and involves neural networks subserving emotional regulation, and include frontotemporal, frontolimbic, and frontostriatal circuits [78]. Dysregulation of mood in bipolar disorder may be associated with diminished prefrontal modulation of subcortical and medial temporal structures within the anterior limbic network (amygdala, anterior striatum, and thalamus) [159]. Similarly as in adults with bipolar disorder, bipolar children and adolescents exhibit increased rates of white matter hyperintensities, most commonly in the prefrontal regions. Volumetric MRI findings were somewhat disparate but they are suggestive of global cerebral developmental abnormalities [36, 37]. Reduced gray matter density and volume associated with pediatric bipolar disorder has been observed in dorsolateral [40] and orbitofrontal [173] prefrontal cortex, anterior cingulate [82], amygdala [21], and left parietal lobe [51]. White matter changes [72], especially involving loss of white matter connectivity within frontal regions [15] also appear to be a central feature of pediatric bipolar disorder [78], and contribute to the neurobehavioral phenotype. Recently, examining resting state functional connectivity, children with bipolar disorder have been identified as having altered task-independent connectivity in fronto-temporal circuits thought to be involved in working memory and learning [39]. The cognitive deficits associated with pediatric bipolar disorder are widespread, however, and involve not only reduced IQ, memory, and learning, but also deficits in executive functions, social cognition, visuospatial skills, and verbal fluency [80].

A 4.2% decreased NAA/Cr ratio was detected in the right but not in the left *dorsolateral prefrontal cortex* in bipolar children and adolescents with parental bipolar disorder [26]. The single voxel ^{1}H MRS study was performed at 3 T, with TR/TE = 2 s/35 ms in 15 euthymic, mostly medicated bipolar patients 9–18 years old and 11 age-matched healthy controls. No differences in Cho/Cr or Ins/Cr ratios were observed [26]. No evidence of group differences in NAA/Cr ratios among bipolar offspring with early onset bipolar disorder ($N=32$, mean age 14.1 ± 3.0 years), bipolar offspring with prodromal symptoms of bipolar disorder ($N=28$, mean age 12.2 ± 2.6 years), and healthy children ($N=26$, mean age 14.2 ± 2.8 years) were detected in a larger study by the same group [54]. While these results do not suggest impairment in neuronal function or integrity in the dorsolateral prefrontal cortex in previously treated children with early onset bipolar disorder, in another single voxel ^{1}H MRS study performed at 1.5 T with TR/TM/TE = 1.5 s/13.6 ms/20 ms in 14 patients with bipolar disorder (mean age 15.5 ± 3 years) in the left dorsolateral prefrontal cortex, a 6.8% lower NAA concentration was detected compared with a control group [146]. Cr and Cho concentrations were within normal values. The study included patients with any subtype of bipolar disorder and at any mood state. Patients with a larger number of previous affective episodes had lower Cho concentrations, which were explained as potential presence of neurodegenerative processes in the prefrontal cortex [146]. In 28 adolescents with bipolar disorder with a depressed episode (mean age 15 ± 1.5 years), concentrations of Cho, Cr, NAA, Ins, and Glx in the left and right ventral lateral prefrontal cortex and concentrations of NAA, Ins, and Glx in the anterior cingulate were higher in patients compared with a control group of healthy adolescents [125, 127]. The study results were interpreted as abnormal brain neurometabolism; however, effects of differences in tissue composition of the spectroscopic voxel, mainly presence of CSF may be considered for explanation of the increase in the concentrations of all metabolites. While all patients were medication free at the time of the study, they were treated previously with psychotropic mediations. The patients were involved in a study of lithium treatment as described below [125–127]. A ^{1}H MRSI study (1.5 T, TR/TE = 1.5 s/272 ms) mapped Cho, Cr, and NAA concentrations in the medial prefrontal cortex, dorsolateral prefrontal cortex, anterior and posterior cingulate, and occipital lobes in a group of 43 children and adolescents with bipolar disorder type I or II (mean age 13.2 ± 2.9 years) and 38 age-matched healthy controls [22]. Some patients had presence of comorbidities including ADHD and anxiety disorders; 12% of patients were not medicated at the time of study. Overall, concentrations of all detected metabolites tended to be lower in the patients, bilaterally, in the medial prefrontal cortex, and the dorsolateral prefrontal regions. Significantly lower NAA concentration was detected in the left and right medial prefrontal cortex and left dorsolateral prefrontal white matter in the patient group. The differences in NAA concentration were in the range from 8.4 to 17.1%. In patients, Cr concentration was lower in the right medial prefrontal cortex and the left dorsolateral prefrontal white matter and Cho concentration was decreased in the medial prefrontal cortex, bilaterally. A previous single voxel MRS study by the same group detected a 3.3% lower NAA concentration in the left dorsolateral prefrontal cortex in pediatric bipolar patients (mean age 13.7 ± 2.6 years) compared with controls [121]. In the subsequent MRSI study, no group differences were detected in the left and right dorsolateral prefrontal gray matter, anterior and posterior cingulate, and the occipital lobe. The results of reduced NAA and Cr concentrations are suggestive of underdevelopment of frontal regions involved in neuropathology of bipolar disorder [22].

In 11 children and adolescents 7–17 years old diagnosed with bipolar disorder, ^{1}H MRS (1.5 T; TR/TE = 3 s/30 ms) of the *anterior cingulate cortex* was performed before and after treatment with lithium [31]. The diagnoses included mixed type and type II bipolar disorder and comorbidities with other neuropsychiatric diseases were also present. The Ins/Cr ratio tended to be higher in bipolar children compared with controls; no other group differences in other detected metabolites were found. Lithium therapy resulted in reduction of the Ins/Cr ratio [31]. Comparison of Ins levels among patients with bipolar disorder type I (6–13 years old; $N = 10$), intermittent explosive disorder (7–15 years old; $N = 10$), and a control group of healthy children and adolescents (mean age 11.7 ± 3.6 years; $N = 13$) revealed a significantly higher anterior cingulate Ins/Cr and Ins concentration in bipolar patients, seven of whom were in the manic phase at the time of scan, compared with both healthy controls and patients with intermittent explosive disorder [32]. Not all patients included in the study were medication naïve. No metabolic differences among groups were detected in a control region, the occipital cortex. Elevated anterior cingulate Ins concentration, by 15.5% on average, was also reported in 9 children 8–12 years old with a mood disorder and at least one parent with bipolar disorder [24]. All children were in the euthymic phase, most were nonmedicated, and five patients had comorbidities with other neuropsychiatric disorders. No group differences in concentrations of NAA, Cr, and Cho were detected. The single voxel MRS study was performed at 1.5 T with TR/TE = 2 s/35 ms in the *anterior cingulate, frontal white matter, and cerebellar vermis*. A trend to lower NAA and Cr concentration was detected in the vermis in patients; no group differences were observed in the frontal white matter [24]. Although the above studies were accomplished with a relatively small number of patients with potential confounding effects of medication and other comorbidities, the results suggest that elevated Ins in the anterior cingulate may be a biological marker for juvenile-onset bipolar disorder [24, 31, 32], considering that Ins concentrations in adult patients with bipolar disorder were reported to be lower or equal to healthy controls [30, 53, 147, 149].

In ten previously treated children with bipolar disorder, 6–12 years old, a higher Glx/Cr ratio in the *frontal lobe* (by 89%) and in the *basal ganglia* (by 98%) was detected after 1 week of drug washout period, compared with a control group [23]. The frontal voxel was centered at the forceps minor white matter and the basal ganglia voxel at the external capsule/insula. The experiments were performed at 1.5 T with TR/TE = 1.5 s/135 ms, a TE not optimal for Glx assessment [23]. In medicated and nonmedicated children and adolescents with bipolar disorder (and other comorbid diagnoses), single voxel ^{1}H MRS at 4 T (TR/TE = 2 s/30 ms) detected lower Gln levels in the anterior cingulate in nonmedicated patients ($N = 6$), by 40.4% compared with stable patients taking medication ($N = 15$) and by 39.5% compared with healthy controls ($N = 10$) [116]. No differences in Glu concentrations were detected among the three groups. It was concluded that abnormal Gln may represent glial pathology of the anterior cingulate cortex in untreated patients in a manic state [116].

^{1}H MRS was successfully applied in follow-up studies that examined the effects of *lithium treatment* on brain metabolism. The first study in pediatric bipolar patients evaluating the effect of lithium treatment on Ins concentrations was the above-mentioned study by Davanzo et al. that detected a 24.9% reduction in the anterior cingulate Ins/Cr ratio after one week of lithium therapy [31]. In contrast, in 28 currently depressed adolescents with bipolar I disorder, no differences in Ins concentration in the medial anterior cingulate cortex, right and left forceps minor were detected between baseline (before lithium treatment) and on the 7th and 42th day of treatment [126]. However, in the anterior cingulate and the right frontal white matter, the mean Ins concentration at day 42 was higher than on day 7 in both regions. In a separate paper, NAA was reported to decrease between baseline and day 42 in the cingulate cortex only [125, 127]. The single voxel ¹H MRS study was performed at 1.5 T with TR/TE = 2 s/35 ms [125–127].

Using the same technical approach and the same regions of interest as the study by Patel et al [126],. the effects of *olanzapine treatment* on frontal NAA levels in 20 adolescents 12–18 years old with bipolar disorder type I, presenting with a manic or mixed episode, were examined at baseline and on the 7th and 28th day of treatment [36, 37]. In successfully treated patients, remission resulted in an increase in anterior cingulate NAA concentration between the baseline and the end point, suggestive of improved neuronal function, while in nonremitters, NAA concentration decreased. Results of Cho analyses included higher baseline Cho concentrations in the anterior cingulate cortex in successfully treated patients and increase in Cho concentration in the anterior cingulate and right forceps minor between baseline and day 7 in manic patients [36, 37]. No effect of *divalproex* on Cho/Cr, NAA/Cr, or Ins/Cr metabolite ratios in the left and right dorsolateral prefrontal cortex was detected after 12 weeks of treatment in 24 children with mood dysregulation but not a fully developed bipolar disorder [27].

In a group of 15–30-year-old *subjects at high risk for type I or II bipolar disorder*, from families with multiple affected members, ¹H MRS (1.5 T, TR/TE = 2 s/30 ms) was performed in the left and right dorsal medial prefrontal and ventromedial prefrontal cortices [70]. No differences in Ins, Cho, Cr, and NAA concentrations were detected between the high-risk affected and unaffected subjects in the analyses including up to 71 subjects in total (21 unaffected, 19 affected, 31 controls). The unaffected group comprised individuals with no lifetime history of psychiatric disorders while the high-risk affected group included offspring who met the criteria for a lifetime diagnosis of mood disorder [70]. The lack of difference in Ins, Cho, Cr, and NAA concentrations in the high-risk group in the medial prefrontal cortex (anterior cingulate) was confirmed in a recent study of children and adolescents, 9–18 years old, at high risk for bipolar disorder [151]. In addition, Glu concentration tended to be lower in offspring with established history of mania ($N = 20$) compared with participants with symptoms subsyndromal to mania ($N = 20$) and healthy controls ($N = 20$). While the subjects in the control group were not previously exposed to psychotropic medication, most of the subjects in the mania groups had previously taken psychotropic medication. The study was performed at 3 T, with TR/TE = 2 s/35 ms [151]. The lack of abnormal findings in Glu, Ins, Cho, Cr, and NAA early in the course of the disease suggests that MRS-detected abnormalities in these metabolites in patient populations may be related to mood state, treatments, or comorbid psychiatric disorders. Altered Glu metabolism in the frontal lobe appears to occur only after full development of mania and does not seem to be associated solely with familiar risk [151]. In a group of 22 children and adolescents (mean age 13.3. ± 2.8 years) with a familial risk for type I or II bipolar disorder, a 3 T ¹H MRS study (TR/TE = 2 s/35 ms) by the same group detected a 12.4% lower Ins and a 14.9% lower Cho concentration in the cerebellar vermis compared with 25 healthy age-matched controls [152]. Low Ins concentration in the vermis was interpreted as possibly associated with altered cellular signaling via second messenger pathways, impairment in regulation of neuronal osmolarity or abnormal metabolism of membrane-bound phospholipids. Low Cho concentration was attributed to disruption in cell membrane synthesis, maintenance, and repair [152].

⁷Li MRS was applied to measure Li concentrations in a group of 9 children and adolescents (mean age 13.4 ± 3.6 years) and in young adults ($N = 18$; mean age 37.3 ± 9.1 years) [115]. Concentrations of Li in the brain and in the serum were positively correlated and the brain-to-serum concentration ratio was positively correlated with age. The group of children and adolescents had a 37% lower brain-to-serum concentration ratio compared with adults, suggesting that younger patients may need higher maintenance serum Li concentrations than adults to reach therapeutic Li concentrations in the brain [115].

In summary, neurochemical abnormalities in pediatric bipolar disorder appear to be localized mainly in the frontal lobes and frontal circuitry (anterior cingulate and dorsolateral prefrontal cortex) and the cerebellar vermis. Future research on neurochemistry and metabolism in pediatric bipolar disorder may be directed at studies of processes mediating emotional development and mood regulation and evaluations of the effects of mood-stabilizing medications.

Obsessive Compulsive Disorder

Obsessive Compulsive Disorder (OCD) involves recurrent patterns of intrusive thoughts (obsessions) that are often accompanied by repetitive acts (compulsions) (2000). There appears to be a bimodal age of onset of OCD, with onset in childhood occurring around 10–12 years [169]. OCD commonly co-occurs with other childhood disorders associated with anomalous frontostriatal development, including ADHD in 10–33% [109] and Tourette syndrome in approximately one-third [68]. OCD is associated with atypical structure and function of the fronto-striatal circuitry, but perhaps in manner distinct from ADHD and Tourette syndrome. Structural brain changes including regional increases and decreases have been observed over the course of childhood OCD [142], although the preponderance of evidence suggests disruption to fronto-striatal circuitry, particularly those involving the orbitofrontal cortex, anterior cingulate, and striatum [5, 108, 133]. Recent shape analysis among individuals with OCD highlights frontostriatal *deformation*, involving shortening of the anterior–posterior dimension of the frontal lobes and basal ganglia, with enlargement of the cerebrospinal fluid spaces near the frontal opercula [134]. Functional imaging studies highlighting reduced activation of the lateral orbitofrontal cortex during tasks requiring mental flexibility among individuals with OCD and their unaffected siblings, suggesting a possible endophenotype [25]. Morphometric MRI, MRS, and DTI studies in OCD provided evidence that gray matter abnormalities are complemented by white matter alterations [50].

Several MRS studies reported data in the *thalamus*. Lower NAA/(Cho + Cr) and NAA/Cho ratios in the medial but not in the lateral thalami were detected with ^{1}H MRSI at 1.5 T (TR/TE = 2.3 s/272 ms) in 8 medication-naïve 8–15-year-old OCD patients compared with a control group [49]. The NAA ratios tended to be more abnormal on the right side; however, only the NAA/Cho ratio in the left medial thalamus was inversely correlated with obsessive (but not compulsive) subscale scores in the patients. A later quantitative MRSI study by the same group including 11 patients explained these findings by a 23.8% and 25.5% higher Cho concentration in the right and left medial thalami, respectively. No group differences in NAA and Cr concentrations and Cho concentrations in the left thalami were found [137]. Two additional papers by the same group reported, first, Cho [153] and, later, Cr concentrations [114] in a group of 27 psychotropic medication-naïve OCD patients 7–16 years old; the papers did not present results on NAA concentrations. Medial thalamic Cho [153] and Cr concentrations [114] were higher bilaterally in the psychotropic medication-naïve OCD patients compared with healthy controls and with pediatric patients with major depressive disorder. Interpretations of the findings included possible disruptions in myelination [153] and in energy metabolism in the medial thalami [114].

In the *dorsolateral prefrontal cortex*, NAA was elevated while Cho and Cr levels were within normal values [143]. A ^{1}H MRSI acquired with the same parameters as the study of the thalamus [49] reported a 20.8% higher NAA concentration in the left but not the right dorsolateral prefrontal cortex in 15 psychotropic mediation-naïve 8–15-year-old OCD patients, compared with controls. These findings may represent neuronal hypertrophy or hyperplasia, reduced glial cell density, or abnormal synaptic/dendritic pruning [143]. As discussed in the paper, the observed laterality in the dorsolateral prefrontal cortex, pointing to an involvement of the left hemisphere in OCD, was in agreement with previous findings of dysregulations of left hemispheric cortical neural networks and may be specific for OCD [143].

Neuroimaging studies provided evidence for the hypothesis of *impaired glutamate neurotransmission* in the frontal–striatal–thalamic model of pediatric OCD [104]. A single voxel 1.5 T MRS study detected a 19% larger Glx concentration (expressed as ratio to the water concentration) in the *left caudate* in medication-naïve OCD patients 11 ± 3 years old, compared with controls; no significant differences were detected in Cho, NAA, and Ins concentrations while Cr tended to be increased in patients. Glx levels normalized after 12 weeks of treatment with paroxetine [138]. No changes in Glx concentration (and concentrations of Cho, Cr, NAA, and Ins) in the left caudate was detected in 21 pediatric OCD patients 6–16 years old after 12–16 weeks of cognitive-behavioral therapy, despite improvement in OCD symptoms [12].

A 15% lower Glx concentration was reported in the *anterior cingulate* region in medication-naïve pediatric OCD patients 10–19 years old without major depressive disorder compared with controls [139]. However, the mean anterior cingulate Glx levels were not different between patients with OCD and with major depressive disorder [139]. Glx reduction in anterior cingulate in OCD is different from findings in other childhood neuropsychiatric disorders: elevated Glx was detected in the anterior cingulate in schizophrenia [165] and in medication-naïve children with bipolar disorder [23] and ADHD [103]. No differences in Glx concentrations or concentrations of other metabolites were detected in the occipital cortex, in a separate group of OCD patients [138]. Evidence is emerging that the Glx neurochemical pattern in childhood OCD may be related to genetic variation [2].

While ^{1}H MRS demonstrated abnormal neurometabolism in several cortical regions, OCD pathophysiology involves broader disruption of brain systems and networks. Morphometric MRI and DTI studies detected abnormalities in white matter adjacent to the frontostriatal regions, corpus callosum, deep white matter, and parietal white matter in pediatric and adult OCD (reviewed in [50]). ^{1}H MRS also detected elevated Cho/Cr in the parietal white matter in previously treated adolescents and young adults with OCD [91]. Thus, future ^{1}H MRS studies may consider including white matter in addition to evaluating specific brain regions of the cortico-striato-thalamo-cortical circuit involved in the complex pathology of OCD.

Childhood Schizophrenia

Schizophrenia is a severe, debilitating, psychiatric disorder that occurs in approximately 1% of adults, with typical onset in the third decade of life. In contrast, early onset schizophrenia (EOS), including childhood-onset (before age 12), and, to a lesser extent, adolescent-onset (between ages 13 and 18) is more rare (less than 1/10,000 and ~14/10,000 respectively), and is considered to reflect a more neurodevelopmental condition [164, 171]. Diagnosis of EOS is considered valid and reliable using the same diagnostic criteria as used for adults [144]. The symptoms manifest in multiple behavioral domains, with delusions (false beliefs that are held in the face of evidence to the contrary) and hallucinations (false sensory perceptions in a conscious and awake state in the absence of external stimuli) as the most typical symptoms. Individuals with schizophrenia may also present with social and cognitive deficits, and with motor and volitional abnormalities [90]. When diagnosed in childhood, EOS shows a stable pattern of behaviors over time [73] and is associated with greater overall disease severity than schizophrenia diagnosed in adulthood [119].

Schizophrenia is viewed as a neurodevelopmental disorder [107]; however, the specific neurobiological deficits and time of onset of maturational deviations are still unknown [29, 87, 157]. Structural MRI detected reduction in overall cerebral volume and in gray matter [56, 57, 163], enlargement of ventricles [56, 57, 96, 135], and white matter structural and growth abnormalities [41, 64]. Compared to adult patients with schizophrenia, the extent of gray and white matter abnormalities is more widespread in EOS, due to a delayed and altered time course of developmental trajectories [41]. Involvement of parietal lobes precedes changes in the temporal and frontal lobes [163]. Underlying neuropathology may include excessive pruning of the prefrontal corticocortical, and corticosubcortical synapses, possibly involving the excitatory glutamatergic inputs to pyramidal neurons [84]. Consistent with excessive synaptic pruning is the reduction in the neuropil in the prefrontal cortex [148].

^{1}H MRS results in COS are in agreement with the theory of a common pathophysiological process specifically affecting mesial temporal-limbic and prefrontal circuitries, as the most common ^{1}H MRS findings in patients with COS include *reduced NAA levels in frontal and temporal brain regions*. A 13% lower NAA/Cr ratio in the left frontal lobe was detected in 16 children (mean age 11.0 ± 1.7 years) with schizophrenia-spectrum disorders, i.e., with some or all symptoms of schizophrenia present compared with a control group [18]. A single voxel 1.5 T ^{1}H MRS study of medial frontal gray matter (TR/TE = 1.5 s/20 ms) detected a 32% reduction in mean NAA/Cr in 13 children and adolescents with schizophrenia (mean age 14 ± 3 years; all patients were medicated), compared with healthy controls [161]. A later ^{1}H MRSI study from the same group explained this finding by higher Cr concentration; a 14.3% higher Cr was detected in the superior anterior cingulate [120]. The study was performed at 1.5 T with TR/TE = 2.3 s/272 ms. NAA, Cho, and Cr concentrations were measured in the superior and inferior anterior cingulate cortex, frontal, parietal, and occipital cortices, head and body of the caudate nucleus, putamen, thalamus, and frontal and parietal white matter 11 in children and adolescents with schizophrenia (mean age 12.3 ± 3.8 years; most patients were medicated) [120]. Of the examined brain regions, the only significant difference in mean NAA concentration between patients and controls was an 11% lower NAA concentration in the left *parietal cortex* [120]. Another ^{1}H MRSI study performed at 1.5 T with TR/TE = 2.2 s/272 ms in 14 patients with COS (mean age 16.4 years) detected bilaterally lower NAA/Cr in the dorsolateral prefrontal cortex and the hippocampus [13]. The NAA/Cr ratios were not correlated with the volumes of the prefrontal lobe and the hippocampus, suggesting that metabolic impairment was not associated with a reduction in tissue volume. NAA levels were also not correlated with the length of illness, suggesting that NAA was not related to progressive pathology [13]. In a single voxel MRS study performed at 1.5 T with TR/TE = 1.5 s/136 ms [178], lower NAA/water ratio (by 10% and 11%, respectively) was detected in the left dorsolateral prefrontal region in 8 adolescents (mean age 15.6 ± 2.1 years) with first-episode schizophrenia with a short illness duration of 14 weeks on average, compared with nonschizophrenia patients with a first episode of psychosis and healthy controls. Normal ratios were detected in the right hemisphere [178]. Normal NAA levels in COS were detected in the thalamus, putamen, caudate, superior temporal gyrus, orbitofrontal cortex, anterior and posterior cingulate, occipital cortex, frontal and parietal white matter [13, 120, 161].

Recent meta-analyses of ^{1}H MRS studies in schizophrenia concluded that NAA reductions in the frontal lobe, temporal lobe, and the thalamus are well documented by literature data [19, 158]. Literature data did not suggest an evidence of differences between first-episode schizophrenia patients and patients with chronic disease [19, 158]. Reductions in NAA may suggest "alterations of neuronal homeostasis, consistent with increasing evidence for the role of NAA in synaptic maintenance, myelination, regulation of cellular osmolarity, and neuronal metabolism" [29]. While MRS findings in COS in some studies are similar to results obtained in adult patients with schizophrenia, other reports finding normal NAA levels in regions including the frontal and temporal lobes in COS [13, 120] suggest that neuronal impairment may develop later in the course of the disease.

In adult schizophrenia patients, *Cho levels* are variable in different brain regions [6, 20, 35, 43, 44]. In COS, no differences in the Cho/Cr ratios between patients and controls were detected by MRSI in cortical and subcortical regions [13]. Normal Cho/water and Cr/water ratios were also reported in the dorsolateral prefrontal cortex [178]. However, one study detected higher Cho concentration in the superior anterior cingulate (by 30.3%), frontal cortex (by 13.3%), and in the caudate (by 13.5%) compared with a control group [120].

Impairment of the Glu–Gln cycle between neurons and astrocytes may contribute to cognitive decline in schizophrenia [93]. ^{1}H MRS, in particular performed at higher magnetic fields, is a highly suitable technique for evaluation of the *glutamatergic metabolism*, implied in schizophrenia [46, 83, 102]. However, compared to number of publications on glutamatergic metabolism in adult schizophrenia [113], studies on neurotransmitters in COS are limited. An early study performed at 1.5 T did not detect any difference in the frontal Glx/Cr ratio but reported a trend to lower occipital Glx/Cr in children and adolescents with schizophrenia, compared with controls [161].

By evaluating if metabolic changes can be detected before the onset of symptoms of schizophrenia, MRS may help to assess risk *factors for development of the schizophrenia*. It has been documented that young relatives at high risk for schizophrenia have neurobehavioral deficits and structural, physiological, and neurochemicals brain abnormalities in early brain development [86, 168]. Literature data suggest that lower thalamic NAA levels can differentiate individuals at risk for schizophrenia from healthy controls [19]. Both ^{1}H and ^{31}P MRS [145] have been applied to studies of children and adolescents at high genetic risk for development of schizophrenia [85, 88, 165]. Single voxel ^{1}H MRS studies at 1.5 T in a left frontal region [71] and the anterior cingulate [88] detected a trend to lower NAA/Cr and Cho/Cr ratios and NAA/Cho ratios, respectively, in children and adolescents at high risk for schizophrenia, compared with control groups of healthy participants. A 3 T single voxel study (STEAM; TR/TM/TE=3 s/30 ms/20 ms) reported a 21.5% higher mean Glx/Cr ratio in the right medial prefrontal cortex in adolescent children (mean age 16.4 years) of schizophrenia patients, possibly suggestive of neurotoxicity. No other metabolic abnormalities were detected compared with a control group [165]. A ^{1}H MRSI study (1.5 T, TR/TE=1/5 s/30 ms) of 40 participants (mean age 15.6±2.9 years) who had at least one parent diagnosed with schizophrenia or schizoaffective disorder reported lower mean NAA concentration (and also lower Cho and Cr concentrations) in the caudate nucleus in the high-risk group compared with healthy controls. NAA levels were higher in the prefrontal white matter and were within control values in the thalamus, prefrontal cortex, and temporal regions [85]. Although there was no group difference in Glu concentration, male subjects in the high-risk group had lower concentrations of Glu in the caudate compared with male counterparts in the control group [85]. While the results of the studies in children and adolescents were in support of the neurodevelopmental theory of schizophrenia, a recent study in young adults (>18 years old) did not detect any differences in NAA/Cr and Cho/Cr ratios in the medial prefrontal cortex, medial anterior cingulate cortex, and left hippocampal region among the groups of subjects at ultra-high risk for schizophrenia, first-episode patients, and healthy controls [167]. The study thus indicated that metabolic abnormalities might not always be present in the early stages of the disease.

^{31}P MRS has been used since the early studies of schizophrenia, although mostly in adult patients. By assessing compounds associated with membrane phospholipids synthesis and degradation, phosphomonoesters (PME) and phosphodiesters (PDE), and high-energy phosphate metabolism, by measuring phosphocreatine (PCr), inorganic phosphate (P_i), ATP, and ADP, ^{31}P MRS has been applied to test the membrane phospholipid hypothesis of schizophrenia [92]. Two ^{31}P MRS studies performed at 1.5 T reported elevated PDE in the frontal lobe of children and adolescents with a familial risk of developing schizophrenia [92, 145]. A ^{31}P MRS study performed bilaterally in a frontal region of 14 adolescents with a high genetic risk for schizophrenia (children and siblings of patients with schizophrenia; mean age of 16.7 years) had 19% lower PME/PDE ratio and an 8% higher mean PDE levels than the control group, suggesting increased breakdown of phospholipids [92]. The results in adolescents are consistent with findings in adults, showing reduced PME and increased PDE in drug-naïve first-episode schizophrenic patients [128]. The later study of the left and right dorsolateral prefrontal regions in 18 adolescents (mean age 16.0±2.5 years) reported a 8.5% higher mean relative levels of PDE and 13.9% lower relative levels of β-ATP in the high-risk group, with no differences between the hemispheres [145]. The main findings of increased PDE are thus similar to observation in patients with schizophrenia, suggestive of impaired metabolism of phospholipids.

In future studies, integration of ^{31}P and ^{1}H MRS into multimodal imaging assessment involving detailed assessment of neurotransmitters (GABA, Glu) and other compounds implied in the pathophysiology of schizophrenia (e.g., glutathione [174]) may help to further elucidate neurometabolic correlates of COS.

Conclusion

^{1}H MRS can detect overall metabolic abnormalities in a variety of neuropsychiatric disorders. However, due to an overlap in metabolic patterns between patients and controls, ^{1}H MRS cannot be applied as a diagnostic tool in individual patients. Similarly, the role of neuroimaging for diagnostic purposes is limited, because of absence of identifiable lesions in neuropsychiatric disorders. In the future, more specific diagnostic information in individual patients may be obtained by integrating multimodal neuroimaging with neuropsychological and genetic evaluations to obtain endophenotypes—biologic markers that are intermediate between genes and behavior [55, 89]. Endophenotypes can potentially distinguish "biologically meaningful subtypes of disorders that may respond to different interventions" [55].

Most of the discussed MRS studies in children and adolescents, typically cross-sectional in design, included limited cohorts of patients and controls. Longitudinal multimodal studies may better identify normal developmental trajectories and developmental pathways that are most sensitive to disruption [160], may help to identify patients who may be the best candidates for novel therapies, follow the course of the disease and assist with evaluation of treatment effects and outcome.

Due to inherent low sensitivity, ^{1}H MRS can detect neurochemicals at concentrations in the high micromolar to millimolar range. Several neurochemicals of interest in studies of psychiatric disorders, such as GABA, Glu, Gln, and glutathione, are difficult or impossible to measure with adequate reliability at low magnetic fields. However, studies at ultra-high fields implementing advanced MRS techniques for detection of these compounds may help to improve measurement accuracy [166]. Novel research approaches combining ultra-high field MRS with multimodal neuroimaging, biological, neuropsychological, and genetic evaluations may lead to better understanding of psychiatric disorders of childhood and adolescence.

References

1. American Psychiatric Association. Diagnostic and statistical manual of mental disorders. 4th ed. Washington, DC: American Psychiatric Association; 2000.
2. Arnold PD, Macmaster FP, Richter MA, Hanna GL, Sicard T, Burroughs E, Mirza Y, Easter PC, Rose M, Kennedy JL, Rosenberg DR. Glutamate receptor gene (GRIN2B) associated with reduced anterior cingulate glutamatergic concentration in pediatric obsessive-compulsive disorder. Psychiatry Res. 2009;172(2):136–9.
3. Arslanoglu A, Bonekamp D, Barker PB, Horska A. Quantitative proton MR spectroscopic imaging of the mesial temporal lobe. J Magn Reson Imaging. 2004;20(5):772–8.
4. Ashtari M, Cervellione KL, Hasan KM, Wu J, McIlree C, Kester H, Ardekani BA, Roofeh D, Szeszko PR, Kumra S. White matter development during late adolescence in healthy males: a cross-sectional diffusion tensor imaging study. Neuroimage. 2007;35(2):501–10.
5. Atmaca M, Yildirim H, Ozdemir H, Tezcan E, Poyraz AK. Volumetric MRI study of key brain regions implicated in obsessive-compulsive disorder. Prog Neuropsychopharmacol Biol Psychiatry. 2007;31(1):46–52.
6. Auer DP, Wilke M, Grabner A, Heidenreich JO, Bronisch T, Wetter TC. Reduced NAA in the thalamus and altered membrane and glial metabolism in schizophrenic patients detected by ^{1}H-MRS and tissue segmentation. Schizophr Res. 2001;52(1–2):87–99.
7. Bak LK, Schousboe A, Waagepetersen HS. The glutamate/GABA-glutamine cycle: aspects of transport, neurotransmitter homeostasis and ammonia transfer. J Neurochem. 2006;98(3):641–53.
8. Baker EH, Basso G, Barker PB, Smith MA, Bonekamp D, Horska A. Regional apparent metabolite concentrations in young adult brain measured by (1)H MR spectroscopy at 3 Tesla. J Magn Reson Imaging. 2008;27(3):489–99.
9. Barker P, Bizzi A, De Stefano N, Gullapalli R, Lin D. Clinical MR spectroscopy. Cambridge, UK: Cambridge University Press; 2010.
10. Barker PB, Szopinski K, Horska A. Metabolic heterogeneity at the level of the anterior and posterior commissures. Magn Reson Med. 2000;43(3):348–54.
11. Barkley RA. Behavioral inhibition, sustained attention, and executive functions: constructing a unifying theory of ADHD. Psychol Bull. 1997;121(1):65–94.
12. Benazon NR, Moore GJ, Rosenberg DR. Neurochemical analyses in pediatric obsessive-compulsive disorder in patients treated with cognitive-behavioral therapy. J Am Acad Child Adolesc Psychiatry. 2003;42(11):1279–85.
13. Bertolino A, Kumra S, Callicott JH, Mattay VS, Lestz RM, Jacobsen L, Barnett IS, Duyn JH, Frank JA, Rapoport JL, Weinberger DR. Common pattern of cortical pathology in childhood-onset and adult-onset schizophrenia as identified by proton magnetic resonance spectroscopic imaging. Am J Psychiatry. 1998;155(10):1376–83.
14. Bonekamp D, Nagae LM, Degaonkar M, Matson M, Abdalla WM, Barker PB, Mori S, Horska A. Diffusion tensor imaging in children and adolescents: reproducibility, hemispheric, and age-related differences. Neuroimage. 2007;34(2):733–42.
15. Brambilla P, Bellani M, Yeh PH, Soares JC, Tansella M. White matter connectivity in bipolar disorder. Int Rev Psychiatry. 2009;21:380–6.
16. Brand A, Richter-Landsberg C, Leibfritz D. Multinuclear NMR studies on the energy metabolism of glial and neuronal cells. Dev Neurosci. 1993;15(3–5):289–98.
17. Brocki KC, Bohlin G. Executive functions in children aged 6 to 13: a dimensional and developmental study. Dev Neuropsychol. 2004;26(2):571–93.
18. Brooks WM, Hodde-Vargas J, Vargas LA, Yeo RA, Ford CC, Hendren RL. Frontal lobe of children with schizophrenia spectrum disorders: a proton magnetic resonance spectroscopic study. Biol Psychiatry. 1998;43(4):263–9.
19. Brugger S, Davis JM, Leucht S, Stone JM. Proton magnetic resonance spectroscopy and illness stage in schizophrenia–a systematic review and meta-analysis. Biol Psychiatry. 2011;69(5):495–503.
20. Bustillo JR, Rowland LM, Lauriello J, Petropoulos H, Hammond R, Hart B, Brooks WM. High choline concentrations in the caudate nucleus in antipsychotic-naive patients with schizophrenia. Am J Psychiatry. 2002;159(1):130–3.
21. Caetano S, Olvera RL, Glahn DC, Fonseca M, Pliszka SR, Soares JC. Fronto-limbic brain abnormalities in juvenile onset bipolar disorder. Biol Psychiatry. 2005;58:525–31.
22. Caetano SC, Olvera RL, Hatch JP, Sanches M, Chen HH, Nicoletti M, Stanley JA, Fonseca M, Hunter K, Lafer B, Pliszka SR, Soares JC. Lower N-acetyl-aspartate levels in prefrontal cortices in pediatric bipolar disorder: a (1)H magnetic resonance spectroscopy study. J Am Acad Child Adolesc Psychiatry. 2011;50(1):85–94.
23. Castillo M, Kwock L, Courvoisie H, Hooper SR. Proton MR spectroscopy in children with bipolar affective disorder: preliminary observations. AJNR Am J Neuroradiol. 2000;21(5):832–8.
24. Cecil KM, DelBello MP, Sellars MC, Strakowski SM. Proton magnetic resonance spectroscopy of the frontal lobe and cerebellar vermis in children with a mood disorder and a familial risk for bipolar disorders. J Child Adolesc Psychopharmacol. 2003;13(4):545–55.
25. Chamberlain SR, Menzies L, Hampshire A, Suckling J, Fineberg NA, del Campo N, Aitken M, Craig K, Owen AM, Bullmore ET, Robbins TW, Sahakian BJ. Orbitofrontal dysfunction in patients with obsessive-compulsive disorder and their unaffected relatives. Science. 2008;321(5887):421–2.
26. Chang K, Adleman N, Dienes K, Barnea-Goraly N, Reiss A, Ketter T. Decreased N-acetylaspartate in children with familial bipolar disorder. Biol Psychiatry. 2003;53(11):1059–65.
27. Chang K, Karchemskiy A, Kelley R, Howe M, Garrett A, Adleman N, Reiss A. Effect of divalproex on brain morphometry, chemistry, and function in youth at high-risk for bipolar disorder: a pilot study. J Child Adolesc Psychopharmacol. 2009;19(1):51–9.

28. Chugani HT. A critical period of brain development: studies of cerebral glucose utilization with PET. Prev Med. 1998;27(2):184–8.
29. Dager SR, Corrigan NM, Richards TL, Posse S. Research applications of magnetic resonance spectroscopy to investigate psychiatric disorders. Top Magn Reson Imaging. 2008;19(2):81–96.
30. Dager SR, Friedman SD, Parow A, Demopulos C, Stoll AL, Lyoo IK, Dunner DL, Renshaw PF. Brain metabolic alterations in medication-free patients with bipolar disorder. Arch Gen Psychiatry. 2004;61(5):450–8.
31. Davanzo P, Thomas MA, Yue K, Oshiro T, Belin T, Strober M, McCracken J. Decreased anterior cingulate myo-inositol/creatine spectroscopy resonance with lithium treatment in children with bipolar disorder. Neuropsychopharmacology. 2001;24(4):359–69.
32. Davanzo P, Yue K, Thomas MA, Belin T, Mintz J, Venkatraman TN, Santoro E, Barnett S, McCracken J. Proton magnetic resonance spectroscopy of bipolar disorder versus intermittent explosive disorder in children and adolescents. Am J Psychiatry. 2003;160(8):1442–52.
33. de Graaf RA, Rothman DL. Detection of gamma-aminobutyric acid (GABA) by longitudinal scalar order difference editing. J Magn Reson. 2001;152(1):124–31.
34. Degaonkar MN, Pomper MG, Barker PB. Quantitative proton magnetic resonance spectroscopic imaging: regional variations in the corpus callosum and cortical gray matter. J Magn Reson Imaging. 2005;22(2):175–9.
35. Deicken RF, Johnson C, Eliaz Y, Schuff N. Reduced concentrations of thalamic N-acetylaspartate in male patients with schizophrenia. Am J Psychiatry. 2000;157(4):644–7.
36. DelBello MP, Adler CM, Strakowski SM. The neurophysiology of childhood and adolescent bipolar disorder. CNS Spectr. 2006;11(4):298–311.
37. DelBello MP, Cecil KM, Adler CM, Daniels JP, Strakowski SM. Neurochemical effects of olanzapine in first-hospitalization manic adolescents: a proton magnetic resonance spectroscopy study. Neuropsychopharmacology. 2006;31(6):1264–73.
38. DeVito TJ, Drost DJ, Pavlosky W, Neufeld RW, Rajakumar N, McKinlay BD, Williamson PC, Nicolson R. Brain magnetic resonance spectroscopy in Tourette's disorder. J Am Acad Child Adolesc Psychiatry. 2005;44(12):1301–8.
39. Dickstein D, Gorrostieta C, Ombao H, Goldberg LD, Brazel AC, Gable CJ, Kelly C, Gee DG, Zuo X-N, Castellanos FX, Milham MP. Fronto-temporal spontaneous resting state functional connectivity in pediatric bipolar disorder. Biol Psychiatry. 2010;68:839–46.
40. Dickstein D, Milham MP, Nugent AC, et al. Frontotemporal alterations in pediatric bipolar disorder: results of a voxel-based morphometry study. Arch Gen Psychiatry. 2005;62:734–41.
41. Douaud G, Mackay C, Andersson J, James S, Quested D, Ray MK, Connell J, Roberts N, Crow TJ, Matthews PM, Smith S, James A. Schizophrenia delays and alters maturation of the brain in adolescence. Brain. 2009;132(Pt 9):2437–48.
42. Durston S, van Belle J, de Zeeuw P. Differentiating frontostriatal and fronto-cerebellar circuits in attention-deficit/hyperactivity disorder. Biol Psychiatry. 2010. doi:10.1016/j.biopsych.2010.07.037.
43. Ende G, Braus DF, Walter S, Henn FA. Lower concentration of thalamic n-acetylaspartate in patients with schizophrenia: a replication study. Am J Psychiatry. 2001;158(8):1314–6.
44. Ende G, Braus DF, Walter S, Weber-Fahr W, Henn FA. Multiregional ^{1}H-MRSI of the hippocampus, thalamus, and basal ganglia in schizophrenia. Eur Arch Psychiatry Clin Neurosci. 2003;253(1):9–15.
45. Ernst M, Mueller SC. The adolescent brain: insights from functional neuroimaging research. Dev Neurobiol. 2008;68(6):729–43.
46. Farber NB, Newcomer JW, Olney JW. The glutamate synapse in neuropsychiatric disorders. Focus on schizophrenia and Alzheimer's disease. Prog Brain Res. 1998;116:421–37.
47. Fields RD. White matter in learning, cognition and psychiatric disorders. Trends Neurosci. 2008;31(7):361–70.
48. Filley CM. White matter and behavioral neurology. Ann N Y Acad Sci. 2005;1064:162–83.
49. Fitzgerald KD, Moore GJ, Paulson LA, Stewart CM, Rosenberg DR. Proton spectroscopic imaging of the thalamus in treatment-naive pediatric obsessive-compulsive disorder. Biol Psychiatry. 2000;47(3):174–82.
50. Fontenelle LF, Harrison BJ, Yucel M, Pujol J, Fujiwara H, Pantelis C. Is there evidence of brain white-matter abnormalities in obsessive-compulsive disorder?: a narrative review. Top Magn Reson Imaging. 2009;20(5):291–8.
51. Frazier J, Ahn MS, DeJong S, Bent EK, Breeze JL, Giuliano AJ. Magnetic resonance imaging studies in early onset bipolar disorder: a critical review. Harv Rev Psychiatry. 2005;13:125–40.
52. Fredericksen KA, Cutting LE, Kates WR, Mostofsky SH, Singer HS, Cooper KL, Lanham DC, Denckla MB, Kaufmann WE. Disproportionate increases of white matter in right frontal lobe in Tourette syndrome. Neurology. 2002;58:85–9.
53. Frey R, Metzler D, Fischer P, Heiden A, Scharfetter J, Moser E, Kasper S. Myo-inositol in depressive and healthy subjects determined by frontal ^{1}H-magnetic resonance spectroscopy at 1.5 tesla. J Psychiatr Res. 1998;32(6):411–20.
54. Gallelli KA, Wagner CM, Karchemskiy A, Howe M, Spielman D, Reiss A, Chang KD. N-acetylaspartate levels in bipolar offspring with and at high-risk for bipolar disorder. Bipolar Disord. 2005;7(6):589–97.
55. Giedd JN. The teen brain: insights from neuroimaging. J Adolesc Health. 2008;42(4):335–43.
56. Giedd JN, Blumenthal J, Jeffries NO, Castellanos FX, Liu H, Zijdenbos A, Paus T, Evans AC, Rapoport JL. Brain development during childhood and adolescence: a longitudinal MRI study. Nat Neurosci. 1999;2(10):861–3.
57. Giedd JN, Jeffries NO, Blumenthal J, Castellanos FX, Vaituzis AC, Fernandez T, Hamburger SD, Liu H, Nelson J, Bedwell J, Tran L, Lenane M, Nicolson R, Rapoport JL. Childhood-onset schizophrenia: progressive brain changes during adolescence. Biol Psychiatry. 1999;46(7):892–8.
58. Giedd JN, Snell JW, Lange N, Rajapakse JC, Casey BJ, Kozuch PL, Vaituzis AC, Vauss YC, Hamburger SD, Kaysen D, Rapoport JL. Quantitative magnetic resonance imaging of human brain development: ages 4–18. Cereb Cortex. 1996;6(4):551–60.
59. Giedd JN, Stockman M, Weddle C, Liverpool M, Alexander-Bloch A, Wallace GL, Lee NR, Lalonde F, Lenroot RK. Anatomic magnetic resonance imaging of the developing child and adolescent brain and effects of genetic variation. Neuropsychol Rev. 2010;20(4):349–61.
60. Gimenez M, Junque C, Narberhaus A, Caldu X, Segarra D, Vendrell P, Bargallo N, Mercader JM. Medial temporal MR spectroscopy is related to memory performance in normal adolescent subjects. Neuroreport. 2004;15(4):703–7.
61. Gimenez M, Soria-Pastor S, Junque C, Caldu X, Narberhaus A, Botet F, Bargallo N, Falcon C, Mercader JM. Proton magnetic resonance spectroscopy reveals medial temporal metabolic abnormalities in adolescents with history of preterm birth. Pediatr Res. 2008;64(5):572–7.
62. Giorgio A, Watkins KE, Chadwick M, James S, Winmill L, Douaud G, De Stefano N, Matthews PM, Smith SM, Johansen-Berg H, James AC. Longitudinal changes in grey and white matter during adolescence. Neuroimage. 2010;49(1):94–103.
63. Giorgio A, Watkins KE, Douaud G, James AC, James S, De Stefano N, Matthews PM, Smith SM, Johansen-Berg H. Changes in white matter microstructure during adolescence. Neuroimage. 2008;39(1):52–61.
64. Gogtay N, Lu A, Leow AD, Klunder AD, Lee AD, Chavez A, Greenstein D, Giedd JN, Toga AW, Rapoport JL, Thompson PM.

Three-dimensional brain growth abnormalities in childhood-onset schizophrenia visualized by using tensor-based morphometry. Proc Natl Acad Sci USA. 2008;105(41):15979–84.
65. Goldstein G, Panchalingam K, McClure RJ, Stanley JA, Calhoun VD, Pearlson GD, Pettegrew JW. Molecular neurodevelopment: an in vivo 31P-¹H MRSI study. J Int Neuropsychol Soc. 2009;15(5):671–83.
66. Govindan RM, Makki MI, Wilson BJ, Behen ME, Chugani HT. Abnormal water diffusivity in corticostriatal projections in children with Tourette syndrome. Hum Brain Mapp. 2010;31(11):1665–74.
67. Govindaraju V, Young K, Maudsley AA. Proton NMR chemical shifts and coupling constants for brain metabolites. NMR Biomed. 2000;13(3):129–53.
68. Grados MA, Mathews CA. Clinical phenomenology and phenotype variability in Tourette syndrome. J Psychosom Res. 2009;67(6):491–6.
69. Haga KK, Khor YP, Farrall A, Wardlaw JM. A systematic review of brain metabolite changes, measured with ¹H magnetic resonance spectroscopy, in healthy aging. Neurobiol Aging. 2009;30(3):353–63.
70. Hajek T, Bernier D, Slaney C, Propper L, Schmidt M, Carrey N, MacQueen G, Duffy A, Alda M. A comparison of affected and unaffected relatives of patients with bipolar disorder using proton magnetic resonance spectroscopy. J Psychiatry Neurosci. 2008;33(6):531–40.
71. Hendren RL, Hodde-Vargas J, Yeo RA, Vargas LA, Brooks WM, Ford C. Neuropsychophysiological study of children at risk for schizophrenia: a preliminary report. J Am Acad Child Adolesc Psychiatry. 1995;34(10):1284–91.
72. Heng S, Song AW, Sim K. White matter abnormalities in bipolar disorder: insights from diffusion tensor imaging studies. J Neural Transm. 2010;117:639–54.
73. Hollis C. Adult outcomes of child- and adolescent-onset schizophrenia: diagnostic stability and predictive validity. Am J Psychiatry. 2000;157(10):1652–9.
74. Horska A, Kaufmann WE, Brant LJ, Naidu S, Harris JC, Barker PB. In vivo quantitative proton MRSI study of brain development from childhood to adolescence. J Magn Reson Imaging. 2002;15(2):137–43.
75. Insel TR. Disruptive insights in psychiatry: transforming a clinical discipline. J Clin Invest. 2009;119(4):700–5.
76. Jackson SR, Parkinson A, Jung J, Ryan SE, Morgan PS, Hollis C, Jackson GM. Compensatory neural reorganization in tourette syndrome. Curr Biol. 2011;21:580–5.
77. Jacobs MA, Horska A, van Zijl PC, Barker PB. Quantitative proton MR spectroscopic imaging of normal human cerebellum and brain stem. Magn Reson Med. 2001;46(4):699–705.
78. James A, Hough M, James S, Burge L, Winmill L, Nijhawan S, Matthews PM, Zarei M. Structural brain and neuropsychometric changes associated with pediatric bipolar disorder with psychosis. Bipolar Disord. 2011;13(1):16–27.
79. Jernigan TL, Trauner DA, Hesselink JR, Tallal PA. Maturation of human cerebrum observed in vivo during adolescence. Brain. 1991;114(Pt 5):2037–49.
80. Joseph M, Frazier TW, Youngstrom EA, Soares JC. A quantitative and qualitative review of neurocognitive performance in pediatric bipolar disorder. J Child Adolesc Psychopharmacol. 2008;18:595–605.
81. Kadota T, Horinouchi T, Kuroda C. Development and aging of the cerebrum: assessment with proton MR spectroscopy. AJNR Am J Neuroradiol. 2001;22(1):128–35.
82. Kaur S, Sassi RB, Axelson D, et al. Cingulate cortex anatomical abnormalities in children and adolescents with bipolar disorder. Am J Psychiatry. 2005;162:1637–43.
83. Keshavan MS. Development, disease and degeneration in schizophrenia: a unitary pathophysiological model. J Psychiatr Res. 1999;33(6):513–21.
84. Keshavan MS, Anderson S, Pettegrew JW. Is schizophrenia due to excessive synaptic pruning in the prefrontal cortex? The Feinberg hypothesis revisited. J Psychiatr Res. 1994;28(3):239–65.
85. Keshavan MS, Dick RM, Diwadkar VA, Montrose DM, Prasad KM, Stanley JA. Striatal metabolic alterations in non-psychotic adolescent offspring at risk for schizophrenia: a (1)H spectroscopy study. Schizophr Res. 2009;115(1):88–93.
86. Keshavan MS, Diwadkar VA, Montrose DM, Rajarethinam R, Sweeney JA. Premorbid indicators and risk for schizophrenia: a selective review and update. Schizophr Res. 2005;79(1):45–57.
87. Keshavan MS, Hogarty GE. Brain maturational processes and delayed onset in schizophrenia. Dev Psychopathol. 1999;11(3):525–43.
88. Keshavan MS, Montrose DM, Pierri JN, Dick EL, Rosenberg D, Talagala L, Sweeney JA. Magnetic resonance imaging and spectroscopy in offspring at risk for schizophrenia: preliminary studies. Prog Neuropsychopharmacol Biol Psychiatry. 1997;21(8):1285–95.
89. Keshavan MS, Prasad KM, Pearlson G. Are brain structural abnormalities useful as endophenotypes in schizophrenia? Int Rev Psychiatry. 2007;19(4):397–406.
90. Kinros J, Reichenberg A, Frangou S. The neurodevelopmental theory of schizophrenia: evidence from studies of early onset cases. Isr J Psychiatry Relat Sci. 2010;47(2):110–7.
91. Kitamura H, Shioiri T, Kimura T, Ohkubo M, Nakada T, Someya T. Parietal white matter abnormalities in obsessive-compulsive disorder: a magnetic resonance spectroscopy study at 3-Tesla. Acta Psychiatr Scand. 2006;114(2):101–8.
92. Klemm S, Rzanny R, Riehemann S, Volz HP, Schmidt B, Gerhard UJ, Filz C, Schonberg A, Mentzel HJ, Kaiser WA, Blanz B. Cerebral phosphate metabolism in first-degree relatives of patients with schizophrenia. Am J Psychiatry. 2001;158(6):958–60.
93. Kondziella D, Brenner E, Eyjolfsson EM, Sonnewald U. How do glial-neuronal interactions fit into current neurotransmitter hypotheses of schizophrenia? Neurochem Int. 2007;50(2):291–301.
94. Krause KH, Dresel SH, Krause J, Kung HF, Tatsch K. Increased striatal dopamine transporter in adult patients with attention deficit hyperactivity disorder: effects of methylphenidate as measured by single photon emission computed tomography. Neurosci Lett. 2000;285(2):107–10.
95. Kreis R, Ernst T, Ross BD. Development of the human brain: in vivo quantification of metabolite and water content with proton magnetic resonance spectroscopy. Magn Reson Med. 1993;30(4):424–37.
96. Kumra S, Giedd JN, Vaituzis AC, Jacobsen LK, McKenna K, Bedwell J, Hamburger S, Nelson JE, Lenane M, Rapoport JL. Childhood-onset psychotic disorders: magnetic resonance imaging of volumetric differences in brain structure. Am J Psychiatry. 2000;157(9):1467–74.
97. Kurlan R. Clinical practice. Tourette's Syndrome. N Engl J Med. 2010;363(24):2332–8.
98. Lebel C, Walker L, Leemans A, Phillips L, Beaulieu C. Microstructural maturation of the human brain from childhood to adulthood. Neuroimage. 2008;40(3):1044–55.
99. Leckman JF, Bloch MH, Smith ME, Larabi D, Hampson M. Neurobiological substrates of Tourette's disorder. J Child Adolesc Psychopharmacol. 2010;20(4):237–47.
100. Lenroot RK, Giedd JN. Brain development in children and adolescents: insights from anatomical magnetic resonance imaging. Neurosci Biobehav Rev. 2006;30(6):718–29.
101. Lewinsohn P, Klein DN, Seeley JR. Bipolar disorders in a community sample of older adolescents: prevalence, phenomenology, comorbidity, and course. J Am Acad Child Adolesc Psychiatry. 1995;34:454–63.
102. Lieberman JA, Sheitman BB, Kinon BJ. Neurochemical sensitization in the pathophysiology of schizophrenia: deficits and dysfunction in neuronal regulation and plasticity. Neuropsychopharmacology. 1997;17(4):205–29.

103. MacMaster FP, Carrey N, Sparkes S, Kusumakar V. Proton spectroscopy in medication-free pediatric attention-deficit/hyperactivity disorder. Biol Psychiatry. 2003;53(2):184–7.
104. MacMaster FP, O'Neill J, Rosenberg DR. Brain imaging in pediatric obsessive-compulsive disorder. J Am Acad Child Adolesc Psychiatry. 2008;47(11):1262–72.
105. Makki MI, Behen M, Bhatt A, Wilson B, Chugani HT. Microstructural abnormalities of striatum and thalamus in children with Tourette syndrome. Mov Disord. 2008;23(16):2349–56.
106. Makki MI, Govindan RM, Wilson BJ, Behen ME, Chugani HT. Altered fronto-striato-thalamic connectivity in children with Tourette syndrome assessed with diffusion tensor MRI and probabilistic fiber tracking. J Child Neurol. 2009;24(6):669–78.
107. Marenco S, Weinberger DR. The neurodevelopmental hypothesis of schizophrenia: following a trail of evidence from cradle to grave. Dev Psychopathol. 2000;12(3):501–27.
108. Marsh R, Maia TV, Peterson BS. Functional disturbances within frontostriatal circuits across multiple childhood psychopathologies. Am J Psychiatry. 2009;166(6):664–74.
109. Masi G, Millepiedi S, Mucci M, Bertini N, Pfanner C, Arcangeli F. Comorbidity of obsessive-compulsive disorder and attention-deficit/hyperactivity disorder in referred children and adolescents. Compr Psychiatry. 2006;47(1):42–7.
110. McAnarney ER. Adolescent brain development: forging new links? J Adolesc Health. 2008;42(4):321–3.
111. Meyer T, Fuhr K, Hautzinger M, Schlarb AA. Recognizing mania in children and adolescents—age does not matter, but decreased need for sleep does. Comp Psychiatry. 2011;52:132–8.
112. Mick E, Spencer T, Wozniak J, Biederman J. Heterogeneity of irritability in attention-deficit/hyperactivity disorder subjects with and without mood disorders. Biol Psychiatry. 2005;58:570–82.
113. Milev P, Miranowski S, Lim K. Magnetic resonance spectroscopy. In: Lajtha A, Javitt D, Kantrowitz J, editors. Handbook of neurochemistry and molecular neurobiology. Heidelberg: Springer; 2009. p. 406–42.
114. Mirza Y, O'Neill J, Smith EA, Russell A, Smith JM, Banerjee SP, Bhandari R, Boyd C, Rose M, Ivey J, Renshaw PF, Rosenberg DR. Increased medial thalamic creatine-phosphocreatine found by proton magnetic resonance spectroscopy in children with obsessive-compulsive disorder versus major depression and healthy controls. J Child Neurol. 2006;21(2):106–11.
115. Moore CM, Demopulos CM, Henry ME, Steingard RJ, Zamvil L, Katic A, Breeze JL, Moore JC, Cohen BM, Renshaw PF. Brain-to-serum lithium ratio and age: an in vivo magnetic resonance spectroscopy study. Am J Psychiatry. 2002;159(7):1240–2.
116. Moore CM, Frazier JA, Glod CA, Breeze JL, Dieterich M, Finn CT, Frederick B, Renshaw PF. Glutamine and glutamate levels in children and adolescents with bipolar disorder: a 4.0-T proton magnetic resonance spectroscopy study of the anterior cingulate cortex. J Am Acad Child Adolesc Psychiatry. 2007;46(4):524–34.
117. Nagae-Poetscher LM, Bonekamp D, Barker PB, Brant LJ, Kaufmann WE, Horska A. Asymmetry and gender effect in functionally lateralized cortical regions: a proton MRS imaging study. J Magn Reson Imaging. 2004;19(1):27–33.
118. Nagy Z, Westerberg H, Klingberg T. Maturation of white matter is associated with the development of cognitive functions during childhood. J Cogn Neurosci. 2004;16(7):1227–33.
119. Nicolson R, Lenane M, Hamburger SD, Fernandez T, Bedwell J, Rapoport JL. Lessons from childhood-onset schizophrenia. Brain Res Brain Res Rev. 2000;31(2–3):147–56.
120. O'Neill J, Levitt J, Caplan R, Asarnow R, McCracken JT, Toga AW, Alger JR. ^{1}H MRSI evidence of metabolic abnormalities in childhood-onset schizophrenia. Neuroimage. 2004;21(4):1781–9.
121. Olvera RL, Caetano SC, Fonseca M, Nicoletti M, Stanley JA, Chen HH, Hatch JP, Hunter K, Pliszka SR, Soares JC. Low levels of N-acetyl aspartate in the left dorsolateral prefrontal cortex of pediatric bipolar patients. J Child Adolesc Psychopharmacol. 2007;17(4):461–73.
122. Ozturk A, Degaonkar M, Matson MA, Wells CT, Mahone EM, Horska A. Proton MR spectroscopy correlates of frontal lobe function in healthy children. AJNR Am J Neuroradiol. 2009;30(7):1308–14.
123. Panigrahy A, Nelson Jr MD, Bluml S. Magnetic resonance spectroscopy in pediatric neuroradiology: clinical and research applications. Pediatr Radiol. 2010;40(1):3–30.
124. Passarotti A, Sweeney JA, Pavuluri MN. Fronto-limbic dysfunction in mania pre-treatment and persistent amygdala over-activity post-treatment in pediatric bipolar disorder. Psychopharmacology. 2010. doi:10.1007/s00213-011-2243-2.
125. Patel NC, Cecil KM, Strakowski SM, Adler CM, DelBello MP. Neurochemical alterations in adolescent bipolar depression: a proton magnetic resonance spectroscopy pilot study of the prefrontal cortex. J Child Adolesc Psychopharmacol. 2008;18(6):623–7.
126. Patel NC, DelBello MP, Cecil KM, Adler CM, Bryan HS, Stanford KE, Strakowski SM. Lithium treatment effects on Myo-inositol in adolescents with bipolar depression. Biol Psychiatry. 2006;60(9):998–1004.
127. Patel NC, DelBello MP, Cecil KM, Stanford KE, Adler CM, Strakowski SM. Temporal change in N-acetyl-aspartate concentrations in adolescents with bipolar depression treated with lithium. J Child Adolesc Psychopharmacol. 2008;18(2):132–9.
128. Pettegrew JW, Keshavan MS, Panchalingam K, Strychor S, Kaplan DB, Tretta MG, Allen M. Alterations in brain high-energy phosphate and membrane phospholipid metabolism in first-episode, drug-naive schizophrenics. A pilot study of the dorsal prefrontal cortex by in vivo phosphorus 31 nuclear magnetic resonance spectroscopy. Arch Gen Psychiatry. 1991;48(6):563–8.
129. Pfefferbaum A, Mathalon DH, Sullivan EV, Rawles JM, Zipursky RB, Lim KO. A quantitative magnetic resonance imaging study of changes in brain morphology from infancy to late adulthood. Arch Neurol. 1994;51(9):874–87.
130. Plessen KJ, Gruner R, Lundervold A, Hirsch JG, Xu D, Bansal R, Hammar A, Lundervold AJ, Wentzel-Larsen T, Lie SA, Gass A, Peterson BS, Hugdahl K. Reduced white matter connectivity in the corpus callosum of children with Tourette syndrome. J Child Psychol Psychiatry. 2006;47(10):1013–22.
131. Posner MI, Rothbart MK. Developing mechanisms of self-regulation. Dev Psychopathol. 2000;12:427–41.
132. Pouwels PJ, Brockmann K, Kruse B, Wilken B, Wick M, Hanefeld F, Frahm J. Regional age dependence of human brain metabolites from infancy to adulthood as detected by quantitative localized proton MRS. Pediatr Res. 1999;46(4):474–85.
133. Pujol J, Soriano-Mas C, Alonso P, Cardoner N, Menchon JM, Deus J, Vallejo J. Mapping structural brain alterations in obsessive-compulsive disorder. Arch Gen Psychiatry. 2004;61(7):720–30.
134. Pujol J, Soriano-Mas C, Gispert JD, Bossa M, Reig S, Ortiz H, Alonso P, Cardoner N, Lopez-Sola M, Harrison BJ, Deus J, Menchon JM, Desco M, Olmos S. Variations in the shape of the frontobasal brain region in obsessive-compulsive disorder. Hum Brain Mapp. 2010;32:1100–8.
135. Rapoport JL, Giedd J, Kumra S, Jacobsen L, Smith A, Lee P, Nelson J, Hamburger S. Childhood-onset schizophrenia. Progressive ventricular change during adolescence. Arch Gen Psychiatry. 1997;54(10):897–903.
136. Rickards H. Functional neuroimaging in Tourette syndrome. J Psychosom Res. 2009;67(6):575–84.
137. Rosenberg DR, Amponsah A, Sullivan A, MacMillan S, Moore GJ. Increased medial thalamic choline in pediatric obsessive-compulsive disorder as detected by quantitative in vivo spectroscopic imaging. J Child Neurol. 2001;16(9):636–41.

138. Rosenberg DR, MacMaster FP, Keshavan MS, Fitzgerald KD, Stewart CM, Moore GJ. Decrease in caudate glutamatergic concentrations in pediatric obsessive-compulsive disorder patients taking paroxetine. J Am Acad Child Adolesc Psychiatry. 2000;39(9):1096–103.
139. Rosenberg DR, Mirza Y, Russell A, Tang J, Smith JM, Banerjee SP, Bhandari R, Rose M, Ivey J, Boyd C, Moore GJ. Reduced anterior cingulate glutamatergic concentrations in childhood OCD and major depression versus healthy controls. J Am Acad Child Adolesc Psychiatry. 2004;43(9):1146–53.
140. Ross AJ, Sachdev PS. Magnetic resonance spectroscopy in cognitive research. Brain Res Brain Res Rev. 2004;44(2–3):83–102.
141. Rostain A. Frontal lobe disorders in pediatric neuropsychology: attention-deficit hyperactivity disorder and Tourette disorder. In: Armstrong C, Morrow L, editors. Handbook of medical neuropsychology. Heidelberg: Springer Science + Business Media, LLC; 2010. p. 251–73.
142. Rotge JY, Guehl D, Dilharreguy B, Tignol J, Bioulac B, Allard M, Burbaud P, Aouizerate B. Meta-analysis of brain volume changes in obsessive-compulsive disorder. Biol Psychiatry. 2009;65(1):75–83.
143. Russell A, Cortese B, Lorch E, Ivey J, Banerjee SP, Moore GJ, Rosenberg DR. Localized functional neurochemical marker abnormalities in dorsolateral prefrontal cortex in pediatric obsessive-compulsive disorder. J Child Adolesc Psychopharmacol. 2003;13 Suppl 1:S31–8.
144. Russell AT. The clinical presentation of childhood-onset schizophrenia. Schizophr Bull. 1994;20(4):631–46.
145. Rzanny R, Klemm S, Reichenbach JR, Pfleiderer SO, Schmidt B, Volz HP, Blanz B, Kaiser WA. 31P-MR spectroscopy in children and adolescents with a familial risk of schizophrenia. Eur Radiol. 2003;13(4):763–70.
146. Sassi RB, Stanley JA, Axelson D, Brambilla P, Nicoletti MA, Keshavan MS, Ramos RT, Ryan N, Birmaher B, Soares JC. Reduced NAA levels in the dorsolateral prefrontal cortex of young bipolar patients. Am J Psychiatry. 2005;162(11):2109–15.
147. Scherk H, Backens M, Schneider-Axmann T, Usher J, Kemmer C, Reith W, Falkai P, Gruber O. Cortical neurochemistry in euthymic patients with bipolar I disorder. World J Biol Psychiatry. 2009;10(4):285–94.
148. Selemon LD, Goldman-Rakic PS. The reduced neuropil hypothesis: a circuit based model of schizophrenia. Biol Psychiatry. 1999;45(1):17–25.
149. Silverstone PH, McGrath BM, Kim H. Bipolar disorder and myo-inositol: a review of the magnetic resonance spectroscopy findings. Bipolar Disord. 2005;7(1):1–10.
150. Singer HS. Discussing outcome in Tourette syndrome. Arch Pediatr Adolesc Med. 2006;160(1):103–5.
151. Singh M, Spielman D, Adleman N, Alegria D, Howe M, Reiss A, Chang K. Brain glutamatergic characteristics of pediatric offspring of parents with bipolar disorder. Psychiatry Res. 2010;182(2):165–71.
152. Singh MK, Spielman D, Libby A, Adams E, Acquaye T, Howe M, Kelley R, Reiss A, Chang KD. Neurochemical deficits in the cerebellar vermis in child offspring of parents with bipolar disorder. Bipolar Disord. 2011;13(2):189–97.
153. Smith EA, Russell A, Lorch E, Banerjee SP, Rose M, Ivey J, Bhandari R, Moore GJ, Rosenberg DR. Increased medial thalamic choline found in pediatric patients with obsessive-compulsive disorder versus major depression or healthy control subjects: a magnetic resonance spectroscopy study. Biol Psychiatry. 2003;54(12):1399–405.
154. Sonuga Barke E, Bitsakou P, Thompson M. Beyond the dual pathway model: evidence for the dissociation of timing, inhibitory, and delay-related impairments in attention-deficit/hyperactivity disorder. J Am Acad Child Adolesc Psychiatry. 2010;49:345–55.
155. Sowell ER, Kan E, Yoshii J, Thompson PM, Bansal R, Xu D, Toga AW, Peterson BS. Thinning of sensorimotor cortices in children with Tourette syndrome. Nat Neurosci. 2008;11(6):637–9.
156. Spear LP. The adolescent brain and age-related behavioral manifestations. Neurosci Biobehav Rev. 2000;24(4):417–63.
157. Stanley JA. In vivo magnetic resonance spectroscopy and its application to neuropsychiatric disorders. Can J Psychiatry. 2002;47(4):315–26.
158. Steen RG, Hamer RM, Lieberman JA. Measurement of brain metabolites by ¹H magnetic resonance spectroscopy in patients with schizophrenia: a systematic review and meta-analysis. Neuropsychopharmacology. 2005;30(11):1949–62.
159. Strakowski SM, Delbello MP, Adler CM. The functional neuroanatomy of bipolar disorder: a review of neuroimaging findings. Mol Psychiatry. 2005;10(1):105–16.
160. Tau GZ, Peterson BS. Normal development of brain circuits. Neuropsychopharmacology. 2010;35(1):147–68.
161. Thomas MA, Ke Y, Levitt J, Caplan R, Curran J, Asarnow R, McCracken J. Preliminary study of frontal lobe ¹H MR spectroscopy in childhood-onset schizophrenia. J Magn Reson Imaging. 1998;8(4):841–6.
162. Thompson PM, Sowell ER, Gogtay N, Giedd JN, Vidal CN, Hayashi KM, Leow A, Nicolson R, Rapoport JL, Toga AW. Structural MRI and brain development. Int Rev Neurobiol. 2005;67:285–323.
163. Thompson PM, Vidal C, Giedd JN, Gochman P, Blumenthal J, Nicolson R, Toga AW, Rapoport JL. Mapping adolescent brain change reveals dynamic wave of accelerated gray matter loss in very early-onset schizophrenia. Proc Natl Acad Sci USA. 2001;98(20):11650–5.
164. Thomsen PH. Schizophrenia with childhood and adolescent onset–a nationwide register-based study. Acta Psychiatr Scand. 1996;94(3):187–93.
165. Tibbo P, Hanstock C, Valiakalayil A, Allen P. 3-T proton MRS investigation of glutamate and glutamine in adolescents at high genetic risk for schizophrenia. Am J Psychiatry. 2004;161(6):1116–8.
166. Tkac I, Oz G, Adriany G, Ugurbil K, Gruetter R. In vivo ¹H NMR spectroscopy of the human brain at high magnetic fields: metabolite quantification at 4 T vs. 7 T. Magn Reson Med. 2009;62(4):868–79.
167. Uhl I, Mavrogiorgou P, Norra C, Forstreuter F, Scheel M, Witthaus H, Ozgurdal S, Gudlowski Y, Bohner G, Gallinat J, Klingebiel R, Heinz A, Juckel G. ¹H-MR spectroscopy in ultra-high risk and first episode stages of schizophrenia. J Psychiatr Res. 2011;45:1135–9.
168. Uhlhaas PJ. The adolescent brain: implications for the understanding, pathophysiology, and treatment of schizophrenia. Schizophr Bull. 2011;37(3):480–3.
169. Valleni-Basile LA, Garrison CZ, Waller JL, Addy CL, McKeown RE, Jackson KL, Cuffe SP. Incidence of obsessive-compulsive disorder in a community sample of young adolescents. J Am Acad Child Adolesc Psychiatry. 1996;35(7):898–906.
170. Vastag B. Imaging studies reveal brain changes in children with bipolar disorder. JAMA. 2003;289(16):2057.
171. Vyas NS, Patel NH, Puri BK. Neurobiology and phenotypic expression in early onset schizophrenia. Early Interv Psychiatry. 2011;5(1):3–14.
172. Whitford TJ, Rennie CJ, Grieve SM, Clark CR, Gordon E, Williams LM. Brain maturation in adolescence: concurrent changes in neuroanatomy and neurophysiology. Hum Brain Mapp. 2007;28(3):228–37.
173. Wilke M, Kowatch RA, DelBello MP, Mills NP, Holland SK. Voxel-based morphometry in adolescents with bipolar disorder: first results. Psychiatry Res. 2004;131:57–69.
174. Wood SJ, Berger GE, Wellard RM, Proffitt TM, McConchie M, Berk M, McGorry PD, Pantelis C. Medial temporal lobe glutathione concentration in first episode psychosis: a ¹H-MRS investigation. Neurobiol Dis. 2009;33(3):354–7.

175. Wozniak J, Biederman J, Kwon A, Mick E, Faraone SV, Orlovsky K. How cardinal are cardinal symptoms in pediatric bipolar disorder?: an examination of clinical correlates. Biol Psychiatry. 2005;58:583–8.
176. Yeo RA, Hill D, Campbell R, Vigil J, Brooks WM. Developmental instability and working memory ability in children: a magnetic resonance spectroscopy investigation. Dev Neuropsychol. 2000;17(2):143–59.
177. Youngstrom EA, Birmaher B, Findling RL. Pediatric bipolar disorder: validity, phenomenology, and recommendations for diagnosis. Bipolar Disord. 2008;10(1 Pt 2):194–214.
178. Zabala A, Sanchez-Gonzalez J, Parellada M, Moreno DM, Reig S, Burdalo MT, Robles O, Desco M, Arango C. Findings of proton magnetic resonance spectometry in the dorsolateral prefrontal cortex in adolescents with first episodes of psychosis. Psychiatry Res. 2007;156(1):33–42.

Magnetic Resonance Spectroscopy Studies of Autistic Spectrum Disorders

17

Jennifer G. Levitt, Joseph O'Neill, and Jeffry R. Alger

In this chapter, we review magnetic resonance spectroscopy (MRS) studies of Autism Spectrum Disorders (ASD). We present a brief clinical overview of autism and related pervasive developmental disorders, and then summarize the neuropathology findings in ASD and neuroimaging investigations of ASD using techniques other than MRS. We then review all published MRS studies of ASD known to us, with some emphasis upon the impact of varying spectroscopic imaging techniques. Finally, we suggest potential future MRS research applications in ASD.

Epidemiology and Diagnosis

Autism is a disorder of development encompassing three primary domains: communication, reciprocal social interactions, and restricted repetitive/stereotyped behaviors and interests [1]. The diagnosis of autism is made based upon symptoms in these domains, typically occurring prior to 3 years of age. Autistic spectrum disorder (ASD) is the broader term that includes autistic disorder, Asperger disorder, Childhood Disintegrative Disorder, atypical autism/pervasive developmental disorders not otherwise specified (PDD-NOS), and Rett syndrome (for review, see Filipek et al.) [2]. Reported prevalence rates vary from 10 [3] to 38.9 [4] per 10,000 for autism, and 60 [5] to 100 [6] per 10,000 for the broader phenotype. Many studies present evidence that prevalence rates have increased dramatically over several decades; however, it is unclear whether this is due to changes in diagnostic practices or an actual increase in the incidence of the disorder. For a review, see King and Bearman [7].

Neuropathology

Despite numerous findings across a variety of investigational methodologies the pathophysiology of autism remains unclear. Neuropathology findings are relatively fewer than imaging, with early studies implicating cerebellar [8–12] and limbic forebrain [8, 13] abnormalities in this disorder of development. These include such findings as decreased numbers of Purkinje cells in the cerebellum [12, 14, 15] and smaller cell size and increased packing density in the hippocampus, amygdala, subiculum, entorhinal cortex, and mammillary bodies [14]. A recent quantitative investigation demonstrating decreased numbers of neurons in the amygdala [16] provides further support for abnormal development of this region in ASD.

Kemper and Bauman [14] demonstrated decreased size and increased packing density of neurons in the anterior cingulate gyrus, and later studies have described wider involvement of the cerebral cortex, with prominent abnormalities of neuronal density and organization, as well as white matter and brain stem irregularities [15]. Disturbance of the normal architecture of cortical minicolumns has been shown as well, with smaller, more compact and more numerous minicolumns in several areas [17].

Similarly, recent immunohistochemical investigations of autopsy subjects have shown variable findings including reductions in GABAa receptor binding in the hippocampus [18], nicotinic receptors in frontal and parietal lobes [19] and cerebellum [20], and increased brain-derived neurotrophic factor in the basal forebrain [19].

J.G. Levitt, M.D. (✉)
Department of Psychiatry, Semel Institute for Neuroscience and Human Behavior, UCLA, Los Angeles, CA, USA

J. O'Neill, Ph.D.
Division of Child and Adolescent Psychiatry, Semel Institute for Neuroscience and Human Behavior, UCLA, Los Angeles, CA, USA

J.R. Alger, Ph.D.
Department of Radiological Sciences, UCLA, Los Angeles, CA, USA

S. Blüml and A. Panigrahy (eds.), *MR Spectroscopy of Pediatric Brain Disorders*,
DOI 10.1007/978-1-4419-5864-8_17,

Structural Magnetic Resonance Imaging in ASD

It is thought that heterogeneity of the disorder has contributed to the disparity in neuropathology findings [11]. Not surprisingly, neuroimaging studies in autism have shown a wide variety of findings as well. Similar to the neuropathology literature, some volumetric studies of ASD support limbic [21–28] and cerebellar abnormalities [29–32] while others have failed to find significant differences from controls in these regions [33].

As noted above, Bailey also found postmortem evidence for neocortical involvement in ASD, including increased frontal cortical neuronal density and cortical dysgenetic lesions [15]. Such lesions may be associated with defective neuronal migration, proliferation, or pruning [34], and reflected in brain structure, such as abnormal organization of the cortical surface [15]. Although nonspecific to autism, qualitative neuroimaging evidence for such surface abnormalities has been demonstrated by Piven et al. [35]. Quantitative neuroimaging evidence for surface abnormalities comes from cortical mapping studies demonstrating irregularities of sulcal anatomy [36] and abnormal gyrification [37].

Volumetric and voxel-based morphometry (VBM) studies have shown abnormalities of both gray and white matter in autistic subjects in a variety of regions throughout the cerebrum, including parietal lobe, left occipito-temporal cortex, right inferior temporal gyrus, left middle temporal gyrus, and left inferior frontal sulcus [22, 38–45]. Reports vary as to direction (increased or decreased) and location of volumetric changes.

Cortical mapping studies have demonstrated displacement of cortical sulci [36], gyrification [36, 37, 46], and cortical thickness including cortical thinning in two studies [47, 48] and primarily increased cortical thickness in one other [49].

Increased head size or overall head circumference [50–52], as well as brain size/volume [26, 45, 53–57] are among the most replicated findings in ASD [39, 52, 55, 58]. The literature suggests that this brain overgrowth occurs in some subjects between 2 and 4 years of age [26, 59], with some cross-sectional studies demonstrating arrest or normalization of this growth in later childhood and adolescence [58, 60]. Other studies, however, have found enlarged brains in older subjects as well [54, 61, 62]. The extent to which gray and white matter contribute to this finding has not been clearly established. While diffusion tensor imaging studies have consistently demonstrated abnormalities of both fractional anisotropy (FA) [63–65] and elevated diffusivity [64, 66], other imaging modalities provide strong evidence for gray matter involvement as well [67, 68].

Functional Neuroimaging in ASD

Similarly, the functional imaging literature indicates varying regional involvement in ASD. Both ^{18}FDG-PET [69] and single photon emission correlated tomography (SPECT) [21, 70] studies provide evidence for abnormal metabolism or perfusion in subjects with ASD. fMRI studies at rest have shown bilateral hypoperfusion of temporal lobe areas [71] in autistic children. Activation studies demonstrate altered activity in cortical regions including the fusiform gyrus [72–74], left middle temporal gyrus [72], inferior temporal gyrus [73], inferior occipital gyrus, and superior temporal sulcus [74] in autistic subjects during face processing tasks; abnormal activation of the superior temporal gyrus (STG) bilaterally during auditory activation tasks [75], and aberrant activity in the right parietal lobe/temperoparietal junction during imitation tasks [76], which may be related to the development of communication skills in autistic children [77].

The above studies demonstrate abnormalities of brain function in regions that subserve language, facial/emotion recognition, and imitation, all of which have been implicated in the primary symptoms of autism [73, 76, 78]. In addition, investigations finding aberrant functional connectivity (FC) in ASD have led to hypotheses that hyper- or hypo-connectivity as a central cause of symptoms in this disorder [78–80].

Magnetic Resonance Spectroscopy in ASD

Magnetic resonance spectroscopy (MRS) provides information on the metabolic aspects of these anatomic and functional abnormalities. Similar to neuropathology, morphometric and fMRI findings, the magnetic resonance spectroscopy research literature in ASD presents a variety of conflicting findings. Some of this is due to heterogeneity of the disorder and some to differences in technique both in acquiring data and in postprocessing. Many of the early studies in the field used ratio evaluation of metabolite content. This approach assumes that the denominator, typically the creatine level, remains constant, which is an assumption that has been repeatedly challenged. In fact, there is evidence that in autism, creatine (Cr) and/or phosphocreatine (PCr) abnormalities may contribute to the disorder [36, 81].

Phosphorous Spectroscopy in ASD

The earliest MRS studies in autism include the only ^{31}P-MRS investigation in this disorder conducted by Minshew and colleagues [82]. ^{31}P MRS measures levels of energy metabolites such as PCr, adenosine di- and triphosphate (ADP, ATP), and inorganic phosphate (Pi). Some membrane phospholipids are also "visible" with ^{31}P MRS. These include phosphomonoesters (PMEs) and phosphodiesters (PDEs) which are, respectively, precursors and breakdown products of membrane phospholipids and provide information about neuronal (and glial) membrane metabolism [83].

The authors examined prefrontal cortex functioning of 11 high-functioning males with autism, aged 12–40 years and controls matched for age, IQ, gender, race, and SES. They found a significant decrease in the content of PCr and esterified ends in the autistic group and an association between these findings and lower test performance on neuropsychological tests including the Wechsler Intelligence scales, Wisconsin Card Sort Test, California Verbal Learning Test, and the Token Test and Test of Language Competence. Minshew and colleagues [82] suggested that these results provide evidence for disturbances of membrane synthesis and metabolism in autism.

Proton Spectroscopy in ASD

Neocortical Spectroscopy Findings in Autism

Here we continue the discussion of neocortical spectroscopy literature in ASD. With the exception of one study finding no abnormalities in any region examined [84], and one finding increased metabolites in subjects with ASD [85], the majority of these investigations have demonstrated reductions of metabolites in the neocortical regions investigated. As we address the amygdala–hippocampus separately, we leave the discussion of the medial temporal lobe (MTL) for that section.

Most spectroscopy studies of ASD have used proton imaging, with early studies focusing on single voxel investigations. Table 17.1 lists MRS and MRSI studies of pediatric ASD in cortical regions. Hashimoto et al. [84] used single voxel proton spectroscopy in 28 subjects with autism (20 male, eight female; age range 2 year 8 months—12 year 2 months), 28 age-matched subjects with mental retardation (MR) (male 22, female 6; age range 2 year to 13 year 3 months), and 25 age-matched healthy children (male 16, female 9; age range from 2 years to 13 years 8 months). The diagnosis of autism was clinical and based on DSM-III-R criteria [86], and the diagnosis of MR was given for an IQ <80 on the Tsumori-Inage and Suzuku-Binet test. The autistic and MR children did not differ in IQ assessment; the control children were not tested. Six of the autistic children and nine of the MR children had epilepsy. Many of the MR and control children less than 6 years of age were administered triclofos sodium for sedation.

The investigators used the chemical shift selective excitation (CHESS) sequence for water suppression and the stimulated echo acquisition mode (STEAM) sequence at a long TE (270 ms). Volumes varied between 8 and 27 cm^3 and were placed in the right parietal region, overlapping both gray and white matter. Using metabolite ratios with either Cho or Cr as the denominator, this group found no differences in the *N*-acetyl-aspartate/choline (NAA/Cho), NAA/Cr + PCr) or Cho/Cr + PCr ratios between subjects with autism and controls in any age group (2 to <5 years of age; 5–<8 years of age, 8–13 years of age).

Although no differences were found between autistic and controls subjects, the groups were well matched and it is possible that the use of ratios to assess outcome negatively affected the investigators' ability to detect differences between subject groups.

However, in another single voxel proton spectroscopy investigation, Hisaoka et al. [87] found significant differences in autistic subjects and controls in the lateral temporal lobes. This was a relatively large study of 55 autistic subjects (ages 2–21 years; 47 male and eight female) and 51 control children (ages 3 months–15 years, 26 boys and 25 girls). Using a point-resolved spectroscopic sequence (PRESS), and a long TE of 135 ms, these investigators found significant reductions of NAA bilaterally in the temporal lobe (presumptive Brodman's areas 41 and 42) ($p<0.05$)—but no differences in frontal or parietal regions, or brain stem. All were single voxels quantified using the water reference method and corrected for T1 and T2 relaxation (although no differences were found in relaxation times between groups).

Murphy et al. [85] also used TE 136 with single voxels to investigate the right frontal and medial parietal lobes in a group of subjects with Asperger's syndrome (AS). Voxels included both gray and white matter, and in this case, as opposed to those previously mentioned studies, the content of gray matter, white matter, and CSF was calculated for each voxel of interest. Data were analyzed both as metabolite concentration based on water reference and also as ratios NAA/Cr + PCr, NAA/Cho, and Cho/Cr + PCr. There were no significant differences in the parietal lobe, but in the frontal lobe NAA, Cr + PCr, and Cho were increased in AS subjects compared to controls, although gray and white matter volumes did not differ between groups. Moreover, prefrontal NAA levels in the AS subjects were positively correlated with scores on the Yale–Brown Obsessive Compulsive Scale [88], and Cho was significantly correlated with the communication domain on the Autism Diagnostic Interview-Revised [89].

Magnetic resonance spectroscopic imaging (MRSI) techniques have further advanced the field, allowing for sampling of multiple brain regions in a single session. Such studies have produced somewhat similar results, although there are differences regarding specific metabolites per region [36, 67, 68, 90]. Figures 17.1 and 17.2 illustrate voxel size and placement in the cingulate gyrus.

Table 17.1 Magnetic resonance spectroscopy (MRS) and magnetic resonance spectroscopic imaging (MRSI) studies of pediatric autism spectrum disorder (ASD) in cortical regions

Reference	MRS technique	Brain regions	Key findings
Hashimoto et al. 1997 [84]	Single Voxel STEAM TR-1500, TE 270	–Right Parietal gray and white	No significant Differences—reported as ratios to Cho and Cr
Hisaoka et al. 2001 [87]	Single Voxel PRESS TR 1300,TE 135	–Frontal, –Parietal –Temporal –Brain Stem	Reduced NAA Temporal lobe
Murphy et al. 2002 [85]	Single Voxel PRESS TR 2000,TE 136 gray/white/CSF segmentation	–Right Frontal –Medial Parietal	– Increased NAA, Cr, Cho Frontal lobe – NAA correlation with Y-BOCS – Cho correlation with ADI-R communication scores
Friedman et al. 2003 [90]	MRSI TR 2,000 TE 20/272 ms Quantitation	Slices placed at the level of: –Temporal lobe –Basal Ganglia	Decreased metabolites throughout See Table 17.2
Levitt et al. 2003 [36]	MRSI TR 2300,TE 272 gray/white/CSF segmentation	Slices placed at the level of: –Supraventricular –Ventricular –Basal Ganglia	– Decreased Cr + PCr –R occipital – Decreased NAA left caudate; left frontal and left parietal white matter; left parietal white matter – Increased Cr + PCr –Caudate – Decreased Cho –Left ACC
Friedman et al. 2006 [67]	MRSI, Gray/white/CSF segmentation	see Friedman et al. 2003	Attributed decreased metabolites in 2003 study primarily to gray
Devito et al. 2007 [68]	3 T MRSI TR 100 TE 135	Slices placed at the level of: –Occipital lobe– Corpus Callosum –Cerebellum–Thalamus	– Decreased NAA frontal and occipital lobes gray – Decreased Glx frontal and occipital gray, and cerebellum – Decreased Cr + PCr left temporal and left occipital gray matter.
Harada et al. 2010 [96]	3 T single voxel –PRESS-TE 68 for GABA –STEAM TE 15 for conventional metabolites	–Frontal lobe –Lenticular Nucleus	Decreased GABA in frontal lobe Decreased GABA/NAA and GABA/Glu in frontal lobe
Bernardi et al. 2011 [95]	3 TMRSI TR 2000 TE 30	–Anterior Cingulate/Thalamus –Temperoparietal	Reduced Glx right anterior cingulate Reduced mI temperoparietal junction
Vasconcelos et al., 2008 [119]	Single Voxel PRESS TR 1500 TE 30	–Cingulate –Left Striatum –Left Frontal lobe –Left cerebellum	Increased mI and Cho anterior cingulate Increased mI/Cr in cingulate and striatum
Oner et al. 2007 [121]	2D-CSI PRESS TR 1500 TE 270	–Right Anterior Cingulate –Right Dorsolateral Prefrontal Cortex	– Increased NAA/Cho ($p = 0.028$) in ACC; – Correlation to Y-BOCS ($p = 0.047$); – Neg correlation Y = BOCS and DLPFC NAA/Cho ($p = 0.015$)
Endo et al. 2007 [148]	Single Voxel PRESS TR 2000 TE 35	–Prefrontal Cortex –Amygdala–hippocampus	Decreased NAA/Cr ASD vs control Decreased NAA/Cr Autism vs PDD-NOS
Kleinhans et al. 2007 [106]	Single Voxel PRESS TR 2000,TE 30 CSF but not gray/white assessed	–Left middle frontal –Left parietal –Occipital cortex –Right cerebellum –Cerebellar vermis	Decreased NAA left frontal lobe middle gyrus.

N-Acetyl (NAA) Compounds, Choline-Containing Compounds (Cho), Creatine + Phosphocreatine (Cr), Myoinositol (MI), Glutamate-glutamine (Glx), Chemical Shift Imaging (CSI)

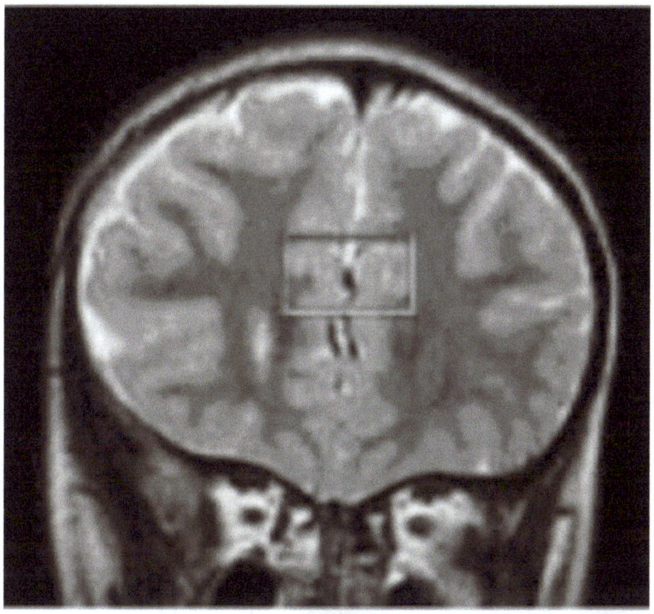

Fig. 17.1 Single voxel study by Hisaoke et al. demonstrating placement bilaterally in the anterior cingulate gyrus. (From Hisaoka S, Harada M, Nishitani H, Mori K. Regional magnetic resonance spectroscopy of the brain in autistic individuals. Neuroradiology 2001;43(6):496–8, with permission.)

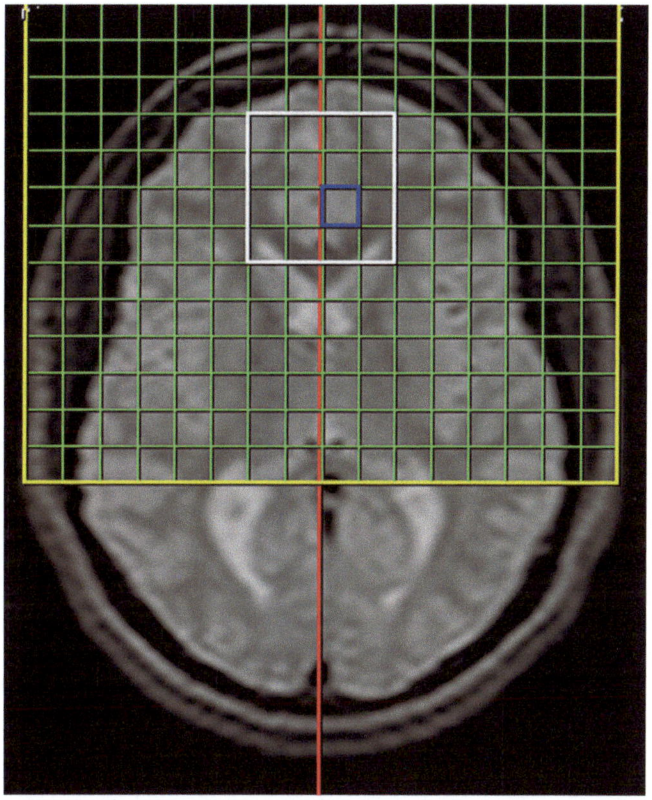

Fig. 17.2 The excited volume of the spectroscopic imaging study area is outlined in white, whereas the smaller voxels within the volume indicate the ROIs for individual voxels. Outlined in blue voxel is a representative ACC voxel. (From Levitt J, O'Neill J, Blanton RE, et al. Proton magnetic resonance spectroscopic imaging of the brain in childhood autism. Biol Psych 54:1355–1366, 2003; with permission.)

Friedman et al. [90] utilized proton echoplanar spectroscopic imaging (PEPSI), two echo times (TE 20/272 ms), and also measured relaxation times in children 3–4 years of age with ASD (38 boys, 7 girls), developmental delay (DD) (6 boys, 9 girls), and typical development (TD) (11 boys, 2 girls). Groups were age matched, but differed in gender distribution, although no covariates were used for this as the authors cited lack of evidence for sex effects on spectroscopy. All autistic and DD children were administered propofol for sedation, while TD children were imaged during sleep and/or after administration of diphenhydramine. Two slices were acquired—one placed atop the temporal lobes and one placed through the basal ganglia. Data was analyzed using the LCModel commercial package [91] for automated fitting and water referencing for metabolite content.

Initial data analysis of averaged metabolite content throughout the slices demonstrated reduced NAA in both autistic and DD children as compared to TD children. The autistic children alone had decreased Cho, Cr+PCr, and myo-inositol (mI) compared to TD subjects. There were no differences in glutamate+glutamine (Glx) between groups. While averaged NAA T2 relaxation time (T2r) was prolonged in the ASD subjects compared to both TD and DD controls, Cr+PCr and Cho T2r were prolonged in ASD subjects compared to DD subjects. The authors suggest, given their findings of prolonged T2r, that proton spectroscopy studies in autism should employ short TE ($\leq$ 30 ms) as the differences in T2r at longer TEs may affect results. Post hoc analysis directed to regional sites demonstrated multiple reductions in proton metabolites, some of which are outlined here and in Table 17.2.

Metabolite differences in the ASD group, not replicated in the DD group, were widespread and affected the thalamus, basal ganglia, cingulate/callosum, and temporal and parietal regions. Metabolite differences that may be attributed to developmental delay in both ASD and DD subjects include the left frontal white matter reduction in NAA and Cr+PCr, and the parietal white matter reduction in NAA.

In an effort to better understand these data, Friedman et al. [67] applied linear regression techniques to analyze the relative contributions of gray and white matter to their findings. In addition, cerebral volume was included as a covariate in these analyses. Their results demonstrated that findings unique to the autistic subjects occurred primarily in gray matter (decreased NAA, Cr, Cho, and mI and prolonged Cho T2r compared to controls), while both AD and DD had reduced white matter NAA and mI (mI at the trend level only in the DD group however) relative to the control subjects. Cho and mI were reduced in AD compared to DD as well.

Table 17.2 Spectroscopic imaging results, Friedman et al. [90]

	Decreased NAA	Decreased Cr + PCr	Decreased Cho	Decreased mI
ASD vs TD	– Right thalamus – Bilateral cingulate	– Left thalamus Anterior Callosum – Left parietal white – Left insula	– Left thalamus – Right medial temporal lobe – Right superior temporal gyrus	– Bilateral caudate – Anterior callosum – Left parietal white – Right insula
ASD and DD vs TD	Left frontal white Right parietal white	Left frontal white		
ASD vs DD	Occipital cortex			

The authors suggest that these findings may provide evidence for a common metabolic abnormality in white matter of both ASD and DD children. However, Levitt et al. [36] also found significant reductions of NAA in left frontal and left parietal white matter in older children with ASD, most of whom had IQ ≥ 70.

In this study, Levitt et al. [36] also used multislice MRSI (TE = 272 ms, Fig. 17.3) to investigate proton metabolites in 22 subjects with autism (4 girls, 18 boys aged 5.4–15.7 years) and 20 age-matched healthy controls (10 girls, 10 boys aged 6.8–16.3 years). Only three of these subjects had IQ < 70, two with full scale IQ scores of 61 and 64, and one scoring 33 verbal and 59 performance on the Mullens Scale of Early Learning [92]. Three 12-mm axial slices were proscribed through (1) the supraventricular region, (2) the ventricles, and (3) the dorsoventral midplane of the basal ganglia. Slices were co-registered to segmented tissue maps, and voxels were selected within manually delineated regions of interest including: the cingulate gyrus, caudate, putamen, and thalamus. Only voxels containing ≥ 75 % gray or white matter were retained in cortical, respectively, regions. Voxels were CSF corrected and absolute quantitation of MRSI metabolite levels was expressed in terms of institutional units (IU), rather than mmol concentrations, because no correction was made for T1 and T2 relaxation effects. Gender was included as a covariate in Levitt et al. [36], but not in Friedman et al. [90].

The findings included decreased Cr + PCr in right occipital cortex ($p = 0.043$), decreased Cho in left anterior cingulate gyrus ($p = 0.003$), and increased Cr + PCr in the left ($p = .0068$) and right ($p = 0.03$) caudate nucleus. Post hoc analyses revealed significantly decreased NAA in autistic subjects in left parietal white matter ($p = 0.019$), left frontal white matter ($p = 0.029$), and left caudate ($p = 0.04$).

As noted above, Friedman et al. [67] suggest that findings of decreased NAA in frontal and parietal white matter may represent a phenomenon common to both subjects with ASD and with DD. However, Levitt et al. [36] found that NAA levels remained significantly reduced in the autistic subjects compared to controls when the analysis was restricted to subjects with full-scale IQ of 83–127. Moreover, a separate single voxel study in 18 month to 7-year-old boys [93] found no significant difference between 25 male subjects with ASD and 12 male subjects with MR or language disorder but not ASD.

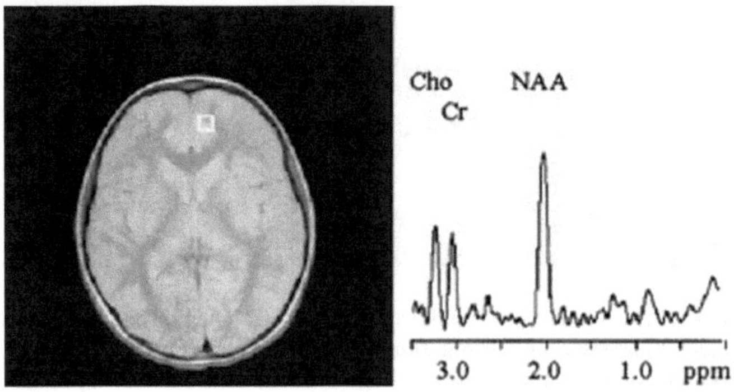

Fig. 17.3 A representative spectrum obtained with MRSI. (From Levitt J, O'Neill J, Blanton RE, et al. Proton magnetic resonance spectroscopic imaging of the brain in childhood autism. Biol Psych 54:1355–1366, 2003; with permission.)

Possible confounds in these studies include the effect of medications in some subjects in both Friedman et al. and Levitt et al., as well as the administration of propofol sedation to some subjects in Levitt et al. [36] and all ASD and DD subjects in Friedman et al. [90]. Levitt et al. [36] examined these potential confounds by excluding medicated and or sedated subjects from the analyses, although this reduced power to detect changes. Significant differences from initial results were found (1) eliminating sedated subjects from the analysis resulted in a loss of Cho findings in the caudate and (2) further analysis of the effect of medication revealed a "normalization" of Cr + PCr content in the right caudate in the medicated subjects. Of note, a proton spectroscopy investigation of obsessive compulsive disorder (OCD) demonstrated a similar effect of selective serotonin inhibitors, producing a normalization of the Glx peak in the caudate of OCD subjects compared to controls [94].

While none of the aforementioned studies detected Glx differences in ASD, all were performed at 1.5 T. De Vito et al. [68] performed the first 3 T study in subjects with ASD, which greatly improves the ability to characterize the Glx peak. Using spectroscopic imaging (TE 135 ms), 2 slices were placed at (1) the lower at the level of the superior cerebellum and thalamus; and (2) through the occipital lobe and splenium of the corpus callosum. This allowed for a sampling of cortical regions except the parietal lobe, in 26 male subjects with autism (6–17 years of age) and 29 controls (6–16 years of age). Eighteen subjects required midazolam for sedation, and 12 were on psychotropic medications. There were no significant group differences in age or nonverbal IQ, although verbal IQ was lower in the subjects with autism.

Voxel gray/white/CSF proportions were calculated based on T1-weighted segmentation data, and metabolites were quantified using phantom metabolite solutions of known concentration. All cortical voxels were pooled for metabolite assessment and, in addition, manually segmented regions were assessed. Based on content of gray and white matter, the regions assessed included: left and right frontal, temporal and occipital gray matter; left and right cerebral white matter; and left and right cerebellum.

Averaged results showed significantly decreased NAA in the autistic subjects, primarily in gray matter ($p=0.006$); regional analysis attributed this to both frontal and occipital lobes and at a trend level, the temporal lobes. NAA was also reduced in white matter in the autistic subjects, but only at the trend level (0.06), and was reduced at the trend level in the ASD group in the cerebellum ($p=0.06$). Glx was significantly decreased in gray matter autistic subjects ($p=0.0007$) in frontal ($p=0.02$) and occipital ($p=0.002$) lobes and in the cerebellum ($p=0.003$), but not in white matter. Cr+PCr was reduced in gray matter in the left temporal ($p=0.04$) and left occipital ($p=0.05$) lobes.

Furthermore, there was a negative correlation found between age and cerebral gray matter NAA ($p=0.002$) and Glx ($p=0.00002$) in frontal, temporal, and occipital gray matter of control subjects, but not in autistic subjects. This negative correlation was found for both groups for NAA in the cerebellum. Analyses of the effects of medication or sedation upon the results did not reveal any significant differences in findings between medicated and unmedicated subjects.

Bernardi et al. [95] also used a 3 T magnet to investigate proton metabolites in the cerebral cortex of 14 adults with ASD and 14 healthy controls matched for age and nonverbal IQ. Using a PRESS sequence (TE = 30 ms) in two slices placed as (1) an axial slice through the anterior cingulate gyrus (ACC) and thalamus and (2) a coronal slice placed approximately along the intraparietal sulcus (IPS) and the temperoparietal junction (TPJ), proton metabolite data was quantified and reported in IU. The investigators found significant reductions in Glx in the right ACC ($p<.006$) and decreased mI in the left temperoparietal junction ($p<.03$). These results are consistent with the previous findings of decreased frontal Glx by DeVito et al. [68]; and as the authors point out, indicate that these changes may be stable into adulthood.

In an investigation designed to examine GABA in ASD, Harada et al. [96] used a 3 T magnet to examine proton metabolites in 12 children with ASD (2–11 years of age) and 10 control subjects (3–12 years of age). Ten of the autistic subjects and nine of the control subjects required sedation with triclofos sodium. The investigators incorporated the MEGA-editing J difference technique [97] into a PRESS sequence (TE = 68 ms) to improve the GABA signal, as well as a STEAM sequence (TE = 15 ms) for the conventional proton metabolites. Single voxels were placed in the frontal lobe and in the lenticular nucleus and were segmented into gray/white/CSF fractions; LCModel [98] was used for metabolite analysis.

Data analysis demonstrated a significant reduction in GABA in the frontal lobe region of the ASD subjects compared to the control subjects ($p<0.01$), and reduced GABA/NAA ($p<0.01$) and GABA/Glu ($p<0.05$). There were no other statistically significant differences. Noting recent research demonstrating irregularities of the $GABA_A$ and $GABA_B$ receptors in subjects with ASD [99, 100], the authors hypothesize that these findings implicate suppression of the GABAergic system and subsequent hyperfunction of glutamate (Glu) during brain development in ASD.

In summary, several proton spectroscopy studies in ASD have found decreased NAA in regions throughout the neocortex in subject groups including very young children [90], children and adolescents [36, 68], and subjects spanning both of these age groups [87]. NAA may be a marker of either neuronal numbers/density, or integrity/function [101, 102], and/or more specifically, of mitochondrial function [103]. Given the evidence outlined above for increased brain volume [58], numbers/density of neurons in the cortex of subjects with autism [15, 17], and cortical thickness [49], these findings seem more consistent with an abnormality of function in the neurons or glia in these regions, and less an indication of reduced neuronal numbers.

Findings of other proton metabolite irregularities in these same cortical regions support this notion. There is evidence for decreased Cr + PCr in occipital gray matter [36, 68], as well as frontal and parietal white matter [90]. The Cr + PCr peak is a marker of cellular energetics that may be driven in part by cytosolic glycolysis [104] and are consistent with earlier fMRI studies demonstrating diminished functional activity in autistic subjects [71, 76, 78] and Harris et al. [105].

Support for a relationship between such abnormalities and the symptom profile of ASD comes from several studies, including a single voxel investigation by Kleinhans et al. [106]. Using short TE (35 ms) PRESS 1 H-MRS in 13 males with ASD (7 autistic, 3 Asperger disorder, and 3 PDD-NOS) and 13 age- and gender-matched controls, these investigators found that reduction of NAA in the left frontal lobe middle gyrus of the subjects with ASD ($p=0.043$) was correlated with the percent of frontal lobe activation on an fMRI test of verbal fluency.

In the temporal lobes, there is also evidence for reduced Cr + Pcr [68] as well as for decreased Cho in the right superior temporal gyrus and reduced mI in the temperoparietal junction [95]. Cho is attributed primarily to membrane constituents, and therefore abnormalities of this metabolite in the STG, a node in the language comprehension network [107], suggest disruption of normal membrane synthesis or degradation [108, 109] in this region. mI is considered to be primarily a marker of glia [101]. Findings of decreased mI in the left temperoparietal junction ($p<.03$) may be evidence of glial abnormalities in this region subserving attention and empathy (see Bernardi et al. for review [95]), and are consistent with Williams et al.'s [76] findings of abnormal metabolic activity in the temperoparietal region during imitation tasks.

In addition, findings of reduced Glx (including both glutamine and glutamate) in frontal, temporal, and occipital lobes [68], as well as decreased GABA in the frontal lobe [96] support hypotheses of disturbed excitation/inhibition in ASD [110]. Taken together, these metabolic changes support and extend neuropathology, morphometric and functional imaging studies outlined above that demonstrate widespread neocortical involvement in the brain in ASD. Similar metabolic abnormalities have been found in many other brain regions in autism, which we discuss below.

The Cingulate Gyrus in Autism

In addition to its well-known role in cognition and attention [111], the anterior cingulate gyrus is centrally involved in processing both cognitive and emotional stimuli [112, 113], and motor responses to these stimuli [114]. Studies implicate this region, as well as the prefrontal cortex, in theory of mind and empathy, which are hypothesized to be central to ASD symptomatology [115, 116]. The ACC is implicated as well in the pathophysiology of obsessive compulsive symptoms [117], which may in some cases be related to the repetitive-stereotyped behaviors symptom domain seen in autism [85, 118].

The findings in the spectroscopy literature regarding the anterior cingulate gyrus in autism are similar to those in the neocortex in that while several investigations provide evidence for metabolic abnormalities in this region, there is variability in the specific metabolic abnormalities found. The spectroscopic imaging investigations outlined above produced evidence for decreased NAA bilaterally in the ACC [90] and decreased Cho in the left ACC [36]. However, Vasconcelos et al. [119] found increased Cho ($p=0.04$) and increased mI ($p=0.02$) in the anterior cingulate using short TE (30 ms) single voxel PRESS in ten boys with autism (median age 9.5 =/–1.8 year) and ten control boys (median age 8.5 ± 1.4 years). Finally, in their 3 T study described above, Bernardi et al. [95] demonstrated decreased Glx in the right ACC.

Decreased levels of Glx in the ACC may be related to receptor abnormalities in this region recently demonstrated by Oblak et al. [120] demonstrating significantly reduced numbers of $GABA_A$ receptors in the ACC in postmortem tissue from subjects with ASD. Corresponding abnormalities of glutamate and/or glutamine may ultimately manifest in aberrant connectivity and function, resulting in disruption of normal ACC function that may lead, at least in part, to the symptomatology of ASD.

Further evidence for the relationship between proton metabolites, functional abnormalities, and symptomatology comes from a study by Oner et al. [121], demonstrating significant correlations between proton metabolites in adult subjects with autism and scores on the Yale–Brown Obsessive Compulsive Scale (Y-BOCS) [88]—a measure of severity of obsessive compulsive symptoms. These investigators used 2D-CSI (Press, TE 270 ms) in both the right ACC and right DLPFC in 14 male patients with AS (17–38 years of age) and in 21 age-, IQ-, and gender-matched control subjects. They found significantly decreased NAA/Cho in the ACC of subjects with autism, as well as a positive correlation between this measure and scores on the Y-BOCS, used as a measure of repetitive and stereotyped behaviors, a cardinal symptom in ASD.

Proton Spectroscopy and the Caudate in ASD

The caudate is also a well-known node in the pathways involved in obsessive compulsive disorder [122–125]; for review, see Maia et al. [126]. Both spectroscopic imaging and single voxel studies describe significant abnormalities in the caudate in subjects with ASD (Table 17.3). Using spectroscopic imaging, Levitt et al. [36] found increased Cr + PCr bilaterally, and decreased NAA (left hemisphere), while Friedman et al. [90] demonstrated decreased mI bilaterally in the caudate. In their single voxel study, Vasconcelos et al. [119] found increased mI/Cr in the striatum.

Between these three studies investigating very young children (3–4 years of age), Friedman et al. [90], as well as older children and adolescents [36, 119], there is a pattern consistent with aberrant Cr + PCr (energy/metabolics) and mI (glial cell) abnormalities in the caudate in ASD. These findings are consistent with PET [127] and fMRI investigations demonstrating abnormalities of functional activation [128, 129] and functional connectivity [130] in this region.

Table 17.3 Proton spectroscopy in anterior cingulate gyrus, caudate, and thalamus in ASD

Reference	MRS technique	Brain regions	Key findings
Friedman et al. 2003 [90]	MRSI TR 2,000 TE 20/272 ms, Quantitation	–Temporal lobe –Basal ganglia	Decreased metabolites throughout See Table 17.2
Levitt et al. 2003 [36]	MRSI TR 2300 TE 272 gray/white/CSF segmentation	–Supraventricular –Ventricular –Basal Ganglia	Increased Cr + PCr–Caudate bilateral Decreased Cho–Left Anterior cingulate Decreased Cr + PCr -R occipital cortex Decreased NAA left caudate; left frontal white matter; left parietal white matter
Bernardi et al. 2011 [95]	3 T MRSI TR 2000 TE 30	–Anterior Cingulate/ Thalamus –Temperoparietal	Reduced Glx right anterior cingulate Reduced mI temperoparietal junction
Vasconcelos et al., 2008 [119]	Single Voxel PRESS TR 1500 TE 30	–Cingulate –Left Striatum –Left Frontal lobe –Left cerebellum	– Increased mI and Cho anterior cingulate – Increased mI/Cr in cingulate and striatum
Oner et al. 2007 [121]	2D-CSI PRESS TR 1500 TE 270	–Right anterior cingulate –Right dorsolateral prefrontal cortex	– Increased NAA/Cho ($p = 0.028$) in ACC; – Correlation to Y-BOCS ($p = 0.047$); – Neg correlation Y = BOCS and DLPFC NAA/Cho ($p = 0.015$)
Hardan et al. 2008 [131]	STEAM CSI TR 1600 TE 20	–Thalamus—bilateral	Decreased NAA right thalamus Left thalamus trend

Proton Spectroscopy and the Thalamus in ASD

Hardan and colleagues [131], interested in investigating the neurophysiology of sensory abnormalities in subjects with autism, examined the thalamus using both morphometry and proton spectroscopy, and correlated their results with scores on the sensory profile questionnaire (SPQ) [132]—a parent report measure of sensory abnormalities.

Using a 2D multivoxel ^{1}H spectroscopy STEAM sequence [133] and chemical shift imaging (TE 20 ms), this group tested 18 boys with ASD and 16 controls boys 8–15 years of age. Significant findings were all in the left hemisphere and included decreased NAA ($p = .006$); PCr + Cr (.022); Cho (expressed as GPC + PC) ($p = .004$); Glx trended to significance ($p = 0.082$). As seen in previous studies of the thalamus in ASD [134–137], no volumetric differences were found between subjects and controls, despite the presence of metabolic or functional effects.

These results are similar to those of Friedman et al. [90] who also found decreased NAA (right $p < 0.05$; left trend), and significantly decreased Cr + PCr and Cho ($p < 0.05$) in the left hemisphere in their ASD subjects aged 3–4 years. In addition, a single voxel study [134] in 31 subjects with autism and 15 control subjects (0–13 years of age) found reduced NAA/PCr + Cr.

These findings, taken together with other proton metabolite abnormalities described above in the ACC and caudate, are consistent with PET [136] and fMRI [129] investigations in ASD that implicate fronto-striato-thalamic circuitry in the pathophysiology of ASD.

Proton Spectroscopy and the Amygdala in ASD

The amygdala has been studied intensively in ASD due to this region's involvement in recognizing and interpreting emotional stimuli [6, 138–141]. Morphologic studies of the amygdala have demonstrated similar growth trajectories to overall brain size in autism, i.e., increased volume in young children [26–28], but normal or reduced size in adolescents and adults [23, 74, 142]. Further evaluation of some of these morphometric abnormalities has demonstrated a relationship between size and severity of symptomatology [28, 142]. Numerous fMRI studies have found abnormalities in this region in AD as well [72, 143–146].

The majority of proton spectroscopy studies in the amygdala/hippocampus region have also produced evidence for significant changes in autistic subjects as compared to controls. These findings include reduced NAA [147], reduced NAA/Cr [147–149], increased Cr and Glx (Page et al. 2006), and increased Cho/Cr and mI/Cr [149]. We review each of these below.

Otsuka et al. [147] studied proton metabolites in the right hippocampus–amygdala and left cerebellar hemisphere in 27 autistic patients 2–18 years old (21 boys and 6 girls) and 10 control children 6–14 years old, (4 boys and 6 girls), using short TE (18 ms) single voxel ($2 \times 2 \times 1.5$ cm^3) STEAM. They found reduced NAA ($p = 0.042$) in the autistic subjects in both regions, using quantitation of proton metabolite levels referenced to water, which may reflect true levels of metabolites more accurately than ratios. The age ranges given differ considerably between groups, which may confound the results, although decreased NAA in the cerebellum was also reported by Chugani et al. [150] in nine autistic children compared to five sibling control subjects ($p = 0.043$).

Endo et al. [148] conducted a short TE (35 ms) single voxel study and reported decreased NAA/Cr ratios in the right MTL—amygdala/hippocampus in 38 subjects with ASD as compared to 16 age-matched control subjects ($p < 0.001$). NAA/Cr was also significantly reduced when the subjects with autism were compared to subjects with PDD-NOS ($p < 0.001$). They further analyzed possible correlations between this data and ratings of autistic symptoms on the childhood autistic rating scale Tokyo version [151] and found negative correlations between NAA/Cr on the right and ratings of symptom severity including the total score ($p = 0.01$), and subscales: emotional response $p = 0.02$ and listening response $p = 0.001$.

Gabis et al. [149] also found decreased NAA/Cr ratios in a single voxel (TE 40 ms) study of the MTL ($p < 0.05$) in subjects with ASD (7 children with PDD-nos, 1 child with autism, and 5 with Asperger's disorder) compared to 8 controls (not matched for gender or IQ). Findings were bilateral and occurred across both language impaired and nonlanguage impaired subgroups. In addition, they found increased mI/Cr in bilateral MTL and in the cerebellum, and increased Cho/Cr in the left MTL and cerebellum. The Cho/Cr findings in the left MTL were attributed largely to the language-impaired subjects in the study.

Page et al. [81] used single voxel PRESS TE 35 ms to investigate proton metabolites in the right amygdala–hippocampus and right parietal lobe in 25 adults with autism and 21 control subjects. MRS metabolite concentrations were corrected for tissue and CSF content, and LCModel was used, plus in-house software, to quantify the results. Cr+PCr as well as Glx was increased significantly in the amygdala/hippocampus region, but not in right parietal lobe. The parietal findings are consistent with a previous ^{1}H-MRS study finding abnormalities in the left, but not right parietal lobe in autistic subjects [36].

These results of increased Cr in the amygdala, quantified using referencing standards, must be taken into account when considering reports of metabolite ratios in this region [148, 149]. While the findings are consistent across the Endo and Gabis studies, e.g., demonstrating decreased NAA/Cr in both, the extent to which increased Cr content may have contributed to these findings renders the results difficult to interpret.

Kleinhans et al. [152] emphasize this point in discussing the results of their bilateral amygdala study using water referencing and quantitative analysis of single voxels at short TE (30 ms). The investigator and colleagues measured proton metabolites in 20 adults with high functioning autism or Asperger's disorder and 19 age- and IQ-matched controls, and found no significant difference between controls and subjects. However, they did find an inverse correlation between measures of NAA and Cr, and symptom severity on the ADI-R. These results are consistent with the findings of an inverse correlation between NAA/Cr and symptom severity in Endo et al. [148], as well as with the studies of amygdala size and severity of symptomatology described above [28, 142], and with a previous fMRI study by Kleinhans et al., [146] demonstrating an inverse correlation between ADI-R severity and functional connectivity between the amygdala and fusiform face area.

Two other studies have also found correlations between symptom severity and proton metabolites in this region in ASD [153, 154]. Sokol et al. [153] reported an association between Cho/Cr+PCr in the hippocampal/amygdala complex and severity of autism as measured by the Children's Autistic Rating Scale (Pearson $r = 0.657$, $p = 0.04$) in ten children with autism, aged 2–12 years. The authors interpreted their results as potentially indicative of increased membrane turnover or cell growth. Results must be interpreted with caution as noted above, Cr+PCr levels may be abnormal in the brains of autistic children, and three of the children had seizures.

Suzuki et al. [154] investigated the hippocampus in relation to aggression in subjects with autism, due to the body of literature demonstrating a modulating influence of the hippocampus upon aggression [155–158]. They used a rectangular voxel, slanted to cover the long axis of the hippocampus on a coronal oblique image, a PRESS sequence (TE = 144 ms) in 12 non-medicated autistic males and 12 age- and gender-matched controls. The investigators found significantly increased concentrations of Cho ($p < 0.001$) and Cr+PCr ($p < 0.001$) in the hippocampal region of autistic subjects as compared to controls, and significantly decreased concentration of NAA in the cerebellum of the autistic subjects. Both Cho and Cr+PCr were related to aggression severity as measured by the Japanese version of the Aggression Questionnaire [159].

Proton Spectroscopy in the Cerebellum in ASD

Three ^{1}H-MRS studies in the cerebellum [106, 119, 149] have found no differences in ASD, while others have found significant decrements in NAA [147, 150, 154] and decreased Glx [68]. Reductions of NAA and Glx in this region may be a marker of decreased Purkinje cells in the cerebellum found in neuropathologic investigations of subjects with ASD [160]. There are reciprocal loops between the cerebellum and sensorimotor regions of the cortex [161], disruption of which might lead to dysfunction of higher cognitive functions involving the cerebellum to some degree [162]. These data support long-standing evidence of a cerebellar contribution to the symptom profile in ASD [163].

Future Directions

The convergence of differing imaging methods demonstrating abnormalities of structure, function, and biochemical metabolites in numerous regions throughout the brain in subjects with ASD provides ample evidence for this being a disorder of diffuse cortical and subcortical involvement. Future studies combining these methodologies in multimodal investigations will greatly enhance our ability to understand the biochemistry underlying functional and structural abnormalities in ASD. Combining such investigations with genetic data should help to elucidate the pathways leading to disruptions of development in this disorder.

References

1. American Psychiatric Association. Diagnostic and statistical manual of mental health disorders. 4th ed. Washington DC: American Psychiatric Association; 1994.
2. Filipek PA, Accardo PJ, Baranek GT, Cook EH, Dawson G, Gordon B, Gravel JS, Johnson CP, Kallen RJ, Levy SE, Minshew NJ, Prizant BM, Rapin I, Rogers SJ, Stone W, Teplin S, Tuchman RF, Volkmar FR. The Screening and Diagnosis of Autistic Spectrum Disorders (1999). J Autism Dev Disord. 1999;29:439–84.
3. Fombonne E. Epidemiology of pervasive developmental disorders. Pediatr Res. 2009;65:591–8.
4. Baird G, Simonoff E, Pickles A, Chandler S, Loucas T, Meldrum D, Charman T. Prevalence of disorders of the autism spectrum in a population cohort of children in South Thames: the Special Needs and Autism Project (SNAP). Lancet. 2006;368:210–15.
5. Fernell E, Gillberg C. Autism spectrum disorder diagnoses in Stockholm preschoolers. Res Dev Disabil. 2010;31:680–5.
6. Baron-Cohen S, Scott FJ, Allison C, Williams J, Bolton P, Matthews FE, Brayne C. Prevalence of autism-spectrum conditions: UK school-based population study. Br J Psychiatry. 2009;194:500–9.
7. King M, Bearman P. Diagnostic change and the increased prevalence of autism. Int J Epidemiol. 2009;38:1224–34.
8. Bauman ML, Kemper TL. Histoanatomic observations of the brain in early infantile autism. Neurology. 1985;35:866–74.
9. Bauman ML, Kemper TL. Neuroanatomic observations of the brain in autism. In: Bauman ML, Kemper TL, editors. The neurobiology of autism. Baltimore: Johns Hopkins University Press; 1994. p. 119–45.
10. Bauman ML, Kemper TL. Observations on the Purkinje cells in the cerebellar vermis in autism. J Neuropathol Exp Neurol. 1996;55:613.
11. Bauman ML, Kemper TL. Neuroanatomic observations of the brain in autism: a review and future directions. Int J Dev Neurosci. 2005;23:183–7.
12. Ritvo ER, Freeman BJ, Scheibel AB, Duong T, Robinson H, Gurthrie D, Ritvo A. Lower Purkinje cell counts in the cerebella of four autistic subjects: initial findings of the UCLA-NSAC Autopsy Research Report. Am J Psychiatry. 1986;143:862–6.
13. Bauman ML, Kemper TL. Developmental cerebellar abnormalities: a consistent finding in early infantile autism. Neurology. 1986;36 Suppl 1:190.
14. Kemper TL, Bauman ML. The contribution of neuropathologic studies to the understanding of autism. Neurol Clin. 1993;11:175–87.
15. Bailey A, Luther P, Dean A, et al. Clinicopathological study of autism. Brain. 1998;121:889–905.
16. Schumann CM, Amaral DG. Stereological analysis of amygdala neuron number in autism. J Neurosci. 2006;26(29):7674–9.
17. Casanova MF, Buxhoeveden DP, Switala AE, Roy E. Minicolumnar pathology in autism. Neurology. 2002;58:428–32.
18. Blatt GJ, Fitzgerald CM, Guptill JT, Booker AB, Kemper TL, Bauman ML. Density and distribution of hippocampal neuro- transmitter receptors in autism. J Autism Dev Disord. 2001;31:537–43.
19. Perry EK, Lee MLW, Martin-Ruiz CM, Court J, Volsen S, Merritt JB, Folly E, Iversen P, Bauman ML, Perry RH, Wenk G. Cholinergic activity in autism: abnormalities in the cerebral cortex and basal forebrain. Am J Psychiatry. 2001;158:1058–66.
20. Lee M, Martin-Ruiz C, Graham A, Court J, Jaros E, Perry E, Iversen P, Bauman M, Perry RH. Nicotinic receptor abnormalities in the cerebellar cortex in autism. Brain. 2002;125:1483–95.
21. Mountz JM, Tolbert LC, Lill DW, Katholi CR, Liu HG. Functional deficits in autistic disorder: characterization by technetium-99 m-HMPAO and SPECT. J Nucl Med. 1995;36(7):1156–62.
22. Abell F, Krams M, Ashburner J, Passingham R, Friston K, Frackowiak R, Happé F, Frith C, Frith U. The neuroanatomy of autism: a voxel-based whole brain analysis of structural scans. Neuroreport. 1999;10(8):1647–51.
23. Aylward EH, Minshew NJ, Goldstein G, Honeycutt NA, Augustine AM, Yates KO, Barta PE, Pearlson GD. MRI volumes of amygdala and hippocampus in nom-mentally retarded autistic adolescents and adults. Neurology. 1999;53(9):2145–50.
24. Haznedar MM, Buchsbaum MS, Wei TC, Hof PR, Cartwright C, Bienstock CA, Hollander E. Limic circuitry in patients with autism spectrum disorders studied with positron emission tomography and magnetic resonance imaging. Am J Psychiatry. 2000;157(12): 1994–2001.
25. Howard MA, Cowell PE, Boucher J, Broks P, Mayes A, Farrant A, Roberts N. Convergent neuroanatomical and behavioral evidence of an amygdala hypothesis of autism. Neuroreport. 2000;11(13):2931–5.
26. Sparks BF, Friedman SD, Shaw DW, Aylward EH, Echelard D, Artru AA, Maravilla KR, Giedd JN, Munson J, Dawson G, Dager SR. Brain structural abnormalities in young children with autism spectrum disorder. Neurology. 2002;59:184–92.
27. Schumann CM, Hamstra J, Goodlin-Jones BL, Lotspeich LJ, Kwon H, Buonocore MH, Lammers CR, Reiss AL, Amaral DG. The amygdala is enlarged in children but not adolescents with autism; the hippocampus is enlarged at all ages. J Neurosci. 2004;24:6392–401.
28. Munson J, Dawson G, Abbott R, Faja S, Webb SJ, Friedman SD, Shaw D, Artru A, Dager SR. Amygdalar volume and behavioral development in autism. Arch Gen Psychiatry. 2006;63(6):686–93.
29. Courchesne E, Yeung-Courchesne R, Press GA, Hesselink JR, Jernigan TL. Hypoplasia of cerebellar vermal lobules VI and VII in autism. N Engl J Med. 1988;318(21):1349–54.
30. Courchesne E, Saitoh O, Yeung-Courchesne R, Press GA, Lincoln AJ, Haas RH, Schreibman L. Abnormality of cerebellar vermian lobules VI and VII in patients with infantile autism: identification of hypoplastic and hyperplastic subgroups with MR imaging. AJR Am J Roentgenol. 1994;162(1):123–30.
31. Kates WR, Mostofsky SH, Zimmerman AW, Mazzocco MM, Landa R, Warsofsky IS, Kaufmann WE, Reiss AL. Neuroanatomical and neurocognitive differences in a pair of monozygous twins discordant for strictly defined autism. Ann Neurol. 1998;43(6):782–91.

32. Carper RA, Courchesne E. Inverse correlation between frontal lobe and cerebellum sizes in children with autism. Brain. 2000;123(4):836–44.
33. Holttum JR, Minshew NJ, Sanders RS, Phillips NE. Magnetic resonance imaging of the posterior fossa in autism. Biol Psychiatry. 1992;32(12):1091–101.
34. Rorke LB. A perspective: the role of disordered genetic control of neurogenesis in the pathogenesis of migration disorders. J Neuropathol Exp Neurol. 1994;53(2):105–17.
35. Piven J, Berthier ML, Starkstein SE, Nehme E, Pearlson G, Folstein S. Magnetic resonance imaging evidence for a defect of cerebral cortical development in autism. Am J Psychiatr. 1990;147:734–9.
36. Levitt JG, Blanton RE, Smalley S, Thompson PM, Guthrie D, McCracken JT, Sadoun T, Heinichen L, Toga AW. Cortical sulcal maps in autism. Cereb Cortex. 2003;13:728–35.
37. Hardan AY, Jou RJ, Keshavan MS, Varma R, Minshew NJ. Increased frontal cortical folding in autism: a preliminary MRI study. Psychiatry Res. 2004;131:263–8.
38. Courchesne E, Press GA, Yeung-Courchesne R. Parietal lobe abnormalities detected with MR in patients with infantile autism. AJR Am J Roentgenol. 1993;160(2):387–93.
39. Carper RA, Moses P, Tigue ZD, Courchesne E. Cerebral lobes in autisjm: early hyperplasia and abnormal age effects. Neuroimage. 2002;16(4):1038–51.
40. Carper RA, Courchesne E. Localized enlargement of the frontal cortex in early autism. Biol Psychiatry. 2005;57:126–33.
41. McAlonan GM, Daly E, Jumari V, Critchley HD, van Amelsvoort T, Suckling J, Simmons A, Sigmundsson T, Greenwood K, Russel A, Schmitz N, Happe F, Howlin P, Murphy DG. Brain anatomy and sensorimotor gating in Asperger syndrome. Brain. 2002;125:1594–606.
42. McAlonan GM, Cheung V, Cheung C, Sucking J, Lam GY, Tai KS, Murphy DG YL, Chua SE. Mapping the brain in autism. A voxel-based MRI study of volumetric differences and intercorrelations in autism. Brain. 2005;128:268–76.
43. McAlonan GM, Suckling J, Wong N, Cheung V, Lienenkaemper N, Cheung C, Chua SE. Distinct patterns of grey matter abnormality in high-functioning autism and Asperger's syndrome. J Child Psychol Psychiatry. 2008;49:1287–95.
44. Amaral DG, Schumann CM, Nordahl CW. Neuroanatomy of autism. Trends Neurosci. 2008;31:137–45.
45. Stanfield AC, McIntosh AM, Spencer MD, Phillip R, Gaur S, Lawrie SM. Towards a neuroanatomy of autism: A systematic review and meta-analysis of structural magnetic resonance imaging studies. Eur Psychiatry. 2008;23:289–99.
46. Jou RJ, Minshew NJ, Keshavan MS, Hardan AY. Cortical gyrification in autistic and asperger disorders: a preliminary magnetic resonance imaging study. J Child Neurol. 2010;25:1462–7.
47. Chung MK, Rbbins SM, Dalton DJ, Davidson RJ, Alexander AL, Evans AC. Cortical thickness analysis in autism with heat kernal smoothing. Neuroimage. 2005;25:256–1265.
48. Hadjikhani N, Joseph RM, Snyder J, Tager-Flusberg H. Anatomical differences in the mirror neuron system and social cognition network in autism. Cereb Cortex. 2006;16:1276–82.
49. Hyde KL, Samson F, Evans AC, Mottron L. Neuroanatomical differences in brain areas implicated in perceptual and other core features of autism revealed by cortical thickness analysis and voxel-based morphometry. Hum Brain Mapp. 2010;31(4):556–66.
50. Kanner L. Autistic disturbance of affective contact. Nerv Child. 1943;2:217–50.
51. Lainhart JE, Piven J, Wzorek M, et al. Macrocephaly in children and adults with autism. J Am Acad Child Adolesc Psychiatry. 1997;36:282.
52. Courchesne E, Carper R, Akshoomoff N. Evidence of brain overgrowth in the first year of life in autism. JAMA. 2003;290:337–44.
53. Piven J, Nehme E, Simon J, Barta P, Pearlson G, Folstein SE. Magnetic resonance imaging in autism: measurement of the cerebellum, pons, and fourth ventricle. Biol Psychiatry. 1992;31(5):491–504.
54. Piven J, Arndt S, Bailey J, Havercamp S, Andreasen NC, Palmer P. An MRI study of brain size in autism. Am J Psychiatry. 1995;152:1145–9.
55. Courchesne E, Karns CM, Davids HR, Ziccardi R, Carper RA, Tigue ZD, Chisum HJ, Moses P, Pierce K, Lord C, Lincoln AJ, Pizzo S, Schreibman L, Haas RH, Akshoomoff NA, Yeung-Courchesne R. Unusual brain growth patterns in early life in patients with autistic disorder. Neurology. 2001;57:245–54.
56. Hardan AY, Minshew NJ, Mallikarjuhn M, Keshavan MS. Brain volume in autism. J Child Neurol. 2001;16(6):421–4.
57. Hazlett HC, Poe M, Gerig G, Smith RG, Provenzale J, Ross A, Gilmore J, Piven J. Magnetic resonance imaging and head circumference study of brain size in autism: Birth through age 2 years. Arch Gen Psychiatry. 2005;62:1366–76.
58. Redcay E, Courchesne E. When is the brain enlarged in autism? A meta-analysis of all brain size reports. Biol Psychiatry. 2005;58(1):1–9.
59. Schumann CM, Bloss CS, Barnes CC, Wideman GM, Carper RA, Akshoomoff N, Pierce K, Hagler D, Schork N, Lord C, Courchesne E. Longitudinal magnetic renonance imaging study of corical development through early childhood in autism. J Neurosci. 2010;30:4419–27.
60. Aylward EH, Minshew NJ, Field K, Sparks BF, Singh N. Effects of age on brain volume and head circumference in autism. Neurology. 2002;59:175–83.
61. Hazlett HC, Poe MD, Gerig G, Smith RG, Piven J. Cortical gray and white brain tissue volume in adolescents and adults with autism. Biol Psychiatry. 2006;59:1–6.
62. Freitag CM, Luders E, Hulst HE, Narr KL, Thompson PM, Toga AW, Krick C, Konrad C. Total brain volume and corpus callosum size in medication-naïve adolescents and young adults with autism spectrum disorder. Biol Psychiatry. 2009;66:316–9.
63. Keller TA, Kana RK, Just MA. A developmental study of the structural integrity of white matter in autism. Neuroreport. 2007;18:23–7.
64. Sundaram SK, Kumar A, Makki MI, Behen ME, Chugani HT, Chugani DC. Diffusion tensor imaging of frontal lobe in autism spectrum disorder. Cereb Cortex. 2008;18:2659–65.
65. Barnea-Goraly N, Lotspeich LJ, Reiss AL. Similar white matter aberrations in children with autism and their unaffected siblings: a diffusion tensor imaging study using tract-based spatial statistics. Arch Gen Psychiatry. 2010;67:1052–60.
66. Lee JE, Bigler EDH, Alexander AL, Lazar M, DuBray MB, Chung MK, Johnson M, Morgan J, Miller JN, McMahon WM, Lu J, Jeong EK, Lainhart JE. Diffusion tensor imaging of white matter in the superior temporal gyrus and temporal stem in autism. Neurosci Lett. 2007;424:127–32.
67. Friedman SD, Shaw DW, Artru AA, Dawson G, Petropoulos H, Dager SR. Gray and white matter brain chemistry in young children with autism. Arch Gen Psychiatry. 2006;63:786–94.
68. DeVito TJ, Drost DJ, Neufeld RW, Rajakumar N, Pavlosky W, Williamson P, Nicolson R. Evidence for cortical dysfunction in autism: a proton magnetic resonance spectroscopic imaging study. Biol Psychiatry. 2007;61(4):465–73.
69. Rumsey JM, Duara R, Grady C, Rapoport JL, Margolin RA, Rapoport SI, Cutler NR. Brain metabolism in autism. Resting cerebral glucose utilization rates as measured with positron emission tomography. Arch Gen Psychiatry. 1985;42:448–55.
70. Ohnishi T, Matsuda H, Hashimoto T, Kuhihiro T, Ishikawa M, Uema T, Sasaki M. Abnormal regional cerebral blood flow in childhood autism. Brain. 2000;123:1838–44.
71. Zilbovicius M, Boddaert N, Belin P, Poline JB, Remy P, Mangin JF, Thivard L, Barthelemy C, Samson Y. Temporal lobe dysfunction in

childhood autism: a PET study. Am J Psychiatry. 2000;157:1988–93.
72. Critchley HD, Daly EM, Bullmore ET, Williams SC, an Amelsvoort T, Robertson DM. The functional neuroanatomy of social behavior: changes in cerebral blood flow when people with autistic disorder process facial expressions. Brain. 2000;123:2203–12.
73. Schultz RT, Gauthier I, Klin A, Fulbright RK, Anderson AW, Volkmar F, Skudlarski P, Lacadie C, Cohen DJ, Gore JC. Abnormal ventral temporal cortical activity during face discrimination among individuals with autism and Asperger syndrome. Arch Gen Psychiatry. 2000;57:331–40.
74. Pierce K, Muller RA, Ambrose J, Allen G, Courchesne E. Face processing occurs outside the fusiform 'face area'in autism: evidence from functional MRI. Brain. 2001;124:2059–73.
75. Boddaert N, Chabane N, Barthelemy C, Bourgeois M, Poline JB, Brunelle F, Samson Y, Zilbovicius M. Bitmeporal lobe dysfunction in infantile autism: positron emission tomography study. J Radiol. 2002;32:1–7.
76. Williams JH, Whiten A, Suddendorf T, Perrett DI. Imitation, mirror neurons and autism. Neurosci Biobehav Rev. 2001;25(4):287–95.
77. Toth K, Munson J. Meltzoff aN, Dawson g. Early predictors of communication development in young children with autism spectrum disorder: joint attention, imitation, and toy play. J Autism Dev Disord. 2006;36:993–1005.
78. Just MA, Cherkassky VL, Keller TA, Minshew NJ. Cortical activation and synchronization during sentence comprehension in high-functioning autism: evidence of underconnectivity. Brain. 2004;127:1811–21.
79. Jones TB, Bandettini PA, Kenworthy L, Case LK, Milleville SC, Martin A, Birn RM. Sources of group differences in functional connectivity: an investigation applied to autism spectrum disorder. Neuroimage. 2010;49:401–14.
80. Welchew D, Ashwin C, Berkouk K, Salvador R, Suckling J. Functional disconnectivity of the medial temporal lobe in Asperger's syndrome. Biol Psychiatry. 2005;57:991–8.
81. Page LA, Daly E, Schmitz N, Simmons A, Toal F, Deeley Q, Ambery F, McAlonan GM, Murphy KC, Murphy DG. In vivo 1 H-magnetic resonance spectroscopy study of amygdala-hippocampal and parietal regions in autism. Am J Psychiatry. 2006;163(12):2189–92.
82. Minshew NJ, Goldstein G, Dombrowski SM, Panchalingam K, Pettegrew JW. A preliminary 31P MRS study of autism: evidence for undersynthesis and increased degradation of brain membranes. Biol Psychiatry. 1993;33:762–73.
83. Arias-Mendoza F, Brown TR. In vivo measurement of phosphorous markers of disease. Dis Markers. 2004;19:49–68.
84. Hashimoto T, Tayama M, Miyazaki M, Yoneda Y, Yoshimoto T, Harada M, Miyoshi H, Tanouchi M, Kuroda Y. Differences in brain metabolites between patients with autism and mental retardation as detected by in vivo localized proton magnetic resonance spectroscopy. J Child Neurol. 1997;12(2):91–6.
85. Murphy DG, Critchley HD, Schmitz N, McAlonan G, Van Amelsvoort T, Robertson D, Daly E, Rowe A, Russell A, Simmons A, Murphy KC, Howlin P. Asperger syndrome: a proton magnetic resonance spectroscopy study of brain. Arch Gen Psychiatry. 2002;59(10):885–91.
86. American Psychiatric Association. Diagnostic and statistical manual of mental health disorders, 3rd edn, revised. Washington DC: American Psychiatric Association; 1987.
87. Hisaoka S, Harada M, Nishitani H, Mori K. Regional magnetic resonance spectroscopy of the brain in autistic individuals. Neuroradiology. 2001;43(6):496–8.
88. Goodman WK, Price LH, Rasmussen SA, et al. The Yale-Brown Obsessive Compulsive Scale. I. Development, use, and reliability. Arch Gen Psychiatry. 1989;46:1006–16.
89. Lord C, Rutter M, Le Couteur A. Autism Diagnostic Interview-Revised: a revised version of a diagnostic interview for caregivers of indiviguals with possible pervasive developmental disorders. J Autsim Dev Disord. 1994;24:659–85.
90. Friedman SD, Shaw DW, Artru AA, Richards TL, Gardner J, Dawson G, Posse S, Dager SR. Regional brain chemical alterations in young children with autism spectrum disorder. Neurology. 2003;60:100–7.
91. Provencher SW. Automatic quantitation of localized in vivo 1 H spectra with LCModel. NMR Biomed. 2001;14:260–4.
92. Mullen E. Mullen Scales of Early Learning TOTAL. Cranston, RI: Child; 1989.
93. Zeegers M, van der Grond J, van Daalen E, Buitelaar J, van Engeland H. Proton magnetic resonance spectroscopy in developmentally delayed young boys with or without autism. J Neural Transm. 2007;114(2):289–95.
94. Rosenberg DR, MacMaster FP, Kehavan MS, Fitzgerald KD. Steward Cm, Moore GJ. Decrease in caudate glutamatergic concentrations in pediatric obsessive-compulsive disorder patients taking paroxetine. J Am Acad Child Adolesc Psychiatry. 2000;39:1096–103.
95. Bernardi S, Anagnostou E, Shen J, Kolevzon A, Buxbaum JD, Hollander E, Hof PR, Fan J. In vivo (1)H-magnetic resonance spectroscopy study of the attentional networks in autism. Brain Res. 2011;1380:198–205.
96. Harada M, Taki MM, Nose A, Kubo H, Mori K, Nishitani H, Matsuda T. Fucntion of the frontal lobe in autistic individuals: a proton magnetic resonance study. J Med Invest. 2010;57:35–44.
97. Mescher M, Merkle H, Kirsch J, Garwood M, Gruetter R. Simultaneous in vivo spectral editing and water suppression. NMR Biomed. 1998;11:266–72.
98. Provencher SW. Estimation of metabolite concentrations from localized in vivo proton NMR spectra. Magn Reson Med. 1993;30:672–9.
99. Fatemi SH, Folsom TD, Reutiman TJ, Thuras PD. Expression of GABA(B) receptors is altered in rains of subjects with autism. Cerebellum. 2009;8:64–9.
100. Fatemi SH, Reutiman TJ, Folsom TD, Thuras PD. GABA(A) receptor downregulation in brains of subjects with autism. J Autism Dev Disord. 2009;39:223–30.
101. Brand A, Richter-Landsberg C, Leibfritz D. Multinuclear NMR studies on the energy metabolism of glial and neuronal cells. Dev Neurosci. 1993;15:289–98.
102. Urenjak J, Williams SR, Gadian DG, Noble M. Proton nuclear magnetic resonance spectroscopy unambiguously identifies different neural cell types. J Neurosci. 1993;13:981–9.
103. Stork C, Renshaw PF. Mitochondrial dysfunction in bipolar disorder: evidence from magnetic resonance spectroscopy research. Mol Psychiatry. 2005;10:900–19.
104. Phelps ME, Huang SC, Hoffman EJ, Selin C, Sokoloff L, Kuhl DE. Tomographic measurement of local cerebral glucose metabolic rate in humans with (F-18)2-fluoro-2-deoxy-D-glucose: Validation of method. Ann Neurol. 1979;6:371–88.
105. Harris GJ, Chabris CF, Clark J, Urban T, Aharon I, Steele S, McGrath L, Condouris K, Tager-Flusberg H. Brain activation during semantic processing in autism spectrum disorders via functional magnetic resonance imaging. Brain Cogn. 2006;61(1):54–68.
106. Kleinhans NM, Schweinsburg BC, Cohen DN, Müller RA, Courchesne E. N-acetyl aspartate in autism spectrum disorders: regional effects and relationship to fMRI activation. Brain Res. 2007;1162:85–97.
107. Turken AU, Dronkers NF. The nueral architecture of the language comprehension network: Converging evidence from lesion and connectivity analyses. Front Syst Neurosci. 2011;5:1.
108. Gill SS, Thomas DG, Van Bruggen N, Gadian DG, Peden CJ, Bell JD, Cox IJ, Menon DK, Iles RA, Bryant DJ, et al. Proton MR spectroscopy of intracranial tumours: in vivo and in vitro studies. J Comput Assist Tomogr. 1990;14:497–504.

109. Speck O, Thiel T, Hennig J. Grading and therapy monitoring of astrocytomas with 1 H-spectroscopy: preliminary study. Anticancer Res. 1996;16:1581–5.
110. Rubenstein JLR, Merzenich MM. Model of autism: Increased ration of excitation/inhibition in key neural systems. Genes Brain Behav. 2003;2:255–67.
111. Pardo JV, Pardo J, Janer KW, Raichle ME. The anterior cingulate cortex mediates processing in the Stroop attentional conflic paradigm. Proc Natl Acad Sci USA. 1990;87:256–9.
112. Lane RD, Reiman EM, Axelrod B, Yun LS, Holmes A, Schwartz GE. Neuroal correlates of levels of emotional awareness. Evidence of an interaction between emotion and attention in the anterior cingulate cortex. J Cogn Neurosci. 1998;10:525–35.
113. Bush G, Luu P, Posner MI. Cognitive and emotional influences in anterior cingulate cortex. Trends Cogn Sci. 2000;4:215–22.
114. Devinsky O, Morrell MJ, Vogt BA. Contributions of anterior cingulate cortex to behaviors. Brain. 1995;118:279–306.
115. Baron-Cohen S. Mindblindness: an essay on autism and theory of mind. Boston: MIT Press/Bradford Books; 1995.
116. Brunet-Gouet E, Decety J. Social brain dysfunctions in schizophrenia: A review of neuroimaging studies. Psychiatry Res: Neuroimaging. 2006;148:75–92.
117. Schlosser RG, Wagner G, Schachtzabel C, Peikert G, Koch K, Reichenbach JR, Sauer H. Fronto-cingulate effective connectivity in obsessive compulsive disorder: a study with fMRI and dynamic causal modeling. Hum Brain Mapp. 2010;31(12):1834–50.
118. Sears LL, Vest C, Mohamed S, Bailery J, Ranson BJ, Piven J. An MRI study of the basal ganglia in autism. Prog Neuropsychopharmacol Biol Psychiatry. 1999;23:613–24.
119. Vasconcelos MM, Brito AR, Domingues RC, da Cruz LC, Jr GEL, Werner Jr J, Gonçalves JP. Proton magnetic resonance spectroscopy in school-aged autistic children. J Neuroimaging. 2008;18(3):288–95.
120. Oblak A, Gibbs TT, Blatt GJ. Decreased GABAA receptors and benzodiazepine binding sites in the anterior cingulate cortex in autism. Autism Res. 2009;2:205–19.
121. Oner O, Devrimci-Ozguven H, Oktem F, Yagmurlu B, Baskak B, Munir KM. Proton MR spectroscopy: higher right anterior Cingulate N-Acetylaspartate/Choline ratio in asperger syndrome compared with healthy controls. Am J Neuroradiol. 2007;28:1494–8.
122. Baxter LR, Saxena S, Brody AL, Ackermann RF, Colgan M, Schwartz JM. Brain mediation of obsessive-compulsive disorder symptoms: evidence from functional brain imaging studies in the human and nonhuman primate. Semin Clin Neuropsychiatry. 1996;1:32–47.
123. Insel TR. Toward a neuroanatomy of obsessive compulsive disorder. Psychiatr Clin North Am. 1992;15:813–24.
124. Modell JG, Mountz JM, Curtis GC, Greden JF. Neurophysiologic dysfunction in basal ganglia/limbic striatal and thalamocortical circuits as a pathogenetic mechanism of obsessive-compulsive disorder. J Neuropsychiatry Clin Neurosci. 1989;1:27–36.
125. Rapoport JL, Wise SP. Obsessive-compulsive disorderL Evidence fo basas ganglia dysfunction. Psychopharmacol Bull. 1988;24:380–4.
126. Maia TV, Cooney RE, Peterson BS. The neural bases of obsessive-compulsive disorder in children and adults. Dev Psychopathol. 2008;20:1251–83.
127. Horwitz B, Rumsey JM, Grady CL, Rapoport SI. The cerebral metabolic landscape in autism: intercorrelations of regional glucose utilization. Arch Neurol. 1988;45:749–55.
128. Shafritz KM, Dichter GS, Baranek GT, Belger A. The neural circuitry mediating shifts in behavioral response and cognitive set in autism. Biol Psychiatry. 2008;63:974–80.
129. Takarae Y, Minshew NJ, Luna B, Sweeney JA. Atypical involvement of frontostriatal systems during sensorimotor control in autism. Psychiatry Res. 2007;156:117–27.
130. Di Martino A, Kelly C, Grzadzinski R, Zuo X, Mennes M, Mairena MA, Lord C, Castellanos FX, Milham MP. Aberrant striatal functional connectivity in children with autism. Biol Psychiatry. 2011;69(9):847–56.
131. Hardan AY, Minshew NJ, Melhem NM, Srihari S, Jo B, Bansal R, Keshavan MS, Stanley JA. An MRI and proton spectroscopy study of the thalamus in children with autism. Psychiatry Res. 2008;163(2):97–105.
132. Dunn W. Performance of typical children on the Sensory Profile: an item analysis. Am J Occup Ther. 1994;48:967–74.
133. Frahm J, Bruhn H, Gyngell ML, Merboldt KD, Hanicke W, Sauter R. Localized high-resolution proton NMR spectrsocopy using stimulated echoes: initial applications to human brain in vivo. Magn Reson Med. 1989;9:79–93.
134. Perich-Alsina J, Aduna de Paz M, Valls A, Munoz-Yanta JA. Thalamic spectrsocopy using magnetic resonance in autism. Rev Neurol. 2002;34:S68–71.
135. Tsatsanis KD, Rourke BP, Klin A, Volkmar FR, Cicchetti D, Schuiltz RT. Reduced thalamic volume in high-functioning individuals with autism. Biol Psychiatry. 2003;15:121–9.
136. Haznedar MM, Buchsbaum MS, Hazlett EA, KiCalzi EM, Cartwright C, Hollander E. Volumetric analysis and three-dimensional glucose metabolic mapping of the striatum and thalamus in patients with autism spectrum disorders. Am J Psychiatry. 2006;163:1252–63.
137. Hardan AY, Girgis RR, Adams J, Gilbert AR, Keshavan MS, Minshew NJ. Abnormal brain size effect on the thalamus in autism. Psychiatry Res. 2006;147:145–51.
138. Adolphs R, Tranel D, Hamann S, Young AW, Calder AJ, Phelps EA, et al. Recognition of facial emotion in nine individuals with bilateral amygdala damage. Neuropsychologia. 1999;37(10):1111–7.
139. Adolphs R. The neurobiology of social cognition. Curr Opin Neurobiol. 2001;11(2):231–9.
140. Adolphs R, Sears L, Piven J. Abnormal processing of social information from faces in autism. J Cogn Neurosci. 2001;13(2):232–40.
141. Bachevalier J, Loveland KA. The orbitofrontal-amygdala circuit and self-regulation of social-emotional behavior in autism. Neurosci Biobehav Rev. 2006;30:87–117.
142. Nacewicz BM, Dalton KM, Johnstone T, Long MT, McAuliff EM, Oakes TR, Alexander AL, Davidson RJ. Amygdala volume and nonverbal social impairment in adolescent and adult males with autis. Arch Gen Psychiarty. 2006;63:1417–28.
143. Wang AT, Dapretto M, Hariri AR, Sigman M, Bookheimer SY. Neural correlates of facial affect processing in children and adolescents with autism spectrum disorder. J Am Acad Child Adolesc Psychiatry. 2004;43:481–90.
144. Dalton KM, Kalin NH, Grist TM, Davidson RJ. Neural-cardiac coupling in threat-evoked anxiety. J Cogn Neurosci. 2005;17:969–80.
145. Ashwin C, Wheelwright S, Baron-Cohen S. Finding a face in the crowd: testing the anger superiority effect in Asperger Syndrome. Brain Cogn. 2006;61:78–95.
146. Kleinhans NM, Richards T, Sterling L, Stegbauer KC, Mahurin R, Johnson LC, et al. Abnormal functional connectivity in autism spectrum disorders during face processing. Brain. 2008;131(4):1000–12.
147. Otsuka H, Harada M, Mori K, Hisaoka S, Nishitani H. Brain metabolites in the hippocampus-amygdala region and cerebellum in autism: an 1 H-MR spectroscopy study. Neuroradiology. 1999;41(7):517–9.
148. Endo T, Shioiri T, Kitamura H, Kimura T, Endo S, Masuzawa N, Someya T. Altered chemical metabolites in the amygdala-hippocampus region contribute to autistic symptoms of autism spectrum disorders. Biol Psychiatry. 2007;62(9):1030–7.
149. Gabis L, Huang W, Azizian A, DeVincent C, Tudorica A, Kesner-Baruch Y, Roche P, Pomeroy J. 1H-magnetic resonance spectroscopy markers of cognitive and language ability in clinical subtypes of autism spectrum disorders. J Child Neurol. 2008;23(7):766–74.

150. Chugani DC, Sundram BS, Behen M, Lee ML, Moore GJ. Evidence of altered energy metabolism in autistic children. Prog Neuropsychopharmacol Biol Psychiatry. 1999;23(4):635–41.
151. Kurita H, Miyake Y, Katsuno K. Reliability and validity of the Childhood Autism Rating Scale- Tokyo version (CARS-TV). J Autism Dev Disord. 1989;19:389–96.
152. Kleinhans NM, Richards T, Weaver KE, Liang O, Dawson G, Aylward E. Brief Report: Biochemical Correlates of Clinical Impairment in High Functioning Autism and Asperger's Disorder. J Autism Dev Disord. 2009;39:1079–86.
153. Sokol DK, Dunn DW, Edwards-Brown M, Feinberg J. Hydrogen proton magnetic resonance spectroscopy in autism: preliminary evidence of elevated choline/creatine ratio. J Child Neurol. 2002;17(4):245–9.
154. Suzuki K, Nishimura K, Sugihara G, Nakamura K, Tsuchiya KJ, Matsumoto K, Takebayahsi K, Isoda H, Sakahara H, Sugiyama T, Tsujii M, Takei N, Mori N. Metabolite alterations in the hippocampus of high-fucntioning adult subjects with autism. Int J Neuropsychopharmacol. 2010;13:529–34.
155. Fontani G, Vegni V. Hippocampal electrical activity during social interactions in rabbits living in a seminatural environment. Physiol Behav. 1990;47:175–83.
156. Tebartz van Elst L, Woermann FG, Lemieux L, Thompson PJ, et al. Affective aggression in patients with temporal lobe epilepsy: a quantitative MRI study of the amygdala. Brain. 2000;123:234–43.
157. Gregg TR, Siegel A. Brain structures and neurotransmitters regulating aggression in cats: implications for human aggression. Prog Neuropsychopharmacol Biol Psychiatry. 2001;25:91–140.
158. Zetzsche T, Preuss UW, Frodl T, Schmitt G, et al. Hippocampal volume reduction and history of aggressive behaviour in patients with borderline personality disorder. Psychiatry Res. 2007;154:157–70.
159. Ando A, Soga S, Yamasaki K, Shimai T, et al. Development of the Japanese version of the Development of the Japanese version of the Buss-Perry Aggression Questionnaire (BAQ) [in Japanese]. Jap J Psychol. 1999;70:384–92.
160. Palmen SJ, van Engeland H, Hof PR, Schmitz C. Neuropathological findings in autism. Brain. 2004;127:2575–83.
161. Schmahmann JD, Pandya DN. There cerebrocerebellar system. In: Schmahmann J, editor. The cerebellum and cognition. San Diego: Academic; 1997. p. 31–60.
162. Ito M. Control of mental activities by internal models in the cerebellum. Nat Rev Neurosci. 2008;9:304–13.
163. Courchesne E, Redcay E, Morgan JT, Kennedy DP. Autism at the beginning: microstructural and growth abnormalities underlying the cognitive and behavioral phenotype of autism. Dev Psychopathol. 2005;17:577–97.

Further Reading

Bluml S, Seymour KJ, Ross BD. Developmental changes in choline- and ethanolamine-containing compounds measured with proton-decoupled (31)P MRS in vivo human brain. Magn Reson Med. 1999;42:643–54.

Castelli F, Frith C, Happe F, Frith U. Autism, Asperger syndrome and brain mechanisms for the attribution of mental states to animated shapes. Brain. 2002;125:1839–49.

Davis MH. Measuring individual differences in empathy: evidence for a multidimensional approach. J Pers Soc Psychol. 1983;44(1):113–26.

Filler A. MR Neurography and Diffusion Tensor Imaging: Origins, history and clinical impact. Neurosurgery. 2009;65:29–43.

Gupta RK, Cloughesy TF, Sinha U, Garakian J, Rubino G, Rubino L, Becker DP, Vinters HV, Alger JR. Relationships between choline magnetic resonance spectroscopy, apparent diffusion coefficient and quantitative histopathology in human glioma. J Neuro-Oncol. 2000;50:215–26.

Hashimoto T, Kawano N, Fukuda K, Endo S, Mori K, Yoneda Y, Yamaue T, Harada M, Miyoshi K. Proton magnetic resonance spectroscopy of the brain in three cases of Rett syndrome: comparison with autism and normal controls. Acta Neurol Scand. 1998;98(1):8–14.

Kahne D, Tudorica A, Borella A, Shapiro L, Johnstone F, Huang W, Whitaker-Azmitia PM. Behavioral and magnetic resonance spectroscopic studies in the rat hyperserotonemic model of autism. Physiol Behav. 2002;75(3):403–10.

Kemper TL, Bauman ML. Neuropathology of infantile autism. J Neuropathol Exp Neurol. 1998;57:645–52.

Langen M, Durston S, Staal WG, Palmen SJ, van Engeland H. Caudate nucleus is enlarged in high-functioning medication-naïve subjects with autism. Biol Psychiatry. 2007;62:262–6.

Minshew NJ, Dombrowski SM. In vivo neuroanatomy of autism: neuroimaging studies. In: Bauman ML, Kemper TL, editors. The neurobiology of autism. Baltimore: Johns Hopkins University Press; 1994. p. 67–85.

Montag C, Schubert F, Heinz A, Gallinat J. Prefrontal cortex glutamate correlates with mental perspective-taking. PLoS One. 2008;3(12):e3890.

Paulus C. Empathie, Kompetenz und Altruismus. 1992. http://www.uni-saarland.de/fak5/ezw/abtell/motiv/paper/empathie.htm.

Pons R, Andreu AL, Checcarelli N, Vilà MR, Engelstad K, Sue CM, Shungu D, Haggerty R, de Vivo DC, DiMauro S. Mitochondrial DNA abnormalities and autistic spectrum disorders. J Pediatr. 2004;144(1):81–5.

Provencher SW. LcModel and LcMgui user's manual. Available at: http://s-provencher.com/pages/lcm-manual.shtml. Accessed January 19, 2000.

Redcay E, Courchesne E. When is the brain enlarged in autism? A meta-analysis of all brain size reports. Biol Psychiatry. 2004;58:1–9.

Rosenberg DR, Keshavan MS, O'Hearn KM, Dick EL, Bagwell WW, Seymour AB, Montrose DM, Pierri JN, Birmaher B. Frontostriatal measurement in treatment-naïve children with obsessive-compulsive disorder. Arch Gen Psychiatry. 1997;54:824–30.

Rosenberg DR, Keshavan MS. AE Bennett Research Award. Toward a neurodevelopmental model of obsessive—compulsive disorder. Biol Psychiatry. 1998;43:623–40.

Rothman DL, Behar KL, Hyder F, Shulman RG. In vivo NMR studies of the glutamate neurotransmitter flux and neuroenergetics: Implications for brain function. Annu Rev Physiol. 2003;65:401–27.

Strauss WL, Unis AS, Cowan C, Dawson G, Dager SR. Fluorine magnetic resonance spectroscopy measurement of brain fluvoxamine and fluoxetine in pediatric patients treated for pervasive developmental disorders. Am J Psychiatry. 2002;159(5):755–60.

Zilbovicius M, Garreau B, Samson Y, Remy P. Delayed maturation of the frontal cortex in childhood autism. Am J Psychiatry. 1995;152:248–52.

18 Magnetic Resonance Spectroscopy Studies of Attention Deficit Hyperactivity Disorder

Joseph O'Neill, Jennifer G. Levitt, and Jeffry R. Alger

This chapter reviews magnetic resonance spectroscopy (MRS) studies of pediatric and adult attention deficit hyperactivity disorder (ADHD). We begin with a brief clinical overview of ADHD. Then we summarize brain findings in ADHD obtained with neuroimaging modalities other than MRS. We suggest conceivable clinical applications of MRS in ADHD. The heart of the chapter is a review of all published MRS studies of ADHD known to us. Drawing from the MRS and other neuroimaging findings, we offer a speculative neurochemical model of the subjective mental symptomatology of ADHD. We identify gaps representing opportunities and make methodological recommendations for future MRS ADHD research.

ADHD as a Psychiatric Disorder

This section briefly overviews clinical aspects of ADHD. For more comprehensive reviews, see Wolraich et al. [1], Cormier [2], Dopheide and Pliszka [3], Bukstein [4], and Wilens and Spencer [5].

J. O'Neill, Ph.D. (✉)
Division of Child and Adolescent Psychiatry, Semel Institute for Neuroscience and Human Behavior, UCLA, Los Angeles, CA, USA
e-mail: joneill@mednet.ucla.edu

J.G. Levitt, M.D.
Department of Psychiatry, Semel Institute for Neuroscience and Human Behavior, UCLA, Los Angeles, CA, USA

J.R. Alger, Ph.D.
Department of Radiological Sciences, UCLA, Los Angeles, CA, USA

Epidemiology, Public Health Impact of ADHD

ADHD is the most commonly diagnosed pediatric psychiatric disorder, affecting ~5% of children and adolescents globally [6, 7]. Prevalence by world region varies 2–12% [7, 8], whereby one should consider that ADHD diagnosis is 3–4 times more likely under DSM-IV (used mainly in North America) than under ICD-10 (used mainly in Europe) criteria [9]. ADHD is diagnosed two to four times more frequently in boys than in girls [10, 11], though it is not established whether males are more susceptible or only more likely to be diagnosed due to social factors [12]. ADHD persists into adulthood in up to 60% of patients [13], whereby the hyperactivity and impulsiveness symptoms of the disease decline with age [14]. Some consider this decline part of the natural history of the disorder, while others view it as symptom masking by compensatory cognitive strategies [15]. The most recent epidemiological data [16] document a striking increase in ADHD prevalence in the last decade across the US and across demographic categories. The CDC speculates that this rise may be due to "shift in the cultural acceptance of ADHD or changes in access to care." We saw no discussion of whether there has been an increase in the true incidence of the disease, due perhaps to environmental, child care, or lifestyle factors, or whether the condition is now being over detected, e.g., "fashionable diagnosis." The economic impact of ADHD resulting from medical treatment, lost productivity, and other costs is estimated in the billions of US dollars [17].

Onset, Symptoms, Diagnosis, Subtypes

Onset and Symptoms

ADHD is a neurobehavioral developmental disorder and per DSM-IV onset of symptoms must come before 7 years of

S. Blüml and A. Panigrahy (eds.), *MR Spectroscopy of Pediatric Brain Disorders*,
DOI 10.1007/978-1-4419-5864-8_18,

Table 18.1 Some possible individual symptoms of attention deficit hyperactivity disorder (ADHD)

Predominantly inattentive symptoms may include
• Be easily distracted, miss details, forget things, and frequently switch from one activity to another • Have difficulty maintaining focus on one task • Become bored with a task after only a few minutes, unless doing something enjoyable • Have difficulty focusing attention on organizing and completing a task or learning something new or trouble completing or turning in homework assignments, often losing things (e.g., pencils, toys, assignments) needed to complete tasks or activities • Not seem to listen when spoken to • Daydream, become easily confused, and move slowly • Have difficulty processing information as quickly and accurately as others
Predominantly hyperactive-impulsive symptoms may include
• Fidget and squirm in their seats • Talk nonstop • Dash around, touching or playing with anything and everything in sight • Have trouble sitting still during dinner, school, and story time • Be constantly in motion • Have difficulty doing quiet tasks or activities.
Predominantly impulsive symptoms may include
• Be very impatient • Blurt out inappropriate comments, show their emotions without restraint, and act without regard for consequences • Have difficulty waiting for things they want or waiting their turns in games

From National Institute of Mental Health (NIMH). Attention deficit hyperactivity disorder (ADHD). NIH Publication No. 08-3572. Bethesda, MD; National Institute of Health. 2008

age [18]. The symptomatic hallmarks of ADHD are inattention, hyperactivity, and impulsivity, each of which may occur alone [18]. Table 18.1 provides a more concrete picture by listing numerous possible individual symptoms [19].

Subtypes

The symptom groups of Table 18.1 lead directly to the three DSM-IV-defined subtypes of ADHD. For patients with the predominantly hyperactive-impulsive subtype (ADHD-HI) (1) most symptoms (six or more) are in the hyperactivity-impulsivity categories; and (2) fewer than six symptoms of inattention are present, although inattention may still be present to some degree. For patients with the predominantly inattentive subtype (ADHD-I) (1) the majority of symptoms (six or more) are in the inattention category and fewer than six symptoms of hyperactivity-impulsivity are present, although hyperactivity-impulsivity may still be present to some degree; (2) children with this subtype are less likely to act out or have difficulties getting along with other children; and (3) they may sit quietly, but they are not paying attention to what they are doing. Therefore, the child may be overlooked, and parents and teachers may not notice symptoms of ADHD. For patients with the combined hyperactive-impulsive and inattentive subtype (ADHC-C) (1) six or more symptoms of inattention and six or more symptoms of hyperactivity-impulsivity are present.

Other Diagnostic Criteria

Other diagnostic criteria of ADHD include the following. Symptoms must continue at least 6 months and must be observed in at least two different settings, e.g., in the classroom, on the playground, at home, in the community, or in social settings. The symptomatic behaviors must be "developmentally inappropriate," meaning the child exhibits more of the untoward behavior than other children of the same age do. And symptoms must not be better explained by another psychiatric or medical disorder.

Neurocognitive Symptoms. Functional and Social Difficulties

Neurocognitive Symptoms

Apart from the core attentional, hyperactive, and impulsive symptoms of ADHD, neurocognitive symptoms often accompanying ADHD include difficulty in problem solving, planning ahead, and understanding others' actions, although there is controversy about whether these symptoms truly form part of the disorder [20].

Functional and Social Difficulties

Difficulties in daily functioning and social interactions commonly go along with ADHD and contribute substantially to poor lifetime outcomes in ADHD patients. These features can lead to difficulties in interpersonal relationships, in maintaining a satisfactory work record, and in enjoying life in general [21]. One study that followed hyperactive boys transitioning to adulthood, for example, found that, when compared to controls, the hyperactive group had lower educational attainment, lower occupational status, more antisocial personality disorder, and more substance abuse [22]. Children with ADHD are at high risk for a wide range of learning problems, substance abuse, psychopathology, and difficulties in their social relationships, work, and marriages. Children with ADHD and early signs of aggressive behavior are at much higher risk than other children with ADHD for later developing poor outcomes including school failure, contact with the criminal justice system, and severe psychopathology including antisocial personality disorder [23]. Similarly, children with ADHD and early signs of anxiety are at higher risk for later depression or other internalizing disorders [24]. Longitudinal studies of outcomes of childhood ADHD in young adults show lower academic and occupational achievement and higher rates of incarceration, mental health problems, and divorce compared with control groups [25, 26]. The path of adolescents with ADHD continues the childhood trend of divergence from that of their peers. They perform worse at school and are at greater risk of suspension or expulsion. Consequently, the occupational achievement of young adults with ADHD is lower than for matched peers [27]. The most disabling aspect of ADHD in adulthood may be the disruption it causes in interpersonal relationships, with increased risk of chronic conflict with work peers, socially inappropriate behaviors, disputes with partners and spouses, and trouble with the law [28]. These repeated findings of multiple negative outcomes reveal the impact of ADHD, the importance of diagnosis and treatment, and opportunity areas for individual case and public health management of the disorder.

Differential Diagnosis. Comorbidities

Differential Diagnosis

Numerous other conditions and situations can trigger ADHD-like behavior. Examples include: problems with schoolwork caused by learning disability, anxiety, or depression; adjustment disorders, for instance in the event of death or divorce in the family or parent's job loss; medical illnesses such as undetected epilepsy, an ear infection causing temporary hearing problems; fetal alcohol syndrome; insufficient or poor quality sleep, or child abuse. Such conditions are ruled out if possible before diagnosing and treating ADHD.

Psychiatric Comorbidities

Associated psychiatric comorbidities [29] are more the rule than the exception in ADHD. Associated conditions include oppositional defiant disorder and conduct disorder, antisocial personality disorder, borderline personality disorder [30], bipolar disorder, depression [31], anxiety disorder (especially in girls; [32]), obsessive-compulsive disorder, and learning disability [29]. In addition to mimicking signs of ADHD leading to possible misdiagnosis as noted above, epilepsy is also often comorbid with ADHD [33, 34]. Co-existing conditions may require other courses of treatment and are diagnosed separately from ADHD. Thus, the presence of one or more of these comorbidities complicates both diagnosis and treatment. The subject samples in the MRS studies reviewed below typically include at least some patients with comorbidities, particularly oppositional defiant disorder.

Etiology

Genetic Factors

The exact cause of ADHD is unknown, but its heritability (~75%) [35] and possible genetic basis have been much emphasized [36, 37]. Candidate genes include those coding for α_{2A} (alpha) adrenergic receptors, dopamine (DA) transporters (DAT) [38], DA D_2/D_3 [39] and DRD_4 [38] receptors, dopamine beta-hydroxylase (DBH TaqI) [40], monoamine oxidase A (MAO_A), cathecholamine-methyl-transferase (COMT), the serotonin transporter (5-HTT) promoter SLC6A4, and the 5-HT_{2A} and 5-HT_{2B} receptors [41]. The broad selection of targets indicates that ADHD does not follow the traditional model of a genetic disease and should therefore be viewed as a complex interaction among genetic and environmental factors. Even though all these genes might play a role, to date no single gene has been shown to make a major contribution to ADHD (Acosta et al. 2004). For other reviews of genetics in ADHD, including recent efforts to link genetics to developmental stages and pharmacotherapy for ADHD, see Galili-Weisstub and Segman [42], Coghill and Banaschewski [43], Banaschewski et al. [44], Faraone et al. [45], Froehlich et al. [46], and Sonuga-Barke and Halperin [47].

Environmental Factors

Proposed nongenetic etiologies include complications during pregnancy and childbirth, including maternal ethanol consumption or tobacco smoking [48]; toxic exposures including environmental lead [49, 50], organophosphates [51], and food additives [52]; early childhood infections including measles, varicella, rubella, enterovirus, and streptococcus [53, 54]; and child rearing conditions including child abuse [55] and institutional deprivation [56].

Developmental Course, Natural History, Prognosis

The proportion of children meeting diagnostic criteria for ADHD drops by ~50% over 3 years after the diagnosis. This occurs independent of treatment [57, 58]. Notwithstanding, children diagnosed with ADHD have difficulties in adolescence, regardless of treatment [59], frequently failing to acquire a college or even high school diploma, often in spite of special education. Those with ADHD as children are at increased risk of adverse life outcomes once they become teenagers, including greater risk of auto crashes, injury and higher medical expenses, earlier sexual activity, and teen pregnancy. ADHD in adults remains a clinical diagnosis, persisting, as mentioned, from childhood in ~60% of cases [13]. As mentioned, the signs and symptoms may differ from those in childhood and adolescence due to acquired coping mechanisms [60]. The fact that such powerful negatives outcomes are observed frequently in subjects who have undergone conventional treatment and/or no longer meet formal diagnostic criteria for ADHD underscores the need to develop superior therapies and for better understanding of brain mechanisms of the disease, perhaps with the aid of MRS research.

Treatment

Stimulant drugs

Both pharmacological and nonpharmacological treatments are used for ADHD. Based on safety, tolerability, and efficacy, CNS stimulants, taken daily orally, represent first-line neuropharmacologic treatment for both pediatric and adult ADHD [61], with methylphenidate (Ritalin, Concerta) being the most commonly prescribed agent [62]. This is the celebrated "paradoxical reaction" whereby stimulant drugs, which typically increase locomotion in healthy subjects, actually relieve hyperactivity in patients with ADHD. Other stimulants prescribed include the amphetamine-based formulations like amphetamine plus dextroamphetamine (Adderall) and dextroamphetamine sulfate (dexedrine). The stimulants increase synaptic DA and noradrenalin (NA) concentrations by inhibiting presynaptic uptake and promoting presynaptic release [63]. Extended-release preparations of stimulants have become popular because they reduce afternoon wear-off and rebound and manifest less abuse potential [64]. FDA approval in adult ADHD is currently only for extended-release stimulants. Untoward effects of stimulants include elevated vital signs, anorexia and weight loss, and stunting of statural growth, although growth is believed to normalize with chronic treatment [65, 66]. Warnings also concern potential cardiovascular events. There is little evidence that patients with ADHD abuse their stimulant medications; however, diversion to non-ADHD youth remains a concern [67, 68]. Modafinil is an additional stimulant, which may alleviate symptoms of pediatric ADHD [69–71]. Methylphenidate has been studied in a number of the MRS investigations reviewed below.

Nonstimulant Drugs

Nonstimulant medications used to treat ADHD include the NAergic agents atomoxetine (Strattera) [72], guanfacine, and clonidine. Oral atomoxetine is usually prescribed once or twice daily for child and adolescent ADHD where it is well tolerated and has efficacy superior to placebo and comparable to methylphenidate [73, 74]. Therapeutic actions of atomoxetine may be ascribed to selective inhibition of presynaptic NA reuptake in prefrontal cortex [75, 76]. Side effects in pediatric ADHD include clinically insignificant tachycardia and hypertension as well as initial loss in expected height and weight, said to return to normal long term [77]. Atomoxetine tends to induce somnolence in contrast to stimulants which tend to induce insomnia [78]. Finally, similar to the serotonin-reuptake inhibitor (SRI) paroxetine, atomoxetine carries a black box warning associating it with suicidal ideation [79]. α (alpha) adrenergic agonists, such as clonidine and guanfacine, have shown some efficacy for core symptoms of ADHD [80, 81]. Extended-release guanfacine is FDA approved for ADHD. Whereas clonidine affects α (alpha) adrenergic receptors nonspecifically, guanfacine is more selective for the α_{2A} (alpha) receptor. Atomoxetine has played a role in a few of the MRS studies reviewed below. Other types of agents used to treat ADHD include the antidepressant bupropion [82–84] and the tricyclic antidepressants as backups for when stimulants fail [85].

Nonpharmacological Treatments

Nonpharmacological, i.e., psychosocial, interventions [5] include support groups (for adults and children), specialized educational planning, educational and home adjustments (increased structure, predicTable routine, learning aids, homework checks, etc.), tutors, parent training, teachers' antecedent and consequent interventions (understanding antecedents to inappropriate behaviors and judicious punishment to encourage appropriate behavior), and classroom accommodations (placing child closer to teacher, eliminating environmental distractions, teaching lessons with more novelty and stimulation than repetition, and others) and have shown efficacy [86, 87]. For adults, several recent studies show efficacy of cognitive and cognitive-behavioral therapies (CBT) for ADHD [88–91]. Mindfulness meditation-based interventions for pediatric and adult ADHD have also recently demonstrated efficacy [92, 93]. Little, if any, MRS investigation of nonpharmacological treatments for ADHD has been carried out.

Brain Bases, Physiological Models

Neuropharmacological Perspectives

The clear symptom amelioration seen in most pediatric and adult cases of ADHD treated with stimulants like methylphenidate fostered the DA theory of ADHD (reviewed by Levy [94, 95]). According to this theory, symptoms of ADHD result from low synaptic DAergic tone in target regions (prefrontal cortex, caudate, putamen, nucleus accumbens) of midbrain DA-synthesizing nuclei (substantia nigra, ventral tegmentum). Via actions such as inhibiting transmitter reuptake and promoting presynaptic release, stimulants increase DA concentrations in the synapse and thereby achieve symptomatic relief. Lesion studies of DA pathways have led to animal models of ADHD [96]. Results of genetic research have also been integrated into the DA hypothesis [97].

Responses of ADHD symptoms to NAergic drugs like atomoxetine, however, indicated a possible role of other cathecholamines in addition to DA. Subsequent modeling and interpretive efforts have sought to explain these therapeutic actions and to outline the specific roles of DA and NA in ADHD [98]. Incorporation of knowledge of the functional neuroanatomy of these transmitters has produced a picture of a DA-NA cortico–striato–thalamo–cortical network for executive function, arousal, attention, and inhibition that is dysfunctional in ADHD [99].

Functional Neuroanatomical Perspectives

Attempts to account for ADHD as the result of a response-inhibition deficit in prefrontal cortex in ADHD [100, 101] were succeeded by the view that ADHD involves dysfunction beyond inhibitory control and executive function [102]. Based on its heavy DAergic innervation, its role in motor response, and volumetric MRI evidence of abnormalities, involvement of the dorsal striatum, in particular the caudate nuclei, was invoked to explain aberrant distribution of reaction times (some very quick, some long-delayed responses) in ADHD children [103]. Involvement of the ventral striatum (nucleus accumbens), heavily implicated in reward and motivation, was suggested by observations that ADHD children exhibit difficulties with delaying gratification, i.e., they prefer to gain a smaller reward now than a larger reward later, and that risky decision making in gambling tasks is associated with hyperactivity-impulsivity [47, 104]. Following this line of thought, some investigators have suggested that subjects with ADHD need a higher level of risk or reward to experience the same level of threat or pleasure as control subjects, producing a more "sensation-seeking" personality. From a neural network point of view, one may speak of prefronto-striatal dysfunction in ADHD [105–107], particularly with respect to response inhibition [108]. Thereby, a differential involvement of the *right* prefronto-striatal system in ADHD has long been supported by some evidence (reviewed by Barkley [109]). Given its role in the temporal aspects of task performance, the cerebellum has also been implicated in ADHD based on deficits in time perception and poor performance on time-estimation and time-discrimination tasks [110, 111]. Most recently, investigators have suggested that the "default network" involving posterior middle cingulate cortex (pMCC), ventral posterior cingulate cortex (vPCC), and precuneus is abnormal in ADHD, leading to lapses in attention associated with failure of suppression of the default network [112, 113]. Thus, an impression is emerging of anatomically widespread functional pathology in the brain in ADHD. It is not yet established, however, whether initial pathology in a single brain region subsequently disrupts function of the others due to shared network participation or whether simultaneous defects in multiple regions are required for symptoms to manifest.

Neurometabolic Perspectives

Russell [114] has worked out a theory of Glu-DA interactions in cortex and nucleus accumbens underlying ADHD symptomatology. In this model, DAergic hypotonia can be a consequence of suboptimal glutamatergic stimulation. A major portion of brain energy is consumed by neuronal activity supporting glutamatergic neurotransmission [115]. Therefore, if Glu is involved in the pathophysiology of ADHD, then brain energy metabolism may be an underlying influence in ADHD and its therapeutic remediation.

The "energy-deficiency" hypothesis of Todd & Botteron [116] and its considerable extension by Russell et al. [117] are of particular interest to MRS ADHD research. These theorists draw on the Magistretti–Pellerin theory of brain energy metabolism [118–121]. Figures 18.1 and 18.2 depict some neurometabolic pathways relevant to these models and to MRS studies of ADHD generally. Magistretti–Pellerin describes metabolic events at and around a glutamatergic cortical synapse after an action potential has arrived. Bordering the synapse are a presynaptic neuron, a postsynaptic neuron, and an astrocyte. The astrocyte is wedged between the neurons and a local capillary—the source of glucose (Glc) for all the cells—enveloping it with its pseudopodia. Hence, the astrocyte gets access to blood-borne Glc before other cells do. When an action potential arrives at the tip of the presynaptic neuron, some of its vesicles fuse with its phospholipid membrane, releasing Glu into the synaptic cleft. As in the conventional picture of neurotransmission, some of these Glu molecules diffuse across the cleft to dock with glutamatergic ionotropic and metabotropic receptors embedded in the membrane of the postsynaptic neuron. Others, however, are taken up by the astrocyte, in part to preserve receptor responsivity and to forestall glutamatergic excitotoxicity. In the astrocyte, Glu is converted to Gln, which is transported into the neighboring neurons for reconversion to Glu in the Glu–Gln cycle. Astrocytic uptake of Glu also consumes energy. According to the model, this energy consumption stimulates the astrocyte to take in more Glc from the capillary. Once in the astrocyte, most of the Glc is converted through anaerobic glycolysis into lactate (Lac), yielding a quick release of a small portion of the total energy of the Glc molecule. The Lac is exported from the astrocyte and taken up by the neurons, which continue the catabolism of Lac down through the Krebs cycle, oxidative phosphorylation, and the electron transport chain, yielding a much larger quantity of energy by completing combustion of the original Glc molecule. Thus, according to Magistretti–Pellerin, the energy-yielding degradation of most Glc is divided between astrocytes and neurons.

Todd and Botteron [116] and Russell et al. [117] propose that a principal metabolic defect in ADHD is that astrocytes fall to supply sufficient Lac to neurons leading to suboptimal neuronal functioning and the symptoms of ADHD. The supply of Lac to oligodendrocytes is also diminished impairing myelin sheath formation worsening cognitive and motor performance over time, e.g., by lengthening reaction times [117]. Bartzokis [122] has a related view of ADHD as dysregulation of myelin development. Husarova et al. [123] have similarly developed a theory of ADHD

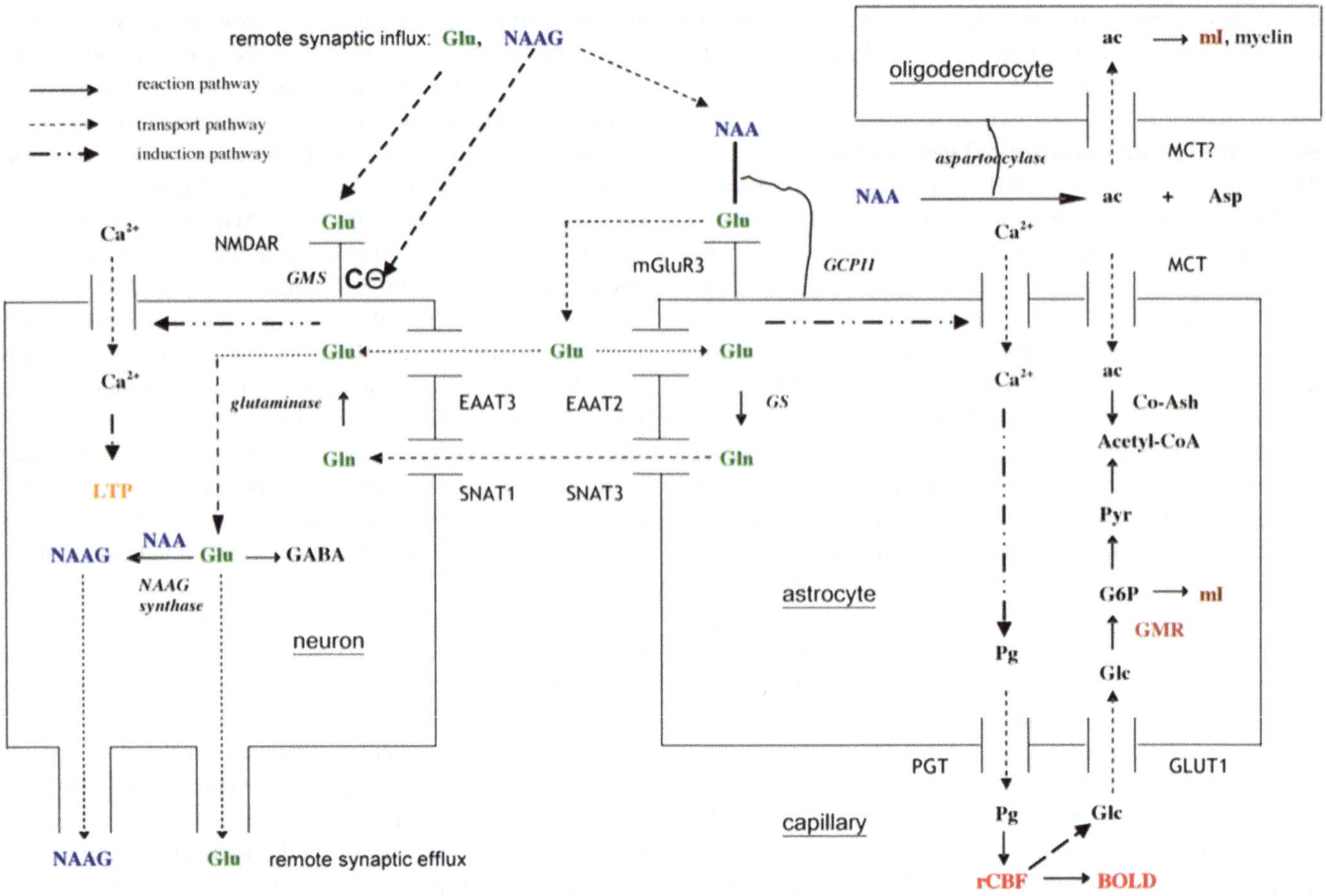

Fig. 18.1 Some neurometabolic reactions (including Glu–Gln cycle and Tricellular NAA cycle) at a cortical glutamatergic synapse relevant to MRS and other neuroimaging studies of ADHD. Glu and NAAG are coreleased from presynaptic neuronal vesicles into the synapse. Glu docks at the primary site of *N*-methyl-D-aspartate receptors (NMDAR) and other glutamatergic receptors on the postsynaptic neuron. If, simultaneously, the neuron plasma membrane is depolarized and the NMDAR Gly modulatory site (GMS) is also occupied, the NMDAR will induce local Ca^{2+} influx leading ultimately to long-term potentiation (LTP), a basis of associative memory formation. The Glu moiety of NAAG is bound by R3 metabotropic glutamatergic receptors (mGluR3) on the astrocyte. There it is cleaved by the neighboring membrane-bound enzyme GCP-II into Glu and NAA. The cleaving action induces Ca^{2+} influx into the astrocyte leading to prostaglandin (Pg) secretion through prostaglandin transporters (PGT) into the capillary circulation. Prostaglandin action on the vasculature increases regional cerebral blood flow (rCBF) detected by $H_2{}^{15}O$-PET and thence the blood oxygenation level-dependent (BOLD) effect detected by fMRI. Capillary blood flow brings glucose (Glc) to the astrocyte through GLUT1 glucose transporters. Phosphorylation of Glc in the first step of glycolysis in the astrocyte (and neuron) generates the glucose metabolic rate (GMR) detected by ^{18}FDG-PET. If the resulting glucose-6-phosphate (G6P) continues down the path of glycolysis it is converted into pyruvate (Pyr) and acetyl-CoA; or it can be diverted to an alternative pathway producing *myo*-inositol (mI). The Glu liberated from NAAG (as well as free synaptic Glu) can enter the astrocyte and the neuron through EAAT2 and EAAT3 Glu transporters, respectively. In the astrocyte, Glu is converted to Gln by glutamine synthase (GS). Gln can leave the astrocyte through SNAT3 and enter the neuron through SNAT2 neutral amino acid transporters. In the neuron, Gln is converted back to Glu by glutaminase. Possible fates of neuronal Glu then include recombination with NAA back into NAAG by NAAG synthase, remote synaptic efflux, conversion to GABA, and consumption by the Krebs cycle. NAA liberated by perisynaptic NAAG lysis is itself lysed by oligodendrocyte membrane-bound aspartoacylase yielding aspartate (Asp) and acetate (ac). ac is taken into the astrocyte by monocarboxylate transporters (MCT) where it is a preferred energetic substrate. It is also taken up (perhaps also via MCT) into the oligodendrocyte, where it can be converted into mI and also used to support myelin synthesis, which ultimately influences diffusion tensor imaging (DTI) indices. Thus, presynaptic discharge prompting vesicular Glu-NAAG release promotes LTP associative memory linkages, Glu-Gln circulation, vascular petition for more Glc and O_2, carbon feeding of astrocytes and oligodendrocytes, and myelination of proximal nerve fibers ("fire together-wire together"). In ADHD, perhaps due to low DAergic tone, synaptic Glu stimulation is thought to be relatively lacking (Russell 2003), hence ADHD patients may have difficulty learning due to failure to attend and may have below-normal myelination of some nerve tracts

based on MRS neurometabolite results. The Todd & Botteron [116] and Russell et al. [117] theories are referenced in a number of the MRS studies reviewed below. One should note that these views are partly dependent on the validity of the original Magistretti–Pellerin model, which, although representing a major contribution to the understanding of brain energetics and glial function, has been challenged [124, 125].

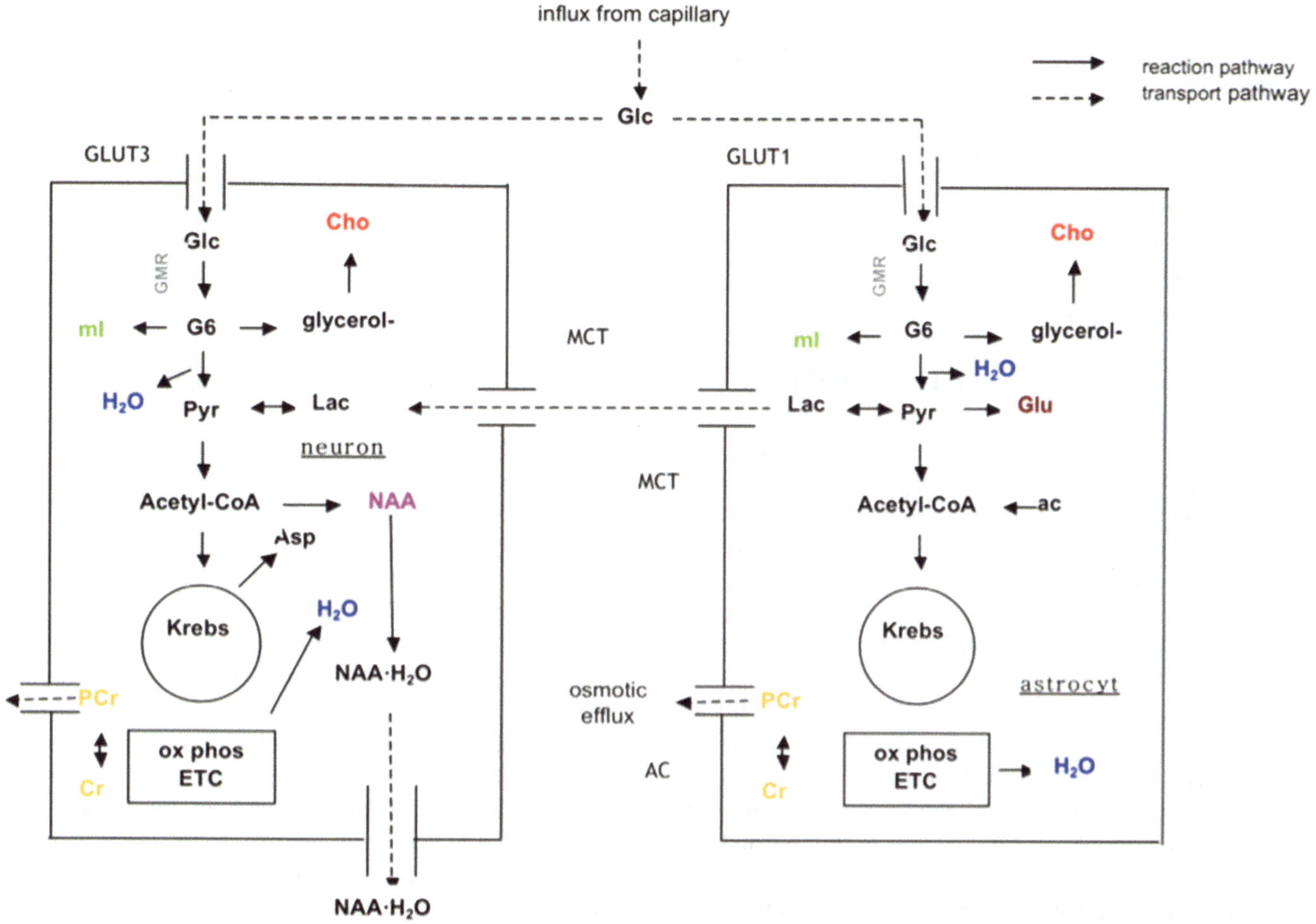

Fig. 18.2 Further MRS-relevant neurometabolic reactions (including energetic catabolism and cell-volume regulation) at a cortical glutamatergic synapse. Capillary Glc enters mainly astrocytes and also neurons (through GLUT3 transporters). In both cell types, Glc is broken down by glycolysis which, together with the subsequent Krebs cycle, oxidative phosphorylation (ox phos), and electron-transport chain (ETC), generates cell energy as ATP and in other forms. Some ATP energy is stored for rapid deployment in the Cr-PCr buffer. Often neglected in metabolic models are the prodigious quantities of *water* produced by energy generation. To preserve function and to prevent phospholipid membrane lysis, the cell regulates its osmotic pressure and thence volume by increasing and decreasing the internal molalities of several small molecular species. These include most of the canonical ^{1}H MRS metabolites, e.g., NAA, Glu, PCr (but not Cr), some of the choline compounds, mI, and Tau. These species leave the cell through anion channels (AC). The neuron, with its long processes, has a very high surface-to-volume ratio leading to high energetic needs and sensitivity to osmotic stresses (high membrane surface for water influx and efflux). Thus, adjunctive water regulation is thought to be provided by a neuron-specific NAA "molecular water pump." Each NAA (and NAAG) molecule can complex with ~50 water molecules. The complexes are then said to be extruded from the neuron by (as yet empirically unverified) water pores in the cell membrane. NAA is formed by acetyl-CoA + Asp, both of which can be diverted from the neuronal Krebs cycle. In the astrocyte, ac can be used for acetyl-CoA synthesis. Early in glycolysis, as mentioned, G6P can be diverted to formation of mI, which is involved in membrane metabolism and other functions. G6P can also be diverted to form glycerol which ultimately is used to form ^{1}H MRS choline-containing compounds. These compounds support membrane synthesis. Thus, both cell types are continually balancing between burning carbon substrate for energy and embedding it into structural membranes and concurrently between "wetter" (expressing H as water) and "dryer" (expressing H as lipid) operating states. Late in glycolysis, astrocytic Pyr can be shuttled into Lac. Lac can leave the astrocyte and enter the neuron via MCT. In the neuron Lac can rejoin the energetic chain through reconversion to Pyr. The Magistretti–Pellerin Theory connects Figs. 18.1 and 18.2 by proposing that Glu import into astrocytes stimulates astrocytic capillary Glc uptake and subsequent Lac transport to neurons. Thus, the burden of feeding the neuron's voracious appetite for energy is shared between the catabolic machinery of the astrocyte (for less energy quicker) and of the neuron (for more energy later). Todd and Botteron (2001) and Russell et al. (2006) hypothesize that Lac shuttling to neurons is deficient in ADHD, perhaps due to suboptimal supply of synaptic Glu

Studies of ADHD With Other Neuroimaging Modalities

This section reviews in summary from published studies of ADHD in neuroimaging modalities other than MRS. The modalities reviewed include structural magnetic resonance imaging (MRI), diffusion tensor imaging (DTI), functional magnetic resonance imaging (fMRI), single-photon emission correlated tomography (SPECT), and positron emission tomography (PET). The findings of such studies motivated many of the MRS studies reviewed below and/or helped to interpret their results. For earlier ADHD neuroimaging reviews, see Giedd et al. [106], Cherkasova and Hechtman [126], Dopheide and Pliszka [3], Konrad and Eickhof [127], Seidman et al. [128], Wilens and Spencer [5].

Structural Magnetic Resonance Imaging (MRI) Studies

Whole-Brain Volume. Cerebral Lobar Volumes

An early MRI finding in ADHD is that whole-brain volume is ~5% smaller than in age- and sex-matched healthy controls [129]. Also, a normal lateral asymmetry, whereby the right anterior brain is slightly larger than the left [130], is less present in ADHD [129, 131, 132]. At the cerebral lobar level, most quantitative MRI studies have found below-normal prefrontal volume and/or cortical thickness in children [129, 132–144] and adults [20, 145] with ADHD. Some studies also found structural abnormalities in the parietal lobes of children [132, 135, 136, 143, 144, 146–148] and adults [145]. Structural imaging has, moreover, documented below-normal temporal-lobe volume [135, 144, 146, 148] or cortical thickness [147] in children and adolescents. The growth trajectories of cortical thickness in children and adolescents with ADHD [147] also imply a delay in cortical maturation in ADHD, most prominently in prefrontal cortex. In children, correlations between frontal and temporal gray matter volume and ADHD symptom rating scale scores have also been noted [135].

These widespread volumetric findings motivate the search with MRS for metabolic abnormalities throughout the cortex. It would be valuable to know if undersized cortex and/or white matter in ADHD are merely quantitatively or also qualitatively different from normal. And if metabolite effects in ADHD presage, accompany, or follow changes in developing brain tissue in ADHD. The ADHD MRS literature to date has only begun to address such questions.

Basal Gangliar Volumes

Numerous studies measuring the volumes of subcortical nuclei in ADHD have found lower volumes of the caudate and globus pallidus [129, 132, 135, 136, 149–154]. A recent meta-analysis [155], incorporating the atlas-space stereotaxic coordinates of effects detected across studies localized a significant defect in subcortical gray matter in ADHD to the right lenticular nucleus (putamen, globus pallidus). Several of the MRS studies reviewed below targeted the basal ganglia, though usually including multiple different nuclei in the same MRS acquisition voxel (partial-voluming problem).

Cerebellar Volume

Cerebellar volumetric abnormalities, in the hemispheres and posterior inferior lobules of the vermis (VIII–X), have been recorded repeatedly in children with ADHD [129, 134, 135, 139, 156–158]. One study [129] included 112 subjects. There is also evidence for progressive developmental cerebellar volume loss in ADHD into adolescence [159]. These findings have helped spur interest in a few MRS studies of the cerebellum in ADHD.

Diffusion Tensor Imaging (DTI) Studies

Structural MRI has found lower whole brain white matter volume in pediatric ADHD compared to age-matched healthy controls [135] and focally smaller anterior corpus callosal volume [160]. A half-dozen studies, typically with under 20 subjects per group, have examined brain white matter in ADHD using DTI. The earliest published study [161] detected below-normal fractional anisotropy (FA) in children with ADHD in the white matter underlying the premotor and left parieto-occipital cortices, as well as in the cerebellum and proximal to the striatum. Combining fMRI data from a Go–No-Go Task with DTI, Casey et al. [162] determined that FA in right prefrontal fiber tracts was correlated with functional BOLD activity in inferior frontal gyrus and caudate in ADHD parents and their children, suggesting a genetic basis for the disturbance of fronto-striatal connections in ADHD. Makris et al. [145] demonstrated abnormalities of the cingulum bundle and superior longitudinal fasciculus in adults with ADHD. Findings of lower FA in the corticospinal tract and the superior longitudinal fasciculus at our center [163] similarly suggested disruption of motor and attention networks in children with ADHD. Abnormalities were also found in ADHD in multiple white matter tracts, including anterior corona radiata, cingulum bundle, superior and inferior longitudinal fasciculi, and internal capsule [164]. Silk et al. [165] identified developmental changes in FA in the caudate with age that were significantly different between ADHD and control subjects. These studies may imply ADHD-related pathology in several widespread white matter brain tracts that might readily be probed with MRS.

Functional Magnetic Resonance Imaging (fMRI) Studies

Prefrontal Cortices

Many fMRI studies have assessed brain function in ADHD during cognitive tasks that test putative inhibitory response and other executive-function deficits. Most frequently used have been the Go–No-Go Task, the Stop-Signal Task, the

Continuous Performance Task (CPT), and variations of the Stroop Task. BOLD fMRI studies of ADHD using the above tasks have consistently reported lower activation in frontal regions [26, 166–175] and anterior middle cingulate cortex (aMCC) [26, 172, 175–178]. In particular, adolescent boys with ADHD showed less BOLD activation in right mesial frontal cortex, right inferior frontal cortex, and left caudate than controls while performing the Stop Task and a motor delay task [166], leading the authors to conclude that the right inferior frontal cortex and the left caudate form a motor response inhibition network that is hypoactive in ADHD.

Parietal Lobes

In the parietal lobes in the resting state, perfusion MRI has signaled hyperperfusion of somatosensory cortex in adults with ADHD that reduces in response to methylphenidate [179]. This suggests below-normal inhibition in sensory areas leading to sensory hyperarousal.

Numerous activation fMRI studies have revealed abnormal parietal BOLD response in ADHD during cognitive tasks testing inhibition, spatial working memory, response switching, selective attention, attention allocation, alertness, episodic memory, and motor function. In adolescent boys with ADHD, event-related fMRI detected lower BOLD activation in the precuneus and vPCC during inhibition failures in the course of the Stop Task [167]. Lower parietal BOLD effect has also been reported during interference suppression in children [180] and during response switching in adolescents [173] with ADHD. Below-normal BOLD effect has also been seen in widespread temporoparietal regions during the visual [181, 182] and auditory [183] Oddball Tasks in boys with ADHD. Below-normal parietal BOLD activity has also been observed in ADHD during tasks of visual selective attention [174], target detection [184], mental rotation [185, 186], and backward digit span [187]. Mostofsky et al. [188] reported below-normal BOLD activation in right superior parietal lobule in children with ADHD during sequential finger tapping. Thus, there is considerable fMRI evidence for parietal hypofunction in ADHD, though the parietal lobes have been relatively little explored with MRS in ADHD.

Temporal Lobes

Some studies have reported compensatory recruitment of lateral temporal cortex in ADHD. Higher BOLD activation of left middle and superior temporal gyri simultaneous with lower aMCC and supplementary motor cortex activation during a Go–No-Go Task was seen in adolescents with ADHD [177]. Higher BOLD activation in left occipito-temporal cortex was measured in adults with ADHD during forward and backward digit span tasks [187]. Elevated BOLD effect in middle temporal cortex was reported in boys with ADHD during mental rotation [165]. Below-normal temporal-lobe BOLD activity, including in the insula and also in the right basal ganglia was found in boys with ADHD during the Oddball Task [182]. Reduced BOLD activation of temporal lobes was also reported in adolescent boys with ADHD during a response-switching task [173]. Lateral temporal cortex has scarcely been examined with fMRI in ADHD.

Striatum (Caudate, Putamen)

The inhibitory and other executive function tasks that induce lower BOLD response in prefrontal cortex also do so in striatum [166, 170, 174, 189, 190] in ADHD subjects compared with control subjects. However, during the Counting Stroop Task, Bush et al. [176] found significant BOLD activation in left caudate, right putamen, right thalamus, left pulvinar, bilateral inferior frontal gyrus, and bilateral insula in adults with ADHD, while matched controls exhibited significant activation of bilateral anterior cingulate alone. Using fMRI during a Go–No-Go task with ADHD and control children on and off methylphenidate, Vaidya et al. [189] found that methylphenidate increased the area of BOLD activation in caudate and putamen in ADHD patients, but had the opposite effect in controls. Patients as well as controls activated significantly larger areas of prefrontal cortex on drug. Note that the patients had been previously exposed to chronic methylphenidate, so it is not known if the striatal effects in patients were acute or chronic. fMRI relaxometry has also detected resting-state hypoperfusion in the striatum in ADHD [191]. These and other neuroimaging findings plus the pharmacologic association with DA have motivated several ADHD MRS studies of the striatum, though the individual nuclei (caudate, putamen) are not often sampled in isolation.

Cerebellum

Prediction of temporal occurrence of events in the cerebellum has been investigated in children and adolescents with ADHD using event-related fMRI and the Go–No-Go Task. Durston et al. [172] showed decreased cerebellar event-related BOLD response to expected (go) stimuli presented at unexpected times, as well as decreased anterior cingulate response to stimuli with unexpected identity (no-go stimuli) presented at expected times. These results support a deficit in predicting the occurrence of future events in ADHD. A second study from the same group [178] extended these findings, suggesting that cerebellar function is sensitive to familial risk for ADHD. Lower BOLD activity in left posterior cerebellum was found in adults with ADHD than in healthy controls during a 2-back working memory task [192]. Another study associated stimulant-related changes in cerebellar BOLD response during a Go–No-Go task to familial risk for ADHD [170]. An fMRI relaxometry study also reported an increase in resting-state BOLD in the cerebellar vermis after acute methylphenidate in children [193]. This all represents reasonable evidence for cerebellar involvement in ADHD and has led to a few MRS investigations.

Tasks Not Directly Related to Core ADHD Symptoms

More recent fMRI studies of ADHD have used tasks investigating such functions as working memory, interference control, decision making, reward processing, and episodic memory. These studies also show below-normal BOLD activation in frontal [180, 183, 184, 194, 195], anterior cingulate [194, 196], and striatal [180, 186, 194, 197–199] regions in ADHD.

Meta-Analysis

A meta-analysis [200] combining 12 prior fMRI and three PET blood-flow studies of ADHD making use of the stereotaxic coordinates of the sites of BOLD activation or blood-flow effects in each study found significant hypoactivity in patients with ADHD in anterior cingulate, dorsolateral prefrontal, and inferior prefrontal cortices, as well as in basal ganglia, thalamus, and parietal cortex. When focusing on response inhibition alone, group differences were limited to inferior prefrontal cortex, mesial frontal regions, and precentral gyrus. Separately, methylphenidate-related increases in frontal [170, 189, 201], anterior cingulate [201], and striatal [170, 189, 197] BOLD activity have been reported in the context of tasks of response inhibition and attention.

Overall, the regional BOLD findings in the various above brain regions have considerably motivated anatomic sampling strategy in MRS studies of ADHD, including pharmacologic studies, and/or informed their interpretation.

Single-Photon Emission Correlated Tomography (SPECT) Studies

Prefrontal Cortex

Most resting-state SPECT studies of ADHD have reported frontal hypoperfusion [202, 204–208] and methylphenidate-related increases in frontal perfusion [205]. Although, for methodological reasons, results of older studies must be enjoyed with caution.

Temporal Cortex

Hypoperfusion at rest has been observed in ADHD children in right middle temporal [209, 210] and occipito-termporal [210] cortices. Lee et al. [210] also reported reductions in occipito-temporal regional cerebral blood flow after a month of methylphenidate treatment, including a further reduction in right middle temporal cortex. Another study, however, found that perfusion in temporal cortex correlated negatively with cognitive and motor impairment in children with ADHD [211].

Striatum

Striatal hypoperfusion was reported in early SPECT studies of ADHD [202, 203, 212] with administration of methylphenidate associated with increased striatal perfusion [202, 208, 212]. The highly selective DA transporter ligand ^{123}I-Altropane was used in a small sample ($n = 6$) of ADHD adults and healthy controls [213]. Striatal binding potential was elevated in all six patients, with each exceeding the control mean by over two standard deviations, strongly indicating increased numbers of local DAT in the ADHD sample.

Cerebellum

Resting-state cerebellar hypoperfusion has been reported using SPECT in children with ADHD [209]. Long-term (4–5 week) methylphenidate treatment did not change this condition [210].

Positron Emission Tomography (PET) Studies

A number of PET studies have been performed in adult ADHD. Notwithstanding the understandable reluctance to perform PET on children, a few studies of pediatric ADHD were also conducted.

^{18}Fluorodeoxyglucose Positron Emission Tomography (^{18}FDG-PET)

^{18}FDG-PET has found below-normal GMR in frontal cortex [214–216] and aMCC [214, 215] in adult ADHD subjects compared with controls. Lower GMR in right posterior temporal lobes was also seen during auditory CPT in adolescents with ADHD [214]. But adolescent girls with ADHD had higher normalized GMR in the hippocampus than control subjects [217].

^{15}O-Water Positron Emission Tomography ($H_2{}^{15}O$-PET)

Activation studies using $H_2{}^{15}O$-PET during cognitive tasks in ADHD have found diminished rCBF in ADHD patients relative to healthy controls in frontal [218] and anterior cingulate [219] cortex. $H_2{}^{15}O$-PET detected above-normal resting-state rCBF in the cerebellar vermis after methylphenidate in adults with ADHD [220, 221], as well as a methylphenidate-related decrease in blood flow during CPT [221].

Other PET Tracers

^{18}Fluorodopa (^{18}F-DOPA) PET was used to label catecholamine terminals in unmedicated adults with ADHD [222]. ^{18}F-DOPA uptake was significantly diminished in left mesial prefrontal cortex of ADHD adults compared to healthy controls. By contrast, in adolescents with

ADHD, ^{18}F-DOPA uptake in right midbrain was significantly elevated compared to controls [223]. These results support the notion that catecholamine dysregulation is central to the pathophysiology of ADHD, and not just to its treatment. They also highlight the proposition that dopaminergic and noradrenergic systems cannot be understood without taking developmental effects into account.

Summary

The above neuroimaging studies vary in scale with cohorts of over 100 for some structural MRI studies and typically smaller groups (10–20 subjects) for the DTI, fMRI, and PET studies. For brevity we suppressed many inconsistent and negative findings, hence a less summary review would expose wider diversity in the data corpus. Nevertheless, these neuroimaging investigations collectively evince certain patterns. There is repeated involvement in ADHD of prefrontal cortex, especially inferior frontal cortex; anterior cingulate cortex, especially the aMCC; striatum, predominantly the caudate; and cerebellum, particularly the vermis. These brain regions tend to be hypoperfused in ADHD. The temporal and parietal (especially precuneal) cortices and white matter are also implicated. Acute and/or chronic methylphenidate does appear to exert effects on regional blood flow and metabolism, typically in the reverse direction of the effects of untreated ADHD. These patterns provide motivation for MRS investigations in these several brain regions and for pharmaco-MRS studies of interventions for ADHD.

Clinical and Neuroscience Motivation for ADHD MRS Studies

At present, there are no solid clinical applications of MRS in the psychiatry of ADHD. We are left with presenting a few sketchy and fanciful ideas for possible future applications in need of refinement, critical testing, and development. Possible contributions of MRS relate to diagnosis, prognosis, and pharmacologic therapy development.

Diagnosis

ADHD is a controversial diagnosis, much more among the lay than the professional public, in part because there is "no valid test for ADHD independent of diagnostic interview." Moreover, ADHD is only invoked as a diagnosis if numerous other psychiatric disorders that might better explain the symptoms are first ruled out. Brain imaging assays employing MRS or other modalities, through the identification of "biomarkers" of disease, offer hope of injecting objective elements into the diagnostic protocol. Thus, MRS may help address the question of the neurophysiological reality of the disorder and inform the general public and public health policy accordingly. In addition to its scientific interest, the brain-reality status of ADHD is highly meaningful for patient management. A stigma can surround ADHD [224], which might be strongly defused if reliable objective neurochemical indices of the condition can be discovered. Additionally, such indices could greatly increase the motivation of patients and families to seek out and to comply with treatment. If a psychiatrist or other therapist is able to present an MR spectrum, a brain map, or other scanner-generated evidence reflecting the patient's condition, this can instill greater confidence and be more convincing (even if in truth not more useful) than an expert opinion or scores on verbal, pencil-and-paper, or even computer-interactive psychometric tests. Thus, MRS endpoint data may conceivably one day be integrated into ADHD clinical management as educational and motivational tools.

Along similar lines, MRS may inform the debate on the clinical validity of the various subtypes of ADHD [225]. A chief obstacle to overcome in using MRS to assess the neurophysiological reality or unreality of ADHD and its subtypes is the possibility of nonrepresentative results arising in small subject samples (Type I error) and the bias towards publication of positive results. Hence, it is important to investigate larger samples. There is also the possibility that traditional formal psychiatric diagnostic categories, such as ADHD, may not be the best way to classify and analyze pathological brain states; approaches based on individual symptoms, cutting across diagnostic boundaries, for example, may turn out to be superior. Such approaches can also be pursued using MRS.

Prognosis, Prediction of Treatment Response

Regarding prognosis, it would be very useful clinically if MRS or other neuroimaging endpoints were predictive of response to stimulants or other therapies. If results of an MRS exam could, within limits of probability, recommend certain treatment courses (e.g., pharmacologic augmentations) as particularly promising or recommend against others as unpromising, this could save time on trials of medications. Such time savings are especially important for inpatients in order to preserve scarce and expensive hospital resources. In the hospital and out, some patients and some families are reluctant to pursue a course of drug treatment even when recommended by a physician, due to concerns over untoward effects of the agent(s) prescribed. Again, effective prediction of response by MRS might allow a practitioner to divide patients into subgroups of those likely to respond to drug treatment, those likely to respond to nonmedicinal therapies, those likely to respond to either, and those likely to respond to neither. And similarly for different classes of drugs for ADHD. This could help avoid unnecessary drug exposures in some cases and in others could help the reluctant agree to auspicious therapies. As stimulants and other agents may be administered daily for years, MRS may also help discover or rule out as yet unknown untoward (or beneficial) effects of chronic treatment on the brain. Prevention of ADHD is relatively little discussed [226], but biomarker-based prediction of the odds or time of onset of ADHD in high-risk subjects, e.g., children with parents and/or siblings with ADHD, represents a further possible field of application for MRS.

Development of Pharmacotherapies

Finally, MRS is capable of assaying regional levels (and with ^{13}C MRS rates of reaction) in the brain of Glu, GABA, and several other metabolites non- or minimally invasively in humans, including children. Neurochemical models that MRS research strives to work out involving these metabolites may be instrumental in identifying novel targets for drug design. For example, should the pharmacologist select agents likely to interact with specific neurotransmitter receptors, enzymes, or transporters that are especially dense in brain regions carrying out certain neurocognitive functions impaired in ADHD? Should, for example, drugs that modulate central glutamatergic systems be pursued? Or drugs that spur glycolytic Lac production in astrocytes? Or myelin synthesis in oligodendrocytes? To the extent that human patient physiology diverges from that of laboratory animals, some human MRS experiments may be more directive for such purposes than certain preclinical studies.

Summary

It is at present unclear if, even in its eventual highest stage of technological evolution, ^{1}H MRS and ^{31}P MRS, hampered by issues of the limited number of different metabolites sampled, reliability and precision of quantitation of metabolite levels, individual-subject heterogeneity, spatial resolution, and others, will contribute decisively and practically to the resolution of outstanding issues in ADHD management and to the elucidation of the underlying brain mechanisms of ADHD and its treatment. (^{13}C MRS with its slightly invasive infusion methodology and ability to measure reaction rates as well as metabolite levels enjoys certain advantages in the elucidation of neurochemical mechanisms in ADHD; although ^{13}C MRS, too, has limitations, notably low spatial resolution.) There are tens of thousands of different biochemical species present in a typical human cell and even ultra-high-field NMR of tissue extracts detects at most a few hundred. Thus, there is no a priori guarantee that the neurochemical factors assessable with MRS will be those most germane to ADHD. There is also the possibility that the most effective biomarkers, when they are discovered, could be associated not with the brain but with other bodily organs [227], though these are also scannable with MRS. But, on the other hand, brain MRS as a field may get lucky; the high abundance, for example, of the few metabolites quantifiable by clinical MRS is also a sign of their high physiologic significance and thus possible disturbance in psychiatric disorders. As MRS, along with PET and SPECT, represents one of our few windows into in vivo human brain metabolism, it is obligatory that at least some workers in the neuroscience community push the technique to its limits in our efforts to restore full quality of life to sufferers with ADHD. The next section reviews MRS results in ADHD to date.

MRS Studies of ADHD

This section reviews published MRS studies of ADHD. A previous review may be found in Perlov et al. [228].

Notes on Anatomical and Spectroscopic Nomenclature

Use of Finer Anatomic Descriptors

When reviewing a paper, we do not always adopt the anatomical nomenclature used in the paper, as when describing placement of MRS voxels in the brain and their contents. We often give voxel locus in terms of smaller brain structures and list more structures and tissues inside the voxel than the paper does. For example, a paper may speak of a "basal ganglia" voxel, whereas we refer to a "left caudate head + putamen" voxel. We have done this for precision and uniformity. In identifying voxel contents, we relied on figures and/or text in the papers. Hence, conclusions regarding localization of effects are only valid to the extent that the text and figures are representative across subjects in the study. This is normally supposed to be the case, but is not always so in practice.

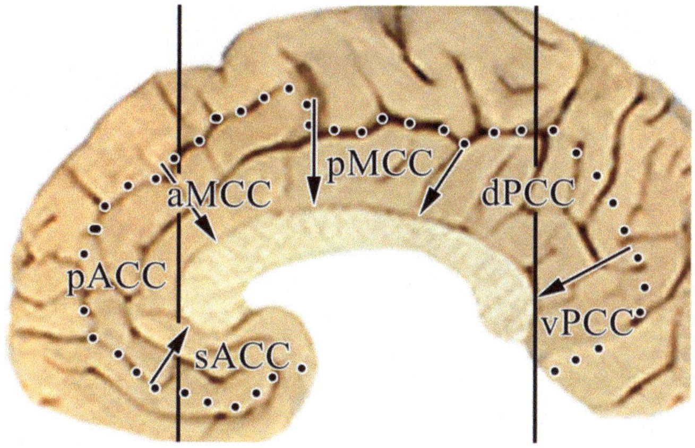

Fig. 18.3 Sagittal section of right cerebral hemisphere showing Eight-Subregion Model of human cingulate cortex. *Black arrows* give rostral-caudal intersubregion boundaries. *sACC* Subgenual anterior cingulate cortex, *pACC* Pregenual anterior cingulate cortex, *aMCC* Anterior middle cingulate cortex, *pMCC* Posterior middle cingulate cortex, *dPCC* Dorsal posterior cingulate cortex, *vPCC* Ventral posterior cingulate cortex. Not shown are the small dorsal and ventral retrosplenial cortices (dRSC, vRSC) inside the callosal sulcus (Modified from O'Neill J, Sobel TL, Vogt BA. Localizing cingulate subregions-of-interest in magnetic resonance images guided by cytological parcellations. In: Vogt BA, ed. Cingulate Neurobiology and Disease. New York, NY: Oxford University Press; 2009:3–30, with permission.)

Use of Eight-Subregion Cingulate Cortex Nomenclature

Frequent changes of nomenclature involve the cingulate cortex, sampled in many of the studies. Most of the studies refer grossly to "anterior cingulate" or "posterior cingulate" using the outdated two-subregion model of human cingulate anatomy; we, in contrast, employ the most recent Eight-Subregion Model [229] (Fig. 18.3), which is in best harmony with the full record of existing histological and neuroimaging data. The subregions coming up most often in the studies are the "pregenual anterior cingulate" (pACC) and the "anterior middle cingulate cortex" (aMCC), both of which are called "anterior cingulate cortex" in most of the papers. "Dorsal anterior cingulate cortex" in the papers frequently wholly or partially overlaps with aMCC in the Vogt nomenclature.

MR Spectroscopic Metabolite Nomenclature

"MRS" and "MRSI" in this review refer to ^{1}H MRS and ^{1}H MRSI unless stated otherwise. We have instituted uniform nomenclature for abbreviations of MRS metabolite resonances, changing any variant designations given in the papers. In particular, many papers use the abbreviation "NAA" without clarifying whether *N*-acetyl-aspartate (NAA) alone or *N*-acetyl-aspartate and *N*-acetyl-aspartyl-glutamate (NAAG) together is meant. In low-field ^{1}H MRS, the contribution of spectrally overlapping NAAG to the combined NAA+NAAG peak is substantial (~25%) [230] and, under the usual conditions of human in vivo spectroscopy, very poorly separable from that of NAA without special pulse sequences [231]. Widely used spectral fitting programs like LCModel [232] do provide both separate and combined values for NAA and NAAG even for conventional pulse sequences; the separate values are not considered reliable by many spectroscopists, though the combined values are. Unfortunately, when a given paper using such a fitting program reports levels of "NAA" it is often uncertain whether the value refers to the fit for NAA alone or for NAA+NAAG. For uniformity, we replaced references to "NAA" in the papers with "total NAA" (tNAA), meaning NAA+NAAG, unless it was clear that NAA alone was appropriate. As glutamate (Glu) and glutamine (Gln) are more often and more easily segregated reliably we do refer to them separately where appropriate. The conditions of most studies, however, do not afford a reliable segregation nor is such claimed by the authors. In such instances, we have retained the abbreviation "Glx" for the sum Glu+Gln. We replace references to "creatine" (Cr) with "creatine+phosphocreatine" (Cr+PCr) in recognition of the fact that these two affine compounds are poorly distinguishable with ^{1}H MRS. Exception is made where the compounds are clearly being mentioned independently, as in the two studies [233, 234] that used ^{31}P MRS, which *does* readily measure a peak for PCr alone. LCModel also reports separate and combined values for Cr and PCr, even where the segregation would not be considered reliable by many spectroscopists. Adriani et al. [235], a high-field animal study, is the only ^{1}H MRS paper reviewed below that reports Cr and PCr separately. We have retained this usage in this isolated case as it is germane to the arguments of the paper, though we do not endorse any conclusions based on these separate values. We abbreviate the choline-containing compounds collectively as "Cho," as in most of the papers cited. This can mean glycerophosphocholine (GPC) plus phosphocholine (PC) or GPC+PC plus (usually smaller) contributions from choline proper and acetylcholine. Some of the papers refer to "inositol compounds" (Ins), which we have uniformly changed to "*myo*-inositol" (mI). Having outlined these conventions, we proceed to review the studies.

MRS Studies of ADHD at Baseline

This section reviews MRS studies of ADHD at baseline. With "baseline" we mean either that the patients enrolled have not been previously treated for ADHD or that they have been or are being treated, but that the treatment per se is incidental to the study, i.e., the focus of these studies is generally on detecting effects of the disorder ADHD itself on regional metabolism.

MRS Studies of Pediatric ADHD at Baseline

Our survey identified 13 published baseline MRS studies of pediatric (child and/or adolescent) ADHD (Table 18.2). In the following, we comment on these studies in chronological order.

Table 18.2 Magnetic resonance spectroscopy (MRS) and magnetic resonance spectroscopic imaging (MRSI) baseline studies of pediatric attention deficit hyperactivity disorder (ADHD)

References	Subjects	MRS Technique	Brain Regions	Key Findings
MacMaster et al. 2003 [236]	9 child + adol ADHD (6 ♂/3 ♀)	1.5 T ^{1}H MRS	R-pACC + PFWM	Glx/Cr + PCr higher in ADHD than in HC; in ADHD, Glx/Cr + PCr correlates positively with age-of-onset
	(8 ADHD-C, 1 ADHD-I)	TR/TE 1500/135 ms		
	(8 stimulants, 1 no meds)	no vox dimensions (4–6 cc)	L-Cdhd + Put + GP	
	9 child + adol HC (6 ♂/3 ♀)			No significant effects
Yeo et al. 2003 [239]	23 child ADHD (17 ♂/6 ♀)	1.5 T ^{1}H MRS	R-PFWM	In ADHD, Cr + PCr correlates positively with CPT score; tNAA, Cr + PCr, Cho correlate positively with R-DLPF volume; in females, tNAA lower in ADHD than in HC
	(18 ADHD-C, 5 ADHD-I)	TR/TE 2000/30 ms		
	(17 stimulants, 1 sertraline, 5 no meds; all off meds 16 h prescan)	no vox dimensions (12.6 cc)		
	24 child HC (16 ♂/8 ♀)			
Courvoisie et al. 2004 [240]	8 child ADHD (7 ♂/1 ♀)	1.5 T ^{1}H MRS	L,R-pACC + SFC + PFWM	On left, tNAA/Cr + PCr, Glu/Cr + PCr higher in ADHD than in HC; in ADHD, mI/Cr + PCr correlates positively with language skills
	(8 ADHD-HI) (8 stimulants)	TR/TE 1600/20 ms		
	8 child HC (7 ♂/1 ♀)	vox: 20 × 20 × 20 mm^3 (8 cc)		On right, tNAA/Cr + PCr, Glu/Cr + PCr, Cho/Cr + PCr higher in ADHD than in HC; in ADHD, tNAA/Cr + PCr correlates positively with sensory motor and memory functioning, mI/Cr + PCr correlates positively with language skills
Sparkes et al. 2004 [241]	8 child ADHD (6 ♂/2 ♀)	1.5 T ^{1}H MRS	L-pACC + PFWM	tNAA/Cr + PCr correlates negatively in ADHD, positively in HC with Go-reaction time
	(8 ADHD-C) (8 no meds)	TR/TE 1500/135 ms		
	6 child HC (4 ♂/2 ♀)	vox: dimensions unstated (4 cc)		
Fayed and Modrego 2005 [242]	8 child + adol ADHD (3 ♂/5 ♀)	1.5 T ^{1}H MRS	L-centrum semiovale	tNAA/Cr + PCr higher in ADHD than in autism or HC
	(? subtype) (8 no meds)	TR/TE 2500/30 ms		
	21 child + adol autism (18 ♂/3 ♀) (21 no meds)	vox: 20 × 20 × 20 mm^3 (8 cc)		
	12 child + adol HC (5 ♂/7 ♀)			
Fayed et al. 2007 [243]	22 child + adol ADHD (18 ♂/4 ♀)	1.5 T ^{1}H MRS	R-aMCC + SFC + PFWM	tNAA/Cr + PCr higher in ADHD than in HC
	(? subtype) (22 drug-naïve)	TR/TE 2500/30 ms	L-centrum semiovale	tNAA/Cr + PCr higher in ADHD than in HC
	8 child + adol HC (4 ♂/4 ♀)	vox: 20 × 20 × 20 mm^3 (8 cc)		
Sun et al. 2005 [244]	20 adol ADHD (20 ♂/0 ♀)	1.9 T ^{1}H MRS	L,R-Put + GP	tNAA/Cr + PCr lower in ADHD-C than in ADHD-I or HC
	(10 ADHC-C, 10 ADHD-I) (20 no meds)	TR/TE 1500/35.5 ms		
	10 adol HC (10 ♂/0 ♀)	vox: 20 × 20 × 20 mm^3 (8 cc)		

Margari et al. 2006 [245]	1 child Sydenham's chorea + ADHD (1 ♂/0 ♀)	1.5 T ^{1}H MRSI	L,R-PFWM	tNAA/Cr + PCr lower, Cho/Cr + PCr higher in Sydenham's + ADHD than HC; "novel" MRS peak claimed
	(1 ADHD-C) (meds unstated)	TR/TE 8002/84.5 ms	L,R-Put	
	1 child "HC" (1 ♂/0 ♀) (migraine)	vox: 20×20×15 mm^3 (8 cc)		
Moore et al. 2006 [246]	15 child + adol ADHD (? ♂/? ♀)	1.5 T ^{1}H MRS	L?R?-antCC-NOS (no picture of voxel)	Glx/Cr + PCr, Glx/mI higher in ADHD than in ADHD + BPD or
	(any ADHD subtype) (3 on meds, 12 no meds)			HC
	8 child + adol ADHD + BPD (? ♂/? ♀) (2 on meds, 6 no meds)	TR/TE 2000/30 ms		
	7 child + adol HC (? ♂/? ♀)	vox: 20×20×12 mm^3 (4.8 cc)		
Stanley et al. 2006 [234]	10 child ADHD (9 ♂/1 ♀)	1.5 T ^{31}P MRSI	L,R-aMCC + SFC + PFWM	PME lower in ADHD than HC
	(7 ADHD-C, 3 ADHD-I) (8 off stimulants 24-h prescan, 2 on stimulants during scan)	TR/TE 2000/1.7 ms	L,R-Cdhd + Put + antTh + WM	PME lower in ADHD than HC
	15 child HC (13 ♂/2 ♀)	vox: 30×45×30 mm^3 (40.5 cc)	L,R-STG + preCG + postCG	No significant effects
Stanley et al. 2008 [233]	31 child ADHD (25 ♂/6 ♀)	1.5 T ^{31}P MRSI	L,R-aMCC + SFC + PFWM	In HC, PME correlate positively with age
	(15 ADHD-C, 16 ADHD-I) (31 drug-naïve)	TR/TE 2000/1.7 ms	L,R-Cdhd + Put + antTh + WM	PME lower in ADHD than HC
	36 child HC (27 ♂/9 ♀)	vox: 30×45×30 mm^3 (40.5 cc)	L,R-STG + preCG + postCG L,R-IPL L,R-PWM L,R-dPCC + precun + cun + OL	No significant effects On right, PME higher in ADHD than HC No significant effects No significant effects
Soliva et al. 2010 [247]	17 child ADHD (15 ♂/2 ♀)	1.5 T ^{1}H MRS	R-MFG	Cr + PCr lower in ADHD than HC
	(14 ADHD-C, 1 ADHD-HI, 2 ADHD-I) (17 off MPH 24-h prescan)	TR/TE 2000/30 ms	L-Cb-Hemi	tNAA, Cr + PCr, mI lower in ADHD than HC
	17 child HC (15 ♂/2 ♀)	vox: 20×20×20 mm^3 (8 cc)		
Yang et al. 2010 [248]	15 adol ADHD (13 ♂/2 ♀)	1.5 T ^{1}H MRS	L,R-pACC + PFWM	On right, tNAA/Cr + PCr higher, Cr + PCr lower in ADHD than in HC
	(9 ADHD-C, 6 ADHD-I) (12 on meds, 3 no meds)	TR/TE 1600/35 ms		
	22 adol HC (14 ♂/8 ♀)	vox: 20×20×20 mm^3 (8 cc)		

The study *MacMaster et al.* [236], the first study, was motivated by prior fMRI and SPECT findings in ADHD in cingulate subregions [166, 176] and striatal nuclei [189, 191, 212]. Nine children and adolescents with ADHD were scanned using single-voxel MRS at a relatively long echo-time (TE) of 135 ms. Eight subjects had been treated with stimulants (6 methylphenidate, 6 dexedrine), but all were off meds (from 48 h to 3 weeks) at time of scan. ADHD patients were compared to 9 sex- and age-matched healthy controls. Two voxels were deployed. One (4 cc in volume) sampled right pACC plus proximal prefrontal white matter; the other (6 cc) sampled left caudate head plus putamen plus globus pallidus. In the right pACC voxel, mean Glx/Cr + PCr was higher in the ADHD than in the control sample. Within the ADHD sample, Glx/Cr + PCr in this voxel correlated positively with age of onset of ADHD. At trend level, mean Glx/Cr + PCr was also higher in the ADHD than in the control sample in the left caudate voxel. The authors suggest that high regional Glx/Cr + PCr may reflect elevation of synaptic Glu that suppresses vesicular DA release via activation of metabotropic Glu receptors [237]. Low DAergic tone in striatal (caudate, putamen, nucleus accumbens) and cortical targets of midbrain DA-synthesizing nuclei (substantia nigra, ventral tegmentum) is hypothesized to foster symptoms of ADHD, e.g., by disrupting ability to inhibit context-inappropriate responses. In the case of cingulate cortex, multiple neurocognitive mechanisms (reviewed in Bush [238]), including impaired target selection, inadequate sensory information filtering, diminished ability to maintain focus, and aberrant linking of rewards or errors to actions, may contribute to ADHD symptomatology. Elevated Glu could be an agent in each of these mechanisms. All have been more solidly localized to aMCC (sampled in some of the studies reviewed below) than to pACC (sampled in this study), although the two regions are neighboring and voxels sampled likely contained some tissue from each.

Limitations of MacMaster et al. [236], acknowledged by the authors, include small number of subjects, stimulant-treatment of nearly all ADHD subjects, and use of ratios rather than absolute metabolite levels. Thus, inference of findings to the general ADHD population must be made cautiously; we do not know if effects are due to ADHD or to chronic stimulant treatment, and we do not know if high Glx/Cr + PCr stems from high Glu, high Gln, low Cr, low PCr, or some combination of these. Also, the long-TE of 135 ms yields a rather small Glx signal. The correlation of Glx/Cr + PCr with age of onset is interesting. If earlier age of onset translates into longer duration of illness in this sample (not possible to tell from the paper), it means that while Glx/Cr + PCr is higher on average in ADHD subjects than in controls, the gap between the two groups decreases with age, especially since Glx/Cr + PCr in the control sample increased with age with near-significance ($p = 0.05$). Perhaps this is a result of treatment or of differing developmental trajectories between the two groups. This investigation provided early evidence of regional metabolic disturbances in pediatric ADHD.

Yeo et al. [249] was the second study. With 23 ADHD children and 24 healthy control children, this was one of the larger studies reviewed. All ADHD patients had been undergoing psychotropic treatment, but were taken off meds 16-h prescan. A single large (12.6 cc) MRS voxel was acquired at short-TE (30 ms) from right prefrontal white matter. Within female subjects only, tNAA was lower in ADHD than in controls. Control females had greater tNAA than control males, while females with ADHD had lower tNAA than males with ADHD. Within the male + female ADHD sample, Cr + PCr correlated positively with scores on the CPT [250] test of selective attention, commonly used in ADHD diagnosis. Mean CPT scores were higher in the ADHD than in the control sample, meaning worse selective attention. Using volumetric MRI, the volumes of left and right "dorsolateral prefrontal" regions were measured in each subject comprising all gray and white matter anterior to the most anterior extension of the corpus callosum on coronal slices and superior to the most inferior extension of the rostral portion of the callosum. In the right cerebral hemisphere only, this dorsolateral prefrontal volume correlated positively with right prefrontal white matter levels of tNAA, Cr + PCr, and Cho and with CPT score.

Yeo et al. [249] suggest that low tNAA in females with ADHD may be related to the especially low GMR measured with ^{18}FDG-PET in females with ADHD [214, 251], as tNAA has been observed to correlate with GMR [252]. PET studies, however, seldom find effects in white matter, where GMR is typically much lower than in gray matter. Yeo et al. [249] also cite reverse lateralization of abnormal frontal α (alpha) EEG power in boys versus girls with ADHD [253]. Thus, bilateral frontal MRS data might help link neurochemical and neuroelectric patterns of sex differences in ADHD. As higher right dorsolateral prefrontal volume was associated with worse selective attention, the authors suggest that ADHD may involve some sort of right frontal hyperactivity. Since, however, it apparently contradicts their prior studies of white matter in normal adults and children showing positive correlations between tNAA and IQ [254] and between Cr + PCr and working memory [239], the authors are reluctant to interpret the correlations found in their ADHD sample between right prefrontal white matter tNAA (trend) and Cr + PCr and worse selective attention as part of this phenomenon. But, of course, they could still be part of this phenomenon as relationships between neurometabolites and cognitive performance need not be the same in ADHD as in normal subjects. This is overall a well-done study. The MRS voxel is large but samples an (ostensibly) homogeneous region of white matter. Interpretation is again limited by chronic, if not acute, treatment with psychotropics (overwhelmingly stimulants) in the ADHD sample. The study yields evidence for sex differences in neurometabolite effects in ADHD and for relationships between regional metabolite levels and neurocognitive performance, in particular the CPT, which continues to play an important clinical and research role in ADHD.

Courvoisie et al. [240], the third study, compared eight children with ADHD (all HI subtype) to eight healthy control children. All ADHD patients were being treated with stimulants, but were off meds 24-h prescan. A pair of MRS voxels sampled left and right pACC plus mesial superior frontal cortex plus vicinal prefrontal white matter. In the left hemisphere, tNAA/Cr+PCr and Glu/Cr+PCr were higher in the ADHD than in the control sample. Within the ADHD sample, mI/Cr+PCr correlated positively with language skills. On the right, tNAA/Cr+PCr, Glu/Cr+PCr, and Cho/Cr+PCr were higher in the ADHD than in the control sample. Within the ADHD sample, tNAA/Cr+PCr correlated positively with sensorimotor and memory functioning and mI/Cr+PCr again correlated positively with language skills.

The authors surmise that the high values of tNAA/Cr+PCr, Glu/Cr+PCr, and Cho/Cr+PCr in their ADHD sample have a diminished Cr+PCr peak as their common source, which in turn is due to a diminished overlapping GABA signal. A diminished Cr+PCr peak may well be the common source, but we question the case for low GABA. Courvoisie et al. [240] cite a 20% decrement in the area of the Cr+PCr peak in their ADHD sample versus their control sample, attributed to lower overlapping GABA. On the Cr+PCr peaks at 3.02 and 3.92 ppm, Courvoisie et al.'s [240] Figs. 2.3 show GABA shoulders for the healthy control subjects only in right pACC that could conceivably constitute 20% of the peak. Yet the same effect is seen for ADHD subjects only in left pACC while the decrement of Cr+PCr is claimed for ADHD bilaterally. Generally, GABA is present in relatively low concentrations in human brain, is highly variable in conventional proton spectra, and is best detected at high field with special pulse sequences [255, 256]. Short-TE proton MR spectra recorded from the pACC at our center yield GABA signals on the order of 10% of Cr+PCr. Does one anticipate the normal presence of twice this amount of GABA and its pathological depletion in ADHD without untoward consequences such as epileptic seizures? Thus, the GABA hypothesis of Courvoisie et al [240] may be tenuous and difficult to test. Simpler alternative explanations suggested by the authors, namely elevated Glu and diminished Cr+PCr per se due to local hypermetabolism, may be more viable. Weaknesses of this study again include small sample size, medication-exposed subjects, and use of metabolite ratios. But the study does add to evidence of neurometabolite abnormalities in pACC in ADHD and of relationships between MRS metabolites and neurocognitive functions.

Sparkes et al. [241] was the fourth study. Here, the left pACC plus proximal white matter was sampled at long-TE in eight nonmedicated children with ADHD and six healthy control children. No between-group differences in metabolite levels were proved, but there was a dissociation in the polarity of the correlation between tNAA/Cr+PCr and the GO-reaction time on the well-known Stop-Signal Task [257]: the correlation was negative for the ADHD group and positive for the control group. The authors interpreted this dissociation in terms of an abnormal preferential use of the sampled cortex on the part of ADHD subjects in response inhibition, as in the Stop-Signal Task. Again we have a study with few subjects and employing metabolite ratios, that once again links pACC metabolites to neurocognitive performance in ADHD.

Fayed and Modrego [242], similar to Yeo et al. [249], sampled white matter, left centrum semiovale, in eight unmedicated ADHD children and adolescents and 12 age- and sex-matched healthy controls using short-TE single-voxel MRS. These groups were compared to each other and to 21 (mainly male) unmedicated children and adolescents with autism. Thus, this was an early MRS study comparing pediatric ADHD with another neuropsychiatric disorder. The major finding was that tNAA/Cr+PCr was higher in the sample with ADHD than in the sample with autism or the control sample. The authors suggested that elevated neuronal density and mitochondrial metabolism may have increased NAA [258] in the ADHD subjects, thence driving up tNAA/Cr+PCr. As these studies go, the sample with autism was large, but the ADHD and control samples were small. Again, the use of metabolite ratios was limiting. Unfortunately, no insights were to be gained in comparing pediatric autism and ADHD.

Fayed et al. [243], the same investigators, conducted a subsequent study of 22 drug-naïve children and adolescents with ADHD, this time only eight controls and no patients with autism. Methodology was similar with the addition of a second MRS voxel placed in right aMCC plus mesial superior frontal cortex plus neighboring prefrontal white matter. Whole-brain diffusion-weighted imaging (DWI) was also performed in these subjects with sampling of the apparent diffusion coefficient (ADC) at four bilateral sites. In both MRS voxels tNAA/Cr+PCr was higher in the ADHD than in the control sample replicating and extending the investigators' prior finding in the smaller ADHD group. The authors again suggest hypersynthesis of NAA in the mitochondrion as an explanation for their findings. There were no between-group differences in ADC; the authors suggested deploying the more sensitive DTI technique to search for effects of ADHD on brain white matter [161]. The limitations here were again small control group and use of ratios. Nonetheless, this paper indicates possible metabolite abnormalities in ADHD in white matter and in a second cingulate subregion much studied by fMRI [238], the aMCC.

Sun et al. [244] acquired MRS from voxels in left and right putamen plus globus pallidus at TE = 35.5 ms and 1.9 T from 20 unmedicated male adolescents with ADHD and ten healthy male adolescent controls. In both voxels they observed that mean tNAA/Cr + PCr was lower in the ten ADHD-C subjects in their sample than in the ten ADHD-I subjects or the controls. They interpret the low ratio in ADHD as driven by low tNAA representing lower neuron density and/or integrity and/or neuronal dysfunction. Such neuronal pathology, in turn, is thought to impair executive function through the shared circuitry of the lenticular nucleus with prefrontal cortices [259]. This study also suffers from the use of ratios, but provides evidence that different subtypes of ADHD may be distinguishable with MRS.

Margari et al. [245], in an example of an MRS investigation of ADHD as a comorbidity to another disorder, presented a case study of a boy with Sydenham's chorea plus ADHD. MRS voxels were scanned at four sites, but as results were compared only to a single healthy control (who might even be disputed as a valid neurological control, since he suffered from migraine headaches), they are scarcely worth discussing. The authors also claim to have discovered a novel metabolite peak in their patient's MR spectra between 3.6 and 4.2 ppm representing sugars and amino acids. New metabolite peaks are (rarely) discovered in clinical MRS, as in cases of metabolic disorders or toxic exposures, but such assignments must be made with great caution. Neither Margari et al. [245] nor the prior MRS case study of Sydenham's they cite [260] discuss how their new peak is distinguished from the quotidian Cr + PCr resonance at 3.92 ppm (presumably straddling and riding underneath it) nor show comparison control spectra.

Moore et al. [246] was another MRS study involving ADHD and comorbidities. Fifteen children and adolescents with ADHD any subtype (mostly no meds) without bipolar disorder (BPD) were compared to eight children and adolescents diagnosed with ADHD plus BPD and to seven age-matched healthy controls. Note that the broad definition of pediatric BPD advocated by certain co-authors of Moore et al. [246] may have influenced patient selection. Single-voxel MRS at TE = 30 ms was acquired from an unspecified part of the anterior cingulate cortex of unspecified laterality. In the ADHD sample, mean Glx/Cr + PCr and Glx/mI in this voxel were higher than in the ADHD + BPD or the control sample. The authors attribute these findings to a possible increase in Glu in ADHD referring to the theory of Russell [114] on Glu-DA interactions in cortex and nucleus accumbens. Elevated Glx/mI may also signal low mI in ADHD patients. The authors take this as further evidence contraindicating drugs such as lithium and valproate that lower brain mI [261] for ADHD [262]. Respecting the limitations of small sample size and use of ratios, the results of this paper add to the mounting evidence of metabolite abnormalities in anterior cingulate cortex in ADHD.

Stanley et al. [233, 234] published the only two studies of ADHD using the ^{31}P nucleus. These were, moreover, ^{31}P MRSI studies, highly innovative at the time. In the first study, 10 children with ADHD and 15 healthy control children were scanned at 1.5 T. All the ADHD children were being treated with stimulants, although eight of the subjects were off meds 24-h prescan. A large cross-section of brain was scanned with 40.5 cc voxels (relatively small for ^{31}P MRS) with data sampled in bilateral aMCC plus superior frontal cortex plus nearby prefrontal white matter, caudate head plus putamen plus anterior thalamus plus white matter, and superior temporal gyrus plus precentral gyrus plus postcentral gyrus. Mean levels of phosphomonoesthers (PME) were lower in the ADHD than in the control sample bilaterally in the aMCC and caudate voxels with no significant metabolite effects in the superior temporal voxels. As PME are molecular building blocks for phospholipid membranes, low levels of these compounds imply below-normal rates of regional cell membrane synthesis in ADHD. The authors make a further inference specifically to synthesis of neuronal processes and synapses in brain regions devoted to attention.

The larger follow-up study [233] included 31 now drug-naïve ADHD and 36 healthy control children with additional brain regions being sampled. These included bilateral inferior parietal lobule, parietal white matter, and dorsal posterior cingulate cortex (dPCC) plus precuneus plus cuneus plus occipital lobe. Below-normal PME were again observed in the ADHD sample bilaterally in the caudate. Within the control sample only in bilateral aMCC, PME correlated positively with age (Fig. 18.4), hinting at a failure of this developmental feature to appear in the ADHD sample. In right inferior parietal lobule only, mean PME were *higher* in the ADHD than in the control sample, suggesting regional variability in the character of phosphorous metabolite abnormalities in ADHD. No significant metabolite effects were found in the superior temporal, parietal white matter, or dPCC voxels. In this paper, the authors present more detailed arguments and evidence relating their PME findings to the formation and also pruning of neurites and synapses. Missing in the discussion is any mention of glial cells, which of course also have phospholipid membranes, the precursors and degradation products of which may also contribute to ^{31}P MRS signals, membrane synthesis being a cardinal function of oligodendroglia in particular. Overall, this pair of studies is rigorous and advances and expands the field of MRS exploration of the brain in ADHD. Using previously unpublished ^{1}H MRSI data from our center, Fig. 18.5 shows two other dissociations between pediatric ADHD patients and healthy

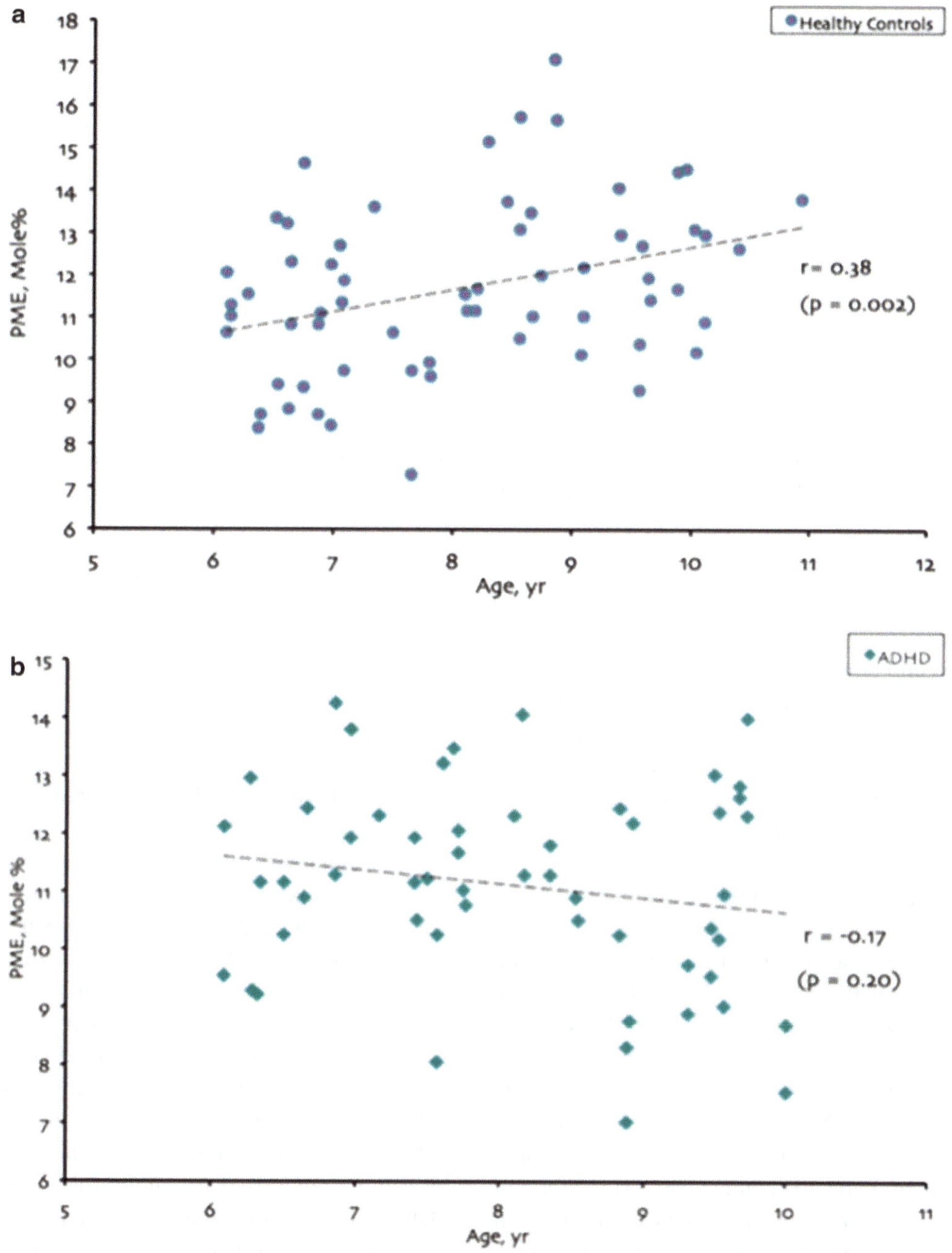

Fig. 18.4 Within a prefrontal region-of-interest, levels of membrane precursor phosphomonoesthers (PME) increased with age for healthy children (A), but decreased with age for children with ADHD suggesting abnormal cell membrane development in the prefrontal brain in ADHD. (Modified from Stanley et al. [233])

controls involving the relationships between regional metabolite levels and age. In right middle frontal gyrus (Fig. 18.5), in a sample of pediatric ADHD patients we noted significant declines in tNAA and Cho with age that were not present in the sex- and age-matched healthy control sample. This is further support for the idea of aberrant regional neurodevelopment in ADHD.

Soliva et al. [247] was a methodologically rigorous ^{1}H MRS study of 17 ADHD children (all off methylphenidate for 24-h prescan) and 17 sex- and age-matched healthy controls. Using single voxels, right middle frontal gyrus and left cerebellar hemisphere were scanned at TE=30 ms (their Figs. 18.1 and 18.2 apparently use neurologic rather than radiologic convention though this is not notated). In right middle frontal gyrus, mean Cr+PCr was lower in the ADHD than in the control sample. In the cerebellum, tNAA, Cr+PCr, and mI were all lower in the ADHD sample. These findings augment structural MRI evidence indicating

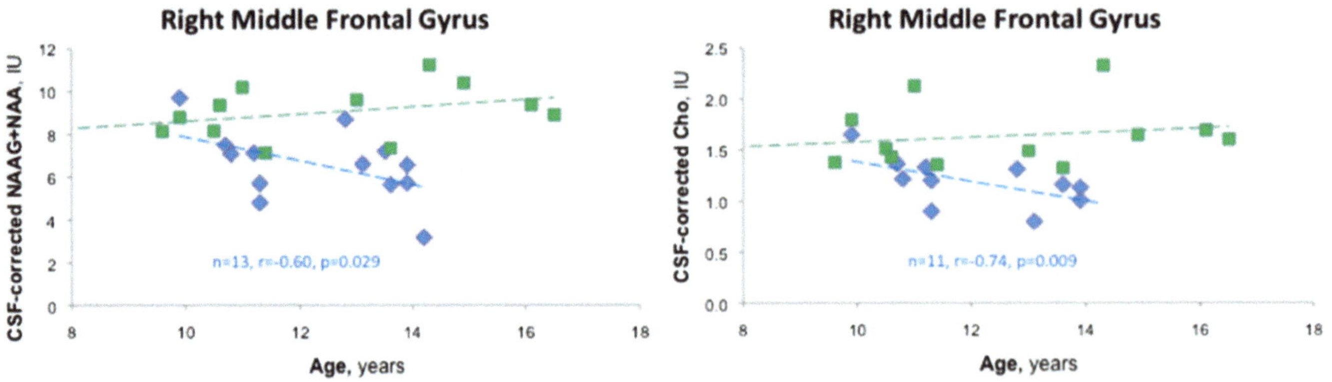

Fig. 18.5 CSF-corrected levels of tNAA ("NAA+NAAG") and Cho acquired in right middle frontal cortex using ^{1}H MRSI at 1.5 T for a series of individual subjects with ADHD (*blue diamonds*) and healthy controls (*green squares*). Significant decline in both tNAA (Spearman, $p<0.05$) and Cho ($p<0.01$) is seen for the ADHD sample but not for controls. This suggests an abnormal neurodevelopmental course in factors influencing these metabolites (brain energetics? membrane metabolism? osmoregulation?) in ADHD. Values are normed to unsuppressed water and given in Institutional Units (IU)

pathology in the cerebellum in ADHD and also point to the middle frontal gyrus as a disturbed region. In interpreting their findings, these authors discuss the associations of NAA with neuronal density [263] and osmoregulation [264] as well as the associations of mI with glial density [265], osmosis, and glucose metabolism [266]. They are reluctant to discuss their Cr+PCr result due to novelty and lower statistical significance, although similar explanatory factors may be invoked.

Yang et al. [248] was the most recently published baseline MRS study of pediatric ADHD. Fifteen adolescents (12 medicated) with ADHD and 22 healthy adolescent controls were scanned at 1.5 T and TE=35 ms using 8-cc single voxels in bilateral pACC and proximal white matter. In the right hemisphere only, tNAA/Cr+PCr was higher and Cr+PCr was lower in the ADHD than in the control sample. Yang et al. [248] interpret their and other prior literature findings in terms of below-normal regional Cr and/or PCr in ADHD. Cr+PCr together are seen as the central energy markers of both neurons and astrocytes [267]. The authors speculate that levels of Cr+PCr may be proportional to the functional activity of a brain area. Lower levels of Cr+PCr may provide neurons with lower energetic resources, thus allowing lower functional autonomy in stressful conditions. The authors postulate that their finding of lower Cr+PCr levels in the right pACC area may provide indirect evidence to support the energetic hypothesis of ADHD of Todd and Botteron [116]. This was a reasonably well-done study.

MRS Studies of Adult ADHD at Baseline

Our survey identified six published baseline MRS studies of adult ADHD (Table 18.3). In the following, we comment on these in chronological order.

Hesslinger et al. [268] was the earliest study, in fact one of the earliest MRS studies of ADHD at all. Ten unmedicated male adults with ADHD were compared to five healthy adult males. ADHD subjects comprised 5 ADHD-C and 5 ADHD-I subtypes. At 2 T, single voxels (8 cc) were acquired at TE=30 ms from left middle frontal gyrus and left caudate head plus putamen. In middle frontal gyrus, tNAA was lower in ADHD-C than in ADHD-I or in controls. No significant effects were detected in the caudate voxel.

The authors take their findings as evidence of subtle left prefrontal neuropathology, particularly of neuron loss or dysfunction in adults with ADHD-C. This is a methodologically fairly well-done study, although after division into the ADHD subtypes one is left with very few subjects per group.

Perlov et al. [269], the same group, published the next MRS study of adult ADHD 6 years later. The more substantial sample comprised 28 adults (now only 17 male) with ADHD all of whom had been off meds for 6 months prescan and 28 sex- and age-matched healthy controls. Subjects were scanned at 1.5 T and 30 ms TE, but with the finer spatial resolution of MRSI (3 cc) in bilateral pACC. In right pACC only, mean Glx/Cr+PCr was lower and Cho/Cr+PCr was higher in the ADHD than in the control sample. The authors provide a detailed analysis of their Glx/Cr+PCr finding in terms of the frontobasal DA-Glu interaction model of Carlsson et al. [270], developed for schizophrenia. The model asserts that the prefrontal cortex modulates the activity of midbrain DA neurons via both an activating ("accelerator") and an inhibitory ("brake") glutamatergic projection pathway, allowing finetuning of DA activity. Following this model, the authors believe their finding of low cingulate Glx/Cr in ADHD could be the consequence of low mesolimbic dopaminergic tone [275]. A comparable discussion of the Cho/Cr+PCr findings

Table 18.3 MRS and MRSI baseline studies of adult attention deficit hyperactivity disorder (ADHD)

Reference	Subjects	MRS technique	Brain regions	Key findings
Hesslinger et al. 2001 [268]	10 ADHD (10 ♂/0 ♀)	2 T ^{1}H MRS	L-MFG	tNAA lower in ADHD-C than in ADHD-I or HC
	(5 ADHD-C, 5 ADHD-I) (10 no meds)	TR/TE 3000/30 ms	L-Cdhd+Put	No significant effects
	5 adult HC (5 ♂/0 ♀)	vox: 20×20×20 mm^3 (8 cc)		
Perlov et al. 2007 [269]	28 adult ADHD (17 ♂/11 ♀)	1.5 T ^{1}H MRSI	L,R-pACC	On right, Glx/Cr+PCr lower, Cho/Cr+PCr higher in ADHD than HC
	(28 6 mn off meds prescan)	TR/TE 1500/30 ms		
	28 adult HC (15 ♂/13 ♀)	vox: 10×20×15 mm^3 (3 cc)		
Colla et al. 2008 [271]	15 adult ADHD (8 ♂/7 ♀)	1.5 T ^{1}H MRSI	L,L+R-aMCC L+R?-aMCC	Cho higher in ADHD than HC; In ADHD, Cho correlates positively with CPT-IP reaction time
	(? subtype) (15 drug-naïve)	TR/TE 1500/135 ms		
	10 adult HC (6 ♂/6 ♀)	vox: 8.75×8.75×15 mm^3 (2.4 cc after apodization)		
Ferreira et al. 2009 [272]	19 adult ADHD (? ♂/? ♀)	1.5 T ^{1}H MRSI	L,R-aMCC	On right, mI/Cr+PCr lower in ADHD-C than n ADHD-I or HC
	(10 ADHD-C, 9 ADHD-I) (19 off meds 6 mn prescan)	TR/TE 1500/30 ms	L,R-Put	On left, Glx/Cr+PCr higher in ADHD-C than n ADHD-I or HC
	12 adult HC (? ♂/? ♀)	vox: 15×15×20 mm^3 (4.5 cc)	L,R-Pul	On left, Cho/Cr+PCr higher in ADHD-C than in ADHD-I or HC
Perlov et al. 2010 [273]	30 adult ADHD (18 ♂/12 ♀)	1.5 T ^{1}H MRSI	L,R-Cb-Hemi	On left, Glx/Cr+PCr higher in ADHD than HC
	(30 no meds)	TR/TE 1500/30 ms	L,R-Cb-verm	
	30 adult HC (15 ♂/15 ♀)	vox: 10×20×15 mm^3 (3 cc)		No significant effects
Rüsch et al. 2010 [274]	14 adult borderline personality disorder+ADHD (0 ♂/14 ♀)	3 T ^{1}H MRS	L-pACC	tNAA, Glu higher, Gln lower in borderline+ADHD than HC
	(14 off meds 2 week prescan)	TR/TE 3000/30 ms	L-Cb-Hemi	
	18 adult HC (0 ♂/14 ♀)	vox: 20×20×20 mm^3 (8 cc)		No significant effects

is not provided. This is one of the better studies methodologically, the principal weakness being the use of ratios. The authors incorrectly imply that quantitation of absolute metabolite levels is firmly established for single-voxel MRS but impossible for MRSI, yet some groups have obtained absolute levels with MRSI since the 1990s and metabolite quantitation remains an incompletely resolved issue for both single-voxel MRS and multivoxel MRSI.

Perlov et al. [273], again the same group, followed-up with a relatively large short-TE MRSI (3 cc voxels) study of the cerebellum in ADHD. Thirty medication-free adult ADHD patients and 30 healthy adult controls were scanned with regions of interest in bilateral cerebellar vermis and cerebellar hemisphere. No significant effects were detected in the vermis but in the left hemisphere, mean Glx/Cr+PCr was higher in the ADHD than in the control sample. This represents evidence for neurometabolite abnormalities in the cerebellum in ADHD, a brain structure in which volumetric abnormalities have repeatedly been demonstrated with structural MRI [134, 135, 156, 159, 178]. The Glx/Cr+PCr finding is again interpreted in terms of the Glu-DA hypothesis of Carlsson [270, 275] and brought in connection with a theory of the cerebellum as a "machine" that models motor and cognitive behavior [276]. Use of metabolite ratios remains a weakness of this otherwise rigorous study.

Colla et al. [271] was the next study. Fifteen drug-naïve adults with ADHD and 10 healthy control adults were scanned with MRSI at 1.5 T. Left and right aMCC were regions of interest and the combination of left and right was also analyzed. Voxel size was 2.4 cc. In left and in left+right aMCC, mean Cho was higher in the ADHD than in the control sample. Within the ADHD sample, Cho correlated positively with CPT reaction time. The authors take their findings as further evidence for anterior cingulate cortex dysfunction in ADHD, including adult ADHD, citing prior ^{18}FDG-PET [214], fMRI [176], and scalp EEG evoked potential [277] results. The authors acknowledge that Cho is a composite MRS signal containing contributions from GPC, PC, and to a lesser extent, free choline itself, molecules that are breakdown products or precursors of membranes [278]. They cite three circumstances that could contribute to pathological elevation of Cho: release of choline-containing compounds accompanying acute damage, membrane biosynthesis associated with new or increased synaptic plasticity, and neoplastic or inflammatory processes. Of these, subtle structural changes associated with membrane turnover and myelination are seen as fitting in with the finding of slowed reaction speeds and the concept of ADHD as a developmental dysregulation of myelination [122]. Despite small subject numbers, this study was important in finding MRS effects in the aMCC, a region multiply linked to ADHD through findings with fMRI and other neuroimaging modalities [238], and MRS effects associated with impaired CPT performance, a common neurocognitive symptom of ADHD.

Ferreira et al. [272] published a short-TE MRSI study (1.5 T, 4.5 cc voxels) of 19 adults with ADHD (10 ADHD-C and 9 ADHD-I) who had been off meds for 6 months prescan and 12 healthy adult controls. Bilateral aMCC, putamen, and pulvinar were sampled. This investigation made use of innovative offline MRSI "voxel-shifting" to optimize anatomical positioning of regions of interest. Apart from Stanley et al. [233, 234] (which also used voxel shifting), this made it the only MRS study of the thalamus in ADHD. In right aMCC, mean mI/Cr+PCr was lower in the ADHD-C than in the ADHD-I or control groups. In left putamen, Glx/Cr+PCr was higher in the ADHD-C than in the ADHD-I or control groups. And in left pulvinar, Cho/Cr+PCr was lower in the ADHD-C than in the ADHD-I or control groups. Thus, this study revealed a variety of MRS metabolite effects of ADHD in different brain regions. It also again showed MRS effects in the ADHD-C subtype that were statistically absent in the ADHD-I subtype. This study did better than most in evading partial-voluming complications, but still suffered from the use of metabolite ratios. The mI/Cr+PCr and Cho/Cr+PCr results were related to the influence of mI and Cho in cell energy and membrane metabolism [246, 279, 280]. An alternative DAergic mechanism was also suggested for the Cho/Cr+PCr excess. The Glx/Cr+PCr result was also related to cell energy metabolism, in particular the lactic acid energy deficit theory of Todd and Botteron [116]. Alternative explanations of the Glx/Cr+PCr elevation included shifts in the interconversion rates of Gln, Glu, and GABA and Glu-DA interactions.

Rüsch et al. [274] was the most recent adult baseline MRS study, a study of borderline personality disorder with comorbid ADHD. At 3 T and TE=30 ms, 14 female patients and 18 healthy female controls were examined. Two voxels were placed (each 8 cc), one in left pACC, the other in left cerebellar hemisphere. No significant effects were detected at the latter site. In left pACC, tNAA and Glu were higher, while Gln was lower in patients versus controls. Note that high field strength facilitated segregation of Glx into Glu and Gln in this investigation. The Glu/Gln imbalance was seen as a possible result of impaired Glu recycling in neuronal-astrocytic metabolism [115], possibly due to ADHD energy deficiency in the sense of Todd and Botteron [116]. As the authors point out, since a simultaneous increase in Glu and decrease in Gln may manifest as unchanged Glx, perhaps it is inadequate to measure only the Glx sum as most MRS studies of ADHD have done. The authors suggest that elevated tNAA may be a consequence of incomplete cortical maturation during adolescence in ADHD [281]. Unexpectedly, the study did not contribute to evidence for cerebellar abnormality in ADHD or borderline personality disorder.

MRS Studies of Interventions for ADHD

This section reviews MRS studies of interventions for ADHD. It deals exclusively with pharmacological treatments, since unfortunately we are aware of no MRS studies of nonpharmacological treatments for ADHD, even though such treatments are common. A further limitation in scope is that most studies reviewed were concerned with stimulant medications, above all methylphenidate, given the widespread application of these agents and their typical success in alleviating symptoms of ADHD.

MRS Studies of Interventions for Pediatric ADHD

Our survey identified five published MRS studies of interventions for pediatric ADHD (Table 18.4). We review these in chronological order.

Jin et al. [282] was the earliest published study. Twelve drug-naïve adolescent boys with ADHD were scanned before and after a single challenge dose of oral methylphenidate. Ten healthy control adolescent boys were also scanned once only. MRS was acquired at 1.9 T and TE=35.5 ms from single voxels (8 cc) placed bilaterally in the globus pallidus with some partial voluming of the putamen. Bilaterally, mean tNAA/Cr+PCr was lower and mean Cho/Cr+PCr was higher in the pretreatment ADHD boys than in the control boys (baseline findings). Within the ADHD sample, Cho/Cr+PCr decreased significantly in response to the methylphenidate challenge. The tNAA/Cr+PCr ratio was unchanged by methylphenidate. There is no mention of follow-up or a third scan to see if Cho/Cr+PCr returned to its prechallenge values. Regarding their baseline tNAA/Cr+PCr finding, the authors state, "The significantly decreased NAA/Cr ratio in globus pallidus indicates that approximately 20–25% of neurons had died or were severely dysfunctional." From our perspective this is quite a premature conclusion. First, the value of tNAA/Cr+PCr may as well be affected by concentrations of

Table 18.4 Magnetic resonance spectroscopy (MRS) and magnetic resonance spectroscopic imaging (MRSI) studies of pharmacologic treatment of attention deficit hyperactivity disorder (ADHD)

Reference	Subjects	MRS technique	Brain regions	Key findings
Treatment studies of pediatric ADHD				
Jin et al. 2001 [282]	12 adol ADHD (12 ♂/0 ♀) (? subtype) (12 drug-naïve) (single challenge dose MPH) 10 adol HC (10 ♂/0 ♀)	1.9 T ^{1}H MRS TR/TE 1500/35.5 ms vox: 20×20×20 mm^3 (8 cc)	L,R-GP+Put	tNAA/Cr+PCr lower, Cho/Cr+PCr higher in pre-Tx ADHD than HC; Cho/Cr+PCr lower in post-Tx than pre-Tx ADHD
Carrey et al. 2002 [283]	4 child ADHD (2 ♂/2 ♀) (3 ADHD-C, 1 ADHD-I) (2 MPH, 2 atomox) (Scan1 predrug baseline; Scan 2 after 14–18 week on meds)	1.5 T ^{1}H MRS TR/TE 1500/135 ms vox: dimensions unstated (4 cc, 7 cc)	R-pACC L-Cdhd+Put	For atomox, Glx/Cr+PCr lower post- than pre-Tx; for MPH, no significant effects Glx/Cr+PCr lower post- than pre-Tx
Carrey et al. 2003 [284]	14 child+adol ADHD (11 ♂/3 ♀) (12 ADHD-C, 2 ADHD-I) (4 MPH, 7 dex, 3 atomox) (Scan1 2–21 days off meds; Scan 2 after ~13 week on meds)	1.5 T ^{1}H MRS TR/TE 1500/135 ms vox: dimensions unstated (4 cc)	R-SFC L-Cdhd+Put+GP	No significant effects Glx/Cr+PCr lower post- than pre-Tx
Carrey et al. 2007 [285]	13 child ADHD (13 ♂/0 ♀) (13 ADHD-C) (13 drug-naïve) (12 rescanned after 8 week MPH)	1.5 T ^{1}H MRS TR/TE 2000/30 ms	R-SFC L-Cdhd+Put	No significant effects Glu, Glx higher in pre- and post-Tx ADHD than in HC; Cr+PCr higher in pre-Tx ADHD than in post-TX ADHD or HC
	10 child HC (10 ♂/0 ♀)	vox: dimensions unstated (4 cc)	L-OWM	No significant effects
Adriani et al.2007 [235]	8 adol MPH rats (8 ♂/0 ♀) 8 adol saline rats (8 ♂/0 ♀) (rats treated as adolescents, MR scanned as adults)	4.7 T ^{1}H MRS TR/TE 4000/23 ms vox: dimensions unstated (0.021–0.056 μl) isofluran sedation	L+R-PFC L+R-dorsal striatum L+R-NAcc	Cr lower, PCr higher in MPH than saline rats Cr+PCr, Cho, Tau higher in MPH than saline rats; in MPH rats, Cr correlates positively with impulsivity score tNAA, Cr+PCr, Tau lower, Gln higher in MPH than saline rats
Treatment study of adult ADHD				
Kronenberg et al. 2008 [286]	7 adult ADHD (5 ♂/2 ♀) (? subtype) (7 drug-naïve) (Scan1 drug-free baseline, Scan2 after 5–6 week MPH)	1.5 T ^{1}H MRSI TR/TE 1500/135 ms vox: 8.75×8.75×15 mm^3 (2.4 cc after apodization)	L+R-aMCC	tNAA higher, Cho lower post- than pre-Tx

Cr and PCr in the denominator as by NAA and NAAG in the numerator. Second, even if levels of NAA and/or NAAG are low, it is not clear whether this stems from slower neuronal synthesis of these amino acids or from their more rapid degradation by astrocytes and oligodendrocytes (Fig. 18.1). (Note that more rapid degradation could be a consequence of higher value of the rate constants for enzymatic degradation, higher enzymatic densities in the astrocyte and oligodendrocyte membranes, and/or higher tissue densities of astrocyte and oligodendrocyte cells.) Third, even if depression of NAA and/or NAAG levels is of neuronal origin, it is not clear whether this results from a small loss of NAA and/or NAAG spread over many neurons or a large loss limited to a few neurons. The authors suggest that elevated baseline Cho/Cr+PCr in the ADHD sample may be due to “imbalance between the dopaminergic and cholinergic systems”. If they mean here the central cholinergic neurotransmitter systems, this explanation may be inadequate. The acetylcholine molecule makes only a small contribution to MRS Cho signal intensity. It might be better to argue, as other authors have done, in terms of disturbances in cell membrane metabolism involving PC and GPC, but these are present in appreciable amounts in both cholinergic and noncholinergic neurons, as well as in glial cells. Although the authors do not discuss the modest postmethylphenidate drop in Cho/Cr+PCr, it is important for future MRS research to note that even a single dose of this agent may bring about an observable change in metabolite levels.

Carrey et al. [283–285] are the next three studies to review. The first [283] was a case series of four children with ADHD, two of whom were treated with methylphenidate and two with atomoxetine. Each child was scanned at predrug baseline, then again after 14–18 weeks of treatment. Scanning was done at 1.5 T and long-TE with one single voxel placed in right pACC (4 cc) and another in left caudate head plus putamen (7 cc). In the pACC, Glx/Cr+PCr decreased markedly (mean 47.5%) post- versus pretreatment for the atomoxetine subjects with no significant metabolite effects for the methylphenidate subjects. In the caudate voxel, Glx/Cr+PCr decreased markedly (mean 56.1%) after treatment for both agents. There were very few patients and no control group in this study. Metabolite ratios were employed and Glx was measured at long-TE. Notwithstanding, this study provided early evidence that striking neurometabolite changes may accompany medicinal treatment for ADHD and/or symptomatic response (all subjects were good responders) and that regional metabolite effects may vary by agent. Carrey et al. [284] followed up with a larger study of 14 children and adolescents with ADHD (4 on methylphenidate, 7 on dextroamphetamine, and 3 on atomoxetine). Each patient was scanned twice: once while 2–21 days off meds, and then again after being *circa* 13 weeks on meds. MR scanning was as in the first study only the two voxels (each 4 cc) were placed in right superior frontal cortex and in left caudate head plus putamen plus globus pallidus. No significant effects were observed in superior frontal cortex. In the caudate voxel, Glx/Cr+PCr was lower after than before treatment. Hence, this replicated, in a larger sample, the major finding of Carrey et al. [283].

In Carrey et al. [285], methods were further improved by excluding adolescents, studying patients of only one sex (13 boys), studying only drug-naïve subjects, and adding a healthy control group (ten boys). Moreover, all patients were the same subtype (ADHD-C). All but one of the patients were scanned before and after an 8-week course of oral methylphenidate (all same drug); controls were scanned only once. TE was reduced to 30 ms and voxel size remained relatively small (4 cc). Absolute metabolite levels rather than ratios were employed and Glu was quantitated separately as well as as the sum Glx. Voxels were placed in right superior frontal cortex, left occipital white matter, and left caudate head plus putamen. No significant effects resulted in the first two voxels. In the caudate voxel, both Glu and Glx were higher in both pre- and posttreatment patients than in controls. Cr+PCr was higher in the pretreatment ADHD sample than in controls. Within the ADHD sample, Cr+PCr decreased to control levels after treatment (Fig. 18.6). The authors refer to prior notions of DA-Glu interactions [114] and suggest that excess Glu (and therefore Glx) in ADHD may result from a failure to deactivate synaptic Glu due to low striatal monoamine levels. This would cause “synaptic spillover” of Glu [287] possibly contributing to symptoms of ADHD. The authors interpret the treatment-responsive Cr+PCr excess in ADHD as a possible consequence of a local cell energetic deficit [116]. They also indicate that Cr may be neuroprotective [288]; hence the ADHD brain may be elevating its Cr levels as attempted compensation for excess excitotoxic Glu. Finally, the authors adduce a possible further link between their Glu and Cr+PCr findings by referring to a PCr-dependent system for Glu uptake into synaptic vesicles [289]. Overall this is a respecTable model for an intervention study with intriguing neurochemical interpretations of results.

Adriani et al. [235] was the last study and the only preclinical animal study to be reviewed here. In an attempt to simulate a common pattern in human ADHD patients, eight rats were exposed to daily i.p. methylphenidate for 14 days as adolescents, then underwent MRS scanning as adults. Another eight rats were similarly exposed to normal saline and scanned. Scanning was performed at high field (4.7 T) with very small voxels in order to fit in the rat brain. Voxels were sampled in midline prefrontal cortex, midline dorsal striatum, and midline nucleus accumbens. This paper reported separate values for Cr and PCr, even though it is a proton MRS study. Even though the standard deviations of the separate Cr and PCr values were implied to be within the

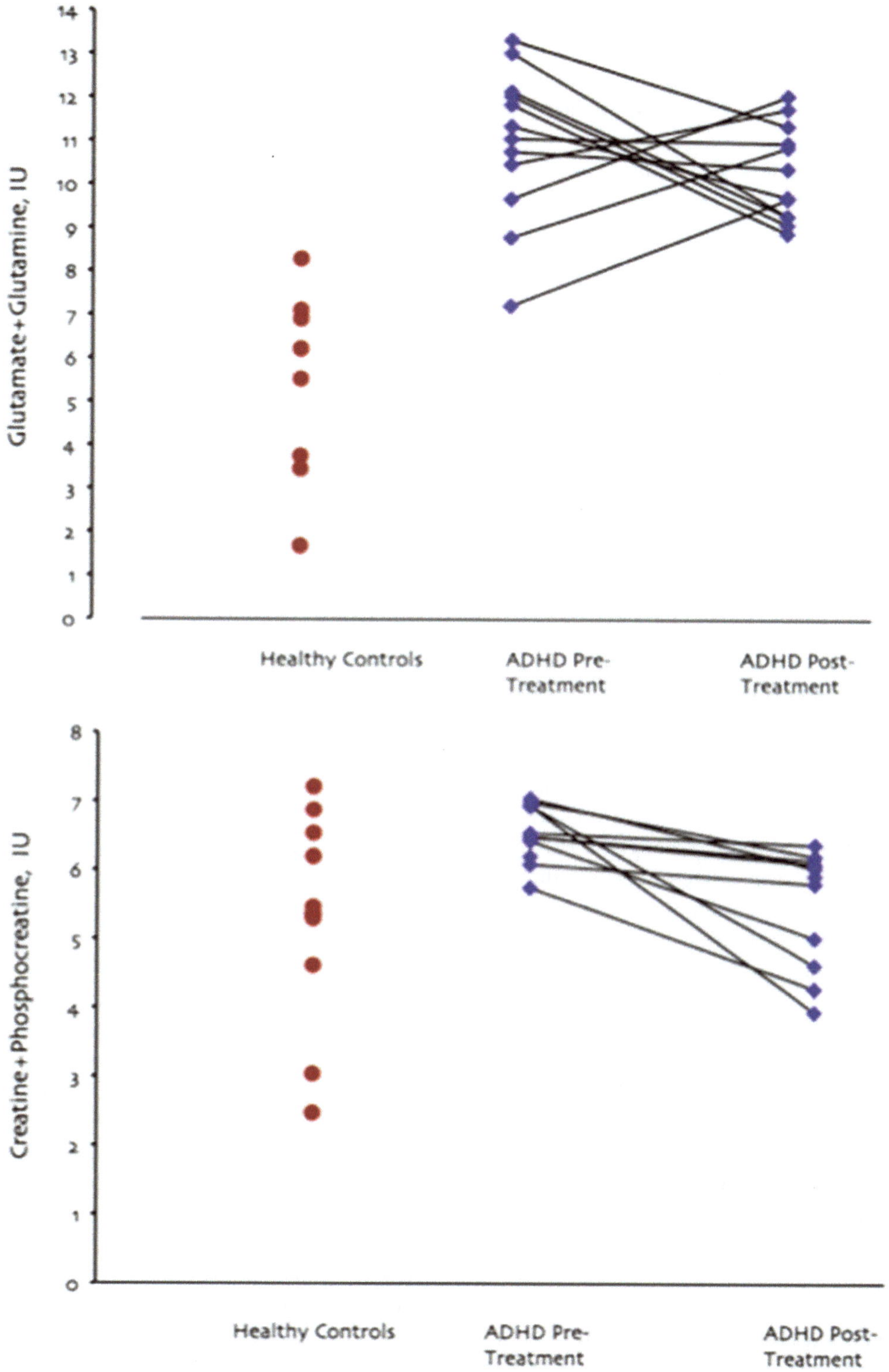

Fig. 18.6 Levels of Glx (upper) and Cr+PCr (*lower*) in a ^{1}H MRS single-voxel sampling left caudate+putamen in a pediatric series of ADHD patients (*circles*) before-and-after 8-week methylphenidate treatment and in a series of healthy controls (filled diamonds) at baseline only. Note substantial baseline elevation of Glx in the ADHD sample, dropping in several subjects after treatment. Also note the more uniform post-treatment fall in Cr+PCr. (Modified from Carrey et al. [285])

20% acceptability threshold of the LCModel program used to fit the data, it is important to note that many spectroscopists would not accept the separate values, contenting themselves with the combined Cr+PCr levels. We agree with those spectroscopists.

In prefrontal cortex, Cr was said to be lower and PCr higher in methylphenidate than in saline rats. In dorsal striatum, Cr+PCr, Cho, and the amino acid taurine (Tau) were all higher in methylphenidate than in saline rats. Within the methylphenidate rats, Cr correlated positively with a behavioral impulsivity score, which itself was lower in the methylphenidate rats. In the accumbens, tNAA, Cr+PCr, and Tau were lower, while Gln was higher in methylphenidate than in saline rats. The authors suggest that Cr and Tau levels in each brain region are proportional to the functional activity of the region and that methylphenidate exposure in adolescence brings about hyperfunction of the dorsal striatum and hypofunction of the accumbens. They also recall the importance of the striatum in habit formation and expression and propose that methylphenidate exposure provides for greater behavioral flexibility and ability to cope with challenging tasks. The tNAA, Gln, and Cho results are not discussed in detail. It is important to keep in mind that normal Wistar lab rats and not ADHD-model rats were treated. Although the authors conclude by warning that methylphenidate treatment in human patients misdiagnosed for ADHD could lead to untoward brain metabolite changes, their overall message seems to be one of positive effects of adolescent methylphenidate exposure on brain and behavior. Studies on larger samples with more extensive outcome measures would be required before extrapolating such conclusions to humans.

The observation of effects on Tau is intriguing. Miller et al. [290] found that Tau was a major osmolyte in the brains of preweaned rats, but declined in concentration in favor of Glu, PCr, and mI as the rats matured to adulthood. Adriani et al. [235] suggest that methylphenidate treatment may alter the normal developmental course of preferred osmotic species in the rodent brain. It is unknown if similar changes take place in human ADHD patients and if these are beneficial.

MRS Study of Intervention for Adult ADHD

Our survey revealed only one MRS intervention study on adult ADHD [286]. In this study, seven drug-naïve adult patients with ADHD were scanned at predrug baseline and then again after 5–6 weeks of daily oral methylphenidate. They were scanned with long-TE MRSI at 1.5 T with a 2.4-cc voxel size. Midline aMCC was the region of interest. In this region, tNAA increased and Cho decreased after treatment. The authors point out that their findings add to evidence linking the aMCC to ADHD and its pharmacological remediation. They interpret both the tNAA increase and the Cho decrease seen in their patients as possible consequences of rise in cellular energy availability brought about by methylphenidate. Mitochondrial synthesis of NAA is energy dependent [258] and oligodendrocyte synthesis of fatty acids and myelin is supported by Lac production [117]. Energy deficiency secondary to DAergic hypotonia in untreated ADHD therefore may lead to low tNAA and high Cho (due to accumulation of unused membrane phospholipid molecular building blocks). This was a reasonably well-done study mainly limited by small subject numbers.

Summary of Findings

Brain Regions Implicated in ADHD By MRS

The above-reviewed MRS studies reveal that significant effects of ADHD and of its pharmacologic treatment can be registered in multiple brain regions, including some of those where such effects were detected using other neuroimaging modalities. Brain structures where effects were repeatedly observed include the pACC and aMCC subregions of the cingulate cortex; the caudate, putamen, and globus pallidus nuclei of the basal ganglia; the vermis and hemisphere of the cerebellum; and different zones of the cerebral white matter; more isolated findings were noted in inferior parietal lobule, the pulvinar, and the middle frontal cortex. Thus, MRS contributes evidence for pathology and/or dysfunction in these regions in ADHD and evidence that these regions may represent anatomic substrata of therapeutic response.

Neurometabolites Implicated in ADHD by MRS

In terms of the metabolites involved, some evidence has been presented for each of the canonical ^{1}H MRS metabolites tNAA, Glx, Cr+PCr, Cho, and mI; most of the findings, however, were expressed as ratios to Cr+PCr. Since some studies [247–249, 285] have uncovered ADHD findings involving Cr+PCr itself, these ratio results are particularly open to ambiguous interpretation. The meta-analysis of Perlov et al. [228] concluded that the most widely reproduced evidence was for elevated regional Cho in ADHD. Although that meta-analysis also substantially included ratio results, its conclusion is at least consistent with the ^{31}P MRS findings [233, 234]. Cho is thought of as reflecting cell phospholipid membrane turnover [291]. Membrane synthesis, however, is an active process, suggesting that Cho levels may also reflect cell energetics [292]. As mentioned in Fig. 18.2, given finite supply, a cell makes trade-off between dedicating carbon substrate to membrane synthesis and burning it for energy. A further consideration is that cell water is produced both by glycolysis and more powerfully by the downstream stages of Glc catabolism. Most of the canonical metabolites, in addition to their other cellular functions, serve as osmolytes [293]. Thus, the cell raises and lowers its intracellular concentrations of these molecules in order to maintain cell volume in the face of changes in the amount of intracellular water. Beyond being osmolytes, NAA and NAAG also have a specific role as "molecular water pumps" and are active in transporting very large quantities of water outside the neuron in proportion to their molar concentration [294]. As much of this water originates from the cell energy chain, essentially all of the canonical metabolites can be linked to energy through water regulation and in other ways. Thus, many results of the ADHD MRS literature to date may directly or indirectly endorse the energetic hypotheses of Todd and Botteron [116] and Russell et al. [117], as is claimed in the discussion sections of several of the papers reviewed.

Fronto-Subcortical Network Loops in ADHD

Many of the above-cited MRS studies add evidence in support of the notion that "prefronto-striatal" neuronal circuit loops are implicated in ADHD. Frequently, the choice of anatomical nomenclature has been self-limiting in these studies. Thus, instead of describing MRS voxel placement as being in a specific rostral subregion of the cingulate cortex (e.g., pACC or aMCC), the authors have referred nonspecifically to "anterior cingulate cortex," to "ventromedial prefrontal cortex," or even to 'prefrontal cortex." Due perhaps to the high intersubject variability in the courses of the human cingulate and paracingulate sulci [295], which makes it hard to distinguish the paracingulate portions of the cingulate from neighboring gyri on MRI, there is a tendency on the part of many investigators to conflate the cingulate and the prefrontal cortices. A further issue is that MRS voxels sampling the basal ganglia frequently contain multiple different nuclei (caudate, putamen, globus pallidus) in the same voxel (partial-voluming problem). Sometimes paired nuclei will be referred to as if they formed a single functional, rather than merely nominal structural, unit, i.e., "striatum" for caudate + putamen, "lenticular nucleus" for putamen + globus pallidus. When citing the MRS studies of ADHD we have substituted more precise nomenclature where tenable. As high-field studies with smaller voxel sizes become more widespread, MRS may yield more critical information on the role of recurrent cortico-basal gangliar loops in ADHD.

Functional Neuroanatomic Model of ADHD

In this section, we take a cingulocentric functional anatomic model involving recurrent cortico-basal gangliar loops recently developed to explain the symptomatic phenomenology of obsessive-compulsive disorder (OCD) and apply it to ADHD. We then speculate on how neurochemical aberrations at the glutamatergic synapse (Fig. 18.1) might be reflected in the temporal dynamics of ADHD and OCD subjective mental experience.

Updated Subcortical Loop Construct and Cingulocentric OCD Theory

Applying the most recent neuropathology and neuroimaging data, Middleton [296] has updated the long-popular concept of recurrent fronto-subcortical neural loops [297]. His updated construct includes loops containing individual subregions of the cingulate and prefrontal gyri. The subcortical nuclei participating in these loops are resolved to the level of subparts of caudate, globus pallidus, thalamus, etc. A cingulocentric model of obsessive-compulsive disorder (OCD) emerges from the updated concept identifying a detailed functional neuroanatomy of the disease. Middleton infers that the same may be done for ADHD, but does not present details. Here we adapt the Middleton [296] model to ADHD by contrasting the condition with OCD.

Loops for OCD Thoughts, Feelings, and Actions

Middleton [296] envisions OCD as driven by a triad of recurrent cortico-subcortical circuits (Fig. 18.7). As in Alexander et al. [297], each circuit forms an excitatory positive feedback loop connecting a series of cortical subregions and subcortical subnuclei. (There are distinctions between "open" and "closed" loops, which we leave aside here.) Glu and GABA are the key neurotransmitters involved. The first loop is the Ideation-Obsessional Thoughts circuit. Neurotransmitter flows in this circuit from the inferior frontal cortex to the caudate to the substantia nigra pars reticulata to the ventral anterior and medial dorsal nuclei of the thalamus back to the cortex. The second loop is the Emotion-Anxiety Depression circuit. It runs from the pACC to the caudate and nucleus accumbens to the substantia nigra pars reticulata and nucleus basalis of Meynert to the ventral anterior and medial dorsal nuclei of the thalamus back to the cortex. The third loop is the Action-Compulsive Behaviors circuit. It flows from the cingulate motor area (in the aMCC) to the putamen to the globus pallidus internal segment to the ventral anterior, ventral lateral, and centromedian thalamic subnuclei back to the cortex.

As their names imply, the Ideation-Obsessional Thoughts and Action-Compulsive Behaviors circuits support the recurrent mental obsession and motor compulsion symptoms of the disease, while the Emotion-Anxiety Depression circuit supports the prevailing affect of the condition, which is perpetual anxiety frequently with comorbid depression. It is envisioned that the positive feedback loops in these three circuits are undergoverned leading them to inject thoughts, feelings, and motor actions repeatedly into consciousness. Functionally, the inferior frontal cortex is implicated in syntax,

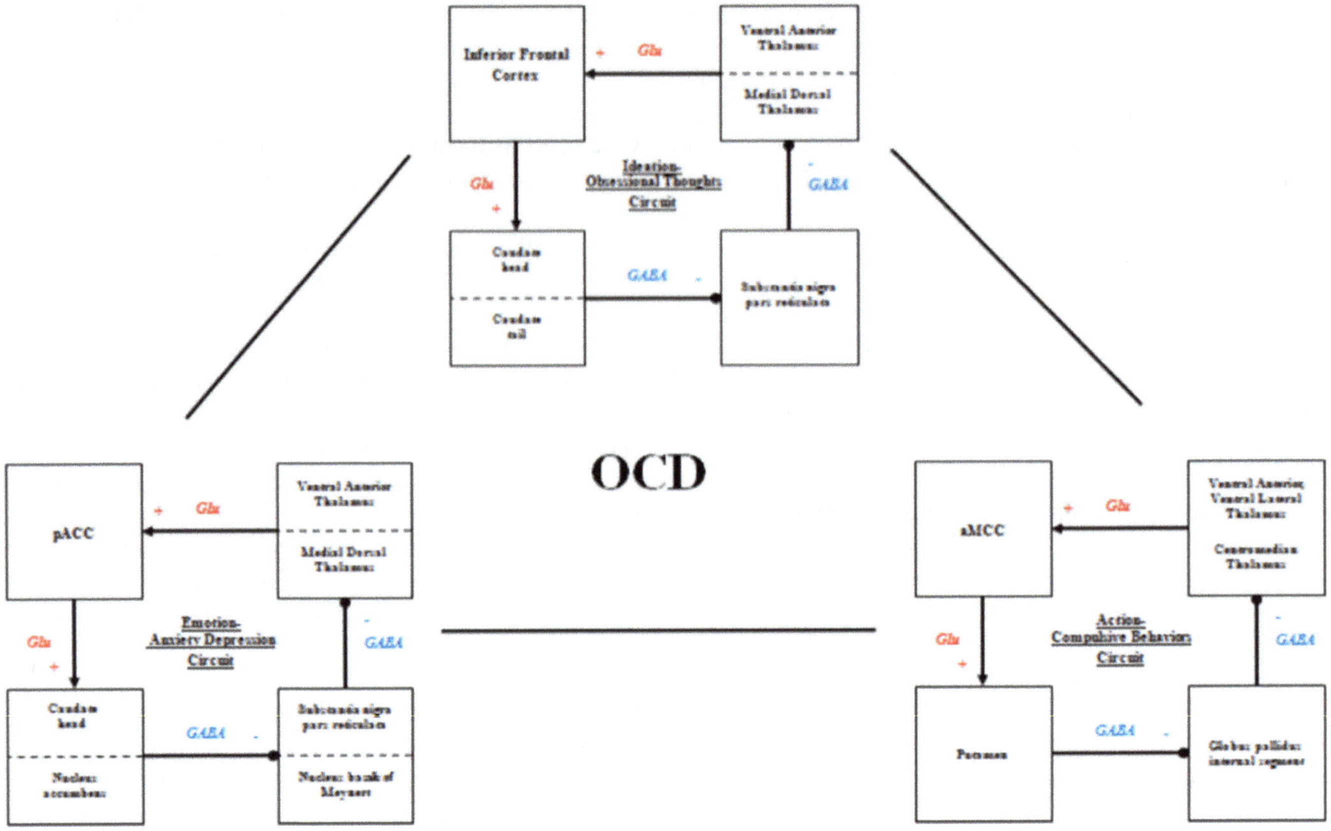

Fig. 18.7 Middleton's (2009) cingulocentric OCD model. Excessive recurrent activity in the three cingulo-subcortical positive feedback loops supports OCD symptoms thoughts, feelings, and actions, respectively. (Modified from Middleton FA. The contribution of anterior cingulate-basal ganglia circuitry to complex behavior and psychiatric disorders. In: Vogt BA, ed. Cingulate Neurobiology and Disease. New York, NY: Oxford University Press; 2009, with permission.)

i.e., serial sequencing of morphemes in building a verbal thought, a subvocalization, or spoken sentence [298–300]. Thus, obsessional thoughts attach to form, i.e., the patient will think or speak the same sentence (or see the same image in consciousness) repeatedly, identically, or with small modifications, in the symptomatic phenomenon known as "getting the right feeling." The pACC is implicated in the emotion of happiness [229]. Hence, pACC dysfunction is associated with anhedonia and depression in OCD and other conditions. Ruminative feelings of dread, of worthlessness, of emptiness, and so on present with a recurring and unshakable character. The aMCC is implicated in will power or voluntary motor control, as well as in fear and pain [229]. The three are closely related as exercise of will power frequently involves overcoming pain, e.g., in weight lifting, or facing up to fears, e.g., in making sales calls. Will power is intimately involved with OCD [301]. The patient must repeatedly exercise will power in choosing how to respond to OCD compulsions: to give in to them, to resist them, to avoid situations that induce them, to do the opposite of what they say (as in CBT exposure therapy), or to note their presence and refocus away from them (as in the Four Steps therapy). This connection with will power also grounds the pervasive guilt often felt in the disorder. Thus, excessive recurrent glutamatergic positive feedback activity in the three loops leads to the thought, feeling, and behavioral action symptoms of OCD.

Egosyntonic Versus Egodystonic

A final concept needed to understand the model is that of "egosyntonic" versus "egodystonic" thoughts, feelings, and behaviors. This concept pair is used in two senses in OCD management and research. In the first sense, egosyntonic mental events are experienced as coming from the self, while egodystonic mental events are experienced as having alien, i.e., outside the self, origin. For example, an unidentified voice in the patient's mind urges him to push grandma down the stairs. In the second sense, egosyntonic simply means something pleasant and egodystonic means something unpleasant. In the following, we will only use these words in

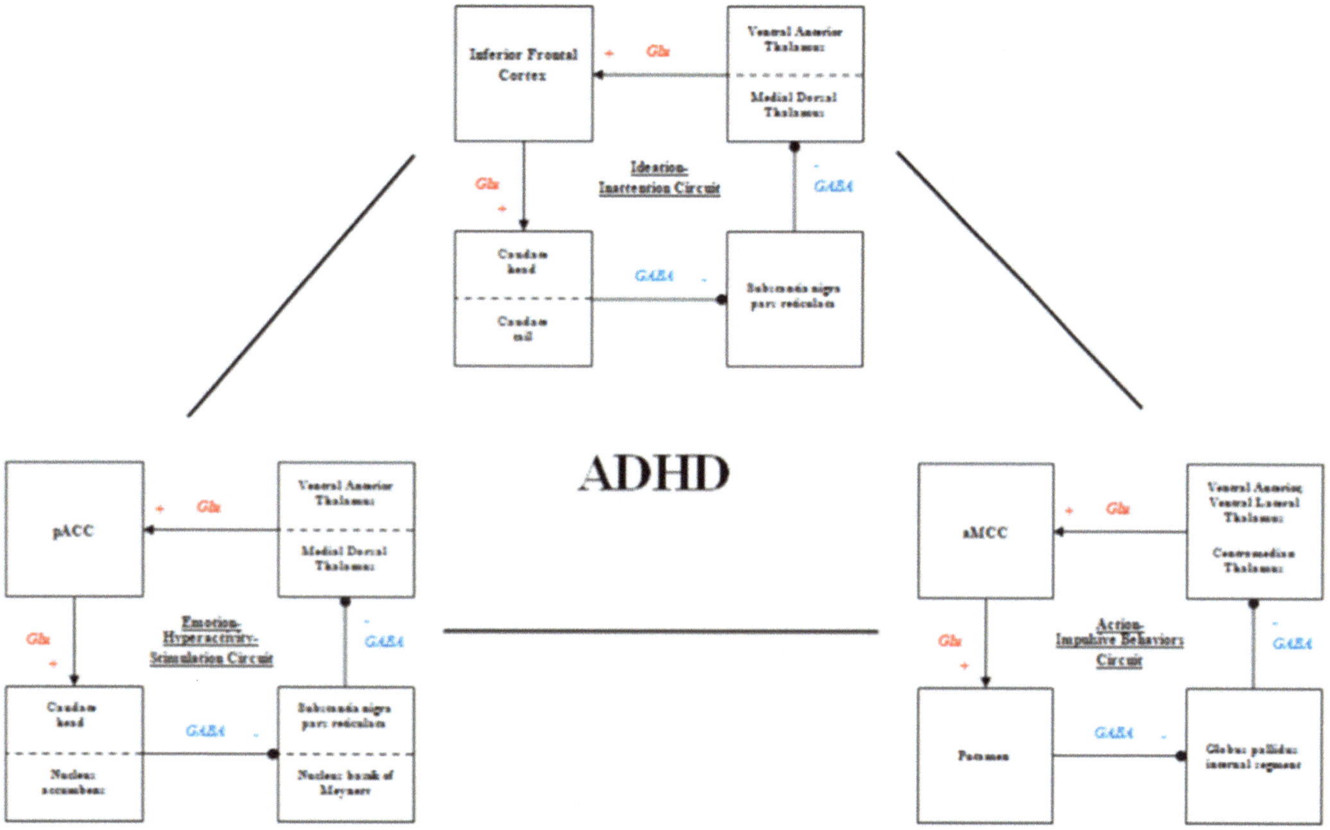

Fig. 18.8 Middleton's (2009) cingulocentric OCD model applied to ADHD. Insufficient recurrent activity in the three loops leads to ADHD symptoms

the second sense. In contrast to, for example, addictive behaviors for substance abuse patients, OCD obsessions and compulsions are pervasively egodystonic in character, i.e., OCD patients do not enjoy the obsessive thoughts that run persistently through their heads nor the compulsive acts they perform over and over; on the contrary, they experience them as highly unpleasant.

Application to ADHD

To describe ADHD, we take the same three OCD circuits form the Middleton [291] model and simply rename them (Fig. 18.8). This yields an Ideation—Inattention circuit, an Emotion-Hyperactivity-(Self)-Stimulation circuit, and an Action-Impulsive Behaviors circuit. We now contrast the way egodystonic mental events are dealt with habitually in OCD versus in ADHD using these three circuits. OCD patients are strongly bound by egodystonic mental events even when these are unwholesome and impractical; ADHD patients are repelled by egodystonic mental events even when these are beneficial and practical. Thus, for example, a patient with OCD counts the panes in a window dozens of times over even though he knows he is wasting time and hates doing it, while a schoolboy with ADHD cannot concentrate on doing his homework because it is boring. An OCD patient's thoughts are continually drawn back to anxiogenic obsessive topics despite stringent mental efforts to flee from them while an ADHD patient's thoughts are drawn away from the unpleasant task at hand and have difficulty coming back (Ideation-Inattention Circuit). For example, an OCD patient cannot drive the thought of licking sandpaper with his tongue out of his mind, while the ADHD schoolboy is distracted from the classroom by sounds of the playground outside and is long in shifting his attention back to the teacher's dull lecture. The OCD patient makes repeated futile attempts at escaping anxious, depressive, ruminative feelings, while the ADHD patient is continually in self-stimulatory pursuit of unfulfilled satisfaction (Emotion-Self-Stimulation Circuit). Responding to drives of inner origin, the OCD patient feels compelled to perform empty rituals; he is over-inhibited in that external stimuli are typically churned over and over-processed within before taking action; the ADHD patient, on the other hand, is typically driven by outward, distracting stimuli; he is underinhibited in that it is difficult for him to return to his inner focus. The above sets of opposite symptoms may be a matter of chronic hyperactivity of the three circuits in OCD versus chronic hypoactivity in ADHD.

Issue of ADHD-OCD Comorbidity

If the two diseases now are polar opposites in terms of their subjective phenomenology and cortico-subcortical loop physiology as described, how is it then that the two are so frequently comorbid? The answer is that it is less of a question of whether the circuits are firing too quickly or too slowly (and thus pushing attention towards or away from an egodystonic focus), but of the stability of the circuits, of their propensity to stay running at an even tempo. In ADHD, Russell et al. [117] have emphasized the importance of the moment-by-moment variability of performance. The effective vesicular supply of Glu, the numbers of active receptors, transporters, enzymes, etc. in a functionally relevant brain region at a given moment may vary, based, for example, on energy supply, allowing different symptomatology to manifest at that moment. Conventional neuropharmacologic treatments for OCD and ADHD may (temporarily) alleviate the dysregulation that fosters instability in these circuits. For example, there is evidence that synaptic serotonin, which is increased by SRIs used to treat OCD, counters Glu actions in many parts of the brain, including suppressing LTP by preventing activation of NMDAR [302]. (Overinduction of LTP may drive the proliferative forging of anxiogenic associations and pathological creativity in OCD.) Thus, SRI treatment for OCD may slow down the three cycling feedback loops. Stimulant treatment for ADHD in contrast increases synaptic DA and the actions of DA at some of its receptors enhance glutamatergic functions, including induction of LTP by NMDAR [303]. Thus, stimulant treatment for ADHD may speed up the three cycling feedback loops. In both cases, the optimal result is a more stabile operating state.

Neurochemical Model of the Mental Dynamics of OCD and ADHD

In modeling energetic interactions at the Glu synapse, Russell et al. [117] use a hydrodynamic analogue [304]. Our speculative theory will instead use a linear electric circuit analogue (Fig. 18.9) to model mass transport of Glu from vesicular release at the presynaptic neuron to ultimate remote synaptic rerelease or consumption in the postsynaptic neuron or astrocyte (as in Fig. 18.1). Although illustrated for a single synapse, the events are meant to occur at numerous, perhaps phase-synchronized, synapses. The electrical analogy is not essential, one can obtain the same results with direct chemical kinetic modeling, but analogues permit us to use existing mathematical solutions immediately and more importantly foster insight and physical intuition.

Electric Current Is Dual to Glu Flux

We model the rate of mass transport or flux of Glu through the synaptic system of Fig. 18.1 as an electric current, i.e., a rate

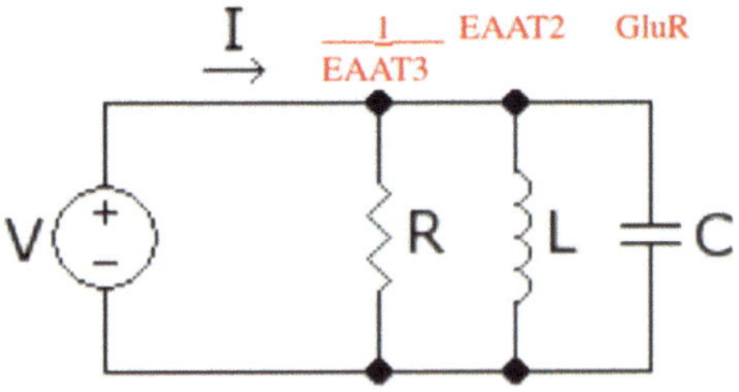

Fig. 18.9 Parallel RLC linear circuit analogue of Glu mass transfer at a cortical synapse in OCD or ADHD. The current I is dual with Glu flux from presynaptic neuron to ultimate remote rerelease or consumption. Capacitance C is dual with surface density and reactivity of neuronal and astrocytic Glu membrane receptors. Inductance L is dual with density and inversely proportional to the density and reactivity of EAAT3 Glu transporters on the postsynaptic neuronal membrane. V is "mass-transfer potential," an amalgam of the Glu concentration gradient due to massing in vesicles and net presynaptic production and delivery minus postsynaptic consumption and clearance

of electric charge transport. To link this to subjective mental experience, we assume that more positive current, i.e., higher Glu flux corresponds to more attention to the thought, feeling, and/or action at hand ("focus"). Negative current corresponds to attention to some *other* thought, feeling, action ("distraction"). Zero current is the default state. In reality, of course, we do not know if higher cortical perisynaptic Glu flux corresponds to greater attention, concentration, mental effort, etc. This assumption, however, is often made in neuroscience and there is some reason to believe it. In particular, $H_2{}^{15}O$-PET [305, 306] and fMRI [307, 308] studies indicate that rCBF and BOLD activation increase both in magnitude and spatial extent across the brain with greater cognitive effort or more difficult tasks. For most (though not all) neuronal synaptic configurations, increases in rCBF and BOLD signify faster neuronal firing [309]. For glutamatergic neurons, the key cortical neurons driving the circuits in our OCD and ADHD loop models, that means higher Glu flux. Thus, we associate higher Glu current in a circuit engaged in a task or holding a scene in consciousness with greater attention to that task or scene. Drawing on our above discussion, we will analyze the case when focus is on an egodystonic (unpleasant) thought, feeling, or action. Our goal will be to compute the time course of the Glu current, and thus of attention to the egodystonic event in consciousness, based on the cellular configuration of Fig. 18.1.

Voltage Is Dual to Glu "Mass-Transfer Potential"

The analogue for electric voltage in the model is less straightforward than for current. One can think of the voltage as a "mass-transfer potential." This means, in part, the concentration gradient in Glu, including the gradient created by massing Glu molecules in vesicles at the terminus of the presynaptic neuron. But additionally the positive pole of the mass-transfer potential represents nonpassive reactive and/or transport forces inside the presynaptic neuron generating and delivering Glu to its terminus; the negative pole represents such forces within the postsynaptic neuron consuming or spiriting away Glu. (As one of several approximations we make, we will ignore Glu ultimate destruction within the astrocyte and oligodendrocyte.) Therefore, we say, the voltage represents an amalgam of concentration gradient and net production and consumption of Glu by the system. The idea is that we have a presynaptic Glu source and a postsynaptic Glu sink that together drive the Glu flow.

The Parallel Electric Circuit Represents the Metabolic Pathway Choices of Synaptic Glu Molecules

In the simplified picture of Fig. 18.1 freshly liberated synaptic Glu molecules of vesicular or NAAG-lytic origin are confronted with multiple simultaneous choices: They can dock with glutamatergic receptors, they can enter astrocytes through EAAT2, or they can enter neurons through EAAT3. Therefore, we have modeled the perisynaptic cell ensemble as a *parallel* electric circuit. In electrical circuits, capacitors create voltage by storing charge, inductors create voltage by storing current (e.g., charge moving in loops), and resistors (also known as conductors) create voltage by allowing charge to pass through them. In our model, therefore, ionotropic and metabotropic Glu receptors (GluR) are analogous to capacitors because they dock with Glu molecules holding them and taking them out of flow for a time. They sustain mass-transfer potential by storing mass of a particular molecular species. The EAAT2 astrocytic Glu transporters are analogous to inductors because they divert synaptic Glu into the Glu–Gln cycle, a mass-flow loop that again delays eventual progress of the Glu from source to sink. Finally, the resistance is represented by 1/EAAT3 (it would be EAAT3 for conductance) as these transporters allow the Glu to pass through to the postsynaptic neuronal sink without reactive time delay. To be more precise, we would say that quantities like EAAT2 are represented by something like their surface density multiplied by some combination of kinetic rate constants for entering and exiting the transporter and so on, but we will leave such details aside for simplicity.

General Solution to the Electric Analogue Equation

For a constant applied voltage, the current through parallel circuit 18-9 is

$$I(t) = A\exp\left(\frac{-1}{2\mathrm{RC}} + \sqrt{\frac{1}{4R^2C^2} - \frac{1}{\mathrm{LC}}}\right)t + B\exp\left(\frac{-1}{2\mathrm{RC}} - \sqrt{\frac{1}{4R^2C^2} - \frac{1}{\mathrm{LC}}}\right)t \qquad (18.1)$$

the exponential prefactory constants A, B being determined by the initial conditions, e.g., was the voltage applied suddenly at time zero by flipping a switch to close the circuit? Was there a nonzero current in the circuit, or perhaps just in the inductor, at time zero? Was the capacitor initially charged? And so on. We will leave such details unspecified for now. In the general case, the shape of the current curve after the switch is flipped, i.e., the time profile of Glu flux after a presynaptic action potential arrives, the shifts in attention once a task is engaged, depends on the values of the circuit elements, in particular the time constants RC and $\sqrt{\mathrm{LC}}$. There are three typical solutions.

Critical Damping. The Healthy Control Condition

The first type of solution is called "critically damped" (and takes the slightly modified form $I(t) = (A + Bt)\exp\left(\frac{-1}{2\mathrm{RC}}t\right)$; Fig. 18.10). This solution applies when $\sqrt{\mathrm{LC}} = 2\mathrm{RC}$. This means there is a balance between harboring of Glu in receptors (C), cycling Glu between astrocytes and neurons (L), and transport of Glu to disposal (R). It is a pure real (i.e., nonoscillatory) solution, a brief rise to a peak value followed by a smooth exponential decay. This corresponds to the healthy control condition in our model. The initial action potential brings on a burst in Glu flux that then returns evenly to baseline with time. The subject applies the requisite strong attention to the egodystonic task straight away, then gracefully leaves it and shifts back to baseline, ready to think about, feel, or do something else without getting distracted.

Underdamping. The OCD Condition

The second type of solution is called "underdamped" (Fig. 18.11; where a slight phase shift is added for the initial peak). It applies when $\sqrt{\mathrm{LC}} < 2\mathrm{RC}$.

That means that the discriminant $\left(\frac{1}{4R^2C^2} - \frac{1}{\mathrm{LC}}\right)$ in (18.1) becomes negative, making the argument of the exponential factors complex, which implies a damped sinusoid waveform. This corresponds to the OCD condition in our model. The inequality in time constants can arise when both EAAT2 and EAAT3 levels are low. That implies a state of low Glu transport and high Glu docking at receptors. The neurons thereby become overstimulated. This induces excess LTP leading to formation of prolific idiosyncratic and anxiogenic associative memory links in OCD. Thus, all kinds of mundane concepts, objects, actions, etc. assume impractically disproportionate importance in the mind of the OCD patient. Excessive stimulation may also contribute to the above-normal GMR multiply documented in OCD; wasteful brain energy expenditure possibly leading to fatigue symptoms. The OCD patient's initial attention does strongly focus on the

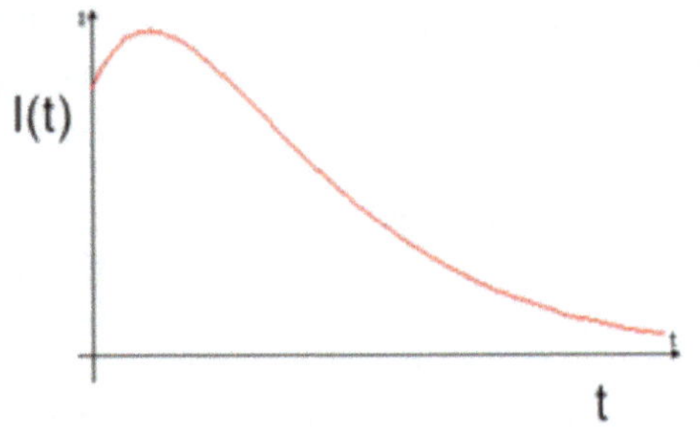

Fig. 18.10 Critically damped = healthy control condition. Plot of current, representing Glu flux and subjective attention to unpleasant task as a function of time. Initial presynaptic depolarization leads to firm burst of Glu flux that then decays smoothly and exponentially to baseline over time. Subject directs the needed attention to the unpleasant task, gradually leveling off, then is done with the task, back to the default mental state

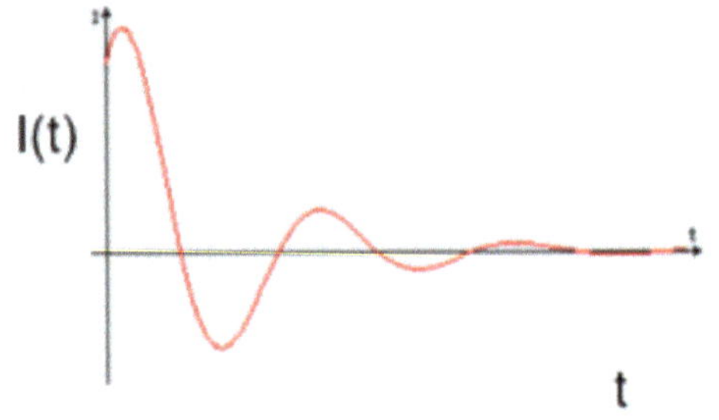

Fig. 18.11 Underdamped = OCD condition. Glu flux shows more rapid initial decay than in the healthy case, and then fluctuates prolongedly about baseline levels. The subject's initial attention to the unpleasant event is strong but too brief to dispense with it adequately. Subsequently, the subject shifts attention to other thoughts but is repeatedly drawn back to the unpleasant matter before settling down to the default state

egodystonic thought, feeling, or action. But he shifts away from it quickly (negative swing of current), really too quickly to process and mentally dispose of the event properly, and thence goes into oscillations in which the egodystonic thought or feeling recurs repeatedly, inbetween flights of attention to other thoughts. The oscillations may be higher and last longer than depicted in Fig. 18.11. Note that CBT exposure therapy for OCD entails having the patient willfully force himself to attend to egodystonic stimuli for longer stretches of time than he is wont. This is equivalent to pushing out the curve of Fig. 18.11 (decreasing the net decay constant) to look more like the healthy curve of Fig. 18.10.

Overdamping. The ADHD Condition

The third solution is "overdamped" (Fig. 18.11). It applies when $\sqrt{LC} > 2RC$, i.e., when levels of both EAAT2 and EAAT3 transporters are high. This corresponds to the ADHD condition in our model. This high Glu transport state implies there is little Glu available for docking with GluR. Thus, neurons are understimulated and induction of

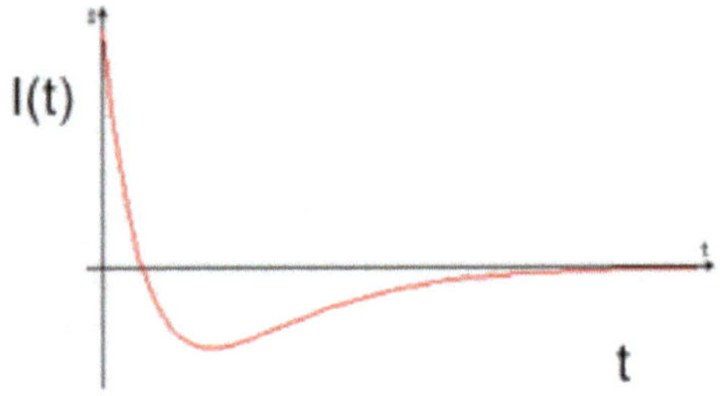

Fig. 18.12 Overdamped = OCD condition. Glu flux decays very rapidly, falling well below baseline, and is slow to recover to baseline. The subject's attention is quickly pulled from the unpleasant task to other, distracting thoughts. It takes a long time for attention to drift back to default

LTP is subnormal. Learning becomes more difficult. The ADHD patient's attention shifts rapidly away from the egodystonic task toward distractors. It returns only slowly to the baseline default state. Note that the negative deflection can be greater and the return to baseline longer than depicted in Fig. 18.12. Because decay is so rapid, motor action is repeatedly reinitiated to try to experience a mental event thoroughly, i.e., to achieve satisfaction (hyperactivity).

Application to Polygenetic Studies of ADHD. Falsification of the Model

Although highly speculative, we hope that the above model at least demonstrates some way that subjective mental phenomena forming clinical symptoms might be linked to neurochemistry. This model might furthermore show one way to approach the issue of multiple susceptibility genes contributing to a psychiatric disorder. For example, in ADHD one might look for simultaneous regional overexpression of the genes coding for EAAT2 and EAAT3, and perhaps aggravated by low expression of genes coding for various GluR; in OCD one could look for the opposite constellation. Hence, particular combinations might cause circuit instability, as opposed to high or low expression of one single gene. The above model might also be falsified by using the rate constants for binding and release of Glu from the various transporters and receptors to try to quantify the curves of Figs. 18.10, 18.12 and 18.13. This could be compared to the behavioral time course of shifts and oscillations of thoughts and rituals in ADHD and OCD. Agreement would tend to support the model, and disagreement would tend to show it is incorrect.

ADHD and OCD as Problems in Neurochemical Stability

In hydrodynamic systems, turbulence or instability becomes highly probable when the operating values of certain dimensionless parameters exceed critical thresholds, e.g., a Reynolds Number >2100 and/or a Mach Number >1 for steady flow of a Newtonian fluid in a smooth cylindrical

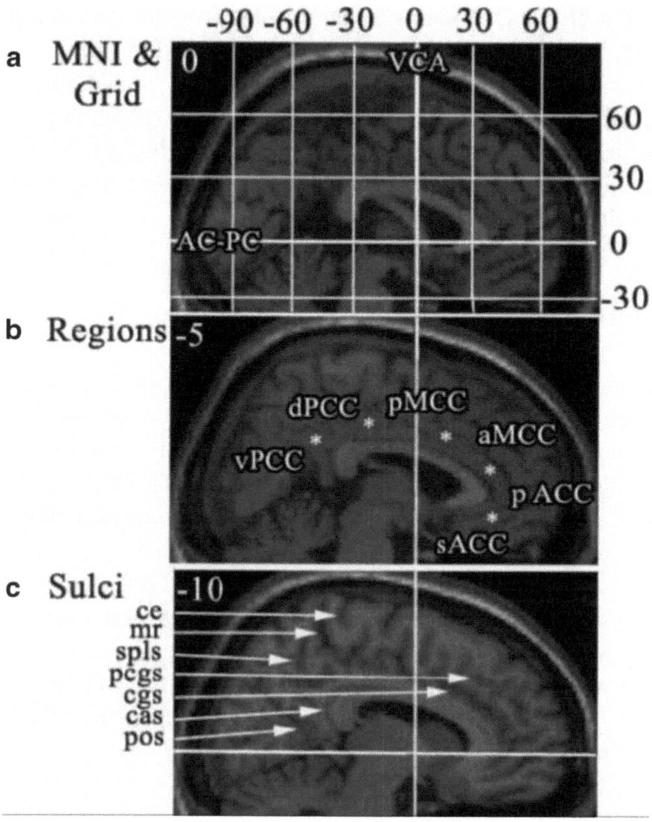

Fig. 18.13 Sagittal MRI section of human brain with yz (anterior-posterior/superior-inferior) grid of Montréal Neurological Institute (MNI) stereotaxic atlas brain overlaid (**a**) Abbreviations (see Fig. 18.3) for six of the cingulate cortical subregions in the Eight-Subregion Model (Vogt 2009) are shown in register (**b**) with *'s marking rostral-caudal subregion borders. In (**c**) *arrows* indicate numerous major cortical sulci for further orientation. This Figure greatly facillitates localization of neuroimaging findings with respect to the standard cingulate subregions when findings are reported in MNI or Talairach coordinates. (Prepared by B. Vogt. Used with permission)

pipe. In the above ADHD-OCD model, the onset and character of "psychiatric instability" is marked by the value of the ratio $\frac{\sqrt{LC}}{RC} \sim \frac{\sqrt{[EAAT2][GluR]}}{[GluR]/[EAAT3]}$. Again, we consider that GluRs are like capacitors that "store" Glu molecules, i.e., take them temporarily out of perisynaptic circulation. At any given time, some fraction of the supply of Glu molecules will be bound up for a time by the GluRs. Once released from these receptors, a Glu molecule may then get caught in the astrocyte-neuron Glu–Gln cycle (EAAT2) and spend some time there or may proceed more directly to be disposed of in the neuron (EAAT3). The dimensionless ratio $\frac{\sqrt{LC}}{RC} \sim \frac{\sqrt{[EAAT2][GluR]}}{[GluR]/[EAAT3]}$ essentially represents the dwell time of Glu cycling through the astrocyte divided by the dwell time of Glu passing through the neuron. A value of the ratio near 2 represents stability, the healthy state. Values dropping below 2 tend towards OCD; values exceeding 2 tend towards ADHD. Thus, one may envision ADHD and OCD as problems in neurochemical mass-transport stability: A transporter-rich synaptic environment and excessive dwell time in the Glu–Gln cycle for ADHD versus a receptor-rich synaptic environment and too short dwell time in the Glu–Gln cycle for OCD. (Such hypotheses might be tesTable with techniques like ^{13}C MRS). The perisynaptic Glu flux seems to correspond to or be a prerequisite of the degree or effort of attention that precedes the possible extraction of an associative memory out of conscious experience. It therefore connects these neurochemical parameters to ADHD and OCD mental symptomatology. The psychiatrist prescribes psychotropics and applies other therapies to fine tune these circuits to stabilize them.

Gaps in the Literature

This section lists several gaps in the ADHD MRS literature, i.e., topics that have been researched little if at all and that may be of interest in future investigations.

Genetic Studies Seeking MRS Biomarkers of ADHD

Given the strong evidence for a genetic contribution to ADHD, future studies will likely attempt to associate specific genetic markers with MRS metabolite endpoints and other neuroimaging variables. Such MRS studies will find it valuable to scan parents and/or affected and unaffected siblings of children with ADHD. This may help identify biomarkers of the disease, identify factors that determine why one sibling comes down with the disease and another does not, and perhaps predict conversion of as yet asymptomatic children. One may also attempt to study "high-risk" children, e.g., children of parents with ADHD or children raised in certain environments to predict onset of ADHD. The MR scanning of very young children is a considerable but nevertheless surmounTable challenge. Such work might lead to an orientation toward and some empirical basis for prophylaxis against ADHD. A lot of work of this type can be done even without assaying specific genetic markers. Although as metabolic models infer involvement of specific receptors, enzymes, and transporters in ADHD, e.g., in the central glutamatergic systems, one may target genes coding for these proteins and compare their variants to specific abnormalities in metabolite levels or reaction rates.

Longitudinal MRS Studies of ADHD

More longitudinal MRS studies of the course of development and treatment in ADHD are in order. Longitudinal studies might help us, among other issues, to determine why many ADHD patients get better over time, whereas many others do not and why hyperactive symptoms tend to recede with age much more than inattentive symptoms do. Few studies have looked at pharmacologically treated subjects after more than about 14 months. Such studies could be important to detect any subtle long-term sequelae (positive or negative) of commonly prescribed long-term treatment. Longitudinal studies will also optimally include healthy control cohorts to account for effects of normal aging and development. Also, relatively old (say over 40 years of age) subjects with ADHD represent a much understudied population.

Noncore Neurocognitive Deficits, Comorbidities, Responders Versus Nonresponders, Nonpharmacologic Therapies

Accompanying neurocognitive deficits apart from the core symptoms represent a significant source of functional impairment in many cases of ADHD. ADHD comorbidities in general, although clinically very common, are understudied, even though they complicate not only diagnosis but also treatment. These represent areas for further investigation with MRS. Although scientifically there is a preference to include only diagnostically pure cases, many studies have found this impractical as well as lacking in external validity. An alternative approach might be to enroll a wider range of patients and examine not diagnostic categories but individual symptoms and symptom domains. Although several studies examined the ADHD subtypes ADHD-HI, ADHD-I, and ADHC-C, few studies have subtyped their ADHD population in terms of responders and nonresponders to treatment, perhaps because treatment response has been very good in most of the studies reviewed. MRS characterization of responsive and refractory cases of ADHD, if feasible, could prove clinically useful and mechanistically insightful. If, as indicated, many cases of ADHD resolve wholly or partly after 3 years, one might acquire MRS from a patient, and matching control, cohort at time of diagnosis then 3 years later to search for predictors of symptomatic resolution. Specific studies of nonpharmacological, i.e., psychosocial treatments, seem to be absent from the ADHD MRS literature, although we can possibly assume that many of the patients in the drug treatment studies received some form of concurrent behavioral treatment. For several reasons, it would be important to isolate the effects of psychosocial treatment alone. One wants to know what drug alone is doing, but more importantly, there are patients and families who refuse pharmacologic treatment, there are noncompliant patients, etc. By demonstrating objective physiological effects of psychosocial treatments, if possible, MRS may help instill confidence in these therapies and uncover their brain mechanisms.

MR Technical Aspects

On the MR technical side, few of the studies reviewed combined MRS with other modalities, not even quantitative structural MRI. Methods are now available for multimodal imaging, i.e., combining MRS data with DTI, fMRI, EEG, etc., results from the same subjects. Such combined analyses will hopefully enrich the picture of regional dysfunction and neuropathology of the brain in ADHD. Other technical gaps include metabolite relaxation studies and long-TE studies to sample Lac, especially since Lac is a key compound in the theories of Todd and Botteron [116] and Russell [117]. Thus, opportunities for future MRS studies of ADHD are ample.

Methodological Recommendations

We turn finally to methodological recommendations for future MRS studies of ADHD. Most of these will be along traditional lines of advising stricter technique. Our advice is biased by our own finite and imperfect laboratory experience, our incomplete reception of the literature, and our opinions.

Subject Sampling

Sedation Usually Not Needed. Fears of Noncompliance Mostly Ungrounded

A positive observation from the above-reviewed studies is that most *were* able to scan reasonable numbers of ADHD children and adults without sedation. This is contrary to skeptical assumptions of poor compliance and excessive movement artifacts, but does largely correspond to our experience in scanning dozens of ADHD subjects in sessions up to 2 h in length. Thereby, allowing subjects to watch a DVD (selected from a library of popular children's films or one of the subject's own brought in) through video goggles during scanning has proved immensely helpful. Despite hyperactivity and inattentive symptoms, it appears feasible to scan most ADHD patients, even off medication. So fear of noncompliance with routine scanning procedures should not be a barrier to future MRS studies of ADHD. Of course, as in any study, it is essential to monitor for and correct or account for movement artifacts.

Medication Issues

Some of the above-reviewed studies have commendably managed to recruit sizable drug-naïve samples with ADHD. In our experience, it is quite challenging to recruit drug-naïve patients given widespread access to stimulants and other agents and the ethical impulses and other factors driving their use in treatment. We believe there are benefits to studying both treated and untreated populations. As both chronic and acute administration of stimulants can affect MRS neurometabolites (Table 18.4), it is wise when preparing reports to at least note drug use in study samples and perhaps to account for it statistically. A rigorous study of drug treatment that, to or knowledge, has not yet been performed, would be to scan an ADHD population three times: once at drug-naïve baseline, once after an initial challenge dose of drug, and a third time after a normal drug trial (i.e., several weeks). One could even add a fourth scan 24–48 h after interruption of chronic drug treatment. Then it might be possible to disentangle acute and chronic effects of drug treatment, as well as to evaluate the validity of the brief washout periods employed in a number of MRS studies that attempt to restore the untreated ADHD brain state. On a related topic, some studies used urine toxicology screens to exclude subjects (patients or controls) who had recently consumed substances of abuse. This is a commendable practice and might even be extended in treatment studies to verify presence of the therapeutic test agent in the blood where compliance could be a factor.

Subject Numbers

Generally, the numbers of patients and controls in MRS studies of ADHD have been rather low (often <20 subjects per group). Several studies despite low numbers still employed conventional inferential statistics that assume normal population distributions (e.g., Student's *T*-test). Also, presumably due to the much higher prevalence of ADHD in boys, sex was not matched in many of the studies, and also not always taken account of statistically. From our own experience, we well recognize the difficulty and expense of recruiting and testing large subject numbers. But given the heterogeneity of ADHD not only in terms of subject sex but also subtype, comorbidities, ongoing and lifetime treatment, and other factors, the field will in all likelihood require larger samples in order to draw valid and reliable conclusions about the neurochemistry of ADHD in its various manifestations. As structural MRI studies of ADHD have already been conducted with over 100 participants, the same is feasible for MRS. Where samples are small (e.g., <20 subjects per group), investigators should opt for the more conservative nonparametric statistics. ADHD and control samples should at least be balanced for sex and if not the imbalance should be accounted for by such means as analyses of male-only and female-only subgroups or use of covariates.

Nomenclature

We will comment at length on the picky topic of nomenclature. The reason is that proper, or at least consistent, nomenclature induces clear thinking and facillitates clear communication. It also helps to predefine the goals and limitations of studies from the outset, setting frameworks for interpretation and theorizing.

MR Spectroscopic Nomenclature

Regarding the labels for MRS metabolite resonances, we recommend against the common proton MRS practice of writing "NAA" to mean both *N*-acetyl-aspartate and *N*-acetyl-aspartyl-glutamate. Instead, we recommend writing "NAA+NAAG" explicitly, or using the abbreviations "tNAA" ("total NAA") or "NA" (for "*N*-acetyl compounds"). Some fitting programs such as LCModel output separate values for NAA, NAAG, and NAA+NAAG. Even for high-field (3–4 T) clinical proton MRS, in the absence of special pulse sequences, many spectroscopists would not consider the separate values for NAA and NAAG output by these programs to be reliable; they would only accept the combined NAA+NAAG value. In reading reports, when the author writes "NAA," it is not always clear whether he or she has read-off the separate (perhaps unreliable) NAA value or has read-off the (reliable) NAA+NAAG value and is calling it "NAA" due to the common abbreviative practice. This is clearly a possible source of error. We recommend only taking the NAA+NAAG value and always calling it NAA+NAAG, tNAA, or NA. "NAA" and "NAAG" may be used separately when one *has* used a special pulse sequence, e.g., MEGA-PRESS [231], to segregate them or when one is referring not to the resonance signal but to the chemical species per se, as when writing chemical equations. Similarly, we advise against the common practice of writing "Cr" to mean "Cr+PCr," unless one is referring to the chemical species or has separated the two, as in ^{31}P MRS which detects PCr alone.

On the matter of Glu and Gln, segregation of the two signals is also difficult with ^{1}H MRS, but is much more feasible than for NAA+NAAG or Cr+PCr. We find both "Glx" and "Glu+Gln" to be useful abbreviations for the combined resonance. One may also wish to add "+GABA" or indicate in the text of the report that GABA is included in the fit, but one should not write "Glu" when Glx is meant, as sometimes happens. We recommend against the occasionally seen usage of "Glu/Gln" for "Glx" or "Cr/PCr" for "Cr+PCr," since they look like ratios.

Neuroanatomic Nomenclature

Cingulate Gyrus As mentioned above, for neuroimaging studies sampling the cingulate gyrus, we recommend the Eight-Subregion Model of Vogt [229] with its subregion designations "sACC, pACC, aMCC, pMCC, dPCC, vPCC, dRSC, vRSC." O'Neill et al. [310] provide instructions for manual parcellation of structural MRI of the cingulate into these subregions (except for the small dRSC and vRSC subregions). A software application for this is in preparation. For those however, who do not wish to invest the time and effort into manual parcellation, the cingulate subregions generated by FreeSurfer2009 are a reasonable approximation to the Vogt subregions. (Fig. 18.13, prepared by B. Vogt, is extremely practical for identifying the cingulate subregions relative to MNI, or its parent Talairach, atlas coordinates.) We hope that use of these subregion designations will facilitate interpretation of MRS results in terms of the histological and functional organization of cingulate cortex.

Dorsolateral Prefrontal Cortex, Etc We do not recommend the very popular use of "dorsolateral prefrontal cortex," "ventrolateral prefrontal cortex," and "ventromedial prefrontal cortex," nor of "dorsomedial prefrontal cortex," which we have never seen. The anatomic definitions of these terms can become vague and diverse. With "dorsolateral prefrontal cortex," for example, we have seen papers that mean superior frontal cortex + middle frontal cortex, middle frontal cortex alone, and only the dorsal half of the middle frontal cortex. We do understand that use of these terms can embody a certain admirable humility with respect to neuroscience's limited knowledge of functional localization and a recognition of the wide intersubject variability in normal gross brain anatomy. Nonetheless, we instead recommend using gross anatomical gyral names (e.g., "middle frontal cortex, inferior frontal cortex…") where possible, perhaps after consulting a radiologist. We also advise against conflating cingulate and noncingulate cortices within umbrella designations such as "ventromedial prefrontal cortex" where possible. Where the two cannot clearly be distinguished or are clearly included in the same voxel, it is preferable to use designations such as "mesial superior frontal cortex + pACC." This is precise, makes the Reader aware of possible anatomical heterogeneity within the sampling, and does not presuppose a functional or structural unity that may or may not be present, even if one is attempting to infer such unity from the findings at hand. We have largely abided by these rules in reviewing the above MRS studies, but were somewhat lax when reviewing the studies in other imaging modalities, due to their lesser relevance and greater burden in disentangling sometimes complex findings.

Reporting Baseline Versus Longitudinal Effects

In comparing metabolite levels and other quantities in ADHD subjects to those in other groups, we recommend against the

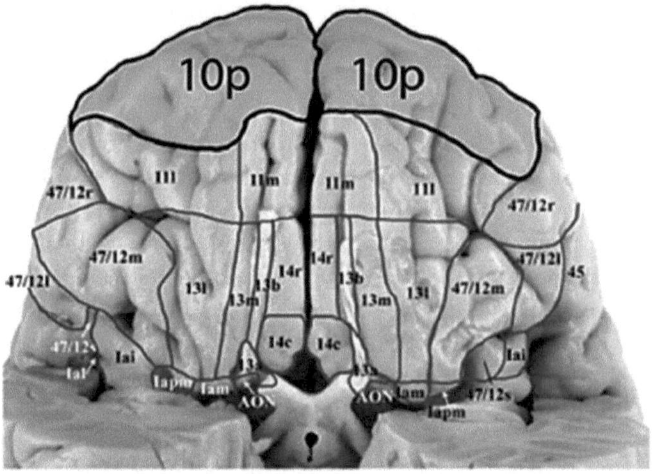

Fig. 18.14 Frontal view of rostral human cerebral cortex with borderlines and markers indicating various cytoarchitectonic areas. Note their profuse number bespeaking cellular, and possibly concomitant functional and metabolic, heterogeneity. This suggests a need for high spatial-resolution in MRS and other neuroimaging studies. (Modified from Dumontheil et al. [324])

common practice of using terms like "increase," "decrease," or "change" to refer to baseline values. Such terms, which carry an implication of time passage, should be reserved for longitudinal studies. When quoting baseline values it is usually not appropriate to write something like, "There was a decrease in tNAA in middle frontal cortex in the ADHD sample." In the absence of additional information, we do not know whether regional tNAA in the patient was once at normal levels, but then fell after the subject contracted ADHD or if tNAA levels never made it up to normal to begin with due to aberrant neurodevelopment. On the other hand, it *is* appropriate to write, "tNAA increased in the ADHD sample following treatment with methylphenidate" for here there is an explicitly identified before-and-after time element. Respecting this distinction particularly avoids confusion in studies that report both baseline and longitudinal effects, as in some of the above-reviewed studies.

Spatial Resolution

The human cerebral cortex, frequently interrogated in MRS studies of ADHD, is divided into a large number of cytoarchitectonic areas, each about the size of a thumbnail or postage stamp. (Figure 18.14 shows the example of the rostral frontal cortex.) The cortex is generally only 3–5 mm thick, though it often folds over on itself. If "forms follows function", each area probably does something different, may contain different concentrations of MRS metabolites, and may respond differently to disease.

Although certain systemic or organ-wide disorders may affect MRS metabolites equally throughout the brain or at least throughout all gray or white matter, a priori we cannot assume that this will always be the case. Therefore, high spatial resolution, perhaps with voxels of 1 cc or less may be necessary to detect metabolite effects on the level that the brain is actually organized. This would tend to recommend MRSI and of course higher field studies. MRSI voxel shifting employed in some of the above-reviewed studies may be an aid. As voxels get smaller and more numerous, it may eventually be fruitful to perfect and deploy an MRSI equivalent of the statistical parametric mapping analysis techniques popular in fMRI, PET, and structural MRI voxel-based morphometry.

Metabolite Quantitation

"Quantitation" is a synonym for "quantification" in MRS jargon. Though some regard it as an objectionable neologism, we identify at least one highly repuTable attestation [311].

Metabolite Ratios

It was very popular in the above-reviewed studies to report metabolite results as ratios to Cr+PCr. There are arguments in favor of this practice, but it remains inherently ambiguous. If regional tNAA/Cr+PCr is lower in ADHD than in control subjects, a priori one cannot know without additional information if this is due to lower tNAA, higher Cr+PCr, or some combination of both. In ADHD in particular, several of the studies reviewed (Tables 18.2, 18.3 and 18.4) found explicit effects of ADHD or of its treatment on Cr+PCr. Hence, exclusive reporting of ^{1}H MRS metabolite results as ratios to Cr+PCr in ADHD studies is under most circumstances inadvisable. An exception is when ratios to Cr+PCr or other ratio combinations exhibit an "amplifier effect." For example, if, simultaneously, tNAA is lower and Cr+PCr is higher in some brain region in ADHD patients, combining the two could yield a stronger signal that is more easily detected and more likely to yield statistically significant results than either of the separate absolute metabolite levels. When an author does opt to use metabolite ratios, we recommend that he or she continue to refer to the full ratio throughout the paper without dropping the denominator for brevity. For example, don't refer to effects on "NAA," "Glu," etc., when one really means effects on "tNAA/Cr+PCr," "Glx/Cr+PCr," etc.

Glutamate and Glutamine

It is desirable and nowadays feasible to go beyond Glx and to quantitate Glu and Gln separately. There is broad consensus among spectroscopists that this is best done at high field (≥3 T). Thereby, the variability (e.g., Cramer–Rao bounds) of the Gln signal is still often too high to be reliable, but the Glu signal usually is reliable. At 4 T, Théberge et al. [312–315] and other groups have repeatedly identified regional brain effects specific to Gln in psychiatric populations. These might also be investigated in ADHD. Some laboratories [316–318] have reported particular success in isolating Glu from Gln using PRESS sequences at TE=80 ms or TE-averaging methodologies [319–321]. Experience in our laboratory is consistent with good segregation of Glu at TE=80 ms. Recently, successful segregation of Glu and Gln has also been obtained using 2D J-coupled MRS [322], although acquisition volumes are typically large with 2D methods. Thus, at high field there are several options to investigate separate regional effects on Glu and Gln in ADHD MRS research. We optimistically expect to see detailed elaboration of effects of ADHD and stimulant treatment on absolute levels of regional Glu and Gln over the next few years.

Voxel Tissue Composition

Most of the studies reviewed did not account for possible between-group and/or between-condition differences in MRS voxel tissue composition. Metabolite ratios are often said to compensate for voxel CSF, but this is not true for voxel gray matter or white matter content. As gray matter and white matter differ substantially in their typical levels of various metabolites, there is a risk of confusing differences in tissue composition for genuine differences in metabolite levels within a particular tissue if one does not deal with tissue composition explicitly. Therefore, MRS studies of ADHD should take account of voxel tissue composition in some form. Ideally, one will measure volume percent gray matter, white matter, CSF, and nonbrain tissue in every voxel of every scan of every subject. Even better, gray matter and white matter can also be determined on a regional level, e.g., vol% "left pACC gray matter" in the voxel. Assuming near zero concentration of the usual metabolites of interest in CSF, one can and should adjust metabolite levels for CSF content. Otherwise, if one reports, for example, that "tNAA is 50% lower in ADHD patients than in controls," it is not clear if this is because the tissue in the ADHD contains half as much tNAA as in the control voxel or if the ADHD voxel happens to contain 50% CSF while the control voxel is 100% tissue.

A few of the above studies examining the cingulate cortex with 15-mm-thick acquisition volumes describe a technique of assuring that their selected MRS voxels contain pure gray matter. The technique is to flip through every MRI slice that intersects the MRS voxel. At our center, we routinely acquire from the cingulate using 9-mm-thick, 0.5-cc voxels and yet we rarely encounter 100% gray matter voxels, including in children, who typically have tightly packed cortex. Therefore, the above investigators may have meticulously selected angle and position of their acquisition volumes to maximize high gray matter content. While we do recommend careful placement and prescan MRI examination of MRS acquisition volumes, we do not recommend relying on this technique without also independently quantifying voxel tissue composition in offline processing.

fMRS. Acute Changes in Neurometabolite Levels

Recently, some investigators (e.g., Zhu and Chen [323]) have revived interest in "functional MRS" (fMRS), analogous to fMRI, i.e., examining very short-term and/or activation-related changes in metabolite levels. Such studies may undermine a, perhaps naïve, assumption behind a good deal of contemporary MRS work, namely that an individual's regional metabolite levels represent more or less static quantities, like the 7.4 pH of blood. That they change on a timescale of days, weeks, and months rather than hours, seconds, and ms. fMRS may reveal that this assumption is incorrect and needs to be tested more thoroughly. As much as it may add to difficulties with recruitment and the rigors of experimental procedure, in order to obtain usable results, it may ultimately be necessary to control for factors such as time of day of scanning, blood sugar level, whether the subject has recently drunk coffee or smoked a cigarette before the scan, etc. Such practices are not yet widespread in MRS research, although they are perfectly routine for certain clinical exams where fasting is required, etc.

Conclusions

ADHD is a prevalent psychiatric disorder in children and adults with high public health impact. Core symptoms include habitual inattention, hyperactivity, and impulsivity. ADHD frequently responds to stimulants and other drugs as well as to psychosocial treatments; core symptoms, especially hyperactivity, often resolve with or without treatment within three years or upon maturing into adulthood. Nonetheless, patients typically suffer multiple chronic functional and social difficulties and poor lifetime outcomes. ADHD has three subtypes and is commonly attended by, often multiple, psychiatric comorbidities which complicate diagnosis and treatment.

There is substantial, though by no means exclusive, evidence for (as yet incompletely characterized) genetic substrates of ADHD. Neurophysiological theories of ADHD have emphasized hypofunction of brain catecholamines, especially DA. More recently, linkages to central Glu disturbances and suboptimal brain energy metabolism have been proposed. Possible brain regions implicated in ADHD include the pACC and aMCC subregions of the cingulate gyrus, middle and inferior frontal cortices, and the caudate, globus pallidus, and other subcortical nuclei, as well as the cerebellum. Multiple neuroimaging modalities, including structural MRI, DTI, fMRI, SPECT, and PET have demonstrated effects of ADHD and its treatment in these regions.

MRS of the brain currently has no direct clinical applications to ADHD but has the potential to make contributions in the areas of diagnosis, prognosis, treatment response, and elucidation of biochemical pathways that may inform development of future pharmacotherapies. MRS studies to date have detected metabolite abnormalities and effects of drug treatment in many of the same brain regions as other neuroimaging modalities. Neurometabolites possibly implicated include mainly tNAA, Glx, Cr + PCr, and Cho. A meta-analysis [228] of MRS studies found effects on Cho most widely measured. Several MRS findings in ADHD are interpreTable as consistent with the astroglial-based brain-energy hypotheses of Todd and Botteron [116] and Russell et al. [117]. Weaknesses of some ADHD MRS studies to date include small subject numbers not always balanced for sex, partial-voluming in MRS acquisition voxels, failure to determine voxel tissue composition, and reporting of metabolite results as ratios to Cr + PCr, especially since some effects of disease or treatment on regional brain Cr + PCr have been documented.

We present an adaptation of Middleton's [296] cingulocentric subcortical loop model of OCD to ADHD, including a speculative effort to link the dynamics of subjective mental and behavioral symptomatology in ADHD to neurochemical processes at cortical glutamatergic synapses. We identify some gaps in the ADHD MRS literature to date and make some methodological recommendations for future work.

Acknowledgments This work was supported by NIMH RC1 MH088507 to Dr. Levitt and NIMH R01MH081864-01A1 to Dr. O'Neill and Dr. John C. Piacentini. Special thanks to Shaila Patel for assistance with figures.

References

1. Wolraich ML, Wibbelsman CJ, Brown TE, Evans SW, Gotlieb EM, Knight JR, Ross C, Shubiner HH, Wender EH, Wilens T. Attention-deficit/hyperactivity disorder among adolescents: a review of the diagnosis, treatment, and clinical implications. Pediatrics. 2005;115:1734–46.
2. Cormier E. Attention deficit/hyperactivity disorder: a review and update. J Pediatr Nurs. 2008;23(5):345–57.
3. Dopheide JA, Pliszka SR. Attention-deficit–hyperactivity disorder: an update. Pharmacotherapy. 2009;29(6):656–79.
4. Bukstein OG. Clinical practice guidelines for attention-deficit/hyperactivity disorder: a review. Postgrad Med. 2010;122(5):69–77.
5. Wilens TE, Spencer TJ. Understanding attention-deficit/hyperactivity disorder from childhood to adulthood. Postgrad Med. 2010;122(5):97–109.
6. Rohde LA, Biederman J, Busnello EA, Zimmermann H, Schmitz M, Martins S, Tramontina S. ADHD in a school sample of Brazilian adolescents: a study of prevalence, comorbid conditions, and impairments. JAACAP. 1999;38:716–22.
7. Polanczyk G, Horta B, Lima M, Biederman J, Rohde LA. The worldwide prevalence of attention-deficit hyperactivity disorder: a systematic review and meta-regression analysis. Am J Psychiatry. 2007;164:942–8.

8. Faraone SV, Mick E. Molecular genetics of attention deficit hyperactivity disorder. Psychiatr Clin N Am. 2010;33(1):159–80.
9. Singh I. Beyond polemics: science and ethics of ADHD. Nat Rev Neurosci. 2008;9(12):957–64.
10. Cantwell DP. Attention deficit disorder: a review of the past 10 years. JAACAP. 1996;35:978–87.
11. Dulcan M. Practice parameters for the assessment and treatment of children, adolescents, and adults with attention-deficit/hyperactivity disorder. JAACAP. 1997;36(10 Suppl):85S–121S.
12. Staller J, Faraone SV. Attention-deficit hyperactivity disorder in girls: epidemiology and management. CNS Drugs. 2006;20(2):107–23.
13. Polanczyk G, Rohde LA. Epidemiology of attention-deficit/hyperactivity disorder across the lifespan. Curr Opin Psychiatry. 2007;20:386–92.
14. Wasserstein J. Diagnostic issues for adolescents and adults with ADHD. J Clin Psychol. 2005;61(5):535–47.
15. Murphy K, Barkley RA. Norms for the DSM-IV symptoms list for ADHD in adults. ADHD Rep. 1995;3:6–7.
16. Center for Disease Control and Prevention. Increasing prevalence of parent-reported attention-deficit/hyperactivity disorder among children: United States, 2003 and 2007. MMWR Morb Mortal Wkly Rep. 2010;59(44):1439–43.
17. Pelham WE, Foster EM, Robb JA. The economic impact of attention-deficit/hyperactivity disorder in children and adolescents. Ambul Pediatr. 2007;7:121–31.
18. Biederman J. Attention-deficit/hyperactivity disorder: a life-span perspective. J Clin Psychiatry. 1998;59 Suppl 7:4–16.
19. National Institute of Mental Health (NIMH). Attention deficit hyperactivity disorder (ADHD). NIH Publication No. 08-3572. Bethesda, MD; National Institute of Health. 2008.
20. Seidman LJ. Neuropsychological functioning in people with ADHD across the lifespan. Clin Psychol Rev. 2006;26:466–85.
21. Newton-Howes G. What happens when children with attention deficit/hyperactivity disorder grow up? J R Soc Med. 2004;97:531–5.
22. Mannuzza S, Klein RG, Bessler A. Adult outcome of hyperactive boys. Arch Gen Psychiatry. 1993;50:565–76.
23. American Psychiatric Association. Practice parameters for the assessment and treatment of children, adolescent and adults with attention-deficit/hyperactivity disorder. JAACAP. 1997;36:085S–121S.
24. Jensen PS, Martin D, Cantwell DP. Comorbidity in ADHD: implications for research, practice and DSM-V. JAACAP. 1997;36:1065–79.
25. Barkley RA, Fischer M, Smallish L, Fletcher K. Young adult outcome of hyperactive children: adaptive functioning in major life activities. JAACAP. 2006;45:192–202.
26. Pliszka SR, Glahn DC, Semrud-Clikeman M, Franklin C, Perez III R, Xiong J, Liotti M. Neuroimaging of inhibitory control areas in children with attention deficit hyperactivity disorder who were treatment naive or in long-term treatment. Am J Psychiatry. 2006;163:1052–60.
27. Slomkowski C, Klien RG, Mannuzza S. Is self-esteem an important outcome in hyperactive children? J Abnorm Child Psychol. 1995;23:303–15.
28. Biederman J, Faraone SV, Spencer T, Wilens T, Norman D, Lapey KA, Mick E, Lehman BK, Doyle A. Patterns of psychiatric comorbidity, cognition and psychosocial functioning in adults with attention deficit hyperactivity disorder. Am J Psychiatry. 1993;150:1792–8.
29. Pliszka SR. Patterns of psychiatric comorbidity with attention-deficit/hyperactivity disorder. Child Adol Psychiatric Clinics North Am. 2000;9(3):525–40.
30. Philipsen A. Differential diagnosis and comorbidity of attention-deficit/hyperactivity disorder (ADHD) and borderline personality disorder (BPD) in adults. Eur Arch Psychiatry Clin Neurosci. 2006;256 Suppl 1:i42–46.
31. Brunsvold GL, Oepen G. Comorbid depression in ADHD: chidlren and adolescents. Psychiatric Times. 2008;25(10).
32. Bauermeister JJ, Shrout PE, Chávez L, Rubio-Stepec M, Ramírez R, Padilla L, García P, Camino G. ADHD and gender: are risks and sequela of ADHD the same for boys and girls? J Child Psychol Psychiatry. 2007;48(8):831–9.
33. Aldenkamp AP, Arzimanoglou A, Reijs R, Van Mil S. Optimizing therapy of seizures in children and adolescents with ADHD. Neurology. 2006;67(12 Suppl 4):S49–51.
34. Tan M, Appleton R. Attention deficit and hyperactivity disorder, methylphenidate, and epilepsy. Arch Dis Childhood. 2005;90(1):57–9.
35. Rietveld MJ, Hudziak JJ, Bartels M, van Beijsterveldt CE, Boomsma DI. Heritability of attention problems in children: longitudinal results from a study of twins, age 3 to 12. J Child Psychol Psychiatry. 2004;45(3):577–88.
36. Smidt J, Heiser P, Dempfle A, Konrad K, Hemminger U, Kathöfer A, Halbach A, Strub J, Grabarkiewicz J, Kiefl H, Linder M, Knölker U, Warnke A, Remschmidt H, Herpertz-Dahlmann B, Hebebrand J. Formalgenetische Befunde zur Aufmerksamkeitsdefizit-/Hyperaktivitätsstörung. Fortschr Neurol Psychiatr. 2003;71:366–77.
37. Freitag CM, Rohde LA, Lempp T, Romanos M. Phenotypic and measurement influences on heritability estimates in childhood ADHD. Eur Child Adolesc Psychiatry. 2010;19:311–23.
38. Swanson JM, Flodman P, Kennedy J, Spence MA, Moyzis R, Schuck S, Moriarity J, Barr C, Smith M, Posner M. Dopamine genes and ADHD. Neurosci Biobehav Rev. 2000;24(1):21–5.
39. Volkow ND, Wang GJ, Kollins SH, Wigal TL, Newcorn JH, Telang F, Fowler JS, Zhu W, Logan J, Ma Y, Pradhan K, Wong C, Swanson JM. Evaluating dopamine reward pathway in ADHD. JAMA. 2009;302(10):1084–91.
40. Acosta MT, Arcos-Burgos M, Muenke M. Attention deficit/hyperactivity disorder (ADHD): complex phenotype, simple genotype? Gen Med. 2004;6(1):1–15.
41. Roman T, Rohde LA, Hutz MH. Polymorphisms of the dopamine transporter gene: influence on response to methylphenidate in attention deficit-hyperactivity disorder. Am J Pharmacogenomics. 2004;4(2):83–92.
42. Galili-Weisstub E, Segman RH. Attention deficit and hyperactivity disorder: review of genetic association studies. Isr J Psychiatry Relat Sci. 2003;40(1):57–66.
43. Coghill D, Banaschewski T. The genetics of attention-deficit/hyperactivity disorder. Expert Rev Neurother. 2009;9(10):1547–65.
44. Banaschewski T, Becker K, Scherag S, Franke B, Coghill D. Molecular genetics of attention-deficit/hyperactivity disorder: an overview. Eur Child Adolesc Psychiatry. 2010;19:237–57.
45. Faraone SV, Sergeant J, Gillberg C, Biederman J. The worldwide prevalence of ADHD: is it an American condition? World Psychiatry. 2003;2(2):104–13.
46. Froehlich TF, McGough JJ, Stein MA. Progress and promise of attention-deficit hyperactivity disorder pharmacogenetics. CNS Drugs. 2010;24(2):99–117.
47. Sonuga-Barke EJ, Dalen L, Daley D, Remington B. Are planning, working memory, and inhibition associated with individual differences in preschool ADHD symptoms? Dev Neuropsychol. 2002;21(3):255–72.
48. Linner KM, Dalsgaard S, Obel C, Wisborg K, Henriksen TB, Rodriguez A, Kotimaa A, Thomsen PH, Olsen J, Jarvelin MR. Maternal lifestyle factors in pregnancy risk of attention deficit hyperactivity disorder and associated behaviors: review of the current evidence. Am J Psychiatry. 2003;160(6):1028–40.
49. Braun JM, Kahn RS, Froehlich T, Auinger P, Lanphear BP. Exposures to environmental toxicants and attention deficit hyperactivity disorder in U.S. children. Environ Health Perspect. 2006;114(12):1904–9.

50. Nigg JT. What causes ADHD? Understanding what goes wrong and why. NY: The Guilford Press; 2006.
51. Bouchard MF, Bellinger DC, Wright RO, Weisskopf MG. Attention-deficit/hyperactivity disorder and urinary metabolites of organophosphate pesticides. Pediatrics. 2010;125:e1270–7.
52. McCann D, Barrett A, Cooper A. Food additives and hyperactive behaviour in 3-year-old and 8/9-year-old children in the community: a randomized, double-blinded, placebo-controlled trial. Lancet. 2007;370(9598):1560–7.
53. Millichap JG. Etiologic classification of attention-deficit/hyperactivity disorder. Pediatrics. 2008;121(2):e358–65.
54. Millichap JG. Attention deficit hyperactivity disorder handbook: a Physician's guide to ADHD. New York, NY: Springer; 2010.
55. Weinstein D, Staffelbach D, Biaggio M. Attention-deficit hyperactivity disorder and posttraumatic stress disorder: differential diagnosis in childhood sexual abuse. Clin Psychol Rev. 2000;20(3):359–78.
56. Stevens SE, Sonuga-Barke EJS, Kreppner JM, Beckett C, Castle J, Colvert M, Groothues C, Hawkins A, Rutter M. Inattention/overactivity following early severe Institutional deprivation: presentation and associations in early adolescence. J Abnorm Child Psychol. 2008;36:385–98.
57. Smucker WD, Hedayat M. Evaluation and treatment of ADHD. Am Fam Phys. 2001;64(5):817–29.
58. Jensen PS, Arnold LE, Swanson JM. 3-year follow-up of the NIMH MTA study. JAACAP. 2007;46(8):989–1002.
59. Molina BS, Hinshaw SP, Swanson JM. The MTA at 8 years: prospective follow-up of children treated for combined-type ADHD in a multisite study. JAACAP. 2009;48(5):484–500.
60. Gentile J. Adult ADHD: diagnosis, differential diagnosis and medication management. Psychiatry. 2004;3(8):24–30.
61. Greenhill LL, Pliszka S, Dulcan MK, Bernet W, Arnold V, Beitman J, Benson RS, Bukstein O, Kinlan J, McClellan J, Rue D, Shaw JA, Stock S, AACAP. Practice parameters for the use of stimulant medications in the treatment of children, adolescents, and adults. JAACAP. 2002;41(2 suppl):26S–49S.
62. Scheffler RM, Hinshaw SP, Modrek S, Levine P. The global market for ADHD medications. Health Aff (Millwood). 2007;26(2):450–7.
63. Wilens T. Mechanism of action of agents used in ADHD. J Clin Psychiatry. 2006;67 suppl 8:32–7.
64. Parasrampuria DA, Schoedel KA, Schuller R, Silber SA, Ciccone PE, Gu J, Sellers EM. Do formulation differences alter abuse liability of methylphenidate? A placebo-controlled randomized, double-blind, crossover study in recreational drug users. J Clin Psychopharmacol. 2007;27(5):459–67.
65. Safer D, Allen R, Barr E. Depression of growth in hyperactive children on stimulant drugs. N Engl J Med. 1972;287(5):217–20.
66. MTA Cooperative Group. National Institute of Mental Health Multimodal Treatment Study of ADHD follow-up: changes in effectiveness and growth after the end of treatment. Pediatrics. 2004;113(4):762–9.
67. Wilens TE, Adler LA, Adamson J, Sgambati S, Rotrosen J, Sawtelle R, Utzinger L, Fusillo S. Misuse and diversion of stimulants prescribed for ADHD: a systematic review of the literature. JAACAP. 2008;47(1):21–31.
68. McCabe SE, Knight JR, Teter CJ, Wechsler H. Non-mdeical use of perscription stimulants among US college students: prevalence and correlates from a national survey. Addiction. 2005;99(1):96–106.
69. Biederman J, Swanson JM, Wigal SB, Boellner SW, Earl CQ, Lopez FA. A comparison of once-daily and divided doses of modafinil in children with attention-deficit/hyperactivity disorder: a randomized, double-blind, and placebo-controlled study. J Clin Psychiatry. 2006;67(5):727–35.
70. Greenhill LL, Biederman J, Boellner SW. A randomized, double-blind, placebo-controlled study of modafinil film-coated Tablets in children and adolescents with attention-deficit/hyperactivity disorder. JAACAP. 2006;45(5):503–11.
71. Biederman J, Pliszka SR. Modafinil improves symptoms of attention-deficit/hyperactivity disorder across subtypes in children and adolescents. J Pediatr. 2008;152(3):394–9.
72. Garnock-Jones KP, Keating GM. Spotlight on atomoxetine in attention-deficit hyperactivity disorder in children and adolescents. CNS Drugs. 2010;24(1):85–8.
73. Kratochvil CJ, Heiligenstein JH, Dittmann R, Spencer TJ, Biederman J, Wernicke J, Newcorn JH, Casat C, Milton D, Michelson D. Atomoxetine and methylphenidate treatment in children with ADHD: a prospective, randomized, open-label trial. JAACAP. 2002;41(7):776–84.
74. Wang Y, Zheng Y, Du Y, Song DH, Shin YJ, Cho SC, Ahn DH, Marquez-Caraveo ME, Gao H, Williams DW, Levine LR. Atomoxetine versus methylphenidate in paediatric outpatients with attention deficit hyperactivity disorder: a randomized, double-blind comparison trial. Aust NZ J Psychiatry. 2007;41(3):222–30.
75. Barton J. Atomoxetine: a new pharmacotherapeutic approach in the management of attention deficit/hyperactivity disorder. Arch Dis Child. 2005;90 Suppl 1:26–9.
76. Ledbetter M. Atomoxetine: a novel treatment for child and adult ADHD. Neuropsych Dis Treat. 2006;2(4):455–66.
77. Spencer TJ, Kratochvil CJ, Sangal RB, Saylor KE, Bailey CE, Dunn DW, Geller DA, Casat CD, Lipetz RS, Jain R, Newcorn JH, Ruff DD, Feldman PD, Furr AJ, Allen AJ. Effects of atomoxetine on growth in children with attention-deficit/hyperactivity disorder following up to five years of treatment. J Child Adolesc Psychopharmacol. 2007;17(5):689–700.
78. Newcorn JH, Kratochvil CJ, Allen AJ, Casat CD, Ruff DD, Moore RJ, Michelson D. Atomoxetine Comparative Study Group. Atomoxetine and osmotically released methylphenidate for the treatment of attention deficit hyperactivity disorder: acute comparison and differential response. Am J Psychiatry. 2008;165(6): 721–30.
79. Bangs ME, Tauscher-Wisniewski S, Polzer J, Zhang S, Acharya N, Desaiah D, Trzepacz PT, Allen AJ. Metaanalysis of suicide-related behavior events in patients treated with atomoxetine. JAACAP. 2008;47(2):209–18.
80. Connor DF, Fletcher KE, Swanson JM. A meta-analysis of clonidine for symptoms of attention-deficit hyperactivity disorder. JAACAP. 1999;38:1551–9.
81. Scahill L, Chappell PB, Kim YS, Schultz RT, Katsovich L, Shepherd E, Arnsten AF, Cohen DJ, Leckman JF. A placebo-controlled study of guanfacine in the treatment of children with tic disorders and attention deficit hyperactivity disorder. Am J Psychiatry. 2001;158:1067–74.
82. Conners CK, Casat CD, Gualtieri CT, Weller E, Reader M, Reiss A, Weller RA, Khayrallah M, Ascher J. Bupropion hydrochloride in attention deficit disorder with hyperactivity. JAACAP. 1996;35(10):1314–21.
83. Wilens TE, Spencer TJ, Biederman J, Girard K, Doyle R, Prince J, Polisner D, Solhkhah R, Comeau S, Monuteaux MC, Parekh A. A controlled clinical trial of bupropion for attention deficit hyperactivity disorder in adults. Am J Psychiatry. 2001;158(2):282–8.
84. Wilens TE, Haight BR, Horrigan JP, Hudziak JJ, Rosenthal NE, Connor DF, Hampton KD, Richard NE, Modell JG. Bupropion XL in adults with ADHD: a randomized, placebo-controlled study. Biol Psychiatry. 2005;57(7):793–801.
85. Spencer T, Biederman J, Wilens T. Pharmacotherapy of attention-deficit/hyperactivity disorder: a life span perspective. In: Dickstein L, Riba M, Oldham J, editors. Review of psychiatry, vol. 16. Washington, DC: American Psychiatric Press; 1998. p. 87–127.
86. Pelham W, Wheeler T, Chronis A. Empirically supported psychosocial treatments for attention-deficit/hyperactivity disorder. J Clin Child Psychol. 1998;27(2):190–205.

87. Chronis AM, Jones HA, Raggi VL. Evidence-based psychosocial treatments for attention deficit hyperactivity disorder. Clin Psychol Rev. 2006;26(4):486–502.
88. McDermott SP, Wilens TE. Cognitive therapy for adults with ADHD. Cognitive therapy for adults with ADHD. In: Brown T, editor. Subtypes of attention deficit disorders in children, adolescents, and adults. Washington, DC: American Psychiatric Press, Inc.; 2000. p. 569–606.
89. Safren SA, Otto M, Sprich S, Winett C, Wilens T, Biederman J. Cognitive-behavioral therapy for ADHD in medication-treated adults with continued symptoms. Behav Res Ther. 2005;43(7): 831–42.
90. Solanto MV, Marks DJ, Mitchell KJ, Kofman MD. Development of a new psychosocial treatment for adult ADHD. J Atten Disord. 2008;11(6):728–36.
91. Toplak ME, Connors L, Shuster J, Knezevic B, Parks S. Review of cognitive, cognitive-behavioral, and neural-based interventions for attention-deficit/hyperactivity disorder (ADHD). Clin Psychol Rev. 2008;28(5):801–23.
92. Smalley SL, Loo SK, Hale TS, Shrestha A, McGough J. Mindfulness and attention deficit hyperactivity disorder. J Clin Psychol. 2009;65(10):1087–98.
93. Zylowska L, Ackerman DL, Yang MH, Futrell JL, Horton NL, Hale TS, Pataki C, Smalley SL. Mindfulness meditation training in adults and adolescents with ADHD: a feasibility study. J Atten Disord. 2008;11:737–46.
94. Levy F. The dopamine theory of attention deficit hyperactivity disorder (ADHD). Aust N Z J Psychiatry. 1991;25:277–83.
95. Levy F. Dopamine vs noradrenaline: inverted-U effects and ADHD theories. Aust N Z J Psychiatry. 2009;43:101–8.
96. Biederman J, Faraone SV. Attention-deficit hyperactivity disorder. Lancet. 2005;366:237–48.
97. Kirley A, Hawi Z, Daly G, McCarron M, Mullins C, Millar N, Waldman I, Fitzgerald M, Gill M. Dopaminergic system senes in ADHD: toward a biological hypothesis. Neuropsychopharmacology. 2002;27:607–19.
98. Levy F. Pharmacological and therapeutic directions in ADHD: Specificity in the PFC. Behav Brain Funct. 2008;4:12.
99. Hale TS, Hariri AR, McCracken JT. Attention-deficit hyperactivity disorder: perspectives from neuroimaging. Ment Retard Dev Disabil Res Rev. 2000;6(3):214–9.
100. Barkley RA. ADHD and the nature of self control. New York: Guildford; 1997.
101. Oosterlaan J, Sergeant JA. Response inhibition and response re-engagement in attention-deficit/hyperactivity disorder, disruptive, anxious and normal children. Behav Brain Res. 1998;94:33–43.
102. Castellanos FX, Sonuga-Barke EJ, Milham MP, Tannock R. Characterizing cognition in ADHD: beyond executive dysfunction. Trends Cogn Sci. 2006;10:117–23.
103. Castellanos FX, Sonuga-Barke EJ, Scheres A, Di Martino A, Hyde C, Walters JR. Varieties of attention-deficit/hyperactivity disorder-related intra-individual variability. Biol Psychiatry. 2005;57:1416–23.
104. Solanto MV, Abikoff H, Sonuga-Barke E, Schacher R, Logan GD, Wigal T, Hechtman L, Hinshaw S, Turkel E. The ecological validity of delay aversion and response inhibition as measures of impulsivity in AD/HD: a supplement to the NIMH multimodal treatment study of AD/HD. J Abnorm Child Psychol. 2001;29:215–28.
105. Himelstein J, Newcorn JH, Halperin JM. The neurobiology of attention-deficit hyperactivity disorder. Front Biosci. 2000;5:D461–478.
106. Giedd JN, Blumenthal J, Molloy E, Casyellanos FX. Brain Imaging of attention deficit/hyperactivity disorder. Ann NYAS. 2001;931:33–49.
107. Stefanatos GA, Wasserstein J. Attention deficit/hyperactivity disorder as a right hemisphere syndrome: selective literature review and detailed neuropsychological case studies. Ann NYAS. 2001;931:172–95.
108. Pliszka SR, McCracken JT, Mass JW. Catecholamines in attention-deficit hyperactivity disorder: current perspectives. JAACAP. 1996;35:264–72.
109. Barkley RA, Grodzinsky G, DuPaul GJ. Frontal lobe functions in attention deficit disorder with and without hyperactivity: a review and research report. J Abnorm Child Psychol. 1992;20(2): 163–88.
110. Rubia K, Noorloos J, Smith A, Gunning B, Sergeant J. Motor timing deficits in community and clinical boys with hyperactive behavior: the effect of methylphenidate on motor timing. J Abnorm Child Psychol. 2003;31:301–13.
111. Toplak ME, Tannock R. Time perception: modality and duration effects in attention-deficit/hyperactivity disorder (ADHD). J Abnorm Child Psychol. 2005;33:639–54.
112. Weissman DH, Roberts KC, Visscher KM, Woldorff MG. The neural bases of momentary lapses of attention. Nat Neurosci. 2006;9:971–8.
113. Castellanos FX, Margulies DS, Kelly C, Uddin LQ, Ghaffari M, Kirsch A, Shaw D, Shehzad Z, Di Martino A, Biswal B, Sonuga-Barke EJ, Rotrosen J, Adler LA, Milham MP. Cingulate-precuneus interactions: a new locus of dysfunction in adult attention-deficit/hyperactivity disorder. Biol Psychiatry. 2008;63:332–7.
114. Russell VA. Dopamine hypofunction possibly results from a defect in glutamate-stimulated release of dopamine in the nucleus accumbens shell of a rat model for attention deficit hyperactivity disorder—the spontaneously hypertensive rat. Neurosci Biobehav Rev. 2003;27:671–82.
115. Rothman DL, Behar KL, Hyder F, Shulman RG. In vivo NMR studies of the glutamate neurotransmitter flux and neuroenergetics: implications for brain function. Annu Rev Physiol. 2003;65:401–27.
116. Todd RD, Botteron KN. Is attention-deficit/hyperactivity disorder an energy deficiency syndrome? Biol Psychiatry. 2001;50:151–8.
117. Russell VA, Oades RD, Tannock R, Killeen PR, Auerbach JG, Johansen EB, Sagvolden T. Response variability in attention-deficit/hyperactivity disorder: a neuronal and glial energetics hypothesis. Behav Brain Funct. 2006;2:30.
118. Magistretti PJ, Sorg O, Yu N, Martin J-L, Pellerin L. Neurotransmitters regulate energy metabolism in astrocytes: implications for the metabolic trafficking between neural cells. Dev Neurosci. 1993;15:306–12.
119. Magistretti PJ, Pellerin L, Rothman DL, Shulman RG. Energy on demand. Science. 1999;283:496–7.
120. Magistretti PJ, Pellerin L. Cellular mechanisms of brain energy metabolism and their relevance to functional brain imaging. Philos Trans R Soc Lond B Biol Sci. 1999;354:1155–63.
121. Pellerin L, Pellegri G, Bittar PG, Charnay Y, Bouras C, Martin J-L, Stella N, Magistretti PJ. Evidence supporting the existence of an activity-dependent astrocyte-neuron lactate shuttle. Dev Neurosci. 1998;20:291–9.
122. Bartzokis G. Acetylcholinesterase inhibitors may improve myelin integrity. Biol Psychiatry. 2006;62(4):294–301.
123. Husarova V, Ondrejka I, Tonhajzerova I. Potential pathomechanisms of ADHD based on neurometabolite changes. Neuro Endocrinol Lett. 2010;31(4):438–45.
124. Hertz L, Swanson RA, Newman GC, Marrif H, Juurlink BH, Peng L. Can experimental conditions explain the discrepancy over glutamate stimulation of aerobic glycolysis? Dev Neurosci. 1998;20(4–5):339–47.
125. Peng L, Swanson RA, Hertz L. Effects of L-glutamate, D-aspartate, and monensin on glycolytic and oxidative glucose metabolism in mouse astrocyte cultures: further evidence that glutamate uptake

is metabolically driven by oxidative metabolism. Neurochem Int. 2001;38(5):437–43.

126. Cherkasova MV, Hechtman L. Neuroimaging in attention-deficit hyperactivity disorder: beyond the frontostriatal circuitry. Can J Psychiatry. 2009;54(10):651–64.
127. Konrad K, Eickhoff SB. Is the ADHD brain wired differently? A review on structural and functional connectivity in attention deficit hyperactivity disorder. Hum Brain Mapp. 2010;31:904–16.
128. Seidman LJ, Valera EM, Makris N. Structural brain imaging of attention-deficit/hyperactivity disorder. Biol Psychiatry. 2005;57:1263–72.
129. Castellanos FX, Giedd JN, Marsh WL, Hamburger SD, Vaituzis AC, Dickstein DP, Sarfatti SE, Vauss YC, Snell JW, Lange N, Krain AL, Ritchie GF, Rajapakse JC, Rapoport N. Quantitative brain magnetic resonance imaging in attention-deficit hyperactivity disorder. Arch Gen Psychiatry. 1996;53:607–16.
130. Weinberger DR, Luchins DJ, Morihisa J, Wyatt RJ. Asymmetrical volumes of the right and left frontal and occipital regions of the human brain. Ann Neurol. 1982;11:97–100.
131. Reiss AL, Abrams MT, Singer HS, Ross JL, Denckla MB. Brain development, gender and IQ in children. A volumetric imaging study. Brain. 1996;119:1763–74.
132. Filipek PA, et al. Volumetric MRI analysis comparing subjects having attention-deficit hyperactivity disorder with normal controls. Neurology. 1997;48:589–601.
133. Hynd GW, Semrud-Clikeman M, Lorys AR, Novey ES, Eliopulos D. Brain morphology in developmental dyslexia and attention deficit disorder/hyperactivity. Arch Neurol. 1990;47:919–26.
134. Castellanos FX, Giedd JN, Berquin PC, Walter JM, Sharp W, Tran T, Vaituzis AC, Blumental JD, Bastain TM, Zijdenbos A, Evans AC, Rapoport JL. Quantitative brain magnetic resonance imaging in girls with attention-deficit/hyperactivity disorder. Arch Gen Psychiatry. 2001;58:289–95.
135. Castellanos FX, Lee PP, Sharp W, Jeffries NO, Greenstein DK, Clasen LS, Blmental JD, James RS, Ebens CL, Walter JM, Zijdenbos A, Evans AC, Giedd JN, Rapoport JL. Developmental trajectories of brain volume abnormalities in children and adolescents with attention-deficit/hyperactivity disorder. JAMA. 2002;288:1740–8.
136. Overmeyer S, Bullmore ET, Suckling J, Simmons A, Williams SC, Santosh PJ, Taylor E. Distributed grey and white matter deficits in hyperkinetic disorder: MRI evidence for anatomical abnormality in an attentional network. Psychol Med. 2001;31:1425–35.
137. Kates WR, Frederikse M, Mostofsky SH, Folley BS, Mazur-Hopkins P, Kofman O, Singer HS, Denckla MB, Pearlson GD, Kaufmann WE. MRI parcellation of the frontal lobe in boys with attention deficit hyperactivity disorder or tourette syndrome. Psychiatry Res: Neuroimaging. 2002;116:63–81.
138. Mostofsky SH, Cooper KL, Kates WR, Denckla MB, Kaufmann WE. Smaller prefrontal and premotor volumes in boys with attention-deficit/hyperactivity disorder. Biol Psychiatry. 2002;52:785–94.
139. Hill DE, Yeo RA, Campbell RA, Hart B, Vigil J, Brooks W. Magnetic resonance imaging correlates of attention-deficit/hyperactivity disorder in children. Neuropsychology. 2003;17:496–506.
140. Sowell ER, Thompson PM, Welcome SE, Henkenius AL, Toga AW, Peterson BS. Cortical abnormalities in children and adolescents with attention deficit hyperactivity disorder (ADHD). Lancet. 2003;362:1699–707.
141. Durston S, Hulshoff Pol HE, Schnack HG, Buitelaar JK, Steenhuis MP, Minderaa RB, Kahn RS, van Engeland H. Magnetic resonance imaging of boys with attention-deficit/hyperactivity disorder and their unaffected siblings. JAACAP. 2004;43:332–40.
142. Shaw P, Lerch J, Greenstein D, Sharp W, Clasen L, Evans A, Giedd JN, Castellanos FX, Rapoport JL. Longitudinal mapping of cortical thickness and clinical outcome in children and adolescents with attention-deficit/hyperactivity disorder. Arch Gen Psychiatry. 2006;63:540–9.
143. McAlonan GM, Cheung V, Cheung C, Chua SE, Murphy DG, Suckling J, Tai KS, Yip KS, Leung P, Ho TP. Mapping brain structure in attention deficit-hyperactivity disorder: a voxel-based MRI study of regional grey and white matter volume. Psychiatry Res. 2007;154:171–80.
144. Wang J, Jiang T, Cao Q, Wang Y. Characterizing anatomic differences in boys with attention-deficit/hyperactivity disorder with the use of deformation-based morphometry. AJNR Am J Neuroradiol. 2007;28:543–7.
145. Makris N, Biederman J, Valera EM, Bush G, Kaiser J, Kennedy DN, Caviness VS, Faraone SV, Seidman LJ. Cortical thinning of the attention and executive function networks in adults with attention-deficit/hyperactivity disorder. Cereb Cortex. 2007;17:1364–75.
146. Carmona S, Vilarroya O, Bielsa A, Trèmois V, Soliva JC, Rovira M, Tomas J, Raheb C, Battle S, Bulbena A. Global and regional gray matter reductions in ADHD: a voxel-based morphometric study. Neurosci Lett. 2005;389:88–93.
147. Shaw P, Gornick M, Lerch J, Addington A, Seal J, Greenstein D, Sharp W, Evans A, Giedd JN, Castellanos FX, Rapoport JL. Polymorphisms of the dopamine D4 receptor, clinical outcome, and cortical structure in attention-deficit/hyperactivity disorder. Arch Gen Psychiatry. 2007;64:921–31.
148. Brieber S, Neufang S, Bruning N, Kamp-Becker I, Remschmidt H, Herpertz-Dahlmann B, Fink GR, Konrad K. Structural brain abnormalities in adolescents with autism spectrum disorder and patients with attention deficit/hyperactivity disorder. J Child Psychol Psychiatry Allied Disc. 2007;48:1251–8.
149. Hynd GW, Hern KL, Novey ES, Eliopulos D, Marshall R, Gonzalez JJ, Voeller KK. Attention deficit hyperactivity disorder and asymmetry of the caudate nucleus. J Child Neurol. 1993;8:339–47.
150. Castellanos FX, Giedd JN, Eckburg P, Marsh WL, Vaituzis AC, Kaysend D, Hamburger SD, Rapoport JL. Quantitative morphology of the caudate nucleus in attention deficit hyperactivity disorder. Am J Psychiatry. 1994;151:1791–6.
151. Castellanos FX, Sharp WS, Gottesman RF, Greenstein DK, Giedd JN, Rapoport JL. Anatomic brain abnormalities in monozygotic twins discordant for attention deficit hyperactivity disorder. Am J Psychiatry. 2003;160:1693–6.
152. Semrud-Clikeman M, Filipek PA, Biederman J, Steingard R, Kennedy D, Renshaw P, Bekken K. Attention-deficit hyperactivity disorder: magnetic resonance imaging morphometric analysis of the corpus callosum. JAACAP. 1994;33:875–81.
153. Aylward EH, Reiss AL, Reader MJ, Singer HS, Brown JE, Denckla MB. Basal ganglia volumes in children with attention-deficit hyperactivity disorder. J Child Neurol. 1996;11:112–5.
154. Mataro M, Garcia-Sanchez C, Junqué C, Estévez-González A, Pujol J. Magnetic resonance imaging measurement of the caudate nucleus in adolescents with attention-deficit hyperactivity disorder and its relationship with neuropsychological and behavioral measures. Arch Neurol. 1997;54:963–8.
155. Ellison-Wright I, Ellison-Wright Z, Bullmore E. Structural brain change in attention deficit hyperactivity disorder identified by meta-analysis. BMC Psychiatry. 2008;8:51.
156. Berquin PC, Giedd JN, Jacobsen LK, Hamburger SD, Krain AL, Rapoport JL, Castellanos FX. Cerebellum in attention-deficit hyperactivity disorder: a morphometric MRI study. Neurology. 1998;50:1087–93.
157. Mostofsky SH, Reiss AL, Lockhart P, Denckla MB. Evaluation of cerebellar size in attention-deficit hyperactivity disorder. J Child Neurol. 1998;13:434–9.
158. Bussing R, Grudnik J, Mason D, Wasiak M, Leonard C. ADHD and conduct disorder: an MRI study in a community sample. World J Biol Psychiatry. 2002;3:216–20.

159. Mackie S, Shaw P, Lenroot R, Pierson R, Greenstein DK, Nugent III TF, Sharp WS, Giedd JN, Rapoport JL. Cerebellar development and clinical outcome in attention deficit hyperactivity disorder. Am J Psychiatry. 2007;164:647–55.
160. Giedd JN, Castellanos FX, Casey BJ, Kozuch P, King AC, Hamburger SD, Rapoport JL. Quantitative morphology of the corpus callosum in attention deficit hyperactivity disorder. Am J Psychiatry. 1994;151:665–9.
161. Ashtari M, Kumra S, Bhaskar SL, Clarke T, Thaden E, Cervellone KL, Rhinewine J, Kane JM, Adesman A, Milanaik R, Maytal J, Diamond A, Szeszko P, Ardekani BA. Attention-deficit/hyperactivity disorder: a preliminary diffusion tensor imaging study. Biol Psychiatry. 2005;57:448–55.
162. Casey BJ, Epstein JN, Buhle J, Liston C, Davidson MC, Tonev ST, Spicer J, Niogi S, Millner AJ, Reiss A, Garrett A, Hinshaw SP, Greenhill LL, Shafritz KM, Vitolo A, Kotler LA, Jarrett MA, Glover G. Frontostriatal connectivity and its role in cognitive control in parent-child dyads with ADHD. Am J Psychiatry. 2007;164:1729–36.
163. Hamilton LS, Levitt JG, O'Neill J, Alger JR, Luders E, Phillips OR, Caplan R, Toga AW, McCracken JT, Narr KL. Reduced white matter integrity in attention-deficit hyperactivity disorder. Neuroreport. 2008;19(17):1705–8.
164. Pavuluri MN, Yang S, Kamineni K, Passarotti AM, Srinivasan G, Harral EM, Sweeney JA, Zhou XJ. Diffusion tensor imaging study of white matter fiber tracts in pediatric bipolar disorder and attention-deficit/hyperactivity disorder. Biol Psychiatry. 2009;65: 586–93.
165. Silk TJ, Vance A, Rinehart N, Bradshaw JL, Cunnington R. White-matter abnormalities in attention deficit hyperactivity disorder: a diffusion tensor imaging study. Hum Brain Mapp. 2009;30:2757–65.
166. Rubia K, Overmeyer S, Taylor E, Brammer M, Williams SC, Simmons A, Bullmore ET. Hypofrontality in attention deficit hyperactivity disorder during higher-order motor control: a study with functional MRI. Am J Psychiatry. 1999;156:891–6.
167. Rubia K, Smith AB, Brammer MJ, Toone B, Taylor E. Abnormal brain activation during inhibition and error detection in medication-naive adolescents with ADHD. Am J Psychiatry. 2005;162:1067–75.
168. Rubia K, Halari R, Smith AB, Mohammed M, Scott S, Giampietro V, Taylor E, Brammer MJ. Dissociated functional brain abnormalities of inhibition in boys with pure conduct disorder and in boys with pure attention deficit hyperactivity disorder. Am J Psychiatry. 2008;165:889–97.
169. Suskauer SJ, Simmonds DJ, Fotedar S, Blankner JG, Pekar JJ, Denckla MB, Mostofsky SH. Functional magnetic resonance imaging evidence for abnormalities in response selection in attention deficit hyperactivity disorder: differences in activation associated with response inhibition but not habitual motor response. J Cogn Neurosci. 2008;20:478–93.
170. Epstein JN, Casey BJ, Tonev ST, Davidson MC, Reiss AL, Garrett A, Hinshaw SP, Greenhill LL, Glover G, Shafritz KM, Vitolo A, Koller LA, Jarrett MA, Spicer J. ADHD- and medication-related brain activation effects in concordantly affected parent-child dyads with ADHD. J Child Psychol Psychiatry. 2007;48:899–913.
171. Durston S, Mulder M, Casey BJ, Ziermans T, van Engeland H. Activation in ventral prefrontal cortex is sensitive to genetic vulnerability for attention-deficit hyperactivity disorder. Biol Psychiatry. 2006;60:1062–70.
172. Durston S, Davidson MC, Mulder MJ, Spicer JA, Galvan A, Tottenham N, Scheres A, Castellanos XF, van Engeland H, Casey BJ. Neural and behavioral correlates of expectancy violations in attention-deficit hyperactivity disorder. J Child Psychol Psychiatry. 2007;48:881–9.
173. Smith AB, Taylor E, Brammer M, Toone B, Rubia K. Task-specific hypoactivation in prefrontal and temporoparietal brain regions during motor inhibition and task switching in medication-naive children and adolescents with attention deficit hyperactivity disorder. Am J Psychiatry. 2006;163:1044–51.
174. Booth JR, Burman DD, Meyer JR, Lei Z, Trommer BL, Davenport ND, Li W, Parrish TB, Gitelman DR, Mesulam MM. Larger deficits in brain networks for response inhibition than for visual selective attention in attention deficit hyperactivity disorder (ADHD). J Child Psychol Psychiatry. 2005;46:94–111.
175. Zang Y-F, Jin Z, Weng X-C, Zhang L, Zeng YW, Yang L, Wang YF, Seidman LJ, Faraone SV. Functional MRI in attention-deficit hyperactivity disorder: evidence for hypofrontality. Brain Dev. 2005;27:544–50.
176. Bush G, Frazier JA, Rauch SL, Seidman LJ, Whalen PJ, Jenike MA, Rosen BR, Biederman J. Anterior cingulate cortex dysfunction in attention-deficit/hyperactivity disorder revealed by fMRI and the Counting Stroop. Biol Psychiatry. 1999;45:1542–52.
177. Tamm L, Menon V, Ringel J, Reiss AL. Event-related fMRI evidence of frontotemporal involvement in aberrant response inhibition and task-switching in attention-deficit/hyperactivity disorder. JAACAP. 2004;43:1430–40.
178. Mulder MJ, Baeyens D, Davidson MC, Casey BJ, van den Ban E, van Engeland H, Durston S. Familial vulnerability to ADHD affects activity in the cerebellum in addition to the prefrontal systems. JAACAP. 2008;47:68–75.
179. O'Gorman RL, Mehta MA, Asherson P, Zelaya FO, Brookes KJ, Toone BK, Alsop DC, Williams SC. Increased cerebral perfusion in adult attention deficit hyperactivity disorder is normalised by stimulant treatment: a non-invasive MRI pilot study. Neuroimage. 2008;42:36–41.
180. Vaidya CJ, Bunge SA, Dudukovic NM, Zalecki CA, Ellioit GR, Gabrielli JD. Altered neural substrates of cognitive control in childhood ADHD: evidence from functional magnetic resonance imaging. Am J Psychiatry. 2005;162:1605–13.
181. Tamm L, Menon V, Reiss AL. Parietal attentional system aberrations during target detection in adolescents with attention deficit hyperactivity disorder: event-related fMRI evidence. Am J Psychiatry. 2006;163:1033–43.
182. Rubia K, Smith AB, Taylor E, Brammer MJ. Linear age-correlated functional development of right inferior fronto-striato-cerebellar networks during response inhibition and anterior cingulate during error-related processes. Hum Brain Mapp. 2007;28:1163–77.
183. Stevens MC, Pearlson GD, Kiehl KA. An fMRI auditory oddball study of combined-subtype attention deficit hyperactivity disorder. Am J Psychiatry. 2007;164:1737–49.
184. Cao Q, Zang Y, Zhu C, Cao X, Sun L, Zhou X, Wang Y. Alerting deficits in children with attention deficit/hyperactivity disorder: event-related fMRI evidence. Brain Res. 2008;1219:159–68.
185. Silk T, Vance A, Rinehart N, Egan G, O'Boyle M, Bradshaw JL, Cunnington R. Fronto-parietal activation in attention-deficit hyperactivity disorder, combined type: functional magnetic resonance imaging study. Br J Psychiatry. 2005;187:282–3.
186. Vance A, Silk TJ, Casey M, Rinehart NJ, Bradshaw JL, Bellgrove MA, Cunnington R. Right parietal dysfunction in children with attention deficit hyperactivity disorder, combined type: a functional MRI study. Mol Psychiatry. 2007;12:826–32.
187. Hale TS, Bookheimer S, McGough JJ, Phillips JM, McCracken JT. Atypical brain activation during simple and complex levels of processing in adult ADHD: an fMRI study. J Atten Disord. 2007;11:125–40.
188. Mostofsky SH, Rimrodt SL, Schafer JGB, Goldberg MC, Pekar JJ, Denckla MB. Atypical motor and sensory cortex activation in attention-deficit/hyperactivity disorder: a functional magnetic resonance imaging study of simple sequential finger tapping. Biol Psychiatry. 2006;59:48–56.
189. Vaidya CJ, Austin G, Kirkorian G, Ridlehuber HW, Desmond JE, Glover GH, Gabrielli JD. Selective effects of methylphenidate in

attention deficit hyperactivity disorder: a functional magnetic resonance study. Proc Natl Acad Sci USA. 1998;95:14494–9.

190. Durston S, Tottenham NT, Thomas KM, Thomas KM, Davidson MC, Eigsti M, Yang Y, Ulug AM, Casey BJ. Differential patterns of striatal activation in young children with and without ADHD. Biol Psychiatry. 2003;53:871–8.
191. Teicher MH, Anderson CM, Polcari A, Glod CA, Maas LC, Renshaw PF. Functional deficits in basal ganglia of children with attention-deficit/hyperactivity disorder shown with functional magnetic resonance imaging relaxometry. Nat Med. 2000;6:470–3.
192. Valera EM, Faraone SV, Biederman J, Poldrack RA, Seidman LJ. Functional neuroanatomy of working memory in adults with attention-deficit/hyperactivity disorder. Biol Psychiatry. 2005;57:439.
193. Anderson CM, Polcari A, Lowen SB, Renshaw PF, Teicher MH. Effects of methylphenidate on functional magnetic resonance relaxometry of the cerebellar vermis in boys with ADHD. Am J Psychiatry. 2002;159:1322–8.
194. Konrad K, Neufang S, Hanisch C, Fink GR, Herpetz-Dahlmann B. Dysfunctional attentional networks in children with attention deficit/hyperactivity disorder: evidence from an event-related functional magnetic resonance imaging study. Biol Psychiatry. 2006;59:643–51.
195. Sheridan MA, Hinshaw S, D'Esposito M. Efficiency of the prefrontal cortex during working memory in attention-deficit/hyperactivity disorder. JAACAP. 2007;46:1357–66.
196. Krauel K, Duzel E, Hinrichs H, Santel S, Rellum T, Baving L. Impact of emotional salience on episodic memory in attention-deficit/hyperactivity disorder: a functional magnetic resonance imaging study. Biol Psychiatry. 2007;61:1370–9.
197. Shafritz KM, Marchione KE, Gore JC, Shaywitz SE, Shaywitz BA. The effects of methylphenidate on neural systems of attention in attention deficit hyperactivity disorder. Am J Psychiatry. 2004;161(11):1990–7.
198. Scheres A, Milham MP, Knutson B, Castellanos FX. Ventral striatal hyporesponsiveness during reward anticipation in attention-deficit/hyperactivity disorder. Biol Psychiatry. 2007; 61:720–4.
199. Ströhle A, Stoy M, Wrase J, Schwarzer S, Schlagenhauf F, Huss M, Hein J, Nedderhut A, Neumann B, Gregor A, Juckel G, Knutson B, Lehmkuhl U, Bauer M, Heinz A. Reward anticipation and outcomes in adult males with attention-deficit/hyperactivity disorder. Neuroimage. 2008;39:966–72.
200. Dickstein SG, Bannon K, Castellanos FX, Milham MP. The neural correlates of attention deficit hyperactivity disorder: an ALE meta-analysis. J Child Psychol Psychiatry. 2006;47(10):1051–62.
201. Bush G, Spencer TJ, Holmes J, Shin LM, Valera EM, Seidman LJ, Makris N, Surman C, Aleardi M, Mick E, Biderman J. Functional magnetic resonance imaging of methylphenidate and placebo in attention-deficit/hyperactivity disorder during the multi-source interference task. Arch Gen Psychiatry. 2008;65:102–14.
202. Lou HC, Henriksen L, Bruhn P. Focal cerebral hypoperfusion in children with dysphasia and/or attention deficit disorder. Arch Neurol. 1984;41:825–9.
203. Lou HC, Henriksen L, Bruhn P. Focal cerebral dysfunction in developmental learning disabilities. Lancet. 1990;335:8–11.
204. Sieg KG, Gaffney GR, Preston DF, Hellings JA. SPECT brain imaging abnormalities in attention deficit hyperactivity disorder. Clin Nucl Med. 1995;20:55–60.
205. Amen DG, Paldi JH. Evaluating ADHD with brain SPECT imaging. Biol Psychiatry. 1993;33:44.
206. Amen DG, Carmichael BD. High-resolution brain SPECT imaging in ADHD. Ann Clin Psychiatry. 1997;9:81–6.
207. Langleben DD, Austin G, Krikorian G, Ridlehuber HW, Goris ML, Strauss HW. Interhemispheric asymmetry of regional cerebral blood flow in prepubescent boys with attention deficit hyperactivity disorder. Nucl Med Commun. 2001;22:1333–40.
208. Kim B-N, Lee J-S, Cho SC, Lee DS. Methylphenidate increased regional cerebral blood flow in subjects with attention deficit/hyperactivity disorder. Yonsei Med J. 2001;42(1):19–29.
209. Kim B-N, Lee J-S, Shin M-S, Cho SC, Lee DS. Regional cerebral perfusion abnormalities in attention deficit/hyperactivity disorder. Eur Arch Psychiatry Clin Neurosci. 2002;252:219–25.
210. Lee JS, Kim BN, Kang E, Lee DS, Kim YK, Chung JK, Lee MC, Cho SC. Regional cerebral blood flow in children with attention deficit hyperactivity disorder: comparison before and after methyphenidate treatment. Hum Brain Mapp. 2005;24:157–257.
211. Gustafsson P, Thernlund G, Ryding E, Rosen I, Cederblad M. Associations between cerebral blood flow measured by single photon emission computed tomography (SPECT), electro-encephalogram (EEG), behaviour symptoms, cognition and neurological soft signs in children with attention-deficit hyperactivity disorder. Acta Paediatr. 2000;89:830–5.
212. Lou HC, Henriksen L, Bruhn P, BÐmer H, Nielsen JB. Striatal dysfunction in attention deficit and hyperkinetic disorder. Arch Neurol. 1989;46:48–52.
213. Dougherty DD, et al. Dopamine transporter density in patients with attention deficit hyperactivity disorder. Lancet. 1999;354:2132–3.
214. Zametkin AJ, Nordahl TE, Gross M, King AC, Semple WE, Rumsey J, Hamburger S, Cohen RM. Cerebral glucose metabolism in adults with hyperactivity of childhood onset. N Engl J Med. 1990;323:1361–6.
215. Zametkin A, Liebenauer L, Fitzgerald G, King AC, Minkunas DV, Herscovitch P, Yamada EM, Cohen RM. Brain metabolism in teenagers with attention deficit hyperactivity disorder. Arch Gen Psychiatry. 1993;50:333–40.
216. Ernst M, Liebenaur LL, King C, Fitzgerald GA, Cohen RM, Zametkin AJ. Reduced brain metabolism in hyperactive girls. J Am Acad Child Adolesc Psychiatry. 1994;33:858–68.
217. Ernst M, Cohen RM, Liebenauer LL, Jons PH, Zamentkin AJ. Cerebral glucose metabolism in adolescent girls with attention-deficit/hyperactivity disorder. JAACAP. 1997;36:1399–406.
218. Schweitzer JB, Faber TL, Grafton ST, Tune LE, Hoffman JM, Kilts CD. Alterations in the functional anatomy of working memory in adult attention deficit hyperactivity disorder. Am J Psychiatry. 2000;157:278–80.
219. Ernst M, Kimes AS, London ED, Matochik JA, Eldreth D, Tata S, Contoreggi C, Leff M, Bolla K. Neural substrates of decision making in adults with attention deficit hyperactivity disorder. Am J Psychiatry. 2003;160:1061–70.
220. Schweitzer JB, Lee DO, Hanford R, Tagamets MA, Hoffman JM, Kilts CD. A positron emission tomography study of methylphenidate in adults with ADHD: alterations in resting blood flow and predicting treatment response. Neuropsychopharmacology. 2003;28:967–73.
221. Schweitzer JB, Lee DO, Hanford RB, Zink CF, Ely TD, Tgamets MA, Hoffman JM, Grafton ST, Kilts CD. Effect of methylphenidate on executive functioning in adults with attention-deficit/hyperactivity disorder: normalization of behavior but not related brain activity. Biol Psychiatry. 2004;56:597–606.
222. Ernst M, Zametkin AJ, Matochik JA, Cohen RM. DOPA decarboxylase activity in attention deficit hyperactivity disorder adults. A [fluorine-18]fluorodopa positron emission tomographic study. J Neurosci. 1998;18:5901–7.
223. Ernst M, Zametkin AJ, Matochik JA, Pascualvaca D, Jons PH, Cohem RM. High midbrain [18 F]DOPA accumulation in children with attention deficit hyperactivity disorder. Am J Psychiatry. 1999;156:1209–15.
224. Kooij JJ, Bejerot S, Blackwell A, Caci H, Casa-Bruqué M, Carpentier PJ, Edvinsson D, Fayyad J, Foeken K, Fitzgerald M, Gaillac V, Ginsberg Y, Henry C, Krause J, Lensing MB, Manor I, Niederhofer H, Nunes-Filipe C, Ohlmeier MD, Oswald P, Pallanti S, Pehlivanidis A, Ramos-Quiroga JA, Rastam M, Ryffel-Rawak D, Stes S, Asherson P. European consensus statement on diagnosis

and treatment of adult ADHD: The European Network Adult ADHD. BMC Psychiatry. 2010;10:67.
225. Rohde LA. Is there a need to reformulate attention deficit hyperactivity disorder criteria in future nosologic classification? Child Adolesc Psychiatr Clin N Am. 2008;17:405–20.
226. Sonuga-Barke EJS, Halperin JM. Developmental phenotypes and causal pathways in attention deficit/hyperactivity disorder: potential targets for early intervention? J Child Psychol Psychiatry. 2010;51(4):368–89.
227. Bradstreet JJ, Smith S, Baral M, Rossignol DA. Biomarker-guided interventions of clinically relevant conditions associated with autism and spectrum disorders and attention deficit hyperactivity disorder. Altern Med Rev. 2010;15(1):15–32.
228. Perlov E, Philipsen A, Matthies S, Drieling T, Maier S, Bubl E, Hesslinger B, Büchert M, Henning J, Ebert D, Tebartz van Elst L. Spectroscopic findings in attention-deficit/hyperactivity disorder: review and meta-analysis. World J Biol Psychiatry. 2009;10(4):355–65.
229. Vogt BA. Regions and subregions of the cingulate cortex. In: Vogt BA, editor. Cingulate neurobiology and disease. New York, NY: Oxford University Press; 2009. p. 3–30.
230. Pouwels PJW, Frahm J. Differential distribution of NAA and NAAG in human brain as determined by quantitative localized proton MRS. NMR Biomed. 1997;10:73–8.
231. Edden RAE, Pomper MG, Barker PB. In vivo differentiation of N-acetyl aspartyl glutamate from N-acetyl aspartate at 3 Tesla. Magn Reson Med. 2007;57:977–82.
232. Provencher SW. Automatic quantitation of localized in vivo ^{1}H spectra with LCModel. NMR Biomed. 2001;14:260–4.
233. Stanley JA, Kipp H, Greisenegger E, MacMaster FP, Panchalingam K, Keshavan MS, Bukstein OG, Pettegrew JW. Evidence of developmental alterations in cortical and subcortical regions of children with attention-deficit/hyperactivity disorder: a multivoxel in vivo phosphorus 31 spectroscopy study. Arch Gen Psychiatry. 2008;65(12):1419–28.
234. Stanley JA, Kipp H, Greisenegger E, MacMaster FP, Panchalingam K, Pettegrew JW, Keshavan MS, Bukstein OG. Regionally specific alterations in membrane phospholipids in children with ADHD: an in vivo ^{31}P spectroscopy study. Psychiatry Res: Neuroimaging. 2006;148:217–21.
235. Adriani W, Canese R, Podo F, Laviola G. ^{1}H MRS-detecTable metabolic brain changes and reduced impulsive behavior in adult rats exposed to methylphenidate during adolescence. Neurotoxicol Teratol. 2007;29:116–25.
236. MacMaster FP, Carrey N, Sparkes S, Kusumakar V. Proton spectroscopy in medication-free pediatric attention-deficit/hyperactivity disorder. Biol Psychiatry. 2003;53:184–7.
237. Verma A, Moghaddam B. Regulation of striatal dopamine release by metabotropic glutamate receptors. Synapse. 1998;28:220–6.
238. Bush G. Dorsal anterior midcingulate cortex: Roles in normal cognition and disruption in attention-deficit/hyperactivity disorder. In: Vogt BA, editor. Cingulate Neurobiology and Disease. New York, NY: Oxford University Press; 2009. p. 245–74.
239. Yeo RA, Hill DE, Campbell RC, Vigil J, Brooks WM. Developmental instability and working memory ability in children: a magnetic resonance spectroscopy investigation. Dev Neuropsychol. 2000;17:143–59.
240. Courvoisie H, Hooper SR, Fine C, Kwock L, Castillo M. Functioning and neuropsychological correlates in children with ADHD-H: preliminary findings. J Neuropsychiatry Clin Neurosci. 2004;16:63–9.
241. Sparkes SJ, MacMaster FP, Carrey NC. Proton magnetic resonance spectroscopy and cognitive function in pediatric attention-deficit/hyperactive disorder. Brain Cogn. 2004;54:173–5.
242. Fayed N, Modrego PJ. Comparative study of cerebral white matter in autism and attention-deficit/hyperactivity disorder by means of magnetic resonance spectroscopy. Acad Radiol. 2005;12:566–9.
243. Fayed N, Modrego PJ, Castillo J, Dávila J. Evidence of brain dysfunction in attention deficit-hyperactivity disorder: a controlled study with proton magnetic resonance spectroscopy. Acad Radiol. 2007;14:1029–35.
244. Sun L, Jin Z, Zang Y-F, Zeng Y-W, Liu G, Li Y, Seidman LJ, Faraone SV, Wang Y-F. Differences between attention-deficit disorder with and without hyperactivity: a ^{1}H-magnetic resonance spectroscopy study. Brain Develop. 2005;27:340–4.
245. Margari L, Ventura P, Portoghese C, Presicci A, Buttiglione M, Cuonzo F. Brain magnetic resonance spectroscopy in Sydenham's chorea and ADHD. Pediatr Neurol. 2006;34:467–73.
246. Moore CM, Biederman J, Wozniak J, Mick E, Aleardi M, Wardrop M, Dougherty M, Harpold T, Hammerness P, Randall E, Renshaw PF. Differences in brain chemistry in children and adolescents with attention deficit hyperactivity disorder with and without comorbid bipolar disorder: a proton magnetic resonance spectroscopy study. Am J Psychiatry. 2006;163:316–8.
247. Soliva JC, Moreno A, Fauquet J, Bielsa A, Carmona S, Gispert JD, Rovira M, Bulbena A, Vilarroya A. Cerebellar neurometabolite abnormalities in pediatric attention/deficit hyperactivity disorder: a proton MR spectroscopic study. Neurosci Lett. 2010; 470:60–4.
248. Yang P, Wu M-T, Dung S-S, Ko C-W. Short-TE proton magnetic resonance spectroscopy investigation in adolescents with attention-deficit hyperactivity disorder. Psychiatry Res: Neuroimaging. 2010;181:199–203.
249. Yeo RA, Hill DA, Campbell RA, Vigil J, Petropoulos H, Hart B, Zamora L, Brooks WM. Proton magnetic resonance spectroscopy investigation of the right frontal lobe in children with attention-deficit/hyperactivity disorder. J Am Acad Child Adolesc Psychiatry. 2003;42(3):303–10.
250. Conners CK. Conners' continuous performance test computer program 3.0. Toronto, ON: Multi-Health Systems; 1994.
251. Ernst M, Zametkin AJ, Matochik JA, Liebenauer L, Fitzgerald GA, Cohen RM. Effects of intravenous dextroamphetamine on brain metabolism in adults with attention-deficit hyperactivity disorder (ADHD). Preliminary findings. Psychopharmacol Bull. 1994;30:219–25.
252. O'Neill J, Eberling JL, Schuff N, Jagust WJ, Reed B, Soto G, Ezekiel F, Klein GJ, Weiner MW. Correlation of ^{1}H MRSI and ^{18}FDG-PET. Magn Reson Med. 2000;43:244–50.
253. Baving L, Laucht M, Schmidt MH. Atypical frontal brain activation in ADHD: preschool and elementary school boys and girls. JAACAP. 1999;38:1363–71.
254. Jung RE, Brooks WM, Yeo RA, Chiulli SJ, Weers DC, Sibbitt Jr WL. Biochemical markers of intelligence: a proton MR spectroscopy study of normal human brain. Proc R Soc Lond B Biol Sci. 1999;266:1375–9.
255. Pouwels PJ, Brockmann K, Kruse B, Wilken B, Wick M, Hanefeld F, Frahm J. Regional age dependence of human brain metabolites from infancy to adulthood as detected by quantitative localized proton MRS. Pediatric Res. 1999;46:474–85.
256. Novotny Jr EJ, Fulbright RK, Pearl PL, Gibson KM, Rothman DL. Magnetic resonance spectroscopy of neurotransmitters in human brain. Ann Neurol. 2003;54 suppl 6:S25–31.
257. Logan GD, Cowan WB, Davis KA. On the ability to inhibit simple and choice reaction time responses: a model and a method. J Exp Psychol Hum Percept Perform. 1984;10:276–91.
258. Clark JB. N-Acetyl aspartate: a marker for neuronal loss or mitochondrial dysfunction. Dev Neurosci. 1998;20:271–6.
259. Barkley RA. Attention-deficit hyperactivity disorder. Sci Am. 1998;279:66–71.
260. Castillo M, Kwock L, Arbelaez A. Sydenham's chorea: MRI and proton spectroscopy. Neuroradiology. 1999;41:943–5.
261. Harwood AJ, Agam G. Search for a common mechanism of mood stabilizers. Biochem Pharmacol. 2003;66:179–89.

262. Popper CW. Pharmacologic alternatives to psychostimulants for the treatment of attention-deficit/hyperactivity disorder. Child Adolesc Psychiatr Clin N Am. 2000;9:605–46.
263. Simmons ML, Frondoza CG, Coyle JT. Immunocytochemical localization of N-acetyl-aspartate with monoclonal antibodies. Neuroscience. 1991;45:37–45.
264. Birken DL, Oldendorf WH. N-acetyl-l-aspartic acid: a literature review of a compound prominent in ^{1}H-NMR spectroscopic studies of brain. Neurosci Biobehav Rev. 1989;13:23–31.
265. Brand A, Richter-Landsberg C, Leibfritz D. Multinuclear NMR studies on the energy metabolism of glial and neuronal cells. Dev Neurosci. 1993;15:289–98.
266. Ross BD. Biochemical considerations in ^{1}H spectroscopy. Glutamate and glutamine: myo-inositol and related metabolites. NMR Biomed. 1991;4:59–63.
267. Bates TE, Strangward M, Keelan J, Davey GP, Munro PM, Clark JB. Inhibition of N-acetylaspartate production: implications for ^{1}H MRS studies in vivo. Neuroreport. 1996;7:1397–400.
268. Hesslinger B, Thiel T, Tebartz van Elst L, Hennig J, Ebert D. Attention-de®cit disorder in adults with or without hyperactivity: where is the difference? A study in humans using short echo ^{1}H-magnetic resonance spectroscopy. Neurosci Lett. 2001;304:117–9.
269. Perlov E, Philipsen A, Hesslinger B, Büchert M, Ahrendts J, Feige B, Bubl E, Henning J, Ebert D, Tebartz van Elst L. Reduced cingulate glutamate/glutamine-to-creatine ratios in adult patients with attention deficit/hyperactivity disorder – A magnet resonance spectroscopy study. J Psychiatr Res. 2007;41:934–41.
270. Carlsson A, Hansson LO, Waters N, Carlsson ML. A glutamatergic deficiency model of schizophrenia. Br J Psychiatry. 1999;37:2–6.
271. Colla M, Ende G, Alm B, Deuschle M, Heuser I, Kronenberg G. Cognitive MR spectroscopy of anterior cingulate cortex in ADHD: elevated choline signal correlates with slowed hit reaction times. J Psychiatr Res. 2008;42:587–95.
272. Ferreira PEMS, Palmini A, Bau CHD, Grevet EH, Hoefel JR, Rohde LA, Anés M, Ferreira EE, Belmonte-de-Abreu P. Differentiating attention-deficit/hyperactivity disorder inattentive and combined types: a ^{1}H-magnetic resonance spectroscopy study of fronto-striato-thalamic regions. J Neural Transm. 2009;116:623–9.
273. Perlov E, Tebartz van Elst L, Büchert M, Maier S, Matthies S, Ebert D, Hesslinger B, Philipsen A. H^{1}-MR-spectroscopy of cerebellum in adult attention deficit/hyperactivity disorder. J Psychiatr Res. 2010;44:938–43.
274. Rüsch N, Boeker M, Büchert M, Glauche V, Bohrmann C, Ebert D, Lieb K, Hennig J, Tebartz van Elst L. Neurochemical alterations in women with borderline personality disorder and comorbid attention-deficit hyperactivity disorder. World J Biol Psychiatry. 2010;11(2):372–81.
275. Carlsson A, Waters N, Carlsson ML. Neurotransmitter interactions in schizophrenia–therapeutic implications. Biol Psychiatry. 1999;46:1388–95.
276. Ito M. Control of mental activities by internal models in the cerebellum. Nat Rev Neurosci. 2008;9:304–13.
277. Fallgatter AJ, Ehlis A-C, Rösler M, Strik WK, Blocher D, Herrmann MJ. Diminished prefrontal brain function in adults with psychopathology in childhood related to attention deficit hyperactivity disorder. Psychiatry Res Neuroimaging. 2005;138(2):157–69.
278. Barker PB, Breiter SN, Soher BJ, Chatham JC, Forder JR, Samphilipo MA, Magee CA, Anderson JH. Quantitative proton spectroscopy of canine brain: in vivo and in vitro correlations. Magn Reson Med. 1994;32(2):157–63.
279. Moore CM, Breeze JL, Gruber SA, Babb SM, Frederick BB, Villafuerte RA, Stoll AL, Hennen J, Yurgelun-Todd DA, Cohen BM, Renshaw PF. Choline, myo-inositol and mood in bipolar disorder: a proton magnetic resonance spectroscopy imaging study of anterior cingulated cortex. Bipolar Disord. 2000;2:207–16.
280. Malhi GS, Valenzuela M, Wen W, Sachdev P. Magnetic resonance spectroscopy and its applications in psychiatry. Aust NZ J Psychiatry. 2002;36:31–43.
281. Halperin JM, Schulz KP. Revisiting the role of the prefrontal cortex in the pathophysiology of attention-deficit/hyperactivity disorder. Psychol Bull. 2006;132:560–81.
282. Jin Z, Zang YF, Zeng YW, Zhang L, Wang YF. Striatal neuronal loss or dysfunction and choline rise in children with attention-deficit hyperactivity disorder: a ^{1}H-magnetic resonance spectroscopy study. Neurosci Lett. 2001;315:45–8.
283. Carrey N, MacMaster FP, Sparkes SJ, Khan SC, Kusumakar V. Glutamatergic changes with treatment in attention deficit hyperactivity disorder: a preliminary case series. J Child Adolesc Psychopharmacol. 2002;12(4):331–6.
284. Carrey N, MacMaster FP, Fogel J, Sparkes S, Waschbusch D, Sullivan S, Schmidt M. Metabolite changes resulting from treatment in children with ADHD: a 1H-MRS study. Clin Neuropharmacol. 2003;26(4):218–21.
285. Carrey N, MacMaster FP, Gaudet L, Schmidt M. Striatal creatine and glutamate/glutamine in attention-deficit/hyperactivity disorder. J Child Adolesc Psychopharmacol. 2007;17(1):11–7.
286. Kronenberg G, Ende G, Alm B, Deuschle M, Heuser I, Colla M. Increased NAA and reduced choline levels in the anterior cingulum following chronic methylphenidate: a spectroscopic test–retest study in adult ADHD. Eur Arch Psychiatry Clin Neurosci. 2008;258:446–50.
287. Barbour B. An evaluation of synapse independence. J Neurosci. 2001;21:7969–84.
288. Brustovetsky N, Brustovetsky T, Dubinsky JM. On the mechanisms of neuroprotection by creatine and phosphocreatine. J Neurochem. 2001;76:425–34.
289. Xu CJ, Klunk WE, Kanfer JN, Xiong Q, Miller G, Pettegrew JW. Phosphocreatine-dependent glutamate uptake by synaptic vesicles. A comparison with ATP-dependent glutamate uptake. J Biol Chem. 1996;271:13435–40.
290. Miller TJ, Hanson RD, Yancey PH. Developmental changes in organic osmolytes in prenatal and postnatal rat tissues. Comp Biochem Physiol A. 2000;125:45–56.
291. Gujar SK, Maheshwari S, Bjorkman-Burtscher I, Sundgren PC. Magnetic resonance spectroscopy. J Neuroophthalmol. 2005;25:217–26.
292. Purdon AD, Rosenberger TA, Shetty HU, Rapoport SI. Energy consumption by phospholipid metabolism in mammalian brain. Neurochem Res. 2002;27:1641–7.
293. Ross B, Blüml S. Magnetic resonance spectroscopy of the human brain. Anat Record (New Anat). 2001;265:54–84.
294. Baslow MH. Evidence supporting a role for *N*-acetyl-l-aspartate as a molecular water pump in myelinated neurons in the central nervous system: an analytical review. Neurochem Int. 2002;40:295–300.
295. Ono M, Kubik S, Abernathey CD. Atlas of the Cerebral Sulci. New York, NY: Georg Thieme Verlag; 1990.
296. Middleton FA. The contribution of anterior cingulate-basal ganglia circuitry to complex behavior and psychiatric disorders. In: Vogt BA, editor. Cingulate neurobiology and disease. New York, NY: Oxford University Press; 2009.
297. Alexander GE, DeLong MR, Strick PL. Parallel organization of functionally segregated circuits linking basal ganglia and cortex. Ann Rev Neurosci. 1986;9:357–81.
298. Embick D, Marantz A, Miyashita Y, O'Neil W, Sakai KL. A syntactic specialization for Broca's area. PNAS. 2000;97(11):6150–4.
299. Caplan D, Chen E, Waters G. Task-dependent and task-independent neurovascular responses to syntactic processing. Cortex. 2008;44(3):257–75.

300. Caplan D, Vijayan S, Kuperberg G, West C, Waters G, Greve D, Dale A. Vascular responses to syntactic processing: event-related fMRI study of relative clauses. Hum Brain Mapp. 2002;15(1): 26–38.
301. O'Neill J, Schwartz JM. OCD Treatment: the role of volition in OCD therapy: neurocognitive, neuroplastic, and neuroimaging aspects. Clin Neuropsychiatry. 2005;1(1):10–8.
302. Ciranna L. Serotonin as a modulator of glutamate- and GABA-mediated neurotransmission: implications in physiological functions and in pathology. Curr Neuropharmacol. 2006;4:101–14.
303. Tseng KY, O'Donnell P. Dopamine–glutamate interactions controlling prefrontal cortical pyramidal cell excitability involve multiple signaling mechanisms. J Neurosci. 2004;24(22):5131–9.
304. Bharucha-Reid AT. Elements of the theory of Markov processes and their applications. New York, NY: McGraw-Hil; 1960.
305. Grady CL, Maisog JM, Horwitz B, Ungerleider LG, Mentis MJ, Salemo JA, Pietrini P, Wagner E, Haxby JV. Age-related changes in cortical blood flow activation during visual processing of faces and location. J Neurosci. 1994;14:1450–62.
306. Raichle ME, Fiez JA, Videen TO, MacLeod AM, Pardo JV, Fox PT, Petersen SE. Practice-related changes in human brain functional anatomy during nonmotor learning. Cereb Cortex. 1994;4(1):8–26.
307. Just MA, Carpenter PA, Keller TA, Eddy WF, Thulborn KR. Brain activation modulated by sentence comprehension. Science. 1996;274:114–6.
308. Bookheimer SY, Strojwas MH, Cohen MS, Saunders AM, Pericak-Vance MA, Mazziotta JC, Small GW. Patterns of brain activation in people at risk for Alzheimer's disease. NEJM. 2000;343(7):450–6.
309. Logothetis NK. The neural basis of the blood-oxygen-level-dependent functional magnetic resonance imaging signal. Phil Trans R Soc Lond B Biol Sci. 2002;357(1424):1003–37.
310. O'Neill J, Sobel TL, Vogt BA. Localizing cingulate subregions-of-interest in magnetic resonance images guided by cytological parcellations. In: Vogt BA, editor. Cingulate neurobiology and disease. New York, NY: Oxford University Press; 2009. p. 3–30.
311. Fawcett DW. Bloom and Fawcett. A textbook of histology. 11th ed. Philadelphia: WB Saunders Company; 1986.
312. Théberge J, Bartha R, Drost DJ, Menon RS, Malla A, Takhar J, Neufelde RWJ, Rogers J, Pavlosky W, Schaefer BA, Densmore M, Al-Semaan Y, Williamson PC. Glutamate and glutamine measured with 4.0 T proton MRS in never-treated patients with schizophrenia and healthy volunteers. Am J Psychiatry. 2002;159:1944–6.
313. Théberge J, Al-Semaan Y, Jensen JE, Williamson PC, Neufelde RWJ, Menon RS, Schaefer B, Densmore M, Drost DJ. Comparative study of proton and phosphorus magnetic resonance spectroscopy in schizophrenia at 4 Tesla. Psychiatry Res: Neuroimaging. 2004;132:33–9.
314. Théberge J, Al-Semaan Y, Williamson PC, Menon RS, Neufelde RWJ, Rajakumar N, Schaefer B, Densmore M, Drost DJ. Glutamate and glutamine in the anterior cingulate and thalamus of medicated patients with chronic schizophrenia and healthy comparison subjects measured with 4.0-T proton MRS. Am J Psychiatry. 2003;160:2231–3.
315. Théberge J, Williamson KE, Aoyama N, Drost DJ, Manhanda R, Malla AK, Northcott S, Menon RS, Neufelde RWJ, Rajakumar N, Pavlosky W, Densmore M, Schaefer B, Williamson PC. Longitudinal grey-matter and glutamatergic losses in first-episode schizophrenia. Br J Psychiatry. 2007;191:335–4.
316. Schubert F, Gallinat J, Seifert F, Rinneberg H. Glutamate concentrations in human brain using single voxel proton magnetic resonance spectroscopy at 3 Tesla. Neuroimage. 2004;21:1762–71.
317. Hancu I, Frye M, Port J. The case of the missing glutamine. Honolulu: Proc ISMRM; 2010.
318. O'Gorman RL, Noible J, Stone JM, Lythgoe DJ, McLean MA, Chowdhury FA, McGuire PK, Richardson MP, Barker GJ. Reliability of in vivo glutamate detection with MRS at 3 T. Honolulu: Proc ISMRM; 2010.
319. Hurd RE, Sailasuta N, Srinivasan R, Vigneron B, Pelletier D, Nelson SJ. Measurement of brain glutamate using TE-averaged PRESS at 3 T. Magn Reson Med. 2004;51:435–40.
320. Hancu I, Zimmerman EA, Sailasuta N, Hurd RE. ^{1}H MR spectroscopy using TE averaged PRESS: a more sensitive technique to detect neurodegeneration associated with Alzheimer's disease. Magn Reson Med. 2005;53:777–82.
321. Sailasuta N, Shriner K, Ross B. Evidence of reduced glutamate in the frontal lobe of HIV-seropositive patients. NMR Biomed. 2009;22(3):326–31.
322. Jensen JE, Licata SC, Öngür D, Friedman SD, Prescot AP, Henry ME, Renshaw PF. Quantification of J-resolved proton spectra in two-dimensions with LCModel using GAMMA-simulated basis sets at 4 Tesla. NMR Biomed. 2009;22:762–9.
323. Zhu X-H, Chen W. Observed BOLD effects on cerebral metabolite resonances in human visual cortex during visual stimulation: a functional ^{1}H MRS study at 4 T. Magn Reson Med. 2001; 46:841–7.
324. Dumontheil I, Burgess PW, Blakemore S-J. Development of rostral prefrontal cortex and cognitive and behavioural disorders. Devel Med Child Neurol. 2008;50:168–181.

Magnetic Resonance Spectroscopy of the Fetal Brain

19

Catherine Limperopoulos

Over the last decade, considerable progress has been made in the care of the developing brain. In spite of these advances, non-invasive methods that reliably assess and monitor the high-risk fetus are not readily accessible. Presently, indirect measures of fetal well-being include the non-stress test, the biophysical profile, and Doppler measures (e.g., middle cerebral artery). However, these measures have been shown to not be very accurate in discriminating between pregnancies requiring delivery to optimize neonatal well-being and those that do not. Similarly, these measures have been shown to have limited specificity for ongoing fetal brain injury that could be potentially prevented by expedited delivery. Direct, non-invasive, and reliable measures of fetal well-being are needed to optimize the care of the compromised fetus.

Proton magnetic resonance spectroscopy (^{1}HMRS) has contributed considerably to our understanding of acute brain injury the high-risk newborn and prediction of outcome. More recently, ^{1}HMRS has been studied in the living fetus and has shown to be a promising non-invasive brain imaging technique for measuring metabolic substrates in brain tissue in the fetus. This chapter provides an overview on the use of ^{1}HMRS to understand normal brain maturation in the living fetus and explore the potential role of ^{1}HMRS in assessing and monitoring the compromised fetus. The advantages and limitations of fetal brain ^{1}HMRS will also be summarized and the emerging role of ^{1}HMRS in high-risk pregnancies will be appraised.

C. Limperopoulos, Ph.D (✉)
Advanced Pediatric Brain Imaging Research Center, Washington, DC, USA

George Washington University Health Center, Washington, DC, USA

Children's National Medical Center, 111 Michigan Avenue, NW, Washington, DC 20010, USA
e-mail: climpero@cnmc.org

In Vivo Fetal Brain ^{1}HMRS

The advent of ultrafast single-shot magnetic resonance imaging (MRI) techniques has greatly facilitated the in vivo study of the developing brain. This in turn has accelerated our understanding of the highly orchestrated developmental processes that underlie normal brain maturation in vivo, and have provided important insights into the timing and progression of acquired brain injury and developmental lesions. Although conventional fetal MRI provides detailed structural information of the immature nervous system and offers reliable cerebral biometry, it does not assess metabolic function of the fetal brain.

More recently, the emerging role of ^{1}HMRS has been explored in the fetus for the evaluation of biochemical tissue in vivo. Fetal brain ^{1}HMRS is based on the similar physiological tents as MRI but provides biochemical information of different metabolites in the brain in the form of a spectrum. The feasibility of ^{1}HMRS in vivo was first examined by Heerschap and van den Berg [1], and has since been increasingly performed in fetuses between 22 and 39 weeks gestational age. To date, most fetal ^{1}HMRS studies have characterized the emergence and progression of metabolic profiles in the developing fetal brain. These studies have provided important, previously unavailable reference brain metabolic information in the second and third trimester of pregnancy. More recently, studies have begun to investigate the application and clinical utility of in vivo ^{1}HMRS in the compromised fetus. These data are summarized below. A brief overview of the technique and current challenges of fetal ^{1}HMRS is first warranted.

Technical Challenges

Fetal ^{1}HMRS is performed on a 1.5-Tesla scanner. The mother lies supine or in side lying if she cannot tolerate lying on her back. A multi-channel torso phased-array coil

S. Blüml and A. Panigrahy (eds.), *MR Spectroscopy of Pediatric Brain Disorders*,
DOI 10.1007/978-1-4419-5864-8_19, © Springer Science+Business Media, LLC 2013

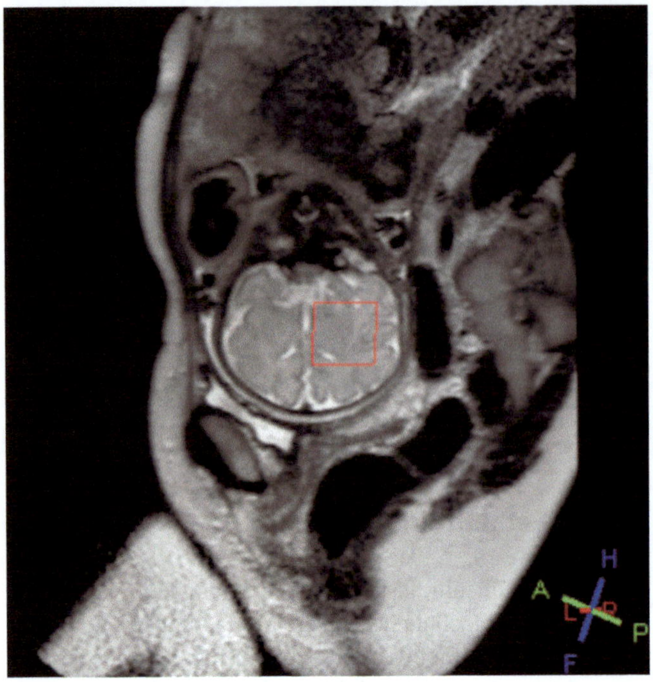

Fig. 19.1 Example of a single 20×20×20 mm³ voxel of interest positioned in the left cerebral hemisphere of a coronal slice in a 33 week gestational age fetus

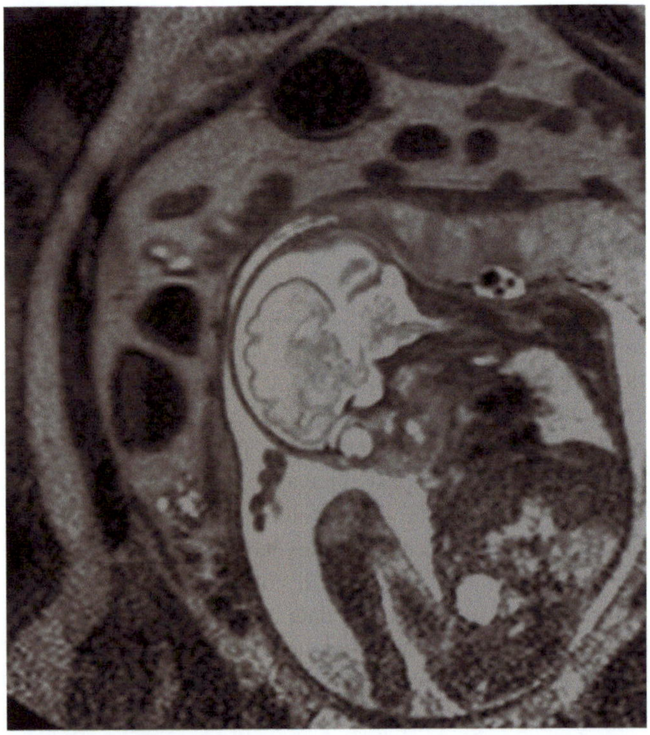

Fig. 19.2 Example of technical challenges of fetal ¹HMRS related to maternal lipid contamination

is used to allow maximal coverage of the fetal head and increased signal-to-noise ratio. Conventional MRI is first carried out to determine the position of the fetal brain. A single voxel fetal ¹HMRS is usually acquired over 3 min using a 20×20×20 mm³ voxel of interest or 20×15×15 mm³ voxel placed in the fetal brain (Fig. 19.1). The location of the voxel is usually placed centrally in the brain, although a more specific anatomical location may be used in older gestational age fetuses [2, 3] given the current challenges of fetal MRI (described below). To date multivoxel ¹HMRS has not been reported in the living fetus.

Fetal ¹HMRS is carried out without sedation. Consequently, a number of factors render the acquisition technically challenging. These include fetal and maternal motion, small head size, lipid contamination (Fig. 19.2), high water content of the fetal brain, low signal to noise (i.e., distance between the receiver coil and the fetal brain), radio frequency receiver coil sensitivities, susceptibility artifacts, and specific absorption rates. Overcoming these challenges and obtaining good quality spectroscopy data relies on a number of considerations which can be summarized as follows (1) identifying the optimal imaging coil, (2) placing the receiver coil as close as possible to the fetus [4], (3) using water suppressions to avoid metabolite signals being flooded by larger water peaks, (4) careful selection of the imaging parameters to optimize the quality of the spectra, and (5) acquiring multiple data sets (e.g., blocks of 3 or 4 averages), in order to eliminate aberrant spectra in the post-processing stage [5]. Some investigators will perform ¹HMRS in fetuses of advanced gestational age only, once the fetal head is engaged in the maternal pelvis to limit fetal motion [4, 6]. We and others have recently reported that over 70% of metabolic spectra acquired are interpretable between 25 and 37 weeks gestational age [3, 5]. Despite these promising preliminary reports, fetal ¹HMRS is presently not routinely incorporated in clinical fetal imaging protocols because of the technical limitations outlined above. Available data are summarized below.

Brain Metabolites in the Developing Fetus

It is well established that the developmental profile of brain metabolites change in the developing brain in utero and ex utero, after birth [2, 3, 7–9]. Prior knowledge of the normal chemical composition of the fetal metabolic spectra is critical in order to understand the corresponding maturational changes that are associated with increases or reductions in the concentrations of these biologically active metabolic substrates in the typically developing fetus in order to "at-risk" fetus.

Single voxel techniques used for fetal ¹HMRS include Stimluated Echo Acquisition Mode (STEAM) and Point Resolved Spectroscopy (PRESS). The fundamental difference between the two techniques is that PRESS uses spin

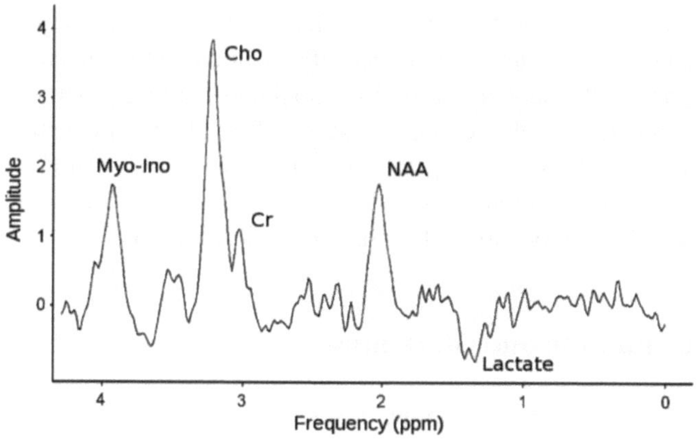

Fig. 19.3 Spectrum acquired in a 32-week gestational age fetus with congenital heart disease using a PRESS sequence (TE = 144 ms). Identifiable peaks include myo-Inositol (Myo-Ino), *N*-acetyl-aspartate (NAA), creatine (Cr), choline (Cho), and Lactate

echo (short echo time of 15 ms or 20 ms) and STEAM uses a stimulated echo sequences (long echo time of 135 ms or 144 ms). Although both techniques have been studied in fetuses, PRESS has been used more commonly in fetal spectroscopic imaging as it provides double the signal compared to the STEAM technique which is extremely valuable in the immature brain [2, 10]. Accordingly, metabolites that have been frequently described in the fetus using ^{1}HMRS include *N*-acetylaspartate, creatine, choline, myo-inositol, and lactate (Fig. 19.3). Other metabolites have also been identified (e.g., glutamate and glutamine) but described less frequently. The emergence and developmental progression of these metabolites are summarized below.

N-acetylaspartate

N-acetylaspartate (NAA) is a neuronal marker and reflects not only the development of dendrites and synapses but also plays a role in oligodendrocyte proliferation and differentiation in early brain development [2, 3, 5]. In vitro studies have shown that NAA is expressed in oligodendrocyte type-2 astrocyte progenitor cells and immature oligodentdrocytes [11]. *N*-acetylaspartate resonates at 2.02 ppm and has the second highest concentration in the human brain after glutamate. *N*-acetylaspartate has been detected as early as 22 week gestational age [2] in vivo and has been shown to increase from 24 to 40 weeks gestational age, [2–4, 10] attaining approximately 50% of adult values at term equivalent. These in vivo studies of the NAA metabolic profile corroborate ex vivo studies in premature infants [8, 12, 13].

Interestingly, postmortem chromatographic analyses comparing full-term and preterm infants have revealed significantly higher regional NAA concentrations in the basal ganglia and thalamus compared to the precentral area and frontal lobe, presumably due to the high density of neuronal tissues, and myelination occurring earlier in the subcortical structures [12]. In fact, NAA has been shown to be a donor of acetyl groups necessary for lipid synthesis in myelin deposition [14]. Indeed, between 32 and 40 weeks gestational age, NAA concentrations remain stable in the perithalamic voxels, where myelination has already begun at 32 weeks [15]. Conversely, NAA increased in the central cerebral white matter where the onset of myelination occurs later [16].

Taken together, these data demonstrate that NAA reflects not only the development of dendrites and synapse, but also oligdentrocyte propagation and differentiation [17]. Postnatally, NAA concentrations reach about half the adult values, and exhibit a slow increase throughout infancy [7, 18].

Myo-Inositol

Myo-Insitol is an osmolyte and a precursor for inositol-derived lipid synthesis and the phosphatidylinosito [19]. Myo-Insitol is important in osmoregulation, cellular nutrition, and detoxification [19]. Myo-Insitol is also an astrocyte marker and plays an important role in the neurulation process [20] including neuronal plasticity and cell growth regulation [21]. Myo-Inositol is located primarily in the glia, functioning as an actrocyte marker and guiding the conduction of nerve pulses [22].

Myo-Inositol resonates at 3.56 ppm and is a dominant resonance in the brain spectrum at short echo time from 22 to 28 weeks gestational age [2]. This likely reflects the high density of glial cells in the white matter at this gestational age range. Girard [2] reported a significant decrease in myo-inositol between 22 and 39 weeks gestational age, similar to the values that Kreis et al. [8], described in preterm infants ex utero. On the other hand, Kok et al. [10], found no significant change in myo-inositol levels over the third trimester of pregnancy. Postnatally, myo-inositol has been shown to markedly decrease in the first weeks, followed by a more gradual reduction in the first year of life [23, 24]. Deficiencies in inositol induces abnormal neurulation and these deficiencies can be reversed by inositol supplementation in mouse embryo [25, 26].

Choline

Choline is composed of several choline-containing compounds, including glycerophosphorylcholine and phospholipids as well as free choline [27]. These compounds are involved in membrane synthesis and degradation [27]. Both glia and neurons are involved in choline uptake [28]. Choline plays a role in myelination and is central to the metabolism of membrane lipids.

Choline resonates at 3.2 pmm. Choline is also dominant resonance at short echo time during the second trimester (i.e., 22–28 weeks gestational age) [2], and undergoes a progressive decline with increasing gestational age at long echo time (TE) [2, 3]. This reduction in choline likely reflects accelerated myelination in the third trimester [10], and during the first postnatal months [8]. The most pronounced decrease in choline happens after 2 years of age, which presumably corresponds to near completion of myelination [7].

The biochemical sequences of integration of different constituents of myelin are identical in the different sites of myelination; at mid-gestation phospholipids are detected first, followed by sphyngomyelin which also contains choline galactocerebrosides and glycoproteins, while at the same time phospholipid concentration is decreased [29]. Therefore, choline likely represents the high levels of substrate needed for the formation of cell membranes, as previously suggested [30] with a gradual reduction as soon as incorporation of lipids has occurred.

During pregnancy, large amounts of choline are delivered to the fetus through the placenta, with a progressive decrease in blood choline concentration that begins in utero, and a high-affinity choline transport early in pregnancy [31]. Choline is needed for neural-tube closure [32] and later in gestation for hippocampal development [33]. Noteworthy is the fact that experimental studies have demonstrated that dietary choline supplementation during pregnancy increases hippocampal progenitor-cell proliferation, decreases apoptosis of the same cells, and enhances long-term potentiation and memory function in rodent off spring.

Creatine

The creatine signal comprises both creatine and phosphocreatine, which are involved in cellular energy metabolism. In vitro studies have demonstrated regional variations in choline with a 2–4 fold higher concentration of creatine in glial cells than in neurons [34]. Similarly, a higher concentration of creatine is present in the gray matter versus white matter and in the cerebellum versus the cerebrum [35].

Creatine is a dominant resonance (3.04 ppm) in the brain spectrum at short echo time from 22 to 28 weeks gestational age. In the living fetus, Girard and colleagues [2] reported a significant increase in total creatine over the second and third trimester (22–39 weeks gestation age), while Kok et al. [10], found not change in creatine levels in the third trimester. Notably, ex utero studies [8] have described higher total concentrations of creatine in preterm infants at term corrected age compared to full-term infants suggesting that intrauterine and extrauterine brain maturation may be different.

Postnatally, creatine increases over the first 2 years of life [8] as well as before and around term. Autopsy reports from preterm and term infants have demonstrated an age-dependent increase and regional specificity in creatine concentrations in the subcortical regions (thalamus and basal ganglia compared to the cortical regions (frontal and precentral areas) [12], suggesting that higher metabolic rates in these subcortical regions where the energy demanding process of myelination occurs earlier than in cortical regions.

Glutamate and Glutamine

Glutamate and glutamine resonate as a composite peak around 3.7 ppm. Glutamate is the principal neurotransmitter and the most profuse amino acid in the brain [36]. In vitro studies have demonstrated that glutamate receptors on neurons are needed for synaptogenesis during normal development [37]. In vitro studies have illustrated glutamate mediated interactions between neurons and glia are also critical for neuronal migration and cerebral cortical development [38], while glutamate and glutamate receptor antagonists regulate proliferation and differentiation of oligodendrocytes [39, 40]. In vivo studies have shown that glutamate and glutamine are visible by 24 weeks gestational age. Although Kreis and colleagues [8] reported a progressive increase in glutamate in ex utero preterm infants with increasing gestational age, this has not been observed in the fetus in vivo at short echo time [2].

Although the function of glutamate in the developing white matter remains controversial, the excitotoxic effects of excessive glutamate release are well established in animal and clinical models of hypoxic–ischemic injury [41, 42]. Glutamate receptor susceptibility to hypoxic ischemic injury has been shown to be age-specific in animal models [43]. Clinical neuroimaging studies support age-and regional dependent areas of vulnerability. For example, in the preterm infant, white matter injury and periventricular leukomalacia are observed, while in the full-term infants, injury primarily affects the cortical areas. However, recent clinical and experimental evidence suggests that this gray–white matter injury distinction is far less discrete [44, 45]. In vitro studies lend further credence to the potential toxic effects of glutamate on oligodendroglia, particularly the premyelinating oligodendrocytes [46, 47].

Lactate

Cerebral lactate is a marker of anaerobic metabolism/glycholysis. Lactate (and NAA) reflects neuronal mitochondrial function and may be valuable measures of brain metabolism [26, 48]. Although a lactate peak is identified at 1.3 ppm, lactate is typically not detected under normal conditions in the mature brain. In the immature brain, a possible role for lactate has been defined as a neuronal energy substrate during physiologic activation. Lactate is considered a fuel for the normal immature brain by using it as an alternative organic substrate it may be elevated in the fetus during starvation or severe hypoglycemia of the mother [49, 50]. Severe dysfunction of the placenta causing hypoxia ischemia may also induce production of lactate in the immature fetal brain (discussed below). Although lactate has been detected in the apparently normal preterm neonatal brain using ^{1}H-MRS, we and others have not found lactate to be present in the healthy fetal brain [2, 3].

The Role of Fetal Brain ^{1}H-MRS in the Compromised Fetus

One of the biggest challenges in fetal medicine is the management of the fetus at risk for brain injury. Importantly, brain morphology may appear normal although brain metabolism may be abnormal. In this respect, ^{1}H-MRS may prove to be useful in monitoring the compromised fetus (e.g., growth restricted fetus) in conjunction with other established instruments for detection of fetal distress. In this regard, ^{1}H-MRS may provide important insights into impaired fetal metabolism resulting fetal growth restriction or other acquired conditions.

The presence of elevated cerebral lactate measures by ^{1}H-MRS in the newborn infants following hypoxic–ischemic insult has been shown to be predictive of both short term adverse outcomes and long term motor and cognitive outcomes [51, 52]. In the fetus, animal models of growth restriction and hypoxia have described the presence of lactate [53–55]. In the living fetus, clinical studies have recently begun to explore the role of ^{1}H-MRS in the compromised fetus. These data are summarized below.

Intrauterine Growth Restriction

Lactate has been described in growth-restricted fetuses in a number of case reports in the literature [48, 56–58]. Robinson [56] reported lactate in the fetal back muscle in a 20 week gestational age fetus and the pregnancy ended with fetal demise the next day. Azpurua and colleagues [57] reported the presence of lactate and a low N-AA/choline index (a metabolic marker for starvation/hypoxia) in a case report of a 25 week fetus with intrauterine growth restriction. The fetus was delivered at 29 weeks and neurologic follow-up after 4 years was reported to be normal. Placental pathology revealed intervillous thrombosis. Additionally, Girard et al. [48], reported increased glutamate+glutamine, low NAA, and total creatine, as well as the presence of lactate in a fetus with intrauterine growth restriction.

More recently, Charles-Edwards [58] reported the quantified fetal cerebral lactate in four third trimester fetuses with intrauterine growth restriction. The concentrations of lactate measured in this study were comparable with levels described in MRS studies of normal preterm infants ex utero [59, 60]. Moreover, concentrations of NAA, total choline, and total creatine were comparable to literature values for normal fetal brain [10]. In a study by Sanz-Cortes and colleagues [61] comparing eight small for gestational age and five matched appropriate for gestational age singleton fetuses at 37 weeks GA with normal umbilical artery Doppler ultrasound scans. SGA fetuses showed a significant increase in inositol/choline ratio, suggesting elevated levels of inositol. A trend towards lower Cho/Cr ratio in small for gestational age fetuses was also observed but did not reach statistical significance, likely due to the small sample size. These data corroborate ex utero postnatal studies in newborn with hypoxic ischemic encephalopathy, in which Ino/Cr ratios were significantly increased during the first postnatal week and correlated with abnormal developmental outcome at 1 year of age [62]. Interestingly, diffusion weighted imaging of the same cohort also showed significantly higher water diffusion (i.e., higher apparent diffusion coefficient values) in the pyramidal tract suggesting delayed brain development and decreased microstructural organization.

Hydrocephalus/Ventriculomegaly

The presence of cerebral lactate has also been reported previously in fetuses with hydrocephalus [13]. Roalants-van Rijn [13] studies six fetuses with hydrocephalus between 29 and 38 weeks gestational age and lactate was present in two fetuses (33%), absent in two and not detectable in the other two because of fetal motion. Additionally, Kok et al. [63], used fetal ^{1}H-MRS in ten hydrocephalic fetuses and compared with healthy controls between 28 and 37 weeks gestational age. Decreased inositol/creatine ratio was reported in fetuses with hydrocephalus versus controls, suggesting a hypo-osmolar state [64]. Interestingly, Girard and colleagues [48] described increased glutamate+glutamine, and a broad NAA peak in a fetus with mild unilateral ventriculomegaly, and germinal matrix hemorrhage. Follow-up brain histology demonstrated ependymal destruction and white-matter gliosis.

Gastroschisis

A single case report by Wolfberg et al. [65] described the presence of lactate in a fetus with gastroschisis at 33 5/7 weeks gestational age. The pregnancy was also complicated by preeclampsia. The authors speculate that the lactate was generated either as a result of transient hypoxia from intermittent torsion of the dilated looks of bowel, or hypoxia related to preeclampsia-induced placental insufficiency. Neurologic follow-up at 4 months was normal.

Congenital Heart Disease

In one of the largest in vivo fetal MRI studies to date, Limperopoulos and colleagues [3] obtained ^{1}H-MRS spectra in 75 fetuses: 36 with congenital heart disease and 39 controls. Cerebral lactate was detected in 20% of fetuses with congenital heart disease, while no control fetuses had detectable lactate. Compared with controls, NAA:choline in CHD fetuses was significantly and progressively lower between 27 and 36 weeks gestational age. The presence of lactate was identified as an independent predictors of lower NAA:choline ratios. Moreover, fetuses with cerebral lactate demonstrated the greatest impairment in volumetric brain growth over the same gestational age time frame. This study presents the first in vivo MRI evidence of progressive third trimester impairment in brain metabolism in fetuses with congenital heart disease, and suggests that an abnormal cardiovascular system fails to support the metabolic demands of accelerated third trimester brain development.

Metabolic Disorders

Studies have also begun to explore the role of ^{1}H-MRS in inherited inborn errors of metabolism enzyme. Specifically, Robinson et al. [66] reported a case of a 31-year-old dichorionic, diamniotic twin pregnancy with a history of two prior infants affected with pyruvate dehydrogenase deficiency. Pyruvate dehydrogenase deficiency comprises a heterogeneous groups of inborn errors of metabolism characterized by mutations in the gene which codes for the $E_{1\alpha}$ subunit of the private decarboxylase complex [67, 68]. This metabolic disorder is associated with early death or profound neurologic sequelae and developmental disability. Magnetic resonance imaging and ^{1}H-MRS were performed on both fetuses at 32 weeks gestational age. The affected fetus had mild ventriculomegaly, increased extracerebrospinal fluid, and decreased cortical sulcation and gyration. The normal fetus had a structurally normal brain. There was no evidence of elevated cerebral lactate levels in either fetus on ^{1}H-MRS. Postnatally, both twins had normal lactate levels at delivery but one twin developed increased lactate levels from 8 h postnatally and died at 3 days of life. Although elevated lactate has been reported in pediatric cases with pyruvate dehydrogenase deficiency [69, 70], the authors speculate that the placental–maternal circulation may provide an efficient mechanism to remove any excess lactate in utero. Further studies are needed to address this intriguing question.

In summary, the long-term neurodevelopmental consequences of fetal cerebral lactate remains unknown and awaits further study. Animal studies suggest that the immature brain has an enhanced capability to metabolize lactate compared with the mature brain as an adaptation to the relatively hypoxemic and hyperlacticacidemic state of the perinatal period [71]. Longitudinal studies are needed to elucidate the role of lactate as a marker for hypoxemia in the prenatal and vulnerable transitional periods in high-risk fetuses.

Conclusions

Fetal ^{1}H-MRS is a promising noninvasive technique for assessing metabolic integrity in the developing brain, and has the potential to open a critical presently unavailable window for antenatal cerebral surveillance in the high-risk pregnancy. However ongoing work is needed to improve the technical success of this emerging technique so as to increase and optimize its utility in the clinical setting. To date in vivo studies have provided important normative data for second and third trimester fetal brain metabolic concentrations in healthy fetuses. Additional studies are needed to elucidate the complex role of these metabolites throughout gestation. This in turn will lay the foundation for the development of clinically meaningful ^{1}H-MRS biomarkers for the accurate assessment of fetal health and well-being. Finally, although a number of studies have performed in vivo spectroscopy studies, the long-term prognostic significance of these acute metabolic findings warrant further study.

References

1. Heerschap A, van den Berg PP. Proton magnetic resonance spectroscopy of human fetal brain. Am J Obstet Gynecol. 1994;170: 1150–1.
2. Girard N, Confort Gouny S, Viola A, et al. Assessment of normal fetal brain maturation in utero by proton magnetic resonance spectroscopy. Magn Reson Med. 2006;56:768–75.
3. Limperopoulos C, Tworetzky W, McElhinney DB, et al. Brain volume and metabolism in fetuses with congenital heart disease: evaluation with quantitative magnetic resonance imaging and spectroscopy. Circulation. 2010;121:26–33.
4. Heerschap A, Kok RD, van der Berg PP. Antenatal proton MR spectroscopy of the human brain in vivo. Childs Nerv Syst. 2003; 19:418–21.
5. Story L, Damodaram MS, Allsop JM, et al. Proton magnetic resonance spectroscopy in the fetus. Eur J Obstet Gynecol. 2011; 158:3–8.
6. Roelants-van Rijn AM, Groenendaal F, Stoutenbeek P, van der Grond J. Lactate in the foetal brain: detection and implications. Acta Paediatr. 2004;93:937–40.
7. Kreis R, Ernst T, Ross BD. Development of the human brain: In vivo quantification of metabolite and water content with proton

magnetic resonance spectroscopy. Magn Reson Med. 1993;30: 424–37.
8. Kreis R, Hofmann L, Kuhlmann B, Boesch C, Bossi E, Huppi PS. Brain metabolite composition during early human brain development as measured by quantitative in vivo ^{1}H magnetic resonance spectroscopy. Magn Reson Med. 2002;48:949–58.
9. Limperopoulos C. Disorders of the fetal circulation and the fetal brain. Clin Perinatol. 2009;36:561–77.
10. Kok RD, van den Berg PP, van den Bergh AJ, Nijland R, Heerschap A. Maturation of the human fetal brain as observed by ^{1}H MR spectroscopy. Magn Reson Med. 2002;48:611–6.
11. Urenjak J, Willliams SR, Gadian DG, Noble M. Specific expression of N-acetylaspartate in neurons, oligodendrocyte-type-2 astrocyte progenitors, and immature oligodendrocytes in vitro. J Neurochem. 1992;59:55–61.
12. Huppi PS, Fusch C, Boesch C, et al. Regional metabolic assessment of human brain during development by proton magnetic resonance spectroscopy in vivo and by high-performance liquid chromatography/gas chromatography in autopsy tissue. Pediatr Res. 1995;37: 145–50.
13. Roelants-van Rijn AM, van der Grond J, Stigter RH, de Vries LS, Groenendaal F. Cerebral structure and metabolism and long-term outcome in small-for-gestational-age preterm neonates. Pediatr Res. 2004;56:285–90.
14. Fenton BW, Lin CS, Macedonia C, Schellinger D, Ascher S. The fetus at term: In utero volume-selected proton MR spectroscopy with a breath-hold technique- A feasibility study. Radiology. 2001;219:563–6.
15. Cady E, Penrice J, Arness P, et al. Lactate, N-acetyl-aspartate, choline and creatine concentrations and spin-spin relaxation in thalamic and occipito-parietal regions of developing human brain. Magn Reson Med. 1996;36:878–86.
16. Huppi PS, Warfield S, Kikinis R, et al. Quantitative magnetic resonance imaging of brain development in premature and mature newborns. Am Neurol. 1998;43:224–35.
17. Bhakoo KK, Pearce D. In vitro expression of N-acetyl-aspartate by oligodendrocytes: Implications for proton magnetic resonance spectroscopy signal in vivo. J Neurochem. 2000;74:254–62.
18. Kreis R, Ernst T, Ross B. Absolute quantification of water and metabolites in the human brain. Part II. Metabolite concentrations. J Magn Reson. 1993;103:9–19.
19. Fisher SK, Novak JE, Agranoff BW. Inositol and higher inositol phosphates in neural tissues: homeostasis, metabolism and functional significance. J Neurochem. 2002;82:736–54.
20. Beemster P, Groenen P, Steegers-Theunissen RPM. The involvement of inositol in reproduction. Nutr Rev. 2002;60:80–8.
21. Kato N. Dependence of long-term depression of postsynaptic metabotropic glutamate receptors in visual cortex. Proc Natl Acad Sci USA. 1993;90:3650–4.
22. Novak JE, Turner RS, Agranoff BW, Fisher SK. Differentiated human NT2-N neurons possess a high intracellular content of myo-inositol. J Neurochem. 1999;72:1431–40.
23. Ross B, Bluml S. Magnetic resonance spectroscopy of the human brain. Anat Rec. 2001;265:54–84.
24. Fisher SK, Novak JE, Agranoff BW. Inositol and higher inositol phosphates in neural tissues: homeostasis, metabolism and functional significance. J Neurochem. 2002;82:736–54.
25. Greene ND, Copp AJ. Inositol prevents folate-resistant neural tube defects in the mouse. Nat Med. 1997;3:60–6.
26. Brighina E, Bresolin N, Pardi G, Rango M. Human fetal brain chemistry as detected by proton magnetic resonance spectroscopy. Pediatr Neurol. 2008;40(5):327–42.
27. Barker P, Breiter S, Soher B, et al. Quantitative proton spectroscopy of canine brain: In vivo and in vitro correlations. Magn Reson Med. 1994;32:157–63.
28. Chugani HT, Phelps ME, Mazziotta JC. Positron emission tomography study of human brain functional development. Ann Neurol. 1987;22:487–97.
29. Stockler S, Holzbach U, Hanefeld F, et al. Creatine deficiency in the brain: a new, treatable inborn error of metabolism. Pediatr Res. 1994;36:409–13.
30. Bizzi A, Bugiani M, Salomons GS, et al. X-linked creatine deficiency syndrome: a novel mutation in creatine transporter gene SLC6A8. Ann Neurol. 2002;52:227–31.
31. Rutherford JM, Moody A, Crawshaw S, Rubin PC. Magnetic resonance spectroscopy in pre-eclampsia: evidence of cerebral ischaemia. Br J Obstet Gynaecol. 2003;110:416–23.
32. Fisher MC, Zeisel SH, Mar MH, Sadler TW. Perturbations in choline metabolism cause neural tube defects in mouse embryos in vitro. FASEB J. 2002;16:619–21.
33. Zeisel SH, Niculescu MD. Perinatal choline influences brain structure and function. Nutr Rev. 2004;64:197–203.
34. Urenjak J, Williams SR, Gadian DG, Noble M. Proton nuclear magnetic resonance spectroscopy unambiguously identifies different neural cell types. J Neurosci. 1993;13:981–9.
35. Jacobs MA, Horska A, van Zijil PC, Barker PB. Quantitative proton MR spectroscopic imaging of normal human cerebellum and brainstem. Magn Reson Med. 2001;46:699–705.
36. Magistretti FG, Pellerin L, Rothman DL, Shulman RG. Energy on demand. Science. 1999;283:496–7.
37. Hutternlocher PR, de Courten C, Garey LJ, Van der Loos H. Synaptogenesis in human visual cortex-evidence for synapse elimination during normal development. Neurosci Lett. 1982;33: 247–52.
38. Gallo V, Ghiani CA. Glutamate receptors in glia: new cells, new inputs and new functions. Trends Pharmacol Sci. 2000;21:252–8.
39. Gallo V, Zhou JM, McBain CJ, Wright PW, Knutson PL, Amstrong RC. Oligodendrocyte progenitor cell proliferation and lineage progression are regulated by glutamate receptor-mediated K^+ channel block. J Neurosci. 1996;16:2659–70.
40. Yuan X, Eisen AM, McBain CJ, Gallo V. A role for glutamate and its receptors in the regulation of oligodendrocyte development in cerebellar tissue slices. Development. 1998;125:2901–14.
41. Benveniste H, Drejer J, Schousboe A, Diemer NH. Elevation of the extra-cellular concentrations of glutamate and aspartate in rat hippocampus during transient cerebral ischemia monitored by intracerebral microdialysis. J Neurochem. 1984;4:1369–74.
42. Hagberg H. Hypoxic-ischemic damage in the neonatal brain: excitatory amino acids. Dev Pharmacol Ther. 2002;18:139–44.
43. Follet P, Deng W, Dai W, et al. Topiramate protection in immature brain injury. J Neurosci. 2004;24:4412–20.
44. Volpe JJ. Encephalopathy of prematurity includes neuronal abnormalities. Pediatrics. 2005;116:221–5.
45. Volpe JJ. Brain injury in premature infants: a complex amalgam of destructive and developmental disturbances. Lancet. 2009;8: 110–24.
46. Itoh T, Beesley J, Itoh A, et al. AMPA glutamate receptor-mediated calcium signaling is transiently enhanced during development of oligodendrocytes. J Neurochem. 2002;81:390–402.
47. Rosenberg PA, Dai W, Gan X, et al. Mature myelin basic protein-expressing oligodendrocytes are insensitive to kainate toxicity. J Neurosci Res. 2003;71:237–45.
48. Girard N, Fogliarini C, Viola A, et al. MRS of normal and impaired fetal brain development. Eur J Radiol. 2006;57:217–25.
49. Vannucci RC, Vannucci SJ. Glucose metabolism in the developing brain. Semin Perinatol. 2000;24:107–15.
50. Khalan S, Parimi P. Gluconeogenesis in the fetus and neonate. Semin Perinatol. 2000;24:94–106.
51. Zarifi MK, Astrakas LG, Poussaint TY, Plessis Ad A, Zurakowski D, Tzika AA. Prediction of adverse outcome with cerebral lactate

level and apparent diffusion coefficient in infants with perinatal asphyxia. Radiology. 2002;225:859–70.
52. Miller SP, Newton N, Ferriero DM, et al. Predictors of 30-month outcome after perinatal depression: role of proton MRS and socioeconomics factors. Pediatr Res. 2002;52:71–7.
53. Loose JM, Miller SL, Supramanian VG, et al. Hypoxia induced activin secretion by the fetoplacental unit: differential responses related to gestation. BJOG. 2004;111:1346–52.
54. van Cappellen van Walsum AM, Heerschap A, Nijhuis JG, Oeseburg B, Jongsma HW. Proton magnetic resonance spectroscopy of fetal lamb brain during hypoxia. Am J Obstet Gynecol. 1998;179:756–7.
55. Dixon JC, Cady EB, Priest AN, Thornton JS, Peebles DM. Growth restriction and the cerebral metabolic response to acute hypoxia of chick embryos in-ovo: a proton magnetic resonance spectroscopy study. Brain Res Dev Brain Res. 2005;160:203–10.
56. Robinson JN, Cleary-Goldman J, Arias-Mendoza F, et al. Detection of fetal lactate with two-dimensional-localized proton magnetic resonance spectroscopy. Obstet Gynecol. 2004;104:1208–10.
57. Azpurua HB, Alvarado A, Mayobre F, Salom T, Copel JA, Guevara-Zuloaga F. Metabolic assessment of the brain using proton magnetic resonance spectroscopy in a growth-restricted human fetus: case report. Am J Perinatol. 2008;25:305–9.
58. Charles-Edwards GD, Jan W, To M, Maxwell D, Keevil SF, Robinson R. Non-invasive detection and quantification of human foetal brain lactate in utero by magnetic resonance spectroscopy. Prenat Diagn. 2010;30:260–6.
59. Leth H, Toft P, Pryds O, Peitersen B, Lou H, Henriksen O. Brain lactate in preterm and growth-retarded neonates. Acta Paediatr. 1995;82:495–9.
60. Cady E. Metabolite concentrations and relaxation in perinatal cerebral hypoxic-ischemic injury. Neurochem Res. 1996;21:1043–52.
61. Sanz-Cortes M, Figueras F, Bargallo N, Padilla N, Amat-Roldan I, Gratacos E. Abnormal brain microstructure and metabolism in small-for-gestational-age term fetuses with normal umbilical artery Doppler. Ultrasound Obstet Gynecol. 2010;36:159–65.
62. Robertson NJ, Lewis RH, Cowan FM, et al. Early increases in brain myo-inositol measured by proton magnetic resonance spectroscopy in term infants with neonatal encephalopathy. Pediatr Res. 2001;50:692–700.
63. Kok RD, Steegers-Theunissen RPM, Eskes TKA, Heerschap A, van den Berg PP. Decreased relative brain tissue levels of inositol in fetal hydrocephalus. Am J Obstet Gynecol. 2003;188(4):978–80.
64. Bluml S, McComb JG, Ross BD. Differentiation between cortical atrophy and hydrocephalus using ^{1}H MRS. Magn Reson Med. 1997;37:395–403.
65. Wolfberg A, Robinson JN, Mulkern R, Rybicki F, Du Plessis AJ. Identification of fetal cerebral lactate using magnetic resonance spectroscopy. Am J Obstet Gynecol. 2007;196:e-9–11.
66. Robinson JN, Norwitz ER, Mulkern R, Brown SA, Rybicki F, Tempany CMC. Prenatal diagnosis of pyruvate dehydrogenase deficiency using magnetic resonance imaging. Prenat Diagn. 2001;21:1053–6.
67. Brown RM, Dahl HHM, Brown GK. X-chromosome localization of the functional gene for the El α (alpha) subunit of the human pyruvate dehydrogenase complex. Genomics. 1989;41:74–81.
68. Brown GK, Otero LJ, Le Gris M, Brown RM. Pyruvate dehydrogenase deficiency. J Med Genet. 1994;31:875–9.
69. Cross JH, Connelly A, Gadian DG, et al. Clinical diversity of pyruvate dehydrogenase deficiency. Pediatr Neurol. 1994;10:276–83.
70. Shevell MI, Matthews PM, Scriver CR, et al. Cerebral dysgenesis lactic academia: an MRI/MRS phenotype associated with pyruvate dehydrogenase deficiency. Pediatr Neurol. 1994;11:224–9.
71. Hernandez MJ, Vannucci RC, Salcedo A, Brennan RW. Cerebral blood flow and metabolism during hypoglycemia in newborn dogs. J Neurochem. 1980;35:622–8.

MRS of the Neonatal Brain: Abnormal Development and Neonatal Pathology

20

Jessica L. Wisnowski, Andre D. Furtado, Niveditha Pinnamaneni, and Ashok Panigrahy

The most frequently encountered intracranial pathologies in the neonatal period include hemorrhage (e.g., germinal matrix/intraventricular hemorrhages (IVH), intraparenchymal hemorrhages or extraaxial hemorrhages), hypoxic–ischemic injuries (i.e., hypoxic–ischemic encephalopathy, stroke), and encephalopathy of prematurity, which includes both focal and diffuse injury to the developing white matter. Less frequently encountered are congenital malformations involving the cerebrum (e.g., diffuse migrational abnormalities, intrahemispheric cysts) or the posterior fossa (e.g., congenital aqueductal stenosis, chiari malformations), infections, trauma, tumors/masses, and early-onset metabolic disorders.

Although it is likely that many of these abnormalities are associated with altered cerebral metabolism in either a relatively discrete region or diffusely throughout the cerebrum or brainstem in line with the neuroanatomic distribution of the underlying cerebral pathology, remarkably little systematic investigation has been conducted in relation to some of the most common intracerebral pathologies of the neonate (e.g., periventricular leukomalacia). Thus, much work remains to be done. In this chapter, we will describe the current state of knowledge pertaining to the application of MRS to pathological processes that affect neonates. Please note that the use of MRS for profound hypoxic–ischemic encephalopathy at term and neonatal non-accidental trauma are described in detail elsewhere in this book (Chaps. 8 and 9) and thus will not be covered in this chapter. Additionally, although normative reference points and knowledge of normal brain maturational processes in late fetal and early postnatal life are essential for understanding and interpreting MRS in neonates, those topics have been covered separately in earlier chapters. This chapter will instead focus on other pathologic processes that affect neonate preterm and term neonates, including hemorrhage, perinatal white matter injury, metabolic diseases, and infections.

Germinal Matrix-Intraventricular Hemorrhage

Hemorrhage into the germinal matrix and/or lateral ventricles is common among preterm infants and can range from a tiny, punctate hemorrhage restricted to the subependymal lining of the lateral ventricles (a Grade I intraventricular hemorrhage or IVH) to a large hemorrhage into the lateral ventricles causing ventricular dilatation (Grade III IVH) and even periventricular infarct secondary to a clogging of the venous outflow (Grade IV IVH, Fig. 20.1). IVH is less common in term infants; however, spontaneous intraparenchymal or intraventricular hemorrhage can be related to venous infarction (venous thrombosis), vascular malformations, and tumors in this population. MRS is generally unnecessary for the diagnosis of intraparenchymal hemorrhage or IVH (MRI or cranial ultrasound are the diagnostic imaging modalities of choice); however, the few MRS studies conducted in preterm infants with IVH have revealed important information regarding the metabolic functions of surrounding "normal appearing" tissues. One study of preterm infants (mean GA 29.3 ± 2.5 weeks) with Grade I–IV IVH demonstrated an elevation in lactate and a decrease in Cr and NAA in the striatal region adjacent to the hemorrhage compared to the striatal region in contralateral hemisphere [1]. By three months

J.L. Wisnowski, Ph.D. (✉)
Brain and Creativity Institute and Dornsife Cognitive Neuroscience Imaging Center, University of Southern California, Los Angeles, CA, USA

A.D. Furtado, M.D.
Division of Pediatric Neuroradiology, Department of Radiology, Children's Hospital of Pittsburgh at UPMC, Pittsburgh, PA, USA

N. Pinnamaneni, B.A., B.S.
Department of Radiology, Children's Hospital of Pittsburgh, University of Pittsburgh Medical Center, Pittsburgh, PA, USA

A. Panigrahy, M.D.
Department of Pediatric Radiology, Children's Hospital of Pittsburgh of UPMC, Pittsburgh, PA, USA

Department of Radiology, University of Pittsburgh School of Medicine, Pittsburgh, PA, USA

S. Blüml and A. Panigrahy (eds.), *MR Spectroscopy of Pediatric Brain Disorders*,
DOI 10.1007/978-1-4419-5864-8_20, © Springer Science+Business Media, LLC 2013

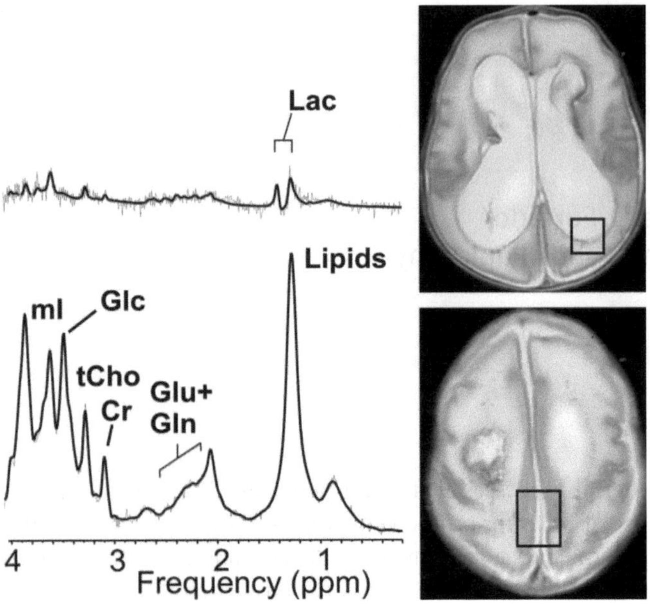

Fig. 20.1 Single voxel MRS (PRESS, TE 35 ms, 1.5 T) of a preterm neonate with Grade IV hemorrhage. The top voxel was placed in the left parietal white matter which part of the voxel overlapping with the CSF in the dilated lateral ventricle. The bottom voxel was placed in the region of the medial posterior parietal lobe. The parietal white matter voxel showed predominately elevated lactate with all other metabolites reduced or depleted. The gray matter voxel showed elevated lipids with reduced NAA. A strikingly high glucose (Glc) signal was observed

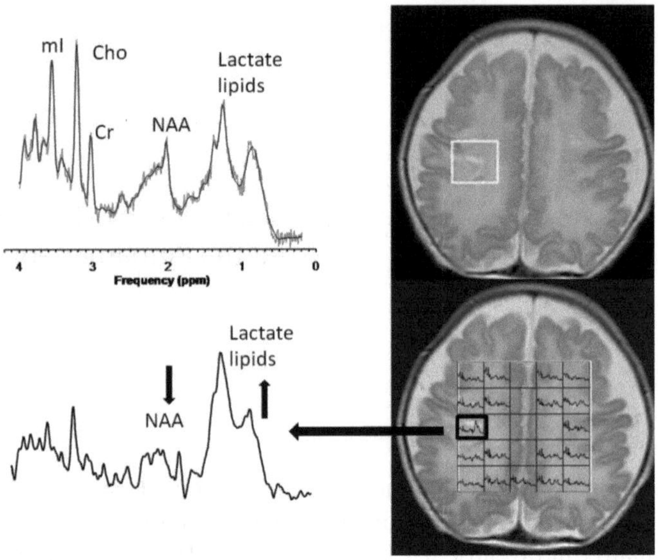

Fig. 20.2 Single voxel MRS (PRESS, TE 35 ms, 1.5 T) (*top*) and multi-voxel long-echo time (*bottom*) MRS of focal white matter necrosis or PVL in the white matter of a preterm neonate. Both spectra showed reduced NAA and elevated lipids and lactate

of age, corrected for GA, conventional MR imaging was largely unremarkable, lactate had disappeared for all but two cases, and NAA had normalized; however, choline was higher in the striatal region ipsilateral to the prior hemorrhage. In general, the pattern of results suggested that metabolism in the adjacent striatial areas is transiently affected in preterm infants with IVH.

In another longitudinal study, high-energy phosphorus metabolites in temporoparietal cortex were compared in preterm infants with grade III/IV IVH to preterm infants without IVH using phosphorous (^{31}P) MRS. Results from that study demonstrated that the ratio of phosphocreatine to adenosine triphosphate was decreased through term-equivalency and that the ratio of phosphocreatine to inorganic phosphate was decreased in the infants with IVH who were less than 30 weeks postconceptional age [2]. In general, much work remains to be done to understand the impact of hemorrhage on cerebral metabolism in the surrounding tissues.

White Matter Injury

White matter injury is the most predominant finding in preterm infants, owing in large part to the intrinsic vulnerabilities of the white matter during the period of rapid development (i.e., axonal outgrowth, development of the oligodendrocyte lineage, onset of myelination) in the late second and early third trimesters of fetal development [3]. Additionally, white matter injury may be observed in term born infants, particularly those with congenital heart disease (especially transposition of the great arteries and hypoplastic left heart syndrome [4, 5], likely due in part to a delay in brain maturation in utero [6, 7], and also in infants with severe cardiopulmonary disorders (e.g., meconium aspiration syndrome, persistent pulmonary hypertension) requiring extracorporeal membrane oxygenation (ECMO).

In general, three patterns of white matter abnormalities are most often described on conventional MR imaging: immature white matter development, focal injury (which includes focal white matter necroses, sometimes referred to as periventricular leukomalacia or PVL, its presumed neuropathological correlate) and diffuse injury (sometimes described as "diffuse excessive high signal intensity" or DEHSI on T2-weighted MR images) [8–10]. While these three patterns can be diagnosed using conventional MR imaging techniques with diffusion, MR spectroscopic techniques are useful adjunctive tools: they provide more information regarding timing of the injury and more detailed metabolic/physiologic information about the integrity of the damaged periventricular white matter (Fig. 20.2).

Early MRS studies of neonates with cystic leukomalacia (also referred to as periventricular leukomalacia or cystic PVL), diagnosed using cranial ultrasound and/or MRI demonstrated a decreased NAA/Cho ratio in preterm and term neonates with grade III or Grade IV lesions (i.e., extensive periventricular or subcortical cystic lesions, respectively), which predicted poorer neurodevelopmental outcome at 18–24 months [11]. However, it should be noted that some of the preterm infants with grade II and grade III lesions had NAA/Cho ratios within normal limits, even when cystic lesions were included in the MRS volume, indicating that a normal NAA/Cho ratio does not preclude injury and that cerebral metabolism may normalize in the chronic epoch after brain injury.

Lactate was detected in more than half of the preterm and term infants included in the study, but did not improve prediction of outcome at 18–24 months [11]. Notably, a low concentration of lactate has also been reported to be a "normal" finding in the brain of preterm infants, increasing with decreasing gestational age [12, 13], and is hypothesized to reflect greater reliance on glycolysis compared to mitochondrial respiration in the fetal/preterm brain [14].

Direct examination of intracellular metabolism using phosphorous MRS in preterm infants with white matter injury/PVL compared to healthy preterm and term born infants has demonstrated that a reduction in the ratio of phosphocreatine (PCr) to inorganic orthophosphate (Pi) may be a strong predictor of adverse outcome in infants with ultrasound evidence of white matter injury [15]. 9/15 infants with white matter injury diagnosed on cranial ultrasound (CUS) found to have a decreased PCr/Pi ratio on MRS conducted 0–8 days later (median 1 day) subsequently died. Moreover, the remaining 6 had evidence of white matter injury on follow-up imaging studies (e.g., cysts, microcephaly) and were neurodevelopmentally abnormal at follow-up. Of the 12 infants with white matter echogenicities on CUS but normal PCr/Pi, all survived and only 3 had subsequent evidence of white matter abnormalities (e.g., cysts, microcephaly) and concomitant abnormal neurodevelopment at follow-up. Of the remaining 9 who did not evidence subsequent white matter abnormalities, 6 were within normal limits at neurodevelopmental follow-up between 16 and 21 months.

White matter injury has also been associated with a shift in the biochemical association among metabolites in cerebral white matter. In one study, myo-inositol/Cr and lactate/Cr were significantly correlated among preterm infants with white matter disease (WMD, resulting primarily from cystic PVL and grade III/IV IVH) but not preterm infants without WMD. Mean lactate/Cr was also higher among preterm infants with WMD, compared to preterm infants without WMD. The ratio of NAA/Cr did not differ among the preterm groups [14]. Another study found similar concentrations of NAA, Cho, and myo-inositol among healthy preterm infants at term equivalency and term-born peers, suggesting that metabolite concentrations are most dramatically altered by cerebral pathology and not early birth, per se [16]. Again, much work remains to be done to understand the precise changes in cerebral metabolism that follow different patterns of white matter abnormalities and the relation between the changes in cerebral metabolism and long-term neurodevelopmental outcome.

Neonatal Metabolic Disorders

Clinically, metabolic disorders in the newborn often present as neonatal encephalopathy and may be difficult to distinguish from other potential cerebral (or systemic) pathologies that cause encephalopathy such as profound hypoxia–ischemia secondary to perinatal asphyxia (covered in Chap. 8) or white matter injury. These disease entities may be classified as either acquired or as inborn error of metabolism. In these instances, MRS may not only provide important information about energy metabolism in the cerebrum or brainstem, it may also provide key diagnostic information.

Acquired Metabolic Disorders

Kernicterus

Kernicterus, or bilirubin encephalopathy, is the result of direct injury to neurons and astrocytes by bilirubin and most often occurs in the context of elevated serum bilirubin, and in particular free bilirubin (rather than bilirubin bound to albumin). Bilirubin is the end product of catabolism of heme, and nearly every term infant undergoes a transient elevation in bilirubin during the first week of life, with healthy, breast-fed infants demonstrating a higher peak and a slower decline compared to formula-fed infants. A variety of conditions in the neonate may lead to further elevations in the concentration of unconjugated bilirubin, which left untreated, may result in a clinical syndrome: kernicterus. On conventional MR images, kernicterus often results in signal abnormalities in the subthalamic nucleus and the globus pallidus [17–21]; however, neuropathological data suggests that other regions may also be damaged, including the hippocampus (CA2 and CA3 sectors), substantia nigra, various brainstem nuclei (particularly the oculomotor, vestibular, auditory, especially the cochlear, and facial nerve nuclei), the reticular formation of the pons, inferior olive, and certain cerebellar nuclei (particularly the dentate) [22–26]. Although diagnosis of kernicterus is typically made based on the clinical presentation and imaging features on conventional MR image (i.e., high T1-signal in the globus pallidum and subthalamic nucleus described above), MRS (Fig. 20.3) may be a useful adjuvant tool to aid in differential diagnosis when the clinical presentation is incomplete (e.g., when serum bilirubin is not

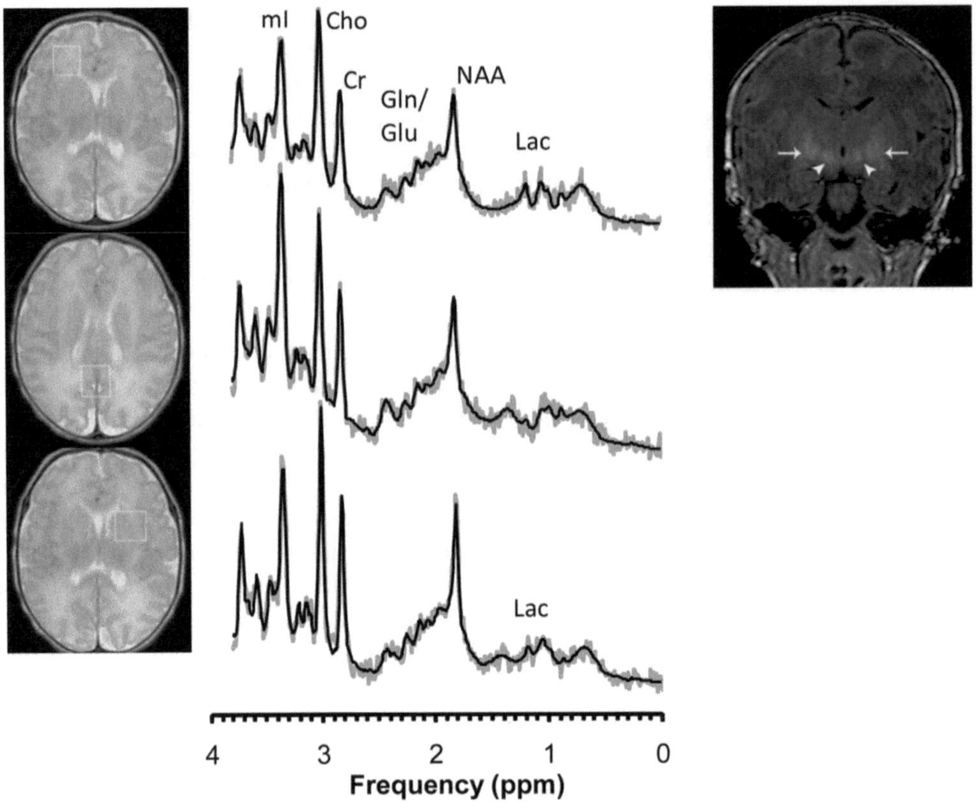

Fig. 20.3 Ex-34 week preterm infant admitted from home at 15-days of age for hyperbilirubinemia and apnea/bradycardia requiring intubation in the emergency room. Baby was subsequently treated with phototherapy in the NICU. MRI at 19-days of age shows mildly increased signal in the globus pallidi (*arrows*) and subthalamic nuclei (*arrowheads*), bilaterally, consistent with kernicterus. Single-voxel PRESS was acquired contemporaneously with the conventional MR imaging and demonstrates mildly above normal lactate (Lac) in frontal white matter and basal ganglia. NAA was close to normal, whereas glutamine/glutamate appeared to be slightly above normal. Myo-inositol (mI) was close to normal or slightly below

significantly elevated), and possibly to assess treatment response, as the neurological deficits are potentially reversible, if treatment is initiated early enough. A possible kernicterus metabolite signature has been proposed using a voxel placed over the basal ganglia: elevations in taurine (Tau), glutamate (Glu), glutamine (Gln), and myo-inositol relative to creatine (mI/Cr), and a decreased choline relative to creatine (Cho/Cr), with no significant elevation of lactate (essentially ruling out a hypoxic–ischemic encephalopathy) [27]. Kernicterus has also been characterized by decreased ratios of NAA/Cho and NAA/Cr [28] and increased Glu + Gln relative to Cr [21, 28].

Hypoglycemia

Glucose is the primary fuel for energy metabolism in the human brain. Additionally, in the neonatal brain, glucose may be used toward the synthesis of amino acids and lipids via the respective biosynthetic pathways. Although the precise threshold is somewhat controversial, neonatal encephalopathy secondary to hypoglycemia occurs when glucose concentrations fall below 30 mg/dl in the term infant or 20 mg/dl in the preterm infant. The clinical presentation of neonatal hypoglycemia includes stupor, jitteriness, seizures, respiratory abnormalities, and hypotonia. MR imaging can show abnormal edema in the occipital lobes, more discernable on DWI than on conventional imaging, which often progresses to cystic lesions in the occipital or occipital white matter [29]. MRS at the time of insult may be useful for discerning the severity of insult, as an increased lactate–lipid peak and a decreased NAA peak have been reported in the involved areas [30] (Fig. 20.4). It remains to be determined whether lactate and NAA concentrations are predictive of long-term neurodevelopmental outcome in this population.

Inborn Errors of Metabolism

Inborn errors of metabolism usually present with signs and symptoms related to the involvement of one or more of the

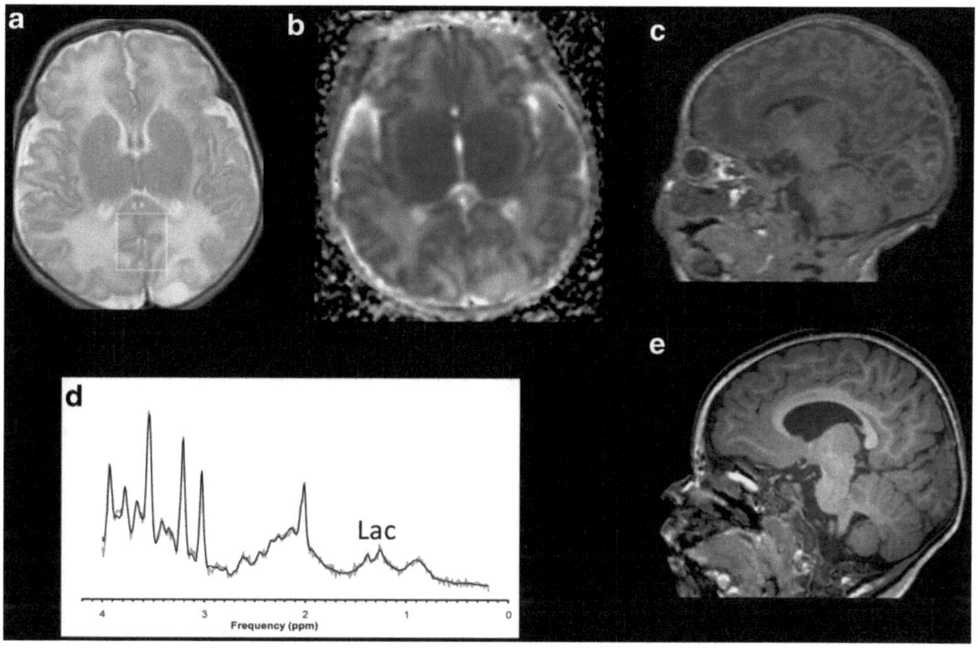

Fig. 20.4 17-day-old ex-36-week preterm infant with history of hypoglycemia and congenital adrenal insufficiency. Conventional MR imaging demonstrates subacute infarcts in the occipital lobes bilaterally, evidenced by low ADC (**b**) and high T1 signal in the pericalcarine cortex and adjacent white matter (**c**). The MR spectrum of "normal" appearing occipital/parietal gray matter rostral and superior to the infarcted cortex showed a slightly above normal lactate (Lac) and below normal NAA. Follow-up imaging at 17 months of age demonstrates a chronic lesion involving the calcarine cortex and subadjacent white matter (**e**)

organ systems, including the central and the peripheral nervous system, the musculoskeletal system, visceral organs (particularly the heart and the liver), and even the skin. Some inborn errors of metabolism exclusively involve the nervous system, but those occur later in life and have not been described in detail in the neonatal period. Inborn errors of metabolism are broadly classified into organic academia, disorders of amino acid oxidation, disorders of fatty acid oxidation, primary lactic acidosis, mitochondria function, lysosomal storage disorders, and peroxisomal disorders [31, 32]. Whereas some inborn errors of metabolism manifest immediately at birth (primary lactic acidosis, type 2 glutaric aciduria, long-chain acyl coenzyme A dehydrogenase, hydroxymethylglutaryl (HMG)-CoA lyase, ornithine transcarbamylase, and carbamyl phosphatase synthetase deficiencies), others take a few days to manifest clinically (isovaleric acidemia, methylmalonic acidemia, propionic acidemia, non-ketotic hyperglycinemia, citrullinemia, argininosuccinic aciduria, and maple syrup urine disease or MSUD).

MRS can provide, as described in more detail for the pediatric population in Chaps. 10–12, valuable information regarding specific metabolites in certain disorders. These include increased branched chain amino acids (l-leucine, l-isoleucine, valine) in MSUD, increased glycine (Gly) in non-ketotic hyperglycinemia, increased NAA in Canavan's disease, and absence of Cr in guanidinoacetate methyltransferase deficiency [33–37].

Peroxisomal disorders that manifest in the neonatal period are primarily due to a failure to form viable peroxisomes, resulting in multiple metabolic abnormalities [38]. Examples of these conditions include Zellweger syndrome and neonatal adrenoleukodystrophy (NALD). Zellweger syndrome is characterized on conventional imaging by delayed myelination, temporal parietal polymicrogyria, and subependymal germinolytic cyst formation in the region of the frontal horns of the lateral ventricles. In NALD, dys- or demyelination in the cerebellar and/or cerebral white matter are characteristic. Given the pathognomonic nature of these findings on conventional radiography, advanced imaging techniques are often not required for a definitive diagnosis of these conditions. In the case of Zellweger syndrome, findings on MRS may include marked decreased NAA in the gray and white matter, thalamus and/or cerebellum. Elevated glutamine and a decreased *myo*-inositol in the gray matter suggest concomitant hepatic dysfunction.

Notably, MRS has detected changes in normal appearing white matter in patients with NALD, suggesting that MRS may be more sensitive than conventional MRI in detecting changes in the white matter associated with disease progression [39], and consequently, better for identifying patients in need of hematopoietic cell transplantation [40].

Neonatal Infection

Infections affecting the neonatal brain can often be distinguished from each other and from their adult counterparts by specific imaging findings [41, 42]. The three major types of neonatal infection are [1] congenital infections (TORCH = *T*oxoplasmosis, *O*ther infections, *R*ubella, *C*ytomegalovirus, *H*erpes simplex), [2] neonatal meningitis, and [3] disseminated fungal infection.

Congenital Infections

TORCH infections are transmitted via direct contact through the birth canal (herpes), hematogenous transplacental transmission (viruses and toxoplasmosis), or by ascending infection from the cervix (bacterial). Their imaging appearance is dependent on the actual timing of infection [41, 42]. For instance, while early gestation infections lead to destructive and developmental lesions, late gestation infections only lead to the former. Cytomegalovirus (CMV), when present at the beginning of the second trimester, is associated with an inflammatory process in the germinal matrix, leading to migration problems and/or a hypoplastic cerebellum. An infection later in pregnancy results in periventricular cystic lesions lined with dystrophic calcification with sparing of the cortex, and is well-visualized on CT. From a neuropathology perspective, the substrates of WMI of prematurity and dysplastic white matter of cytomegalovirus appear to be similar. Congenital CMV infection and WMI of prematurity affect the cerebral white matter in the same developmental period, in which the oligodendrocytes are immature and particularly vulnerable. Both demonstrate increased ADC values, reduced FA values and magnetization transfer ratios, and reduced concentrations of total NAA and Cho; slightly increased myo-inositol concentrations may also be present (Fig. 20.5), which is suggestive of axonal losses, lack of myelin deposition due to oligodendrocytic losses and/or astrogliosis [43].

In a toxoplasmosis infection, calcifications and signal abnormalities are present in the basal ganglia and the periventricular white matter. In contrast, congenital HIV infections are characterized by calcifications in the cortical–subcortical junction and the basal ganglia, which are typically not present at birth. HSV (herpes simplex virus) 2 infection results in severe meningo-encephalitis with ischemic and hemorrhagic infarction which can be detected by diffusion MR imaging. Rubella infection can manifest in a variety of ways, including migration abnormalities, abnormal periventricular signal intensities, cerebellar hypoplasia, and basal ganglia calcifications. Much remains to be discovered about how these lesions impact cerebral metabolic functions in these regions. An example of MRS of a patient with acute HSV encephalitis is shown in Fig. 20.6.

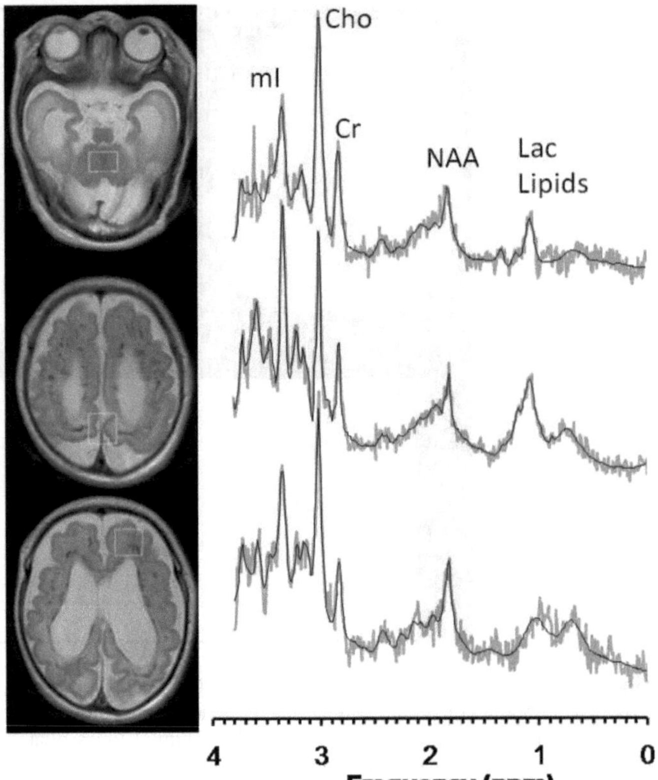

Fig. 20.5 Single voxel MRS (PRESS, TE 35 ms, 1.5 T) of a 1-week-old premature-born (33 weeks gestational age) with a congenital CMV infection

Bacterial Infections

The most common form of CNS bacterial infection in the newborn is bacterial meningitis. [44]. Group B streptococcus and Escherichia coli are the most common pathogens; other pathogens include *Staphylococcus aureus*, *Pseudomonas aeruginosa*, and *Listeria monocytogenes*. As part of this infection, there is irritation of the leptomeninges with subsequent ventriculitis and arachnoiditis. The inflammatory reaction can extend to the vasculature leading to a vasculitis and

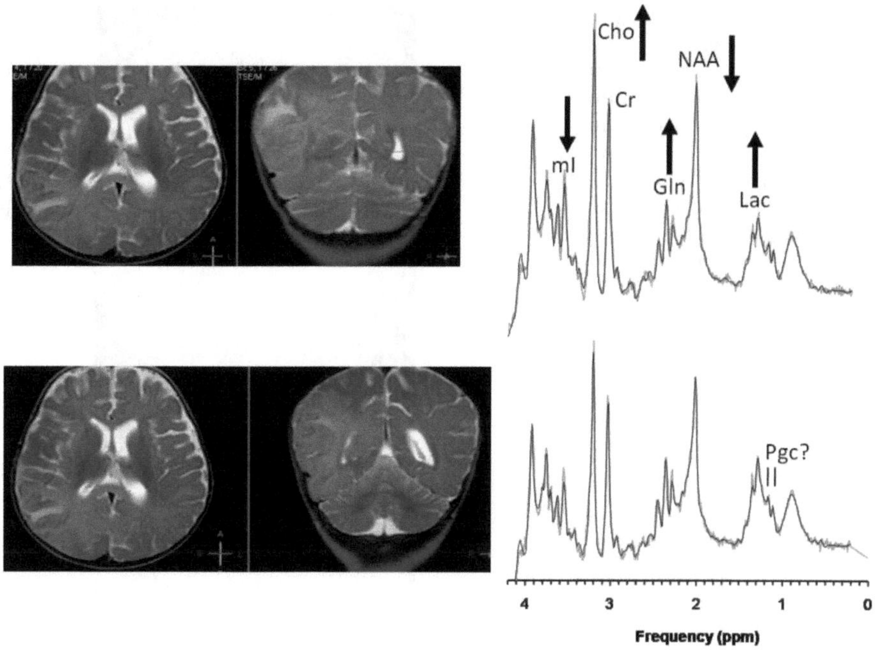

Fig. 20.6 Single voxel MRS (PRESS, TE 35 ms, 3 T) of an 11-month-old baby with acute HSV encephalitis and an associated right lateral temporoparietal infarct. Spectra acquired from non-infarcted tissue in the medial parietooccipital gray matter and left parietal white matter both demonstrate elevated lactate, Gln, and Cho relative to Cr, whereas NAA and mI appear to be reduced. A doublet next to the Lac doublet at approximately 1.1 ppm is consistent with propylene glycol, possibly used as a solvent for drugs administered to this patient

resulting infarction. Diffusion imaging is a useful tool in detecting infarction secondary to meningitis. MRS has not yet been shown to provide additional information in the differential diagnosis or understanding of meningitis in neonates. One study demonstrated a mild elevation in lactate with normal levels of creatine, choline, NAA, and myo-inositol in a patient with meningitis [45]. In our experience, MRS is useful in determining whether meningitis is associated with additional parenchymal involvement (encephalitis) and in the differential diagnosis of intraparenchymal abscess from other intracranial lesions.

Disseminated Fungal Infection

Candida albicans is the most common systemic infection affecting the newborn, affecting 3–5% of low-birth weight infants, with CNS involvement in 64% of cases. Meningitis, ependymitis, and brain parenchymal microabscesses are associated with this infection. These microabscesses can be detected with contrast, T1-weighted imaging and diffusion imaging and usually involve the subcortical, periventricular, and basal ganglia regions. Later stages of this infection can entail severe cavitation of the periventricular white matter. Experimental MRS studies suggest that these lesions might demonstrate elevated lipids and lactate [46].

Migration Disorders

During brain development, neurons that arise at the germinal ventricular zone at the surface of the lateral ventricles migrate to their final locations in the brain. Migration disorders are birth defects where abnormal migration resulted in structurally abnormal or missing areas of the brain. Migration disorders are rarely encountered and very few MR spectroscopy studies have been carried out in this population. In a case report, Shiroishi et al. [47] present data from a 5-day-old neonate with *hemimegalencephaly*. MRI of this patient demonstrated an enlarged right cerebral hemisphere and diffused volume loss in the contralateral hemisphere. MRS of these two hemispheres was distinctly different with relatively higher NAA in right frontal white matter whereas in the contralateral white matter lactate appeared elevated (Fig. 20.7). Spectra obtained from individual patients diagnosed with *holoprosencephaly* and *lissencephaly* are shown in Figs. 20.8 and 20.9. Clearly, more studies are needed to determine whether MRS has a role for a better characterization of migration disorders of the developing brain.

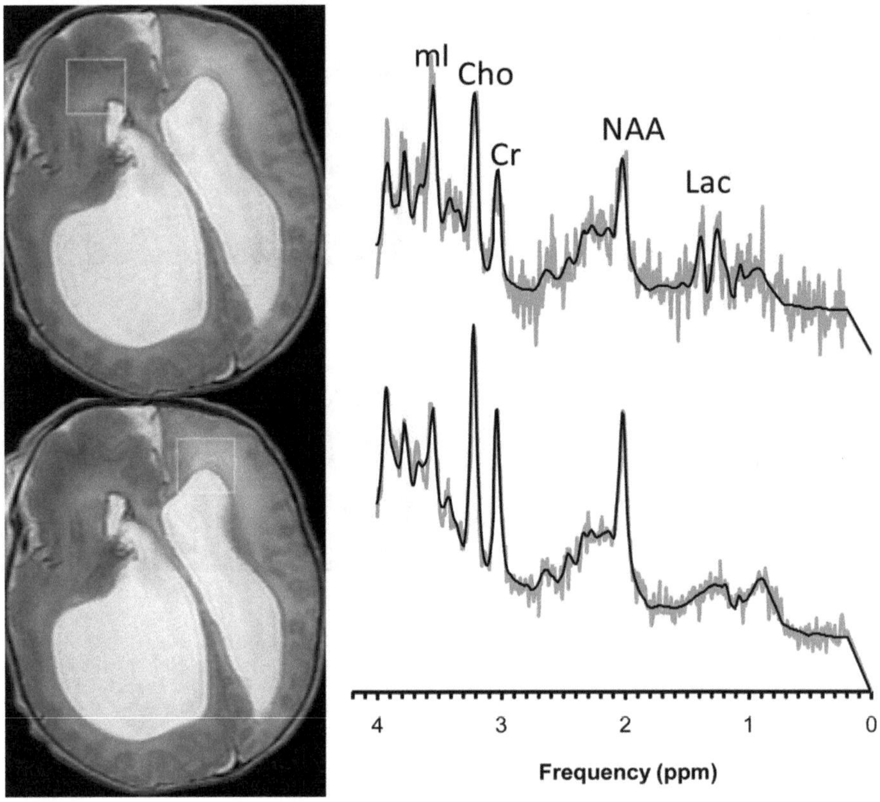

Fig. 20.7 MRI of a patient with hemimegalencephaly demonstrated an enlarged right cerebral hemisphere and diffuse volume loss in the contralateral hemisphere. MRS of these two hemispheres was distinctly different with relatively higher NAA in right frontal white matter whereas in the contralateral white matter lactate appeared elevated

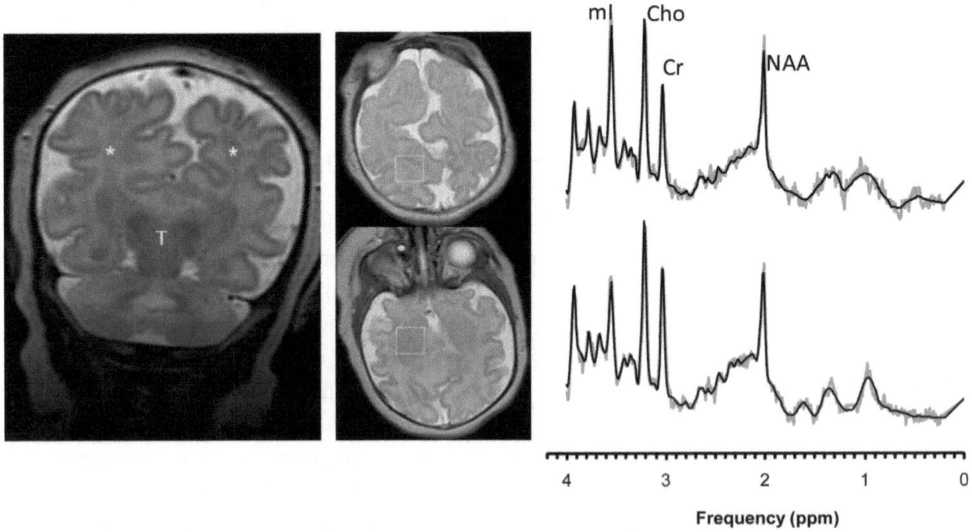

Fig. 20.8 16-day-old term infant with middle hemispheric variant of holoprosencephaly (syntelencephaly). Note the fused thalami (T) and the abnormally migrating cells in the middle of the parietal white matter (*). Single voxel MRS in this patient showed no major abnormalities. Different levels of myo-inositol (mI) in the white matter and basal ganglia spectra are normal

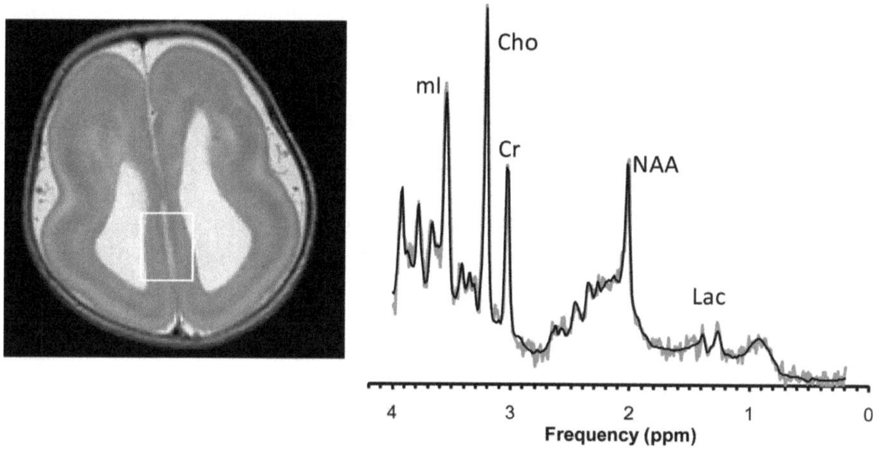

Fig. 20.9 15-day-old ex-36-week preterm with lissencephaly. Note the smooth gyration pattern and abnormal migration pattern. Despite the profoundly abnormal MRI, the MR spectrum is rather unremarkable, except possibly a slightly elevated lactate signal

References

1. Toft PB, Leth H, Peitersen B, Lou HC. Metabolic changes in the striatum after germinal matrix hemorrhage in the preterm infant. Pediatr Res. 1997;41:309–16.
2. Younkin D, Medoff-Cooper B, Guillet R, Sinwell T, Chance B, Delivoria-Papadopoulos M. In vivo 31P nuclear magnetic resonance measurement of chronic changes in cerebral metabolites following neonatal intraventricular hemorrhage. Pediatrics. 1988; 82:331–6.
3. Volpe JJ. Cerebral white matter injury of the premature infant-more common than you think. Pediatrics. 2003;112:176–80.
4. Miller SP, McQuillen PS, Vigneron DB, Glidden DV, Barkovich AJ, Ferriero DM, Hamrick SE, Azakie A, Karl TR. Preoperative brain injury in newborns with transposition of the great arteries. Ann Thorac Surg. 2004;77:1698–706.
5. Beca J, Gunn J, Coleman L, Hope A, Whelan LC, Gentles T, Inder T, Hunt R, Shekerdemian L. Pre-operative brain injury in newborn infants with transposition of the great arteries occurs at rates similar to other complex congenital heart disease and is not related to balloon atrial septostomy. J Am Coll Cardiol. 2009;53: 1807–11.
6. Miller SP, McQuillen PS, Hamrick S, Xu D, Glidden DV, Charlton N, Karl T, Azakie A, Ferriero DM, Barkovich AJ, Vigneron DB. Abnormal brain development in newborns with congenital heart disease. N Engl J Med. 2007;357:1928–38.
7. Licht DJ, Shera DM, Clancy RR, Wernovsky G, Montenegro LM, Nicolson SC, Zimmerman RA, Spray TL, Gaynor JW, Vossough A. Brain maturation is delayed in infants with complex congenital heart defects. J Thorac Cardiovasc Surg. 2009;137:529–36. discussion 536–7.
8. Barkovich AJ. MR imaging of the neonatal brain. Neuroimaging Clin N Am. 2006;16:117–35. viii-ix.
9. Maalouf EF, Duggan PJ, Rutherford MA, Counsell SJ, Fletcher AM, Battin M, Cowan F, Edwards AD. Magnetic resonance imaging of the brain in a cohort of extremely preterm infants. J Pediatr. 1999;135:351–7.
10. Dyet LE, Kennea N, Counsell SJ, Maalouf EF, Ajayi-Obe M, Duggan PJ, Harrison M, Allsop JM, Hajnal J, Herlihy AH, Edwards B, Laroche S, Cowan FM, Rutherford MA, Edwards AD. Natural history of brain lesions in extremely preterm infants studied with serial magnetic resonance imaging from birth and neurodevelopmental assessment. Pediatrics. 2006;118:536–48.
11. Groenendaal F, van der Grond J, Eken P, van Haastert IC, Rademaker KJ, Toet MC, de Vries LS. Early cerebral proton MRS and neurodevelopmental outcome in infants with cystic leukomalacia. Dev Med Child Neurol. 1997;39:373–9.
12. Leth H, Toft PB, Pryds O, Peitersen B, Lou HC, Henriksen O. Brain lactate in preterm and growth-retarded neonates. Acta Paediatr. 1995;84:495–9.
13. Cady EB, Penrice J, Amess PN, Lorek A, Wylezinska M, Aldridge RF, Franconi F, Wyatt JS, Reynolds EO. Lactate, N-acetylaspartate, choline and creatine concentrations, and spin-spin relaxation in thalamic and occipito-parietal regions of developing human brain. Magn Reson Med. 1996;36:878–86.
14. Robertson NJ, Kuint J, Counsell TJ, Rutherford TA, Coutts A, Cox IJ, Edwards AD. Characterization of cerebral white matter damage in preterm infants using 1 H and 31P magnetic resonance spectroscopy. J Cereb Blood Flow Metab. 2000;20:1446–56.
15. Hamilton PA, Hope PL, Cady EB, Delpy DT, Wyatt JS, Reynolds EO. Impaired energy metabolism in brains of newborn infants with increased cerebral echodensities. Lancet. 1986;1:1242–6.
16. Huppi PS, Schuknecht B, Boesch C, Bossi E, Felblinger J, Fusch C, Herschkowitz N. Structural and neurobehavioral delay in postnatal brain development of preterm infants. Pediatr Res. 1996;39: 895–901.
17. Penn AA, Enzmann DR, Hahn JS, Stevenson DK. Kernicterus in a full term infant. Pediatrics. 1994;93:1003–6.
18. Govaert P, Lequin M, Swarte R, Robben S, de Coo R, Weisglas-Kuperus N, de Rijke Y, Sinaasappel M, Barkovich J. Changes in globus pallidus with (pre)term kernicterus. Pediatrics. 2003;112: 1256–63.
19. Coskun A, Yikilmaz A, Kumandas S, Karahan OI, Akcakus M, Manav A. Hyperintense globus pallidus on T1-weighted MR imaging in acute kernicterus: is it common or rare? Eur Radiol. 2005; 15:1263–7.
20. Gkoltsiou K, Tzoufi M, Counsell S, Rutherford M, Cowan F. Serial brain MRI and ultrasound findings: relation to gestational age, bilirubin level, neonatal neurologic status and neurodevelopmental outcome in infants at risk of kernicterus. Early Hum Dev. 2008; 84:829–38.
21. Kamei A, Sasaki M, Akasaka M, Soga N, Kudo K, Chida S. Proton magnetic resonance spectroscopic images in preterm infants with bilirubin encephalopathy. J Pediatr. 2012;160:342–4.
22. Norman MG. Perinatal brain damage. Perspect Pediatr Pathol. 1978;4:41–92.
23. Ahdab-Barmada M, Moossy J. Kernicterus reexamined. Pediatrics. 1983;71:463–4.

24. Ahdab-Barmada M, Moossy J. The neuropathology of kernicterus in the premature neonate: diagnostic problems. J Neuropathol Exp Neurol. 1984;43:45–56.
25. Turkel SB, Miller CA, Guttenberg ME, Moynes DR, Godgman JE. A clinical pathologic reappraisal of kernicterus. Pediatrics. 1982;69: 267–72.
26. Friede R. Developmental neuropathology. New York: Springer; 1989.
27. Oakden WK, Moore AM, Blaser S, Noseworthy MD. 1 H MR spectroscopic characteristics of kernicterus: a possible metabolic signature. AJNR Am J Neuroradiol. 2005;26:1571–4.
28. Wang X, Wu W, Hou BL, Zhang P, Chineah A, Liu F, Liao W. Studying neonatal bilirubin encephalopathy with conventional MRI, MRS, and DWI. Neuroradiology. 2008;50:885–93.
29. Filan PM, Inder TE, Cameron FJ, Kean MJ, Hunt RW. Neonatal hypoglycemia and occipital cerebral injury. J Pediatr. 2006;148: 552–5.
30. Kim SY, Goo HW, Lim KH, Kim ST, Kim KS. Neonatal hypoglycaemic encephalopathy: diffusion-weighted imaging and proton MR spectroscopy. Pediatr Radiol. 2006;36:144–8.
31. Wolf MJ, Wolf B, Beunen G, Casaer P. Neurodevelopmental outcome at 1 year in Zimbabwean neonates with extreme hyperbilirubinaemia. Eur J Pediatr. 1999;158:111–4.
32. Volpe JJ. Neurology of the newborn. Philadelphia: Saunders Elsevier; 2008.
33. Barker PB, Bryan RN, Kumar AJ, Naidu S. Proton NMR spectroscopy of Canavan's disease. Neuropediatrics. 1992;23:263–7.
34. Grodd W, Krägeloh-Mann I, Petersen D, Trefz FK, Harzer K. In vivo assessment of N-acetylaspartate in brain in spongy degeneration (Canavan's disease) by proton spectroscopy. Lancet. 1990;336:437–8.
35. Ensenauer R, Thiel T, Schwab KO, Tacke U, Stockler-Ipsiroglu S, Schulze A, Hennig J, Lehnert W. Guanidinoacetate methyltransferase deficiency: differences of creatine uptake in human brain and muscle. Mol Genet Metab. 2004;82:208–13.
36. Schulze A, Hess T, Wevers R, Mayatepek E, Bachert P, Marescau B, Knopp MV, de Deyn PP, Bremer HJ, Rating D. Creatine deficiency syndrome caused by guanidinoacetate methyltransferase deficiency: diagnostic tools for a new inborn error of metabolism. J Pediatr. 1997;131:626–31.
37. Stöckler S, Holzbach U, Hanefeld F, Marquardt I, Helms G, Requart M, Hänicke W, Frahm J. Creatine deficiency in the brain: a new, treatable inborn error of metabolism. Pediatr Res. 1994;36: 409–13.
38. Bruhn H, Kruse B, Korenke GC, Hanefeld F, Hänicke W, Merboldt KD, Frahm J. Proton NMR spectroscopy of cerebral metabolic alterations in infantile peroxisomal disorders. J Comput Assist Tomogr. 1992;16:335–44.
39. Oz G, Tkác I, Charnas LR, Choi IY, Bjoraker KJ, Shapiro EG, Gruetter R. Assessment of adrenoleukodystrophy lesions by high field MRS in non-sedated pediatric patients. Neurology. 2005;64: 434–41.
40. Moser HW, Barker PB. Magnetic resonance spectroscopy: a new guide for the therapy of adrenoleukodystrophy. Neurology. 2005;64:406–7.
41. Barkovich AJ, Lindan CE. Congenital cytomegalovirus infection of the brain: imaging analysis and embryologic considerations. AJNR Am J Neuroradiol. 1994;15:703–15.
42. Kubota T, Ito M, Maruyama K, Kato Y, Miyajima Y, Ogawa A, Kuno K, Okumura A, Watanabe K. Serial diffusion-weighted imaging of neonatal herpes encephalitis: a case report. Brain Dev. 2007;29:171–3.
43. van der Voorn JP, van der Voom JP, Pouwels PJ, Pouweis R, Vermeulen RJ, Barkhof F, van der Knaap MS, van der Knaap M. Quantitative MR imaging and spectroscopy in congenital cytomegalovirus infection and periventricular leukomalacia suggests a comparable neuropathological substrate of the cerebral white matter lesions. Neuropediatrics. 2009;40:168–73.
44. Weisman LE, Stoll BJ, Cruess DF, Hall RT, Merenstein GB, Hemming VG, Fischer GW. Early-onset group B streptococcal sepsis: a current assessment. J Pediatr. 1992;121:428–33.
45. Ashwal S. Neurologic evaluation of the patient with acute bacterial meningitis. Neurol Clin. 1995;13:549–77.
46. Himmelreich U, Somorjai RL, Dolenko B, Daniel HM, Sorrell TC. A rapid screening test to distinguish between Candida albicans and Candida dubliniensis using NMR spectroscopy. FEMS Microbiol Lett. 2005;251:327–32.
47. Shiroishi MS, Jackson HA, Nelson MD, Bluml S, Panigrahy A. Contralateral hemimicrencephaly in neonatal hemimegalencephaly. Pediatr Radiol. 2010;40:1826–30.

Multinuclear MRS in Children

21

Stefan Blüml

MR imaging and ^{1}H MRS are based on the magnetic moments of the nuclei of hydrogen atoms. However, also other nuclei of atoms with an uneven number of nucleons (protons and neutrons) do have a spin and a detectable magnetic moment when brought into a magnetic field (Table 21.1). Because in vivo MR spectroscopy today is dominated by proton MRS, it is hard to imagine that in the early days of MRS other nuclei, particularly phosphorous (^{31}P) MRS, received far more attention. However, the need for additional expensive equipment, special expertise (PhD on site), the relative low sensitivity (= long scan times), and the ever increasing competition from well-reimbursed clinical MR imaging have pushed MRS methods other than ^{1}H MRS to the side. On the other hand, there is currently a shift from 1.5 T to 3 T or even higher field strengths MR scanners and an effort by manufacturers to provide multinuclear MRS capabilities with *proton-decoupling.*[1] Multinuclear spectroscopy (MNS) benefits from higher field strength and from proton-decoupling considerably and it is therefore expected that there will be a renewed interest in studying important medical and biological question with MNS in the future. Still, because of the additional expertise and resources required, it needs to be emphasized that the use of MNS will almost certainly be limited to a small number of academic centers.

Phosphorous (^{31}P) MRS

The phosphorous nucleus (^{31}P) has 100% natural abundance and approximately 6.63% of the sensitivity of the hydrogen nucleus (Table 21.1). With ^{31}P MRS the energy metabolites adenosine triphosphate ATP, by many biologists considered the most important molecule for life, phosphocreatine (PCr) and inorganic phosphate (Pi) can be measured. From the chemical shift difference between the PCr and Pi peaks the pH of the tissue can be measured quite accurately non-invasively. ^{31}P MRS also allows the observation of phosphomonoesters (PME) and phosphodiesters (PDE). Using a technology termed *proton-decoupling* the phosphomonoesters phosphorylcholine (PC) and phosphorylethanolamine (PE) and the phosphodiesters glycerophosphorylcholine (GPC) and glycerophosphorylethanolamine (GPE) can be observed individually (Fig. 21.1). ^{31}P MRS has been mostly used to study muscle metabolism. Despite the low physiological concentration of ^{31}P in tissue, using surface coils, skeletal muscles have been studied rested and during exercise with a time resolution of a few seconds [1, 2]. Also in the brain, ^{31}P MRS has been used long before ^{1}H MRS became available.

Interestingly, clinical MRS in the human brain began with ^{31}P MR spectroscopy of newborns using smaller magnets not suitable for adults in the mid eighties. Several studies showed that hypoxic–ischemic disease of the brain could be monitored by the changes in high-energy phosphates, Pi and pH [3–5]. These studies also showed that the outcome after severe hypoxic–ischemic injury is determined by the intracerebral pH and Pi/ATP ratio. Wide-bore high-field magnets eventually permitted extension to adults and infants beyond a few weeks of age. ^{31}P MRS in adult stroke exactly mirrored the findings in hypoxic–ischemic disease of newborns, and even appears to offer predictive value through intracellular pH and Pi/ATP [6, 7]. In the subsequent years, also other areas of human neuropathology have been studied by ^{31}P MRS. Oberhaensli et al [8]. overturned three decades of thought about brain tumors in particular, showing their intracellular pH to be generally alkaline not acidic. More recently,

[1] As a result of *J-coupling* (see Chap. 2) between spins, signals are commonly split into *multiplets*. Such multiplets can be collapsed into single lines by applying irradiation at the resonance frequency of the nuclei to which the spins of interest are coupled. Decoupling significantly simplifies the interpretation of spectra and increases the ***S/N***. This can involve considerable irradiation power. Several techniques are described in the literature that allow sufficient decoupling to be carried out without excessive power requirements. Additional S/N gain is achieved by the build-up of a nuclear Overhauser effect (***NOE***). Spin decoupling is most commonly used in ^{13}C MRS.

S. Blüml (✉)
Department of Radiology, Children's Hospital Los Angeles,
Keck School of Medicine, University of Southern California,
Los Angeles, CA, USA
e-mail: SBluml@chla.usc.edu

S. Blüml and A. Panigrahy (eds.), *MR Spectroscopy of Pediatric Brain Disorders*,
DOI 10.1007/978-1-4419-5864-8_21, © Springer Science+Business Media, LLC 2013

Table 21.1 Properties of some of the more commonly observed nuclei

Nucleus	Spin	Gyromagnetic ratio (rel. to ^{1}H)	Frequency at 1.5 T (MHz)	Natural abundance (%)	Sensitivity (rel. to ^{1}H)[a]
^{1}H	½	1	63.86	99.98	1
^{31}P	1/2	0.405	25.85	100	6.63×10^{-2}
^{13}C	½	0.252	16.06	1.11	1.76×10^{-5}
^{19}F	½	0.941	60.08	100	0.83

[a]The sensitivity is proportional to (gyromagnetic ratio)$^3\times$natural abundance

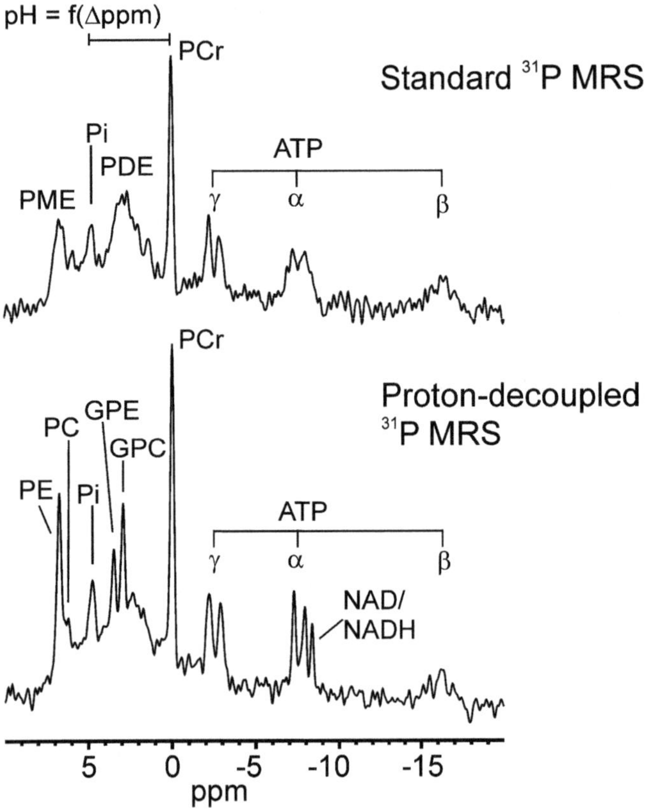

Fig. 21.1 Standard ^{31}P MRS of the brain (*top*) and a ^{31}P MRS spectrum acquired with proton-decoupled of the same volume of tissue with the same acquisition sequence (*bottom*). Standard ^{31}P MRS allows the detection of the energy metabolites phosphocreatine (PCr), adenosine triphosphate (ATP), and inorganic phosphate (Pi). From the chemical shift difference between PCr and Pi, the pH of the tissue can be determined. In addition, broad peaks of phosphomonoesters (PME) and phosphodiesters (PDE) can be observed. Using proton-decoupling, the PME and PDE resonances are resolved and their individual components phosphoethanolamine (PE), phosphocholine (PC) and glycerophosphoethanolamine (GPE), glycerophosphocholine (GPC) can be observed sitting on top of a broader baseline signal, likely membrane phospholipids. Spectra were acquired with a spinecho sequence with a self-refocusing radiofrequency (RF) pulse, an echo time of TE = 2.5 ms, and a repetition time of TR = 2 s. A WALTZ-4 sequence was used for broadband proton-decoupling with a decoupling bandwidth of 500 Hz. The irradiation by WALTZ-4 pulses was continued at a tenfold reduced power level during the recovery period to generate signal enhancement due to the Nuclear Overhauser Effect (NOE). Data were acquired at Children's Hospital Los Angeles

proton-decoupled ^{31}P MRS in pediatric patients (Fig. 21.2) confirmed this observation [9]. Indeed, the pH of untreated tumors was slightly higher (more alkaline) than the pH of normal brain tissue. Proton-decoupled ^{31}P MRS also revealed more details about the composition of the PME and PDE peaks in the ^{31}P spectra of tumors and their relation with the choline peak observed with ^{1}H MRS. It was shown that the PE/GPE and PC/GPC ratios were significantly higher in medulloblastoma than in control tissue or other tumors. Also, mean PC/PE was elevated in tumors relative to normal tissue but there was no difference between medulloblastoma and other tumors. Total choline concentration determined with quantitative ^{1}H MRS was significantly elevated while creatine was reduced in tumors. A quantitative comparison of total phosphorylated cholines (PC + GPC)/ATP measured with ^{31}P MRS and total choline measured with ^{1}H MRS showed that in tumors a large fraction of the choline signal was not accounted for by PC and GPC. The fraction of unaccounted choline was particularly large in medulloblastoma.

The ^{31}P spectrum also undergoes considerable age-dependent changes [10, 11]. Van der Knapp et al. [12] correlated the changes in the ^{31}P PME and PDE and long echo time ^{1}H MRS with the development of myelination. They found decreasing levels of PME and increasing PDE as the brain matures. Using proton-decoupled ^{31}P MRS the individual components of PME and PDE resonances, PE, PC and GPE, GPC, were studied in the developing brain [13].

In the neonate, PE dominated the spectrum and decreased with age along with PC, whereas GPE, GPC, and PCr increased in concentration with postnatal age. Whereas in the newborn the majority of the choline peak detectable by ^{1}H MRS is PC, in the mature brain, GPC accounts for close to 2/3 and PC for 1/3 of total choline. ATP slightly decreased with age whereas inorganic phosphate and the pH did not show significant developmental changes (Fig. 21.3).

Proton-decoupled ^{31}P was also used to study a rare leukodystrophy termed Van der Knaap syndrome [14]. In this disease, extreme rarefaction of white matter is caused by mutations in one of the five subunits of the translation initiation factor 2B (eIF2B). ^{31}P MRS showed that of the metabolites involved in biosynthesis and catabolism of membrane phospholipids, GPE

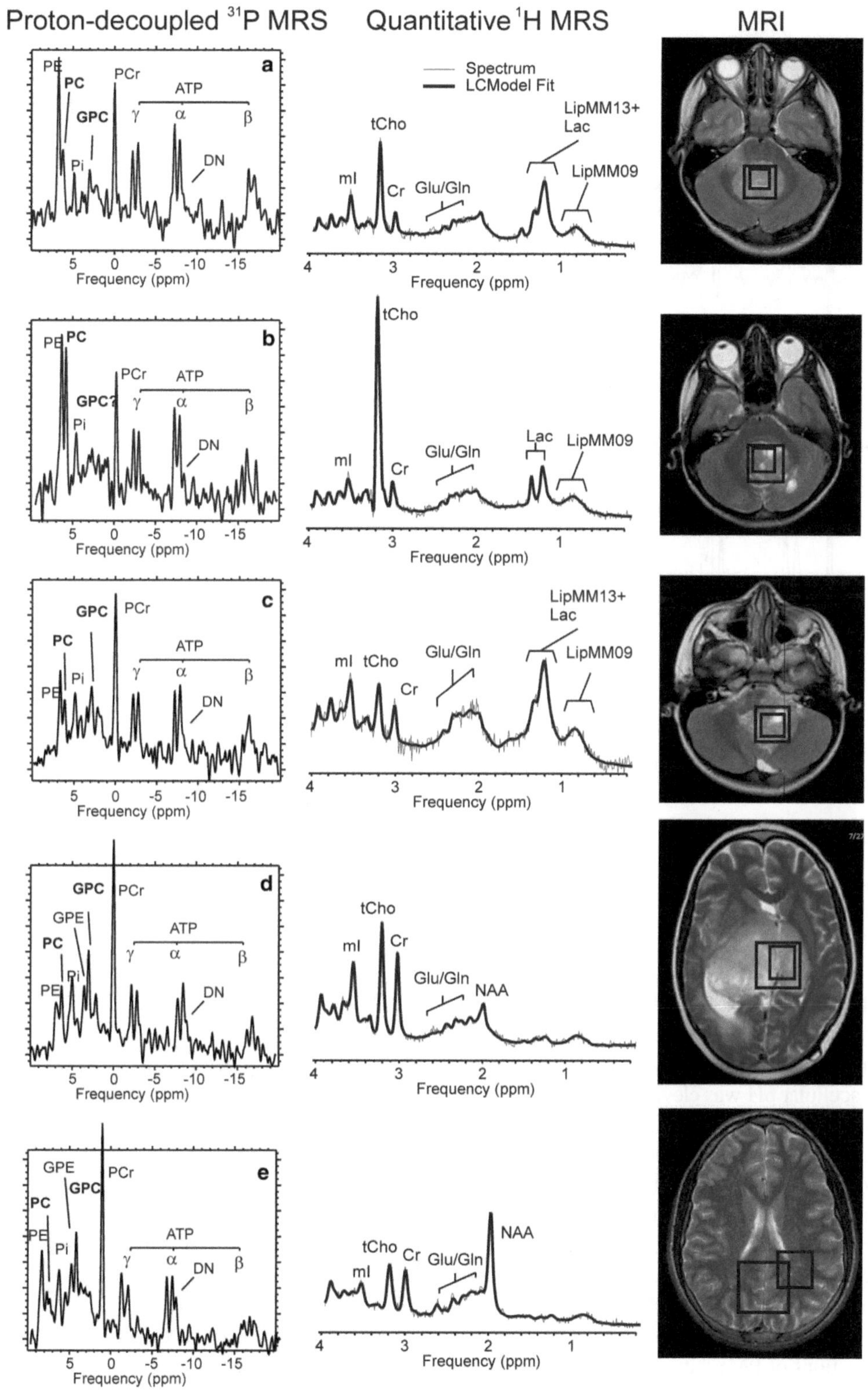

Fig. 21.2 Proton-decoupled ^{31}P MRS, ^{1}H MRS, and MRI of cerebellar medulloblastoma (**a+b**), anaplastic ependymoma (**c**), anaplastic astrocytoma (**d**), and mixed gray/white matter of a control (patient with minor indication for MRI) (**e**). ^{31}P spectra are scaled to ATP as an internal reference. ^{1}H spectra are scaled to measure absolute concentrations to allow direct comparison with each other. Areas or amplitudes of ^{31}P and ^{1}H spectra cannot be directly compared. All spectra were acquired on a clinical 1.5 T scanner. A custom-designed dual tuned head coil was used for clinically indicated MR imaging, proton MRS, and for experimental ^{31}P MRS. The total examination time was approximately 70 min and ^{1}H and ^{31}P acquisitions were integrated in routine pre-operative work-up of patients. ROIs for ^{1}H (*small box*) and ^{31}P are marked on MRI, respectively. *PC* phosphocholine, *GPC* glycerophosphocholine, *PE* phosphoethanolamine, *GPE* glycerophosphoethanolamine, *Pi* inorganic phosphate, *PCr* phosphocreatine, *DN* dinucleotides, *NAA N*-acetyl-aspartate, *mI* myo-inositol (peak may also comprise small amounts of glycine), *tCho* total choline (= PC+GPC+free choline), *Cr* total creatine (= PCr+free Cr), *LipMM13* lipid and macromolecule signal at 1.3 ppm (–CH2- groups), *LipMM09* lipid and macromolecule signal at 0.9 ppm (–CH3 groups), *Lac* lactate. All data were acquired at Children's Hospital Los Angeles

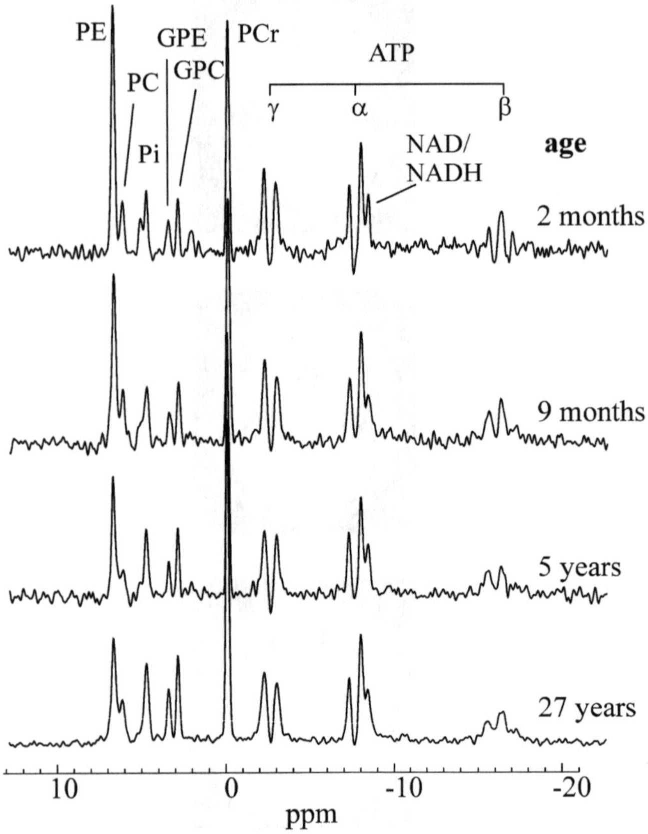

Fig. 21.3 Whereas in the newborn the majority of the choline peak detectable by ^{1}H MRS is PC, in the mature brain, GPC accounts for close to 2/3 and PC for 1/3 of total choline. ATP slightly decreased with age whereas inorganic phosphate and the pH did not show significant developmental changes

was reduced and PE was increased, while the choline containing phosphorylated metabolites, PC and GPC, were unchanged. ATP and inorganic phosphate was reduced and PCr was elevated whereas intracellular pH was elevated (Fig. 21.4).

Minshew et al. [15] studied high-functioning autistic children and adolescents with ^{31}P MRS. They found significantly abnormal levels of phosphorylated metabolites such as PCr. In addition, they found a correlation between test performance and PME and PDE. Specifically, PME was decreasing and PDE was increasing with declining performance scores. In another study by the same group, offspring at risk for schizophrenia or schizoaffective disorder were examined with 31P MRS [16]. Subjects at risk showed reductions of PME but showed signal increases for the broad signal underlying the PME and PDE peaks. However, follow-up studies are needed to determine whether these findings are indeed of predictive value.

Several groups have used ^{31}P MRS to monitor treatment of patients where the biosynthesis of creatine is impaired [17]. The combination of ^{1}H MRS and ^{31}P MRS allows not only monitoring of increasing levels of total creatine and phosphocreatine but at the same time, by monitoring directly Cr and PCr in the brain, the optimum (minimum) dose of Cr intake can be determined for different types of creatine deficiency (e.g., deficient creatine transport versus deficient de novo synthesis of creatine) [18, 19].

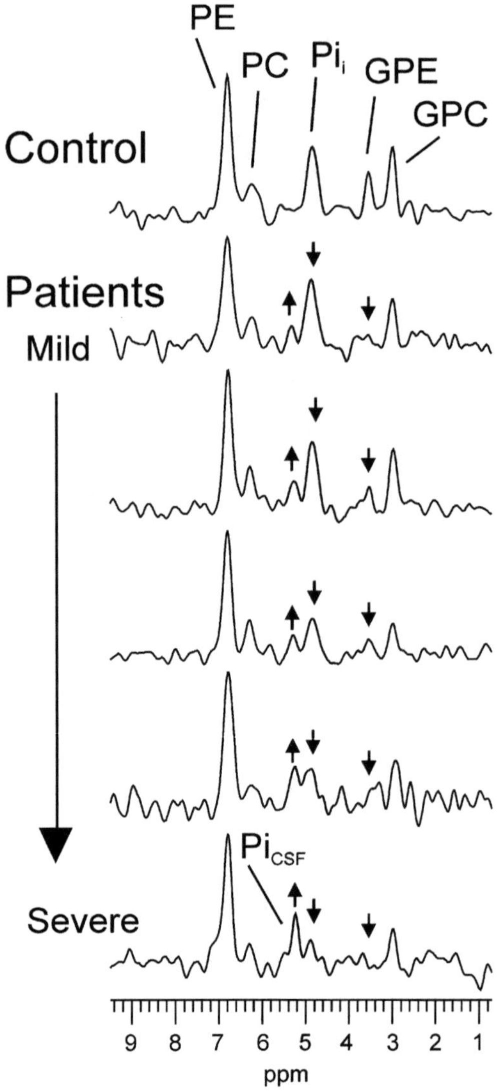

Fig. 21.4 Phosphomonoester/diester region of proton-decoupled ^{31}P MR spectra of individual Van der Knaap syndrome patients and a control. Two peaks from inorganic phosphate are labeled. The inorganic phosphate peak Pi_{CSF} at a chemical shift consistent with a pH of 7.35 of extracellular water and cerebrospinal fluid increases with the severity of the disease quantified here as the extent by which CSF replaced brain tissue in the region of interest. The Pi_i peak is consistent with the Pi peak observed in controls. All data were acquired at Huntington Medical Research Institutes, Pasadena

Carbon (^{13}C) MRS

The application of ^{13}C MRS for basic research/medical applications is challenging and, despite being available for more than twenty-five years, only a few groups have attempted ^{13}C MRS in vivo. ^{13}C MRS has a much lower sensitivity than ^{1}H

MRS (Table 21.1) and the natural abundance of ^{13}C is only 1.1% whereas most of the carbon in tissue is MR-invisible ^{12}C. Although there might be applications for in vivo natural abundance ^{13}C MRS, possibly outside the brain as a noninvasive tool to assess lipid composition [20], to harvest the full potential of ^{13}C MRS, enrichment of metabolites with ^{13}C via intra-venous (i.v.) or oral administration of ^{13}C labeled substrates is necessary.

Glucose is the principal substrate for energy metabolism for both neurons and glia cells in the brain and facilitates the de novo synthesis of many neurochemicals. In normal brain, ^{13}C -labeled glucose (^{13}C-Glc) passes the blood–brain barrier and is readily metabolized through glycolysis and in the tricarboxylic acid (TCA) cycle. ^{13}C enrichment of individual carbon atoms of glutamate, glutamine, aspartate (Asp), NAA, γ-amino butyric acid (GABA), lactate, alanine (Ala), and bicarbonate (HCO_3^-) follows [21–26] (Figs. 21.5 and 21.6). From repeated ^{13}C MR spectra acquired during studies over 2–3 h, the in vivo rates of several of the principal bioenergetic pathways of normal adult brain have been determined [22, 23, 27]. The interested reader is referred to an entire issue of NMR in Biomedicine [28] for more details about the methods and recent advances of ^{13}C MRS.

The future role of ^{13}C glucose MRS as a clinical tool to study *diseased brain* remains a matter of speculation considering the technical challenges. Only a very small number of patient studies have been performed. In adults, striking abnormalities in glucose metabolism and glutamate and glutamine label accumulation were observed in patients with chronic hepatic encephalopathy. In children, glucose oxidation was reduced in a juvenile with hypoxic injury and in a premature infant. Abnormalities were also detected in pediatric patients with leukodystrophies and in children with mitochondrial disorders [25, 26]. The information obtained from following the fate of ^{13}C labeled glucose goes beyond that of providing a rate for energy production. A tight coupling between cerebral glucose metabolism and glutamate neurotransmitter flux in humans has been proposed by Magistretti et al [29]. Aspartate (a neurotransmitter?) can be studied in vivo in humans by its ^{13}C label accumulation. The role of NAA in mammalian brain, a neuronal/axonal marker which is central for its diagnostic power in ^{1}H MRS, is incompletely understood. NAA synthesis can be measured with ^{13}C MRS after glucose infusion in a clinical setting. Moreno et al [30]. reported that the NAA synthesis rate in children with Canavan disease is lower than in normal brain.

The application of ^{13}C MRS after substrate infusion is by no means limited to glucose. Glucose is convenient because of its rapid oxidation and the fast appearance of ^{13}C label in its metabolites and its non-toxicity even at extremely high concentrations. However, the use of other substrates may further enhance the potential of ^{13}C MRS as a research and diagnostic tool in human brain disease. The candidate next best to glu-

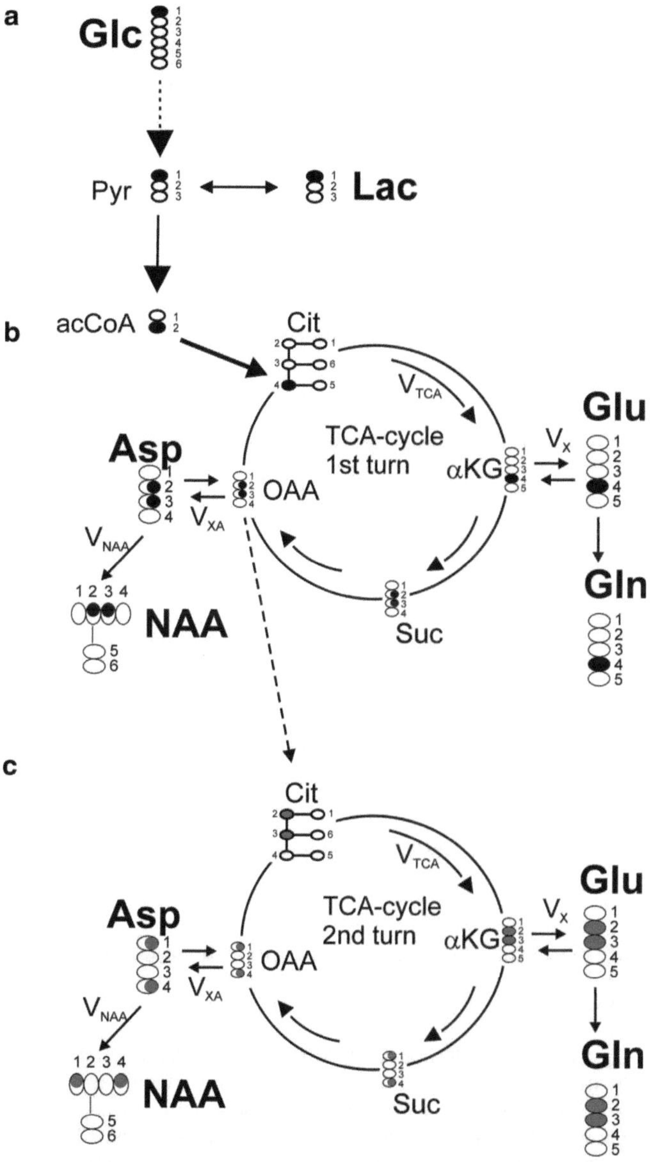

Fig. 21.5 The breakdown of glucose and ^{13}C label accumulation in glucose breakdown products is illustrated for a glucose molecule where the ^{12}C at C1-position of the molecule has been replaced with ^{13}C (1-^{13}C-Glc). Glycolysis breaks down the glucose molecule into two pyruvate molecules (**a**). One of the two pyruvate molecules is labeled at the C_1-position, the other pyruvate molecule is unlabled. From there the ^{13}C labeled can be transferred to lactate (detectable if there is a significant concentration of lactate in tissue). The ^{13}C label enters the TCA-cycle at the C_4-position of citrate (**b**). From there the label is transferred to the C_4-position α-ketoglutarate (α-KG) which is in fast exchange with glutamate C_4.In vivo concentrations of glutamate are high and glutamate C_4 is generally the first peak detectable in this particular experiment using 1-^{13}C-Glc. From glutamate C_4 the ^{13}C-label moves to glutamine C_4. Within the TCA-cycle, is transferred with equal probability from the asymmetric α-KG C_4 to the C_2 and C_3 positions of succinate (Suc) and than oxaloacetate (OAA). From there, 13C label can go to aspartate (Asp) and NAA C_2 and C_3. ^{13}C label remaining in the TCA-cycle will start the second turn at the C_2 and C_3 positions of citrate (**c**). Label accumulation at α-KG $C_{2,3}$, glutamate $C_{2,3}$, glutamine $C_{2,3}$ follows. During the 2nd turn of the TCA-cycle also other positions of Asp and NAA accumulate label. ^{13}C label leaves the TCA-cycle during the third turn (not shown) as bicarbonate when also the C_1 positions of glutamate and glutamine accumulate label

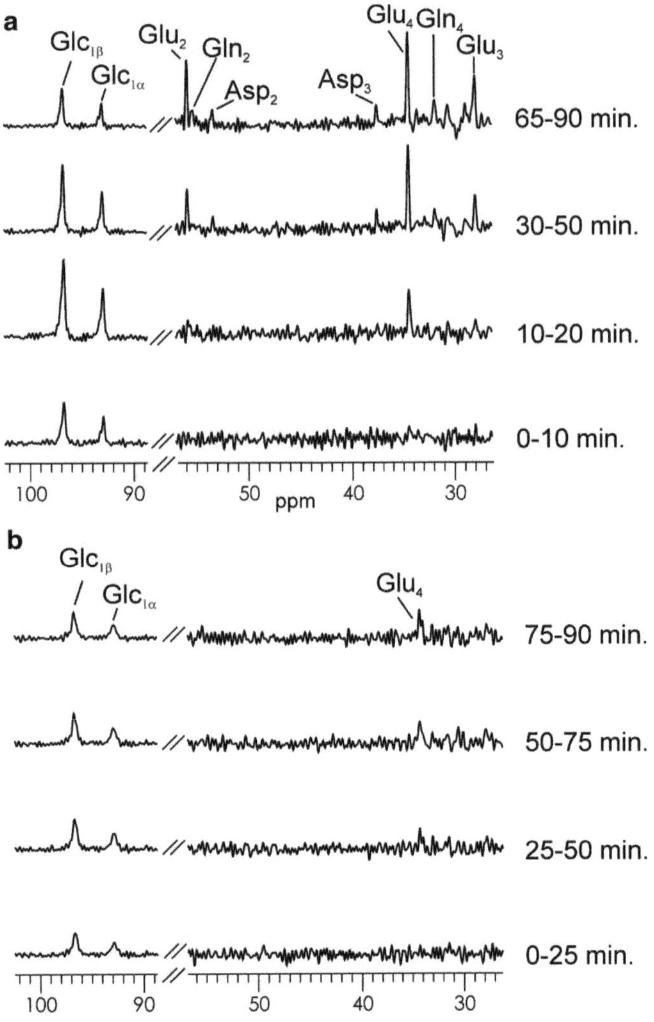

Fig. 21.6 Proton-decoupled ^{13}C MR spectra of adult (**a**) and newborn (**b**) after 1-^{13}C labeled glucose infusion are shown. As ^{13}C-enriched glucose enters the brain, peaks of the two isomers of glucose appear in the spectra within a few minutes after the (here intra-venous) administration of the substrate. Thereafter peaks form the various carbons of glutamate, glutamine, and aspartate become detectable. In this particular experiment, the glutamate C_4 carbon accumulates label in the first turn of the TCA-cycle (cf. Fig. 5) and is thus detected first. In the premature infant, retrospectively classified as neurologically normal, glucose uptake is markedly prolonged and its breakdown slowed-down when compared with an adult control. All spectra were acquired on a 1.5 T scanner using a home-built dual-tuned ^{13}C–^{1}H surface coil arrangement. Using a pulse-and-acquire sequence, baseline spectra and spectra during and after infusion of ^{13}C-enriched glucose were obtained. Difference spectra were calculated to remove the prominent lipid signal and to highlight the ^{13}C label accumulation at the various positions of TCA-cycle intermediates. Peak heights can be converted to concentrations of ^{13}C labeled compounds. From concentration vs. time curves, metabolic flux rates can be determined. All data were acquired at Huntington Medical Research Institutes, Pasadena

cose appears to be acetate [31, 32]. Acetate (Ac) is metabolized to acetyl-CoA only in the glial compartment [33]. Using the same MR technique as for ^{13}C-glucose, glial acetate metabolism can be investigated in normal and diseased brain. ^{13}C label accumulation in HCO_3, in Glu C_5 and Gln C_5 (first turn of the TCA-cycle), and in Glu C_1 and Gln C_1 (second turn) can be observed after [1-^{13}C] Ac in fusion. The rate of Ac oxidation in human brain was estimated to be ≈20% of the total neuronal/glial TCA-cycle rate in fasted human brain [31, 32]. Recently it was demonstrated that Glu C_5 and Gln C_5, which are primarily derived from acetate in the glial compartment, accumulated more in patients on ketogenic diet (KD) than in controls, whilst accumulation of bicarbonate was similar or lower [31] (Fig. 21.7). These results are consistent with altered glutamate–glutamine neutrotransmitter cycling and adaptation to ketogenic diet with up-regulation of acetate oxidation relative to glucose oxidation. KD is a treatment option for epileptic patients, which is particularly effective in children. The biochemical mechanisms why KD improves seizure activity are incompletely understood. In vivo ^{13}C MRS may elucidate a possibly biochemical basis for reduction in seizures during KD therapy. These studies indicate that ^{13}C MRS is an appropriate tool to investigate diseases which are believed to originate in glial cells. Together with data from glucose infusion experiments this could result in a more complete understanding of cerebral metabolism in normal and diseased human brain.

Read This Before Attempting ^{13}C MRS

^{13}C MRS requires expensive additional equipment and considerable technical expertise. Even when technical obstacles have been resolved, the investigator still needs to plan any study very carefully. In vivo ^{13}C studies, in particular of humans requiring large amounts of ^{13}C labeled substrates, are expensive, lengthy, and the subsequent data analysis requires a considerable effort. To avoid frustration and jeopardizing the success of a ^{13}C experiment, all "peripheral" steps of a study need to be planned with due diligence as the acquisition of the ^{13}C spectra. Depending on the biological question, it needs to be decided what substrate should be infused for how long and in what fashion. For some applications oral administration may be appropriate [34, 35], which would simplify the procedure considerably because one inter-venous (i.v.) infusion line could be eliminated. For studies of humans, i.v. administered substrates need to be prepared with great care, kept refrigerated, and used within a couple of days. It is usually necessary to determine fractional ^{13}C enrichment of the substrate in plasma. Therefore the drawing, storage, and analysis of blood samples need to be planned. A new investigator is advised to carefully read the "Methods" sections of previous publications [22, 23, 36] and references therein.

With the dramatically improved stability of MR systems other approaches to dynamic MRS might be feasible. Recently, it has been demonstrated that standard FDA approved proton MRS can be used to monitor ^{13}C label accumulation after ^{13}C glucose administration [37] (Fig. 21.8). No additional hardware or special MR sequences are required. However, it is acknowl-

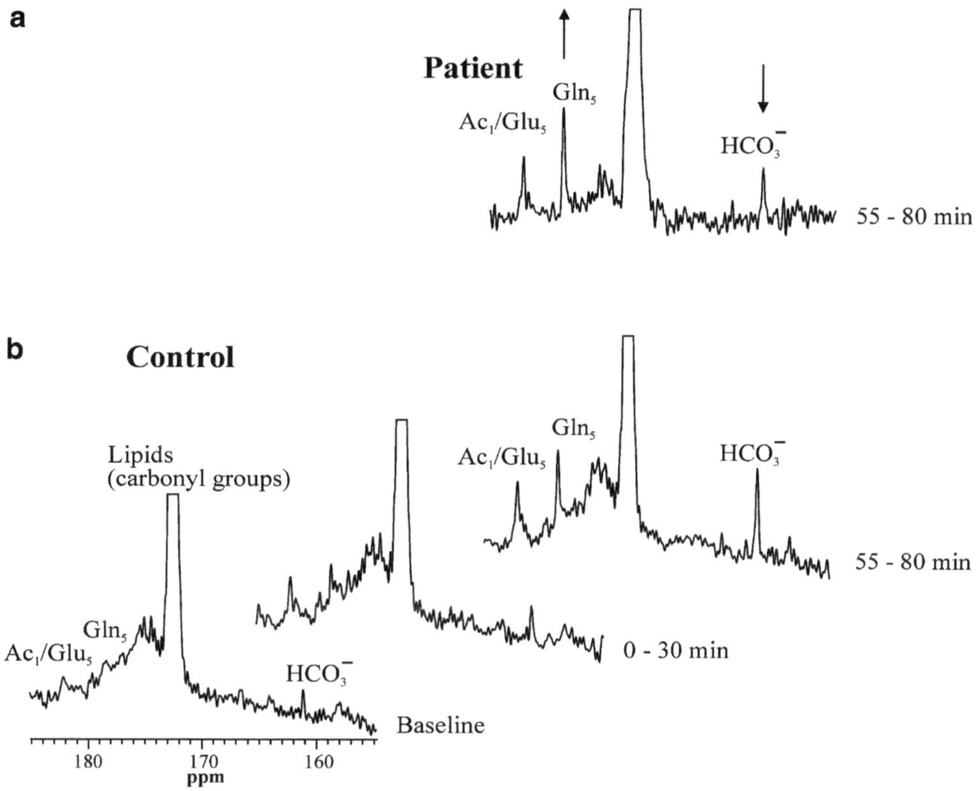

Fig. 21.7 Shown are proton-decoupled ^{13}C spectra acquired before (**a**, *bottom*) and after infusion of 1-^{13}C-acetate (**a**, *middle and upper trace*) in a control and pediatric patient with seizures on ketogenic diet. Infusion of 1-^{13}C-Ac results in label accumulation in glutamate C_5 and glutamine C_5 and bicarbonate. There appears to be more ^{13}C label accumulation in glutamine C_5 in the patient than in the control. All data were acquired at Huntington Medical Research Institutes, Pasadena

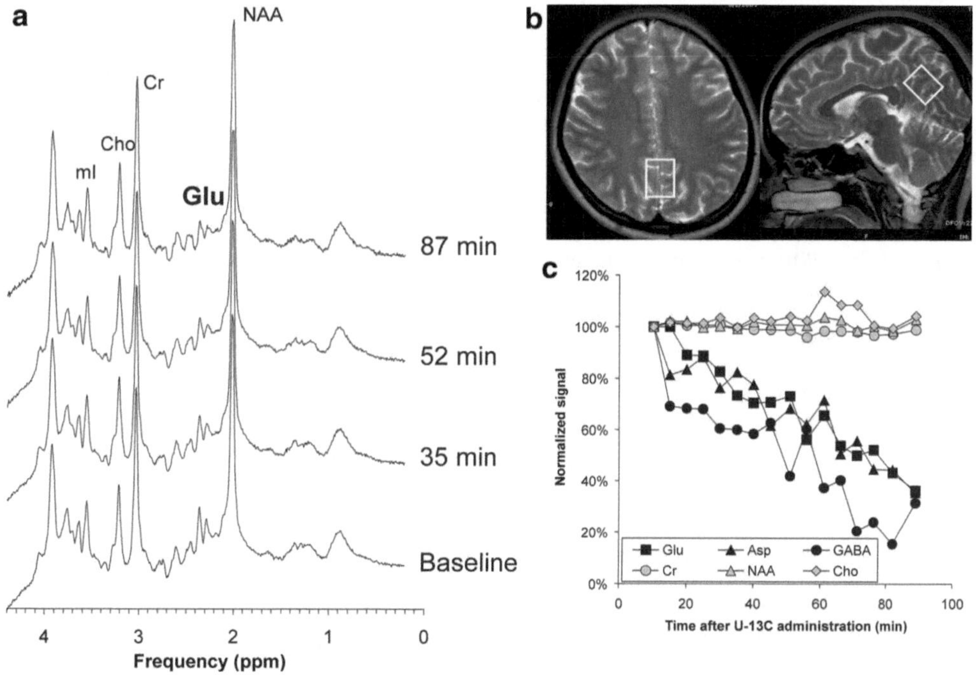

Fig. 21.8 Illustrated is the indirect detection of ^{13}C label accumulation with standard ^1H MRS. Shown are spectra obtained from mostly occipital gray matter (**a**, **b**) at baseline and after oral ^{13}C-labeled glucose administration. ^{13}C label accumulated in breakdown products of Glc, such as glutamate. Due to heteronuclear ^{13}C–^1H J-coupling, intensity is spread to sidebands and ^{13}C accumulation can be detected indirectly as an apparent reduction of the proton glutamate, aspartate, GABA signal (**c**). Data were acquired at Children's Hospital Los Angeles

edged that the simplicity of this approach comes at the cost of a vastly inferior specificity when compared with more advanced approaches such as direct ^{13}C detection, polarization transfer, and methods that employ more complex editing for indirect detection (1–4) [25, 38–40]. Still, this method may be useful to answer important biological questions in clinical settings where the logistical challenges of more advanced methods cannot be overcome.

Fluorine (^{19}F)

Fluorine (^{19}F) has 100% natural abundance and the sensitivity of ^{19}F MRS is comparable with that of ^{1}H MRS. On the other hand, the physiological concentration of ^{19}F in tissue is practically zero. Thus, ^{19}F MRS is only feasible after administration of ^{19}F containing compounds. This has the advantage that the metabolism of these compounds can be observed practically without any background signal. In this context, a possible application is the monitoring of chemotherapies with 5-Fluorouracil (5FU) with ^{19}F MRS in cancer [41–43] outside of the brain. To the best of our knowledge, ^{19}F MRS studies of the brain in children have not been performed.

References

1. Ross BD, Radda GK, Gadian DG, Rocker G, Esiri M, Falconer-Smith J. Examination of a case of suspected McArdle's syndrome by 31P nuclear magnetic resonance. N Engl J Med. 1981;304(22):1338–42.
2. Gadian D, Radda G, Ross B, et al. Examination of a myopathy by phosphorus nuclear magnetic resonance. Lancet. 1981;2(8250):774–5.
3. Hamilton PA, Hope PL, Cady EB, Delpy DT, Wyatt JS, Reynolds EO. Impaired energy metabolism in brains of newborn infants with increased cerebral echodensities. Lancet. 1986;1(8492):1242–6.
4. Cady EB, Costello AM, Dawson MJ, et al. Non-invasive investigation of cerebral metabolism in newborn infants by phosphorus nuclear magnetic resonance spectroscopy. Lancet. 1983;1(8333):1059–62.
5. Hope PL, Costello AM, Cady EB, et al. Cerebral energy metabolism studied with phosphorus NMR spectroscopy in normal and birth-asphyxiated infants. Lancet. 1984;2(8399):366–70.
6. Levine SR, Welch KM, Helpern JA, et al. Prolonged deterioration of ischemic brain energy metabolism and acidosis associated with hyperglycemia: human cerebral infarction studied by serial 31P NMR spectroscopy. Ann Neurol. 1988;23(4):416–8.
7. Martin GB, Paradis NA, Helpern JA, Nowak RM, Welch KM. Nuclear magnetic resonance spectroscopy study of human brain after cardiac resuscitation. Stroke. 1991;22(4):462–8.
8. Oberhaensli RD, Hilton-Jones D, Bore PJ, Hands LJ, Rampling RP, Radda GK. Biochemical investigation of human tumours in vivo with phosphorus-31 magnetic resonance spectroscopy. Lancet. 1986;2(8497):8–11.
9. Albers MJ, Krieger MD, Gonzalez-Gomez I, et al. Proton-decoupled (31)P MRS in untreated pediatric brain tumors. Magn Reson Med. 2005;53(1):22–9.
10. Boesch C, Gruetter R, Martin E, Duc G, Wuthrich K. Variations in the in vivo P-31 MR spectra of the developing human brain during postnatal life. Work in progress. Radiology. 1989;172(1):197–9.
11. Longo R, Ricci C, Dalla Palma L, et al. Quantitative 31P MRS of the normal adult human brain. Assessment of interindividual differences and ageing effects. NMR Biomed. 1993;6(1):53–7.
12. van der Knaap MS, van der Grond J, van Rijen PC, Faber JA, Valk J, Willemse K. Age-dependent changes in localized proton and phosphorus MR spectroscopy of the brain. Radiology. 1990;176(2):509–15.
13. Bluml S, Seymour KJ, Ross BD. Developmental changes in choline- and ethanolamine-containing compounds measured with proton-decoupled (31)P MRS in in vivo human brain. Magn Reson Med. 1999;42(4):643–54.
14. Bluml S, Philippart M, Schiffmann R, Seymour K, Ross BD. Membrane phospholipids and high-energy metabolites in childhood ataxia with CNS hypomyelination. Neurology. 2003;61(5):648–54.
15. Minshew NJ, Goldstein G, Dombrowski SM, Panchalingam K, Pettegrew JW. A preliminary 31P MRS study of autism: evidence for undersynthesis and increased degradation of brain membranes. Biol Psychiatry. 1993;33(11–12):762–73.
16. Keshavan MS, Stanley JA, Montrose DM, Minshew NJ, Pettegrew JW. Prefrontal membrane phospholipid metabolism of child and adolescent offspring at risk for schizophrenia or schizoaffective disorder: an in vivo 31P MRS study. Mol Psychiatry. 2003;8(3):316–23. 251.
17. Bianchi MC, Tosetti M, Fornai F, et al. Reversible brain creatine deficiency in two sisters with normal blood creatine level. Ann Neurol. 2000;47(4):511–3.
18. Bianchi MC, Tosetti M, Battini R, et al. Treatment monitoring of brain creatine deficiency syndromes: a 1 H- and 31P-MR spectroscopy study. AJNR Am J Neuroradiol. 2007;28(3):548–54.
19. Stöckler S, Holzbach U, Hanefeld F, et al. Creatine deficiency in the brain: a new, treatable inborn error of metabolism. Pediatr Res. 1994;36(3):409–13.
20. Moonen CT, Dimand RJ, Cox KL. The noninvasive determination of linoleic acid content of human adipose tissue by natural abundance carbon-13 nuclear magnetic resonance. Magn Reson Med. 1988;6(2):140–57.
21. Beckmann N, Turkalj I, Seelig J, Keller U. 13C NMR for the assessment of human brain glucose metabolism in vivo. Biochemistry. 1991;30(26):6362–6.
22. Mason GF, Gruetter R, Rothman DL, Behar KL, Shulman RG, Novotny EJ. Simultaneous determination of the rates of the TCA cycle, glucose utilization, alpha-ketoglutarate/glutamate exchange, and glutamine synthesis in human brain by NMR. J Cereb Blood Flow Metab. 1995;15(1):12–25.
23. Gruetter R, Seaquist ER, Kim S, Ugurbil K. Localized in vivo 13C-NMR of glutamate metabolism in the human brain: initial results at 4 tesla. Dev Neurosci. 1998;20(4–5):380–8.
24. Pan JW, Stein DT, Telang F, et al. Spectroscopic imaging of glutamate C4 turnover in human brain. Magn Reson Med. 2000;44(5):673–9.
25. Bluml S, Moreno A, Hwang J-H, Ross BD. 1-(13)C glucose magnetic resonance spectroscopy of pediatric and adult brain disorders. NMR Biomed. 2001;14(1):19–32.
26. Blüml S, Moreno-Torres A, Ross B. [1-13C]glucose MRS in chronic hepatic encephalopathy in man. Magn Reson Med. 2001;45(6):981–93.
27. Shen J, Petersen KF, Behar KL, et al. Determination of the rate of the glutamate/glutamine cycle in the human brain by in vivo 13C NMR. Proc Natl Acad Sci USA. 1999;96(14):8235–40.
28. NMR Biomed. 2003;16(6–7):301–457.
29. Magistretti PJ, Pellerin L, Rothman DL, Shulman RG. Energy on demand. Science. 1999;283(5401):496–7.
30. Moreno A, Ross B, Blüml S. Direct determination of the N-acetyl-L-aspartate synthesis rate in the human brain by (13)C MRS and [1-(13)C]glucose infusion. J Neurochem. 2001;77(1):347–50.
31. Bluml S, Moreno-Torres A, Shic F, Nguy CH, Ross BD. Tricarboxylic acid cycle of glia in the in vivo human brain. NMR Biomed. 2002;15(1):1–5.

32. Lebon V, Petersen KF, Cline GW, et al. Astroglial contribution to brain energy metabolism in humans revealed by 13C nuclear magnetic resonance spectroscopy: elucidation of the dominant pathway for neurotransmitter glutamate repletion and measurement of astrocytic oxidative metabolism. J Neurosci. 2002;22(5):1523–31.
33. Muir D, Berl S, Clarke DD. Acetate and fluoroacetate as possible markers for glial metabolism in vivo. Brain Res. 1986;380(2):336–40.
34. Watanabe H, Umeda M, Ishihara Y, et al. Human brain glucose metabolism mapping using multislice 2D (1)H-(13)C correlation HSQC spectroscopy. Magn Reson Med. 2000;43(4):525–33.
35. Moreno A, Blüml S, Hwang J, Ross B. Alternative 1-(13)C glucose infusion protocols for clinical (13)C MRS examinations of the brain. Magn Reson Med. 2001;46(1):39–48.
36. Mason GF, Falk Petersen K, de Graaf RA, et al. A comparison of (13) C NMR measurements of the rates of glutamine synthesis and the tricarboxylic acid cycle during oral and intravenous administration of [1-(13)C]glucose. Brain Res Brain Res Protoc. 2003;10(3):181–90.
37. Nagasunder AC, Panigrahy A, Boumezbeur F, Nelson MD, Bluml S. Serial proton MRS of the human brain after oral administration of 12C and 13C enriched glucose. Paper presented at: International Society of Magnetic Resonance in Medicine (ISMRM)2011; Montreal, Canada.
38. Gruetter R, Novotny EJ, Boulware SD, et al. Localized 13C NMR spectroscopy in the human brain of amino acid labeling from D-[1-13C]glucose. J Neurochem. 1994;63(4):1377–85.
39. Rothman DL, Behar KL, Hetherington HP, et al. 1 H-Observe/13C-decouple spectroscopic measurements of lactate and glutamate in the rat brain in vivo. Proc Natl Acad Sci USA. 1985;82:1633–7.
40. Gruetter R, Adriany G, Merkle H, Andersen PM. Broadband decoupled, 1 H-localized 13C MRS of the human brain at 4 Tesla. [erratum appears in Magn Reson Med 1997 Feb;37(2):267]. Magn Reson Med. 1996;36(5):659–64.
41. Stevens AN, Morris PG, Iles RA, Sheldon PW, Griffiths JR. 5-fluorouracil metabolism monitored in vivo by 19 F NMR. Br J Cancer. 1984;50(1):113–7.
42. Wolf W, Albright MJ, Silver MS, Weber H, Reichardt U, Sauer R. Fluorine-19 NMR spectroscopic studies of the metabolism of 5-fluorouracil in the liver of patients undergoing chemotherapy. Magn Reson Imaging. 1987;5(3):165–9.
43. Semmler W, Bachert-Baumann P, Gückel F, et al. Real-time follow-up of 5-fluorouracil metabolism in the liver of tumor patients by means of F-19 MR spectroscopy. Radiology. 1990;174(1):141–5.

Part III

Case Reports: Introduction

22 Case Reports

Stefan Blüml and Ashok Panigrahy

This section consists of a selection of individual cases we deem to be interesting and educational examples for the use of MR spectroscopy in a clinical or research environment. Some of the case studies are complex including follow-up with several MRS studies whereas often only a single study was available for review. There are a few caveats for the reader. First, findings in individual patients may be incidental and thus should not be generalized. When selecting the cases we did not always look for the most typical studies but for the more striking cases. Second, whenever available, final diagnoses/outcomes are provided. Still, in a substantial number of cases that information, as of today, is not available. We nevertheless decided to include such cases. Under the head Interpretation/Discussion, the findings as filed in the medical records of a patient at the time of the study are summarized. This may also include interpretations that turned out to be incorrect (which we acknowledge)—illustrating pitfalls and opportunities. In addition, essentially for all spectra, absolute concentrations of metabolites were available and used for the original interpretation of MRS. We have omitted information about absolute concentrations whenever we deemed absolute quantitation not essential to arrive at a final interpretation. MRS remains a technically challenging modality. For that reason we also included cases where MRS studies were incomplete or failed for technical or other reasons. The "natural" strategy for the interpretation of MRS, in our opinion, is to consider clinical information and to look at the MRI first, followed by reviewing spectra. We have generally followed this strategy when presenting the cases. Essentially all spectra were acquired and processed using the same methodology, which simplifies the interpretation of the studies. All cases were selected from a database of more than 3,000 pediatric cases studied at Children's Hospital Los Angeles between 2001 and 2011.

Case 1: Classic Medulloblastoma, Typical and Atypical

Clinical Background

Three pediatric patients with newly diagnosed, untreated tumors of the posterior fossa.

MRS Method

1.5 T, single-voxel PRESS, TE 35 ms, lesion.

Interpretation/Discussion

All three lesions were subsequently resected and the tissue samples were interpreted to be consistent with *classic medulloblastoma.* These cases are shown to illustrate the metabolic/biologic heterogeneity even within medulloblastomas of the *same subtype*. The framed spectrum in the center is the most typical and most likely appearance of a classic medulloblastoma (Fig. 22.1). It is possible to observe spectra that are substantially different in their appearance. Here medulloblastoma spectra with very low and very high Tau are shown. The inset shows the histogram of Tau concentrations measured at Children's Hospital LA in classic medulloblastoma. As expected, it follows a normal (Gaussian)

S. Blüml (✉)
Department of Radiology, Children's Hospital Los Angeles, Keck School of Medicine, University of Southern California, Los Angeles, CA, USA

A. Panigrahy
Department of Pediatric Radiology, Children's Hospital of Pittsburgh of UPMC, Pittsburgh, PA, USA

Department of Radiology, University of Pittsburgh School of Medicine, Pittsburgh, PA, USA

S. Blüml and A. Panigrahy (eds.), *MR Spectroscopy of Pediatric Brain Disorders*, DOI 10.1007/978-1-4419-5864-8_22, © Springer Science+Business Media, LLC 2013

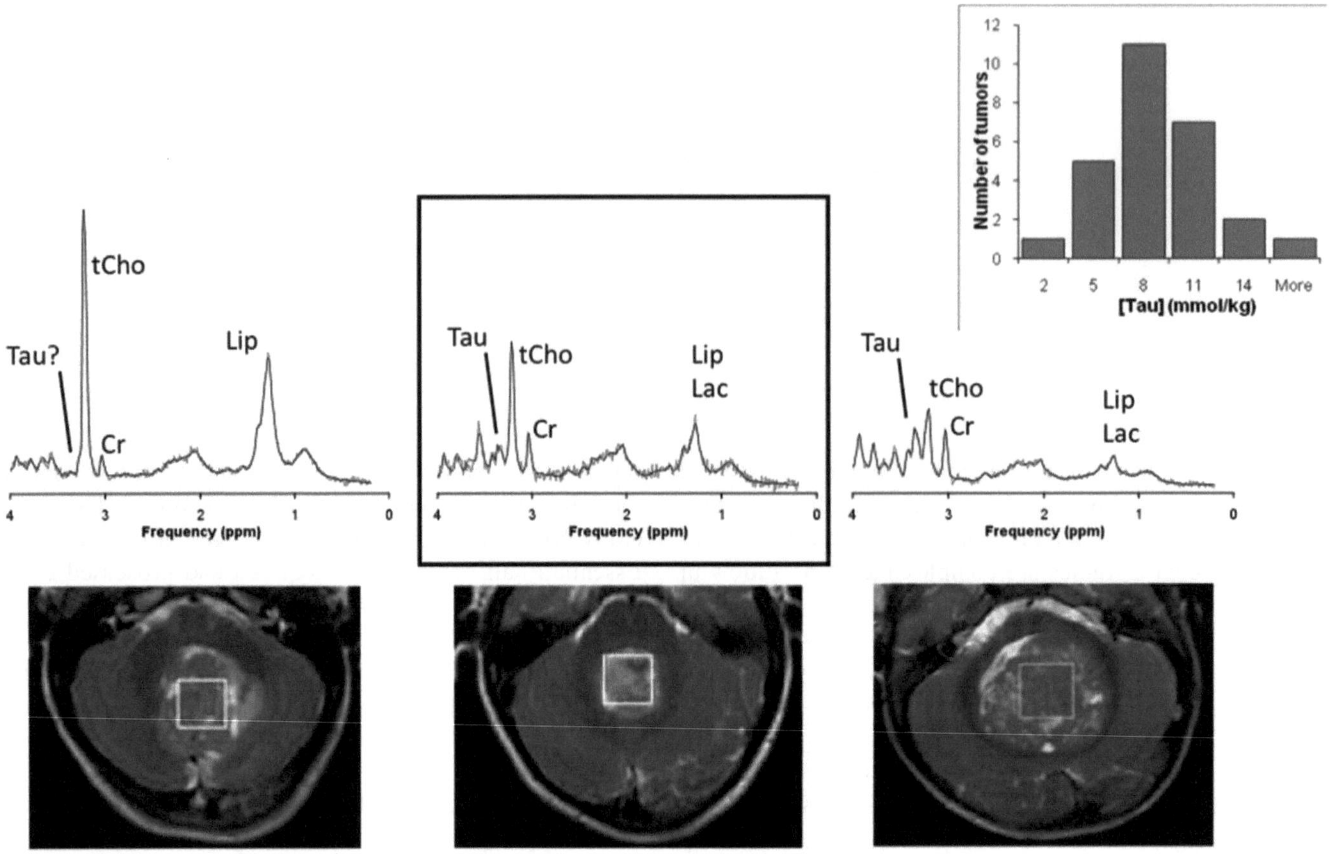

Fig. 22.1 Classic Medulloblastoma, Typical and Atypical

distribution. As several groups have shown [1, 2], the elevated Tau is a very good indicator for medulloblastoma, however, not in 100% of the cases. Despite the low Tau of the spectrum on the left, this tumor was nevertheless diagnosed correctly, as the very high absolute concentration of Cho is not typical for ependymoma (or pilocytic astrocytoma). Of note, most medulloblastoma will demonstrate restricted diffusion or low ADC on diffusion-weighted imaging. It is worth noting that these three patients all fell in the same risk class and were treated equally. One may wonder whether the quite different metabolic profile correlates with different biological behavior, which could (some day in the future) be exploited to optimize therapies.

Conclusions

The metabolic profiles of medulloblastoma can vary significantly, although elevated taurine can be seen in a large subset with classic histology.

Case 2: Medulloblastoma, Anaplastic

Clinical Background

8-year-old male with cerebellar mass.

MRS method

1.5 T, SV-PRESS TE 35 ms, lesion.

Interpretation/Discussion

MRI showed a heterogeneous solid/cystic mass consistent with a medulloblastoma. The MR spectrum showed prominent lipids (and lactate), depleted NAA, and below normal tissue levels Cr (Fig. 22.2). Cho was prominent and significantly above normal tissue levels. Tau was detected and mI was above normal. MRS was consistent with

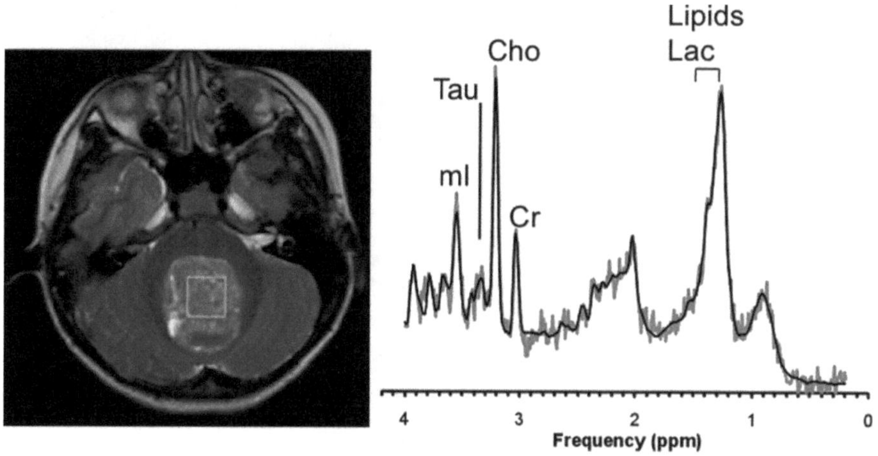

Fig. 22.2 Medulloblastoma, Anaplastic

medulloblastoma. Anaplastic medulloblastoma is a subtype of medulloblastoma and is believed to be more aggressive than classic medulloblastoma. Extensive leptomeningeal disease spread was observed in the patient within 1 year after initial diagnosis.

Conclusions

MRS features of anaplastic medulloblastoma are comparable with features observed in classic medulloblastoma, including elevated Tau.

Case 3: Medulloblastoma, Large Cell, Disseminated

Clinical Background

8-year-old male with cerebellar mass.

MRS Method

1.5 T, SV-PRESS TE 35 ms, lesion.

Interpretation/Discussion

MRI showed a mass adjacent to the roof of the fourth ventricle and extending into the left medial cerebellar parenchymal region (Fig. 22.3). There was evidence of diffuse leptomeningeal metastases involving the leptomeninges surrounding the cerebellum and brainstem and basilar cisterns. The MR spectroscopy demonstrates elevated lipids. There was residual NAA, possibly due to small partial volume of surrounding tissue with the ROI. Cr was close to normal tissue levels whereas Cho was slightly elevated. Tau was readily detectable and mI was slightly below normal levels. Large cell medulloblastoma is a subtype of medulloblastoma and is believed to be more aggressive than classic medulloblastoma. Extensive leptomeningeal disease spread was observed in the patient already at initial diagnosis. Clinical course was poor.

Conclusions

MRS features of anaplastic medulloblastoma are comparable with features observed in classic medulloblastoma including elevated Tau.

Case 4: Medulloblastoma, Desmoplastic I

Clinical Background

2-year-old male with posterior fossa mass.

MRS Method

1.5 T, SV-PRESS TE 35 ms, lesion.

Interpretation/Discussion

The MRI showed a homogeneously enhancing lobulated mass centered in the fourth ventricle with mass effect on the dorsal pons (Fig. 22.4). MRI was interpreted as consistent with a highly cellular tumor such as a medulloblastoma. The MR spectrum showed only slightly elevated lactate and lipids. NAA was depleted and Cr was well below normal tissue levels. Cho was prominent and

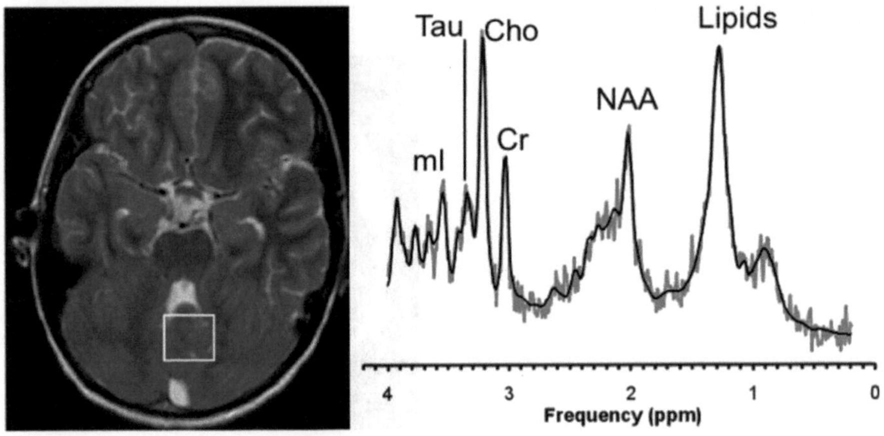

Fig. 22.3 Medulloblastoma, Large Cell, Disseminated

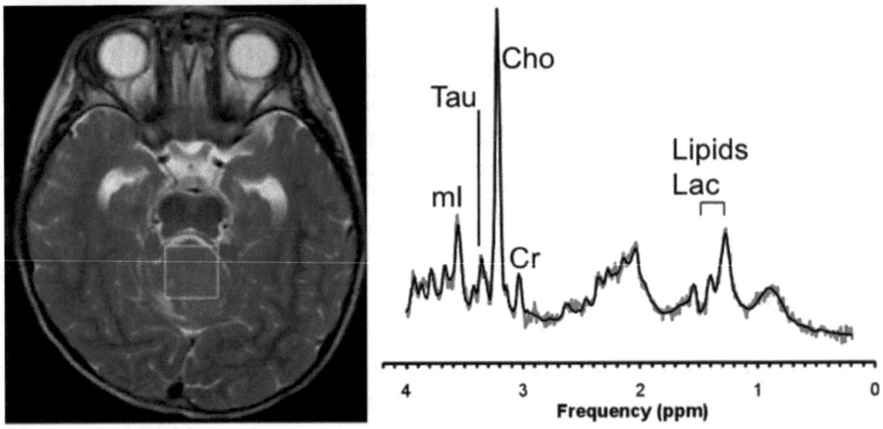

Fig. 22.4 Medulloblastoma, Desmoplastic I

significantly above normal tissue levels. Tau was readily detectable and mI was above normal. MRS was consistent with medulloblastoma. This lesion was resected and classified as a desmoplastic medulloblastoma, a subtype of medulloblastoma believed to have more favorable outcomes. It is our impression that Tau levels are lower in the desmoplastic subtype compared to other medulloblastoma histological types. However, due to biological variations and overlap, Tau does not appear a good predictor for subtype in individual cases. This patient has been stable for more than 4 years after diagnosis.

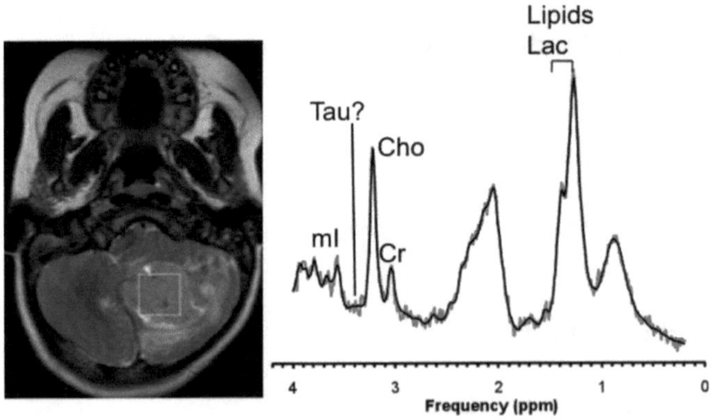

Fig. 22.5 Medulloblastoma, Desmoplastic II

Conclusions

MRS features of desmoplastic medulloblastoma are comparable with features observed in classic medulloblastoma.

Case 5: Medulloblastoma, Desmoplastic II

Clinical Background

3-year-old female with left cerebellar mass.

MRS Method

1.5 T, SV-PRESS TE 35 ms, lesion.

Interpretation/Discussion

The MRI showed a left parenchymal-based inferior cerebellar hemisphere hypercellular mass (Fig. 22.5). Due to the lateral placement, a desmoplastic type medulloblastoma was suggested. The MR spectrum showed prominently elevated lactate and lipids. NAA was depleted and Cr was well below normal tissue levels. Cho was prominent and significantly above normal tissue levels. There was no evidence for Tau in this case and mI was below normal. MRS was consistent with medulloblastoma. The desmoplastic subtype was subsequently confirmed. There has been only limited follow-up of this patient.

Conclusions

MRS features of desmoplastic medulloblastoma are comparable with features observed in classic medulloblastoma. There is a significant heterogeneity of the metabolic profiles among desmoplastic medulloblastoma (cf. *Case 4*).

Case 6: CNS Primitive Neuroectodermal Tumor (PNET)

Clinical Background

4-year-old female with right occipital mass.

MRS Method

1.5 T, SV-PRESS TE 35 ms and TE 144 ms, lesion.

Interpretation/Discussion

MRI showed a right occipital mass heterogeneously enhancing mass that was interpreted as possibly intraventricular (Fig. 22.6). Spectroscopy indicated elevated lactate and possibly the presence of alanine (Ala). NAA was depleted and Cr was below normal. Cho was elevated and Tau was readily detectable. mI was also elevated. Inverted peaks consistent with lactate and alanine were observed in the spectrum acquired at a long echo time of 144 ms (upper trace). Medulloblastoma and CNS PNET are the same type of tumor distinguished in name only by their different location within the brain.

Conclusions

A CNS PNET demonstrated elevated Tau.

Case 7: Atypical Rhabdoid/Teratoid Tumor (AT/RT), Recurrent, Serial MRS

Clinical Background

18-month-old male with lethargy/vomiting with CT showing right frontoparietal intraparenchymal mass with calcification.

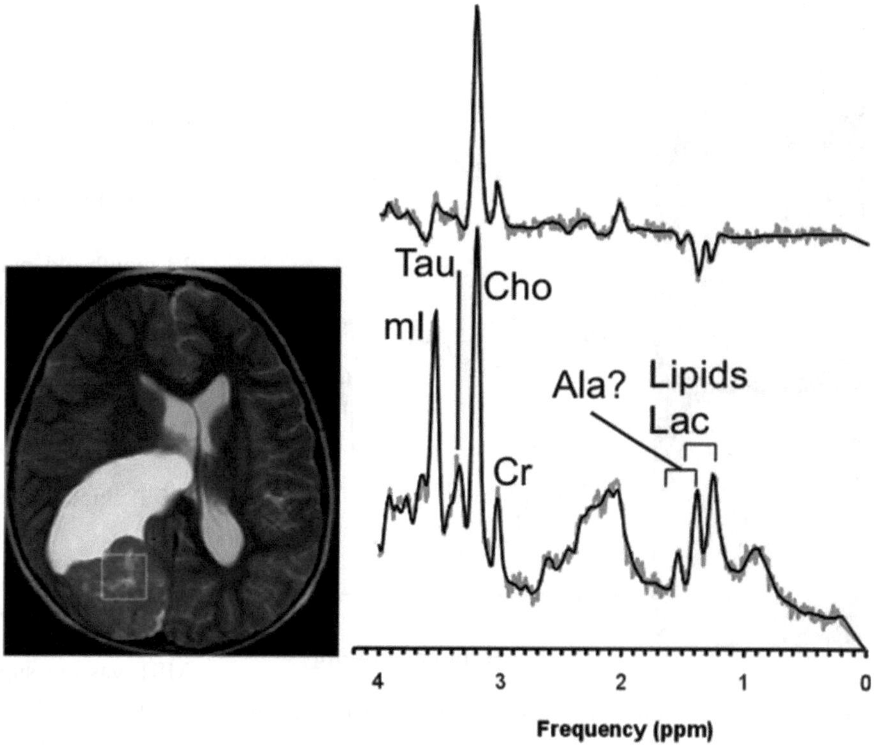

Fig. 22.6 CNS Primitive Neuroectodermal Tumor (PNET)

MRS Method

1.5 T, single-voxel PRESS, TE 35 ms, of lesion, subsequently of areas at risk/suspicious for residual/recurrent tumor.

Interpretation/Discussion

At initial diagnosis (A), the MRI showed a large heterogeneously enhancing mass centered in the right temporal lobe with extension into the region of the right basal ganglia (Fig. 22.7). The lesion appeared to be likely paraventricular in location with both parenchymal and intraventricular components.

The lesion demonstrated restricted diffusion, which would be suggestive of a hypercellular tumor. The MRI report suggested as this to be a glial tumor, primitive neuroectodermal tumor (PNET), or an ependymoma. The MRS showed elevated lipids and lactate whereas NAA was depleted. Cr was close to normal tissue levels whereas Cho was slightly elevated. mI was also above normal. Tau was not detectable. Prominent lipids and lactate in MRS have been associated with tumors that are more aggressive. However, in case of an aggressive astrocytoma, Cho levels would have been expected to be more prominent as well. Lactate was unusually prominent for ependymoma. On the other hand, Tau has been observed frequently in PNET/medulloblastoma. Thus, this spectrum was slightly atypical for the three tumor types mentioned in the MRI report. No specific tumor type was suggested from the pattern of the spectrum. The lesion was subsequently resected and an AT/RT was diagnosed. AT/RTs are the subtype among embryonal tumors (other embryonal tumors are medulloblastoma and CNS PNETs) with the worst prognoses. Five months after resection (B), MRS was performed of a small area suspicious for residual/recurrent disease. The MRS showed features comparable with profile of the untreated tumor at initial diagnosis and was reported as consistent with tumor. A MRI/S study 10 months after diagnosis provided further evidence for recurrent disease (C). A final study at 12 months after initial diagnosis showed progressive disease and an MR spectrum consistent with an aggressive tumor (D).

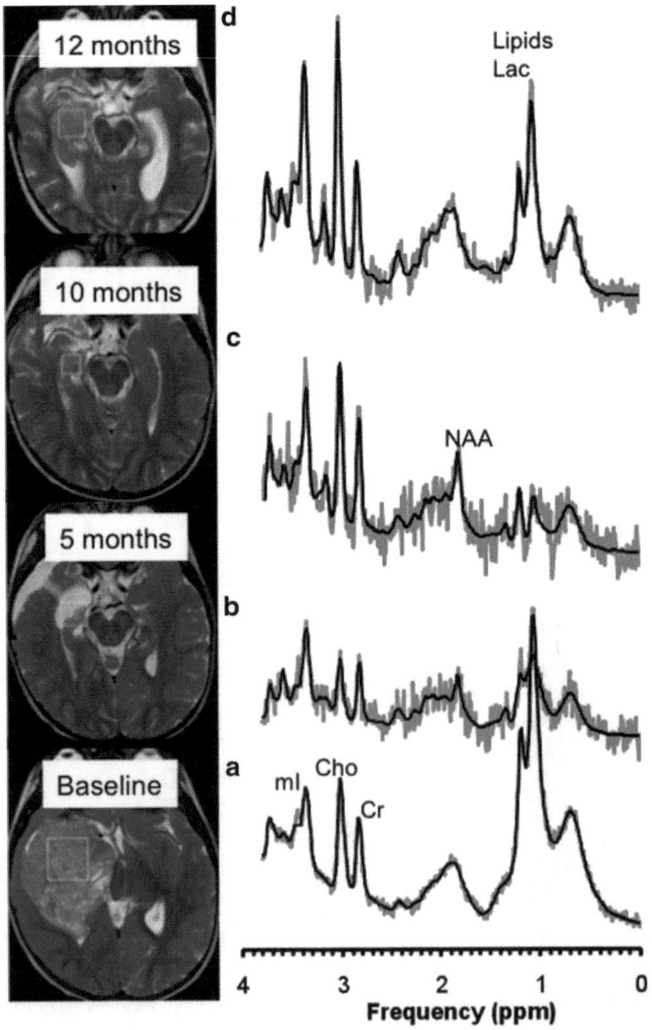

Fig. 22.7 Atypical Rhabdoid/Teratoid Tumor (AT/RT), Recurrent, Serial MRS

Conclusions

MRS of an AT/RT, tumors with very poor prognoses, showed moderate Cho signal but high lactate and lipids at diagnosis. At progression, a spectrum with more prominent Cho was observed. Tau, frequently observed in other primitive embryonal tumors, was not detectable at baseline or at progression.

Case 8: Atypical Rhabdoid/Teratoid Tumor (AT/RT), Intraventricular

Clinical Background

13-month-old male with mass in left lateral ventricle and hydrocephalus, previous CT interpreted as choroid plexus papilloma.

MRS Method

1.5 T, single-voxel PRESS, TE 35 ms, lesion, two locations.

Interpretation/Discussion

MRI was not suggestive for a choroid plexus tumor as the lesion was only minimally enhancing and showed restricted diffusion consistent with a hypercellular tumor. MRS showed elevated lipids and lactate, NAA was depleted, Cr was reduced, and Cho was elevated (Fig. 22.8). mI was also above normal and Tau was not detectable. Based on MRI findings and the MRS pattern an atypical rhabdoid/teratoid tumor was suggested as the most likely tumor type. This was subsequently confirmed after the lesion was resected.

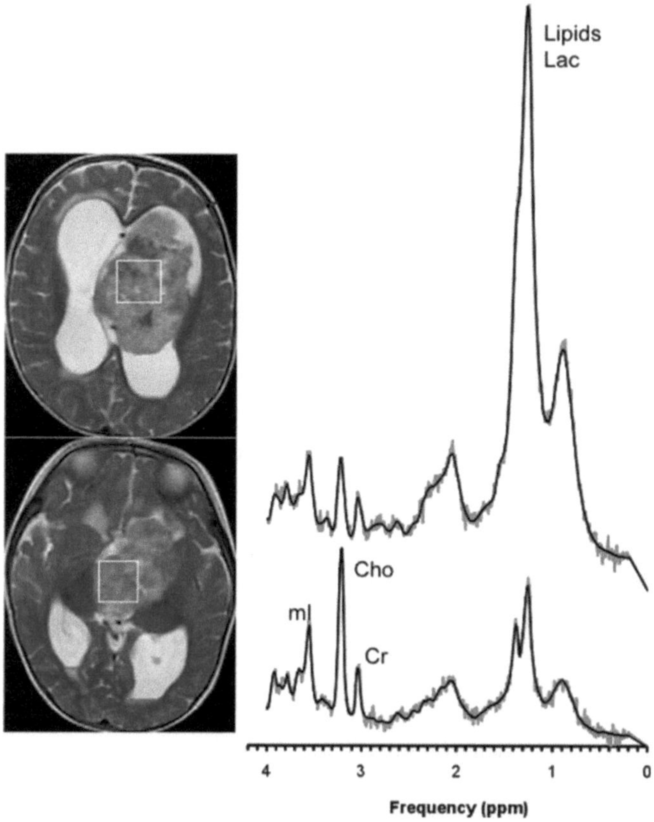

Fig. 22.8 Atypical rhabdoid/teratoid tumor (AT/RT), intraventricular

Conclusions

MRS in conjunction with MRI may narrow differential of tumors and improve initial diagnosis.

Case 9: Medulloblastoma After Surgery, Residual Tumor Versus Postoperative Changes

Clinical Background

6-year-old male with a medulloblastoma. MRI performed immediately after resection was inconclusive. There were concerns for residual tumor.

MRS Method

1.5 T, single-voxel PRESS, TE 35 ms, of original lesion and of suspicious tissue after resection.

Interpretation/Discussion

The preoperative MRS (A) showed a spectrum consistent with a medulloblastoma. Lactate was present, NAA was depleted, Cr was reduced, Cho was prominent, and Tau was observed (Fig. 22.9). Postoperatively, within the posterior fossa thick and bulky T2 heterogeneous material along the margins of the resection cavity was observed on MRI. Because of the relatively mild enhancement of the tumor preoperatively the assessment of residual tumor was difficult. It was suggested that some of these changes might be postoperative in etiology. Still, there were concerns of residual tumor. MR spectroscopy

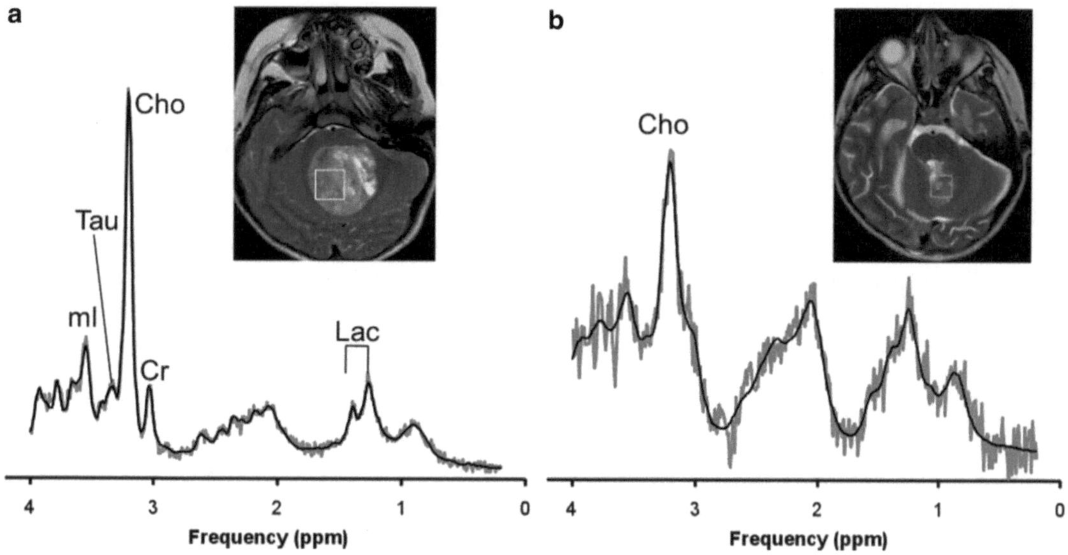

Fig. 22.9 Medulloblastoma after surgery, residual tumor versus post-operative changes

was recommended to evaluate suspicious tissue. The subsequently performed MRS study was compromised in its quality probably because of blood products. Nevertheless, a prominent Cho peak was noted suggestive for residual tumor.

Conclusions

MRS can be useful to distinguish between treatment-related changes and residual tumor.

Case 10: Recurrent Medulloblastoma

Clinical Background

4-year-old female found to have hydrocephalus and posterior fossa mass.

MRS Method

3 T, single-voxel PRESS, TE 35 ms, of untreated lesion at initial diagnosis, of recurrent tumor 19 months after diagnosis and complete resection of initial mass.

Interpretation/Discussion

At initial diagnosis (A), the MRI showed a large mass centered within the fourth ventricle extending inferiorly through the foramen of Magendie and foramen magnum into the upper cervical spine with associated mass effect on the cervicomedullary consistent with a medulloblastoma (Fig. 22.10). The MRS showed elevated lipids and lactate, NAA was depleted, Cr was close to normal tissue levels, Cho was significantly elevated, and mI was reduced. Tau was prominent and the MRS was interpreted to be consistent with medulloblastoma. The lesion was resected with no residual disease detectable on several follow-up studies. However, at 19 months recurrent disease was noted (B). MRS at that time showed a spectrum that was slightly altered when compared with the baseline scan. Lipids and lactate were less prominent. Also, absolute Cho and Cho relative to Cr were less prominent. However, Tau was clearly detectable.

Conclusions

MRS of a recurrent medulloblastoma showed a metabolic profile that was slightly different than what has been observed at initial diagnosis. Recurrent medulloblastoma is associated with elevated Tau.

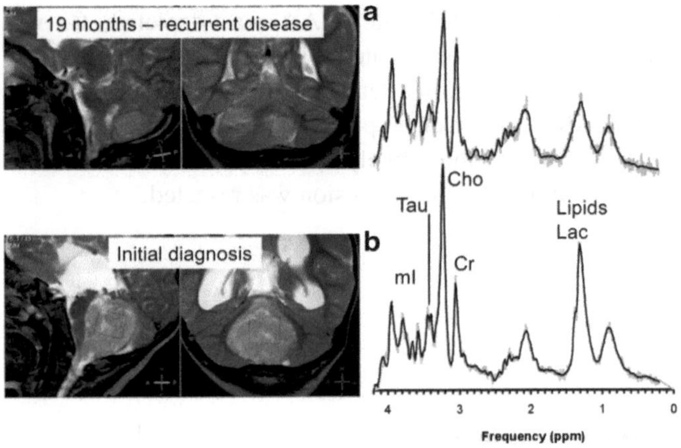

Fig. 22.10 Recurrent Medulloblastoma

Case 11: Pilocytic Astrocytoma, Infratentorial

Clinical Background

2-year-old male presenting with cyclical vomiting, concerning for hydrocephalus and brain tumor based on CT.

MRS Method

3 T, SV-PRESS TE 35 ms, lesion.

Interpretation/Discussion

The MRI showed a large, complex cystic and solid mass arising from the right cerebellar hemisphere with supratentorial extension. Imaging findings were most consistent with a pilocytic astrocytoma. The MR spectrum showed elevated lactate and lipids (Fig. 22.11). There was a residual peak consistent with NAA, despite the fact that the ROI was placed carefully to exclude any partial volume of surrounding tissue. Cr was significantly below normal tissue concentrations. Cho, albeit appearing prominent was only slightly above levels observed in normal tissue. mI was below normal tissue levels. The MRS was interpreted to be consistent with a pilocytic astrocytoma subsequently confirmed after resection. Low absolute metabolite concentrations of this tumor were consistent with a globally hypocellular lesion when compared to other tumor types.

Conclusions

Pilocytic astrocytoma may have a peak consistent with NAA. Cho may appear prominent, albeit pilocytic astrocytomas are WHO grade I tumors.

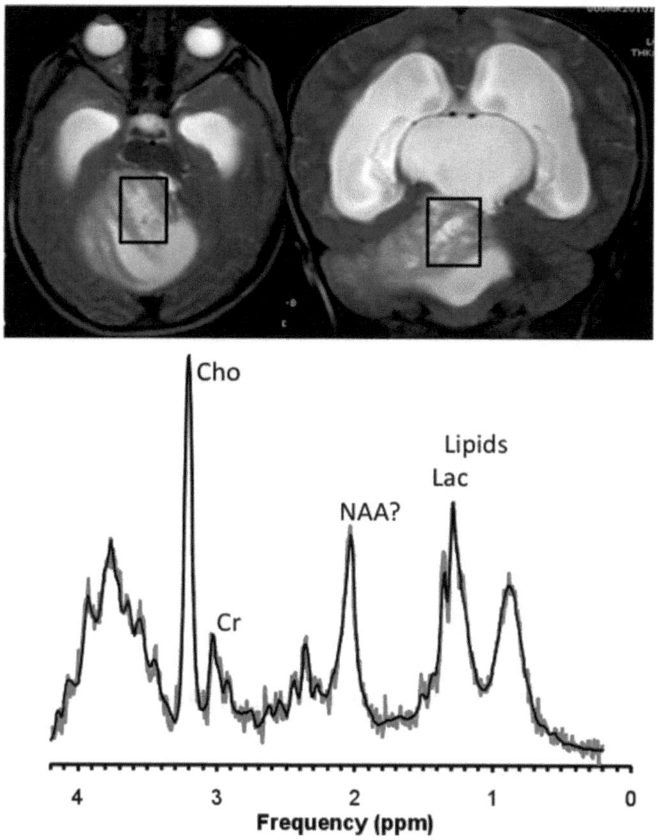

Fig. 22.11 Pilocytic astrocytoma, infratentorial

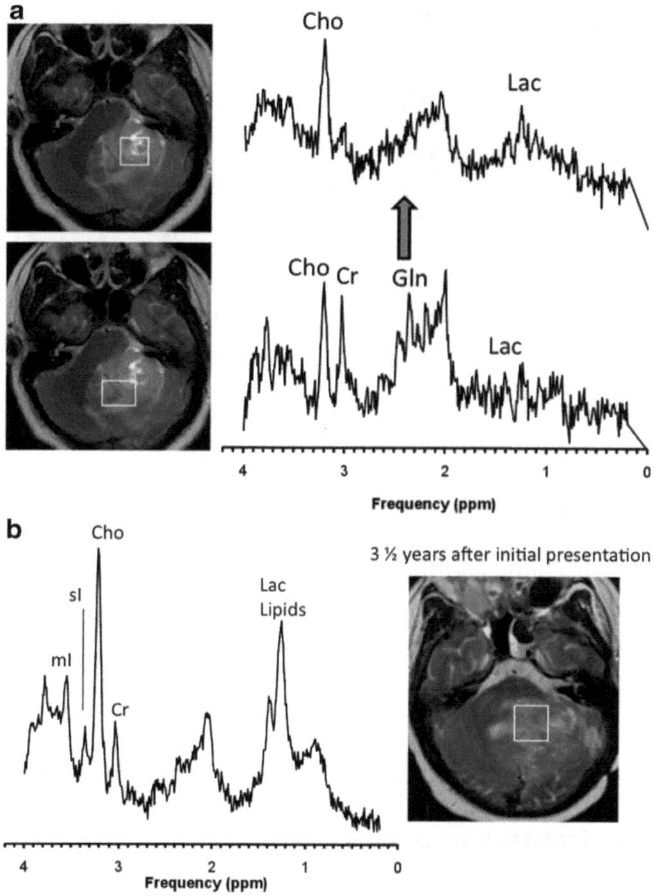

Fig. 22.12 Pilocytic Astrocytoma (WHO I) with aggressive behavior

Case 12: Pilocytic Astrocytoma (WHO I) with Aggressive Behavior

Clinical Background

16-year-old female with vertigo and vomiting, assess intracranial mass.

MRS Method

1.5 T, single-voxel PRESS, TE 35 ms, of lesion.

Interpretation/*Discussion*

On MRI, at diagnosis (A) a left cerebellar mass with central necrosis and a moderate amount of edema and mass effect was seen. In addition, mild hydrocephalus of the third and lateral ventricles was noted (Fig. 22.12). Based on MRI, it was felt that the lesion was likely a glioma, probably anaplastic astrocytoma. The MRS profile (upper trace) was not typical for a regular astrocytoma. Cr levels were very low. Cho appeared prominent, albeit absolute concentration Cho was close to normal tissue levels. mI was low, which is also not typical for regular astrocytoma. MRS was more consistent with a pilocytic astrocytoma, which was subsequently confirmed after surgical resection of the tumor. However, a second spectrum acquired from a different part of the lesion showed a pattern that was not consistent with pilocytic astrocytoma. Indeed, the spectrum showed elevated lactate, considerable residual NAA, elevated (likely) Gln, unremarkable Cr and Cho, and below normal mI. This pattern is not typical for tumors. Instead, similar patterns have been observed in edema and hypoxic/ischemic injury. In addition, acute infection and acute hepatic encephalopathy may sometime present with similar MRS profiles. Clinical course was very atypical for this patient. Pilocytic astrocytomas are WHO grade I tumors and rarely progress. In this case, however, clinicians were unable to control the disease despite two surgeries, radiation, and chemotherapies. The diagnosis of a pilocytic astrocytoma was confirmed by the second surgery. A spectrum obtained shortly before the patient died showed, when compared with the baseline scan, much higher metabolite levels consistent with a more cellular lesion at that time. Specifically, Cho concentration was approximately three times higher than at baseline.

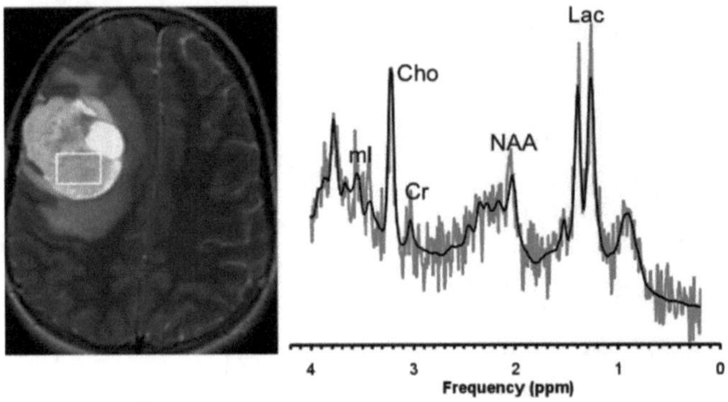

Fig. 22.13 Pilocytic Astrocytoma, MRI unusual

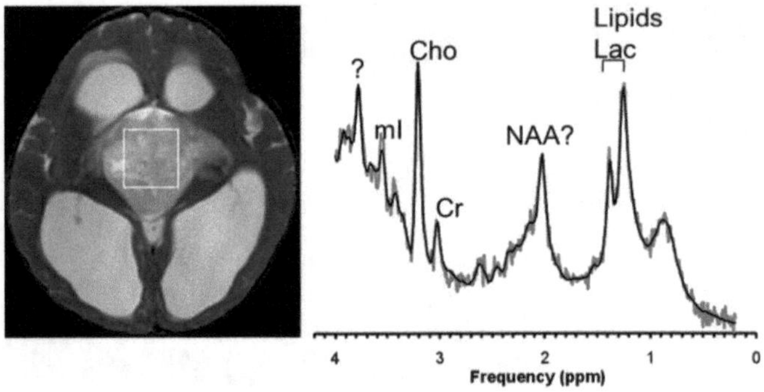

Fig. 22.14 Pilocytic Astrocytoma, Supratentorial

Conclusion

Albeit considered low grade, some pilocytic astrocytoma may show aggressive behavior. Presently, it is unclear whether there are any metabolic indicators that would allow identifying individual patients at risk at an early stage.

Case 13: Pilocytic Astrocytoma, MRI Unusual

Clinical Background

13-year-old female with right cerebral mass seen on previous CT obtained at different hospital.

MRS Method

1.5 T, SV-PRESS TE 35 ms, lesion.

Interpretation/Discussion

The MRI was interpreted as showing a presumed extra-axial mass displacing the posterior right frontal lobe. There was surrounding edema and effacement of the right lateral ventricle. The mass had multiple ring enhancing areas within the tumor (Fig. 22.13). There were multiple cysts seen within the lesion and the overall signal on T2 was relatively low. The MRI differential diagnosis included peripheral PNET, sarcoma, metastasis, and less likely an intrinsic glial tumor. The MRS showed prominent lactate, reduced NAA, and very low Cr. Cho was the most prominent peak. However, absolute Cho was low. mI was low as well. The MRS was interpreted to be consistent with pilocytic astrocytoma subsequently confirmed when the lesion was resected.

Conclusions

MRS can improve accuracy of initial diagnoses.

Case 14: Pilocytic Astrocytoma, Supratentorial

Clinical Background

19-month-old female with new hypothalamic mass and hydrocephalus on CT.

MRS Method

1.5 T, SV-PRESS TE 35 ms, lesion.

Interpretation/Discussion

The MRI showed a large enhancing mass centered in the suprasellar region/third ventricle with secondary obstructive hydrocephalus. There was no evidence for metastatic disease. The characteristics were most suggestive of glial tumor/astrocytoma. The MR spectrum showed elevated lactate and lipids (Fig. 22.14). There was a residual peak consistent with NAA, despite the fact that the ROI was placed carefully to exclude any partial volume of surrounding tissue. Cr was significantly below normal tissue concentrations. Cho, albeit appearing prominent was close to levels observed in normal tissue. mI was below normal tissue levels. The MRS was interpreted to be consistent with a pilocytic astrocytoma subsequently confirmed after resection. Low absolute metabolite concentrations of this tumor were consistent with a globally hypocellular lesion when compared to other tumor types.

Conclusions

Pilocytic astrocytoma may have a peak consistent with NAA. Cho may appear prominent, albeit pilocytic astrocytomas are WHO grade I tumors.

Case 15: Pilocytic Astrocytoma, Supratentorial, Partially Cystic/Necrotic

Clinical Background

2-year-old female with hypothalamic pilocytic astrocytoma.

MRS Method

1.5 T, SV-PRESS TE 35 ms, solid appearing part of lesion and necrotic appearing part.

Interpretation/Discussion

The MRI showed a large mixed cystic solid mass consistent with a hypothalamic pilocytic astrocytoma. The mass had increased in size when compared to an earlier study from a different hospital. The MR spectrum of the more solid part of the lesion (A) showed elevated lactate and lipids (Fig. 22.15). There was a residual peak consistent with NAA and Cr was virtually undetectable. Cho was prominent and was slightly above normal tissue levels. mI was below normal tissue levels. The MRS including partially necrotic tissue showed more prominent lipids but had otherwise a comparable profile (B). The MRS profile was typical for pilocytic astrocytoma.

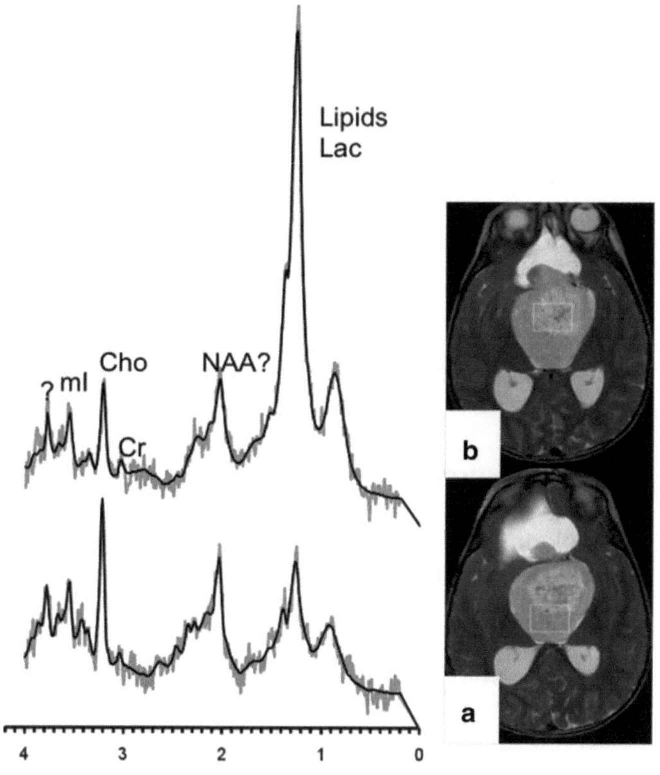

Fig. 22.15 Pilocytic Astrocytoma, Supratentorial, Partially Cystic/Necrotic

Conclusions

Pilocytic astrocytoma may have a peak consistent with NAA. Cho may appear prominent, albeit pilocytic astrocytomas are WHO grade I tumors. Lipids might be prominent in the spectrum if necrotic parts of the lesion are enclosed in the region of interest.

Case 16: Pilocytic Astrocytoma, Supratentorial, Partially Cystic/Necrotic, High mI

Clinical Background

3-year-old male with mass in brain demonstrated on CT with neurological changes with hydrocephalus.

MRS Method

1.5 T, SV-PRESS TE 35 ms, solid appearing part of lesion and necrotic appearing part.

Interpretation/Discussion

The MRI showed a partly cystic partly solid mass with heterogeneous contrast accumulation centered in the suprasellar cistern extending into the midbrain, right basal ganglia, and thalamus.

MRI was interpreted as consistent with either pilocytic astrocytoma or a diffuse astrocytoma. The MR spectrum of the more solid part of the lesion (A) showed elevated lactate and lipids. There was a residual peak consistent with NAA and Cr was very low (Fig. 22.16). Cho was prominent and was moderately above normal tissue levels. mI was also elevated. Lipids were more prominent in the MRS that included partially necrotic tissue (B). mI was, however, not prominent in this spectrum. The MRS was reported to be consistent with a pilocytic astrocytoma albeit the very prominent mI was considered slightly unusual.

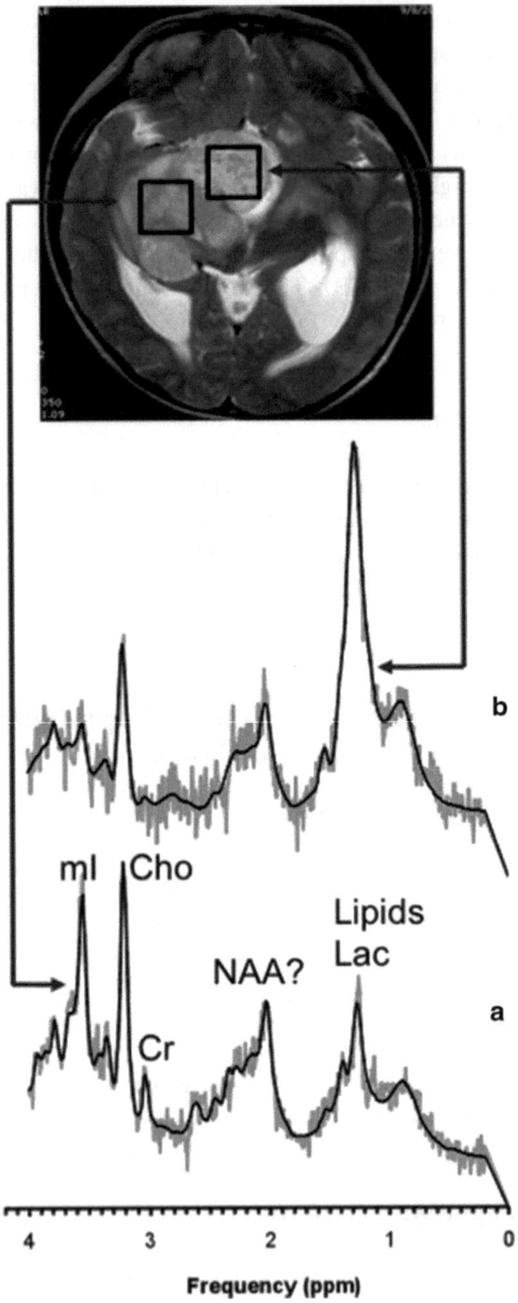

Fig. 22.16 Pilocytic Astrocytoma, Supratentorial, Partially Cystic/Necrotic, High mI.

Conclusions

A suprasellar pilocytic astrocytoma shows unusually prominent mI but is otherwise consistent with a pilocytic lesion.

Case 17: Unusual Peak at 2.8 ppm: Pilocytic Astrocytoma

Clinical Background

3-year-old male with a pilocytic astrocytoma, evaluate for progression.

MRS Method

3 T, single-voxel PRESS, TE 35 ms and 144 ms of lesion.

Interpretation/Discussion

The MRI showed a large hypothalamic pilocytic astrocytoma. MRS demonstrated elevated lipids and lactate (Fig. 22.17). There was also a peak consistent with NAA (note: no partial volume with surrounding tissue) in both long TE and short TE MRS. Cr levels were very low and Cho, albeit prominent relative to Cr, was at or below normal levels. There was an unknown peak at ≈2.8 ppm in the short TE spectrum. The origin and significance of this peak is unknown. There have been reports in the literature that polyunsaturated fatty acids (PUFA) may have a peak in this part of the spectrum (1). Despite pilocytic astrocytoma being a low-grade WHO I tumor, the lesion kept on growing and the patient died from the disease.

Conclusions

An unusual peak, possibly from PUFA, was observed in a spectrum of a hypothalamic pilocytic astrocytoma.

Case 18: Pilocytic Astrocytoma, Supratentorial, Serial MRS

Clinical Background

2-year-old male with optic pathway pilocytic astrocytoma, diagnosed several months earlier, undergoing chemotherapy.

MRS Method

1.5 T, SV-PRESS TE 35 ms, lesion, follow-up MRS studies.

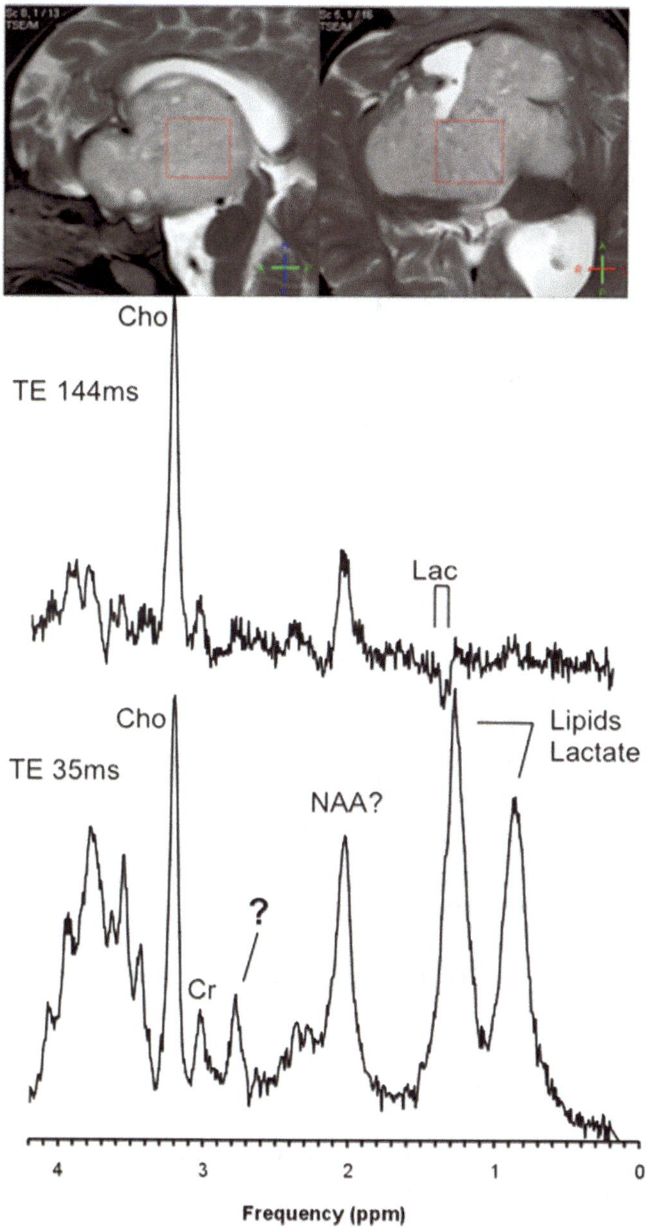

Fig. 22.17 Unusual Peak at 2.8 ppm: Pilocytic Astrocytoma

Interpretation/Discussion

The MRI showed a large optic chiasmal glioma with extension along both left and right optic tracts to the mesial temporal lobes and thalami, which had slightly increased in size when compared with an earlier study (no MRS at that time). The first MRS study (A) showed elevated lactate and lipids (Fig. 22.18). NAA was significantly reduced or depleted and Cr was virtually undetectable. Cho was prominent with absolute Cho concentrations slightly above normal. mI was significantly increased relative to normal tissue (cf. *Case 16*). The MRS was interpreted as consistent with pilocytic astrocytoma although the mI peak was unusually prominent. It is unclear whether this could be associated with treatment, which had commenced at the time of the study. In subsequent studies, a reduction of the lesion volume was observed on MRI (B-D). Spectroscopy showed an increase of NAA and Cr whereas Cho and mI decreased. It was noted that this process was already apparent when the MRS region of interest enclosed clearly abnormal appearing tissue (cf. A–C). The final spectrum (D), acquired from an area with essentially normal MRI features, was consistent with mostly normal tissue having replaced large parts of the pathologic tissue.

Conclusions

Serial MRS shows dramatic changes of the metabolic profile of a pilocytic lesion after therapy.

Case 19: Ependymoma I

Clinical Background

22-month-old female with suspicion for brain tumor.

MRS Method

1.5 T, single-voxel PRESS, TE 35 ms, lesion.

Interpretation/Discussion

On MRI, a patchy enhancing mass filling the fourth ventricle, growing out the left lateral recess crossing into the spinal canal was noted. MRI was consistent with an ependymoma or medulloblastoma. MRS showed elevated lactate and depleted NAA (Fig. 22.19). Cr was close to normal tissue levels and Cho was only slightly above normal levels. mI was prominent and Tau was not detectable. MRS was not consistent with pilocytic astrocytoma with respect to the high Cr peak and the lack of hypocellularity. The very moderate Cho levels and the absence of any evidence for Tau were not typical for medulloblastoma. MRS was suggestive for an ependymoma. A grade II ependymoma was confirmed after resection of the lesion.

Conclusions

MRS can help narrowing the differential from MRI of posterior fossa lesions.

Fig. 22.18 Pilocytic Astrocytoma, Supratentorial, Serial MRS

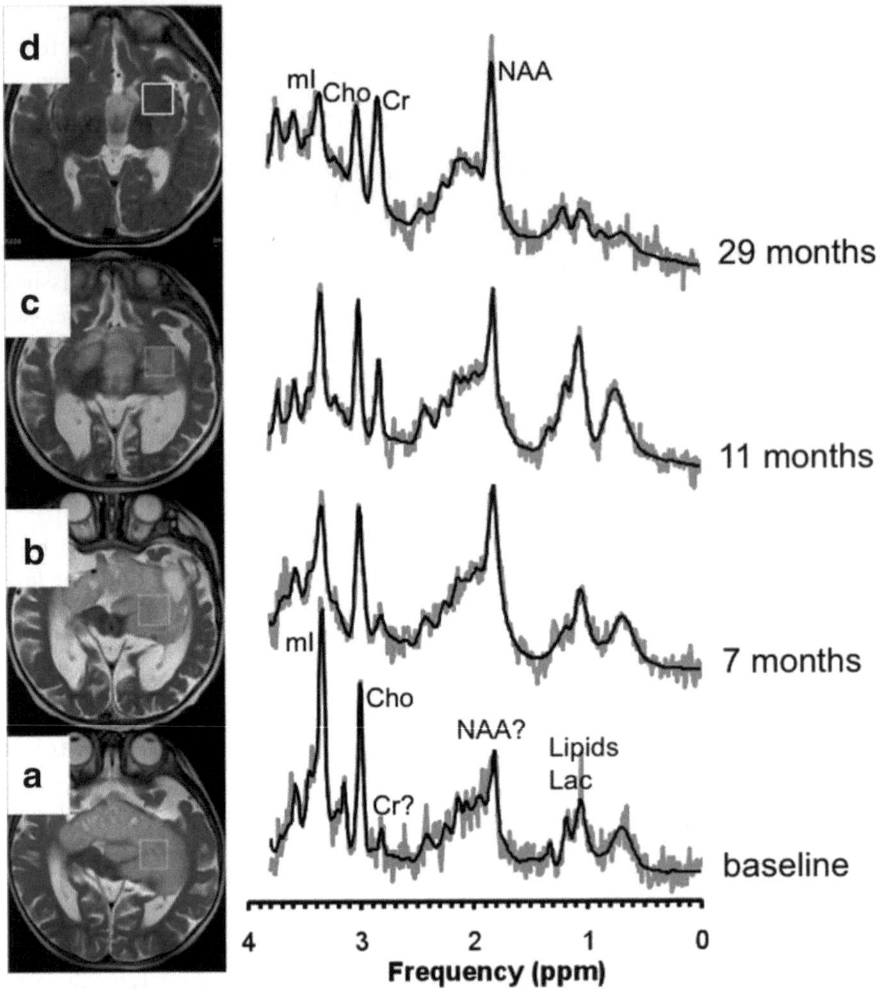

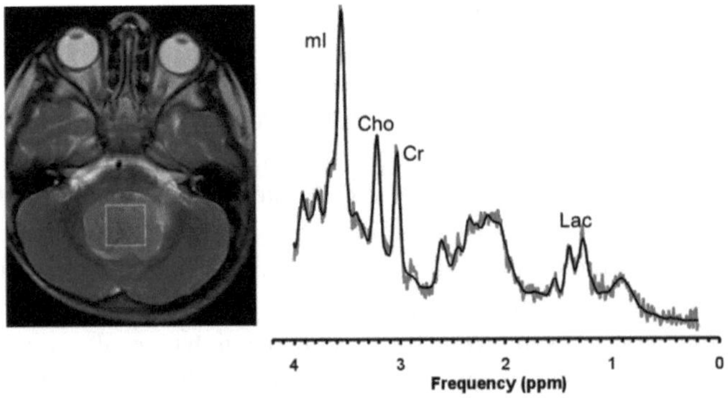

Fig. 22.19 Ependymoma I

Case 20: Ependymoma II

Clinical Background

4-month-old female with suspicion for brain tumor.

MRS Method

1.5 T, single-voxel PRESS, TE 35 ms, lesion, baseline and follow-up at 16 months after diagnosis.

Interpretation/Discussion

At diagnosis (A), a large posterior fossa mass was noted. It showed mostly peripheral enhancing. CT (not shown) indicated possibly hemorrhagic areas (Fig. 22.20). The MRI differential included ependymoma as the most likely tumor type. Medulloblastoma and choroid plexus tumors were also mentioned. The MR spectrum was of low quality, likely because of the hemorrhages. Particularly, the linewidth was poor. Prominent lipid signal was detected. Cr and Cho peaks were questionable. MRS did not add specific information that would have improved the reading of MRI alone in this case. After resection, an ependymoma was confirmed. Recurrent tumor was noted at 16 months after diagnosis (B).

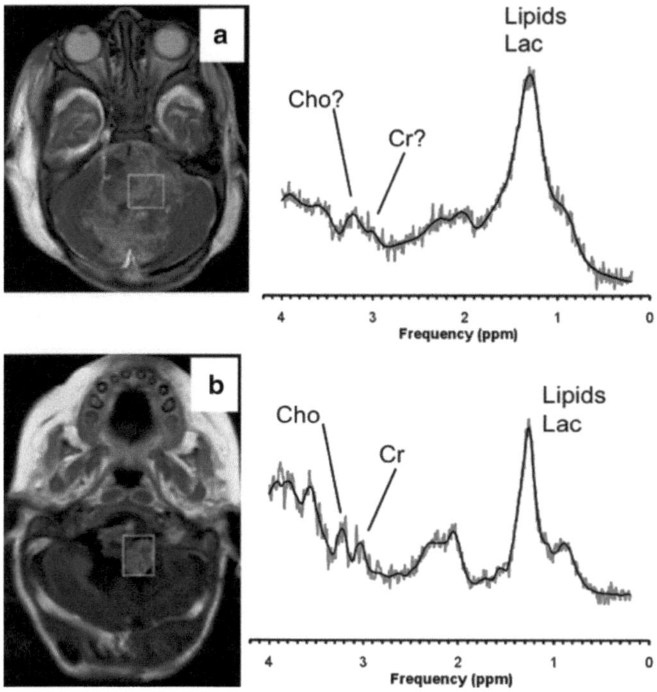

Fig. 22.20 Ependymoma II

At that time a slightly better quality MRS was obtained with prominent lipids and Cho and Cr peaks detectable.

Conclusions

The presence of blood products may render the interpretation of MRS difficulty. Correlation with CT imaging and blood sensitive sequences (including GRE and SWI) maybe useful to exclude the possibility of blood compromising the quality of the voxel.

Case 21: Anaplastic Ependymoma I

Clinical Background

5-year-old male with new posterior fossa tumor.

MRS Method

1.5 T, single-voxel PRESS, TE 35 ms, lesion.

Interpretation/Discussion

On MRI, there was an inhomogeneously enhancing mass centered in the fourth ventricle growing out the lateral recess to the foramen magendie (Fig. 22.21). The impression from MRI was that this lesion was consistent with an ependymoma and less likely a medulloblastoma. The MR spectroscopy demonstrates elevated lipids. NAA was depleted and Cr was slightly below normal tissue levels. Cho and mI were slightly elevated. The relatively higher level of mI is more suggestive of an ependymoma compared to a medulloblastoma. It is unclear whether there is a Tau signal. MRS was interpreted at being more typical for ependymoma albeit an unusual medulloblastoma with comparably low Cho could not be ruled out. A grade III anaplastic ependymoma was confirmed after resection of the lesion. This tumor turned out to be highly aggressive and progressed within two years after initial diagnosis despite complete resection and chemotherapy.

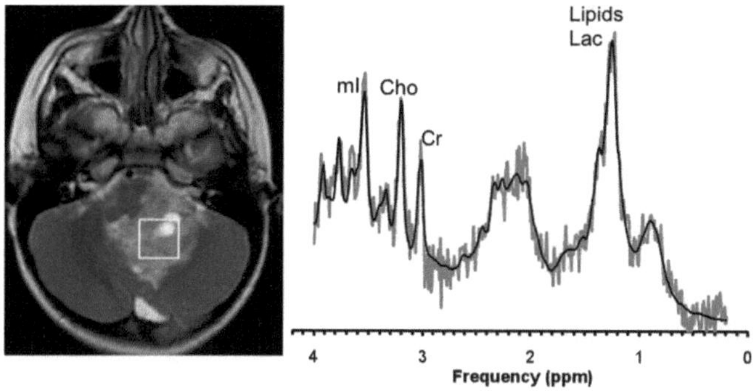

Fig. 22.21 Anaplastic Ependymoma I

Conclusions

MRS of an anaplastic ependymoma with poor outcome is shown.

Case 22: Anaplastic Ependymoma II

Clinical Background

9-year-old male with large posterior fossa mass.

MRS Method

1.5 T, single-voxel PRESS, TE 35 ms, lesion.

Interpretation/Discussion

The MRI scanned showed a fourth ventricular posterior fossa mass in the midline with calcifications and heterogeneous attenuation with heterogeneous enhancement following contrast administration (Fig. 22.22). The lesion was contiguous

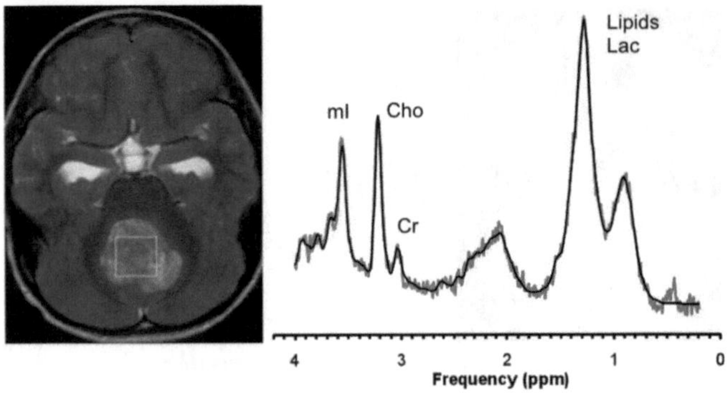

Fig. 22.22 Anaplastic Ependymoma II

with both floor and the roof of the fourth ventricle. The MRI differential included ependymoma and PNET. The MR spectroscopy showed undetectable levels of Tau. The Cr level was low and the Cho to Cr ratio was high. A large mI peak and elevated lipids and lactate were noted. MR spectroscopy supported ependymoma. After resection an anaplastic ependymoma was diagnosed.

Conclusions

MRS can help narrowing the differential from MRI. There is a significant metabolic heterogeneity within ependymoma of the same grade (cf. *Case 21*).

Case 23: Diffuse Pontine Glioma I, Homogeneous, Nonenhancing

Clinical Background

10-year-old female with new pontine mass.

MRS Method

1.5 T, single-voxel PRESS, TE 35 ms, lesion at diagnosis and at disease progression (final study).

Interpretation/Discussion

At baseline (A), the MRI showed a T2-hyperintense, nonenhancing mass within the center of the pons with a slightly infiltrative superior border (Fig. 22.23). There was partial encasement of the basilar artery. MRS showed no evidence for elevated lipids. However, there was evidence of elevated lactate, reduced NAA, reduced Cr, and total Cho below normal levels for brainstem. The mI was elevated. The presence

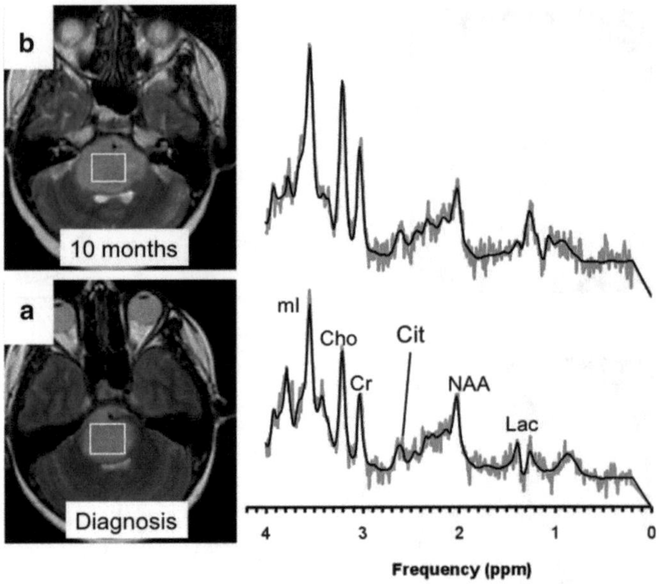

Fig. 22.23 Diffuse Pontine Glioma I, Homogeneous, Nonenhancing

of citrate was noticed. Both MRI and MRS were highly suggestive for a diffuse intrinsic pontine glioma. This patient was subsequently treated with radiation therapy and chemotherapy and improved clinically. At 10 months after diagnosis, the patient relapsed. The MRI performed at that time (B) showed a nonenhancing lesion increased in size when compared with previous studies (not shown in detail). The MRS pattern was very comparable with the initial scan.

Conclusions

Overall, MR spectra acquired at baseline and at progression (10 months) showed spectra that were not typical for high-grade gliomas, which typically feature elevated lipids and lactate and prominent Cho. The metabolic features of the tumor did not change significantly.

Case 24: Diffuse Pontine Glioma II, Homogeneous, Nonenhancing, Enhancing at Progression

Clinical Background

9-year-old male with pontine mass.

MRS Method

1.5 T, single-voxel PRESS, TE 35 ms, lesion at diagnosis and at disease progress (final study).

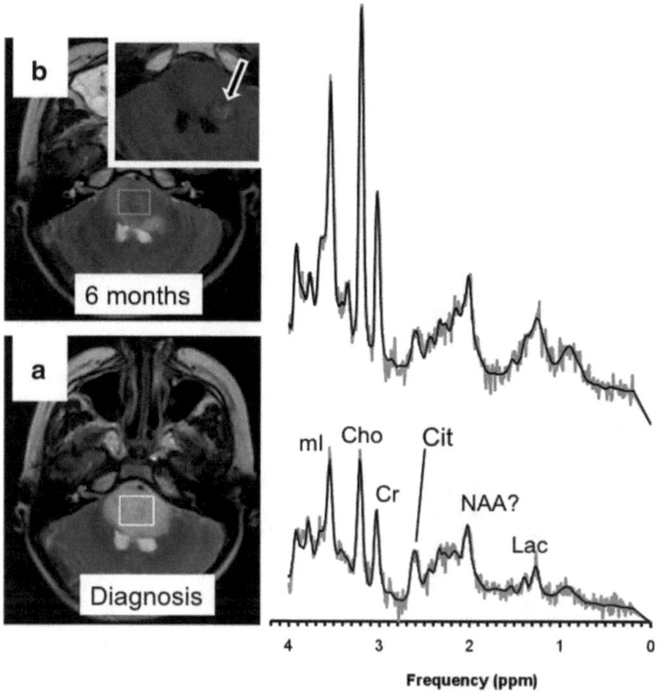

Fig. 22.24 Diffuse Pontine Glioma II, Homogeneous, Nonenhancing, Enhancing at Progression

At baseline (A), the MRI showed a T2-hyperintense, nonenhancing mass within the center of the pons consistent with diffuse pontine glioma (Fig. 22.24). MRS showed elevated lactate, reduced NAA, reduced Cr, and total Cho below normal levels for brainstem. The mI was elevated and the presence of citrate was noted. MRS was consistent with a diffuse intrinsic pontine glioma. This patient was subsequently treated with radiation therapy and chemotherapy and improved clinically temporarily. Six months after initial diagnosis the patient relapse and an MRI study performed at that time showed a new focus of enhancement (B, arrow). The lesion appeared now less T2-hyperintense. The MRS, acquired from the nonenhancing part of the lesion, showed generally increased metabolite levels with the exception of citrate, which appeared to be reduced. Cho appeared to be more prominent relative to Cr and mI when compared with the baseline scan.

Conclusions

Mild to moderate changes of the metabolic profile were observed in a pontine glioma from baseline to progression. Cho/Cr ratios tend to be higher in higher grade gliomas.

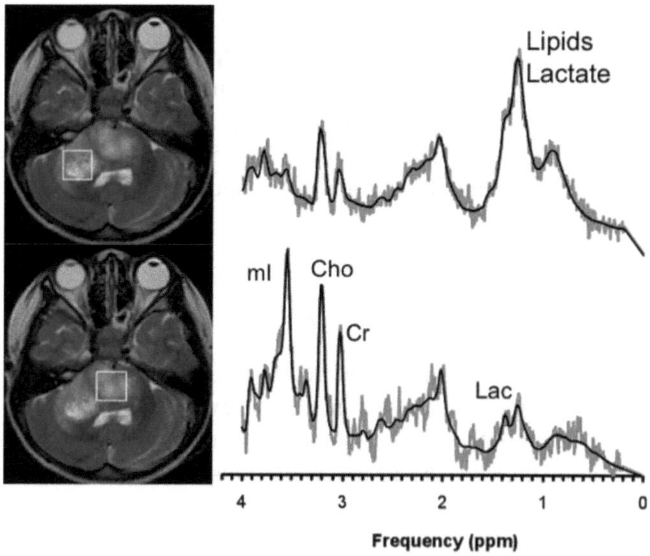

Fig. 22.25 Diffuse Pontine Glioma III, Enhancing

Case 25: Diffuse Pontine Glioma III, Enhancing

Clinical Background

6-year-old female with ataxia and weakness, evaluate for brain mass.

MRS Method

1.5 T, single-voxel PRESS, TE 35 ms, nonenhancing and enhancing part of lesion.

Interpretation/Discussion

On MRI the lesion showed heterogeneously low signal on T1-weighted and heterogeneously high signal on T2-weighted MRI (Fig. 22.25). The lesion was largely centered in the right portion of the pons but extended superiorly to the midbrain and superior cerebral peduncle, inferiorly into the medulla, and laterally into the cerebellopontine angle and the right cerebellar hemisphere. A portion of this lesion in the right middle cerebellar peduncle demonstrated cystic appearance and mild peripheral enhancement suggesting necrosis. The MR spectrum acquired from the more solid nonenhancing part of the lesion (lower trace) showed elevated lactate. NAA was depleted whereas Cr and Cho were both below normal levels for the brainstem. mI was elevated.

The MRS from the more cystic/necrotic appearing and enhancing area showed elevated lipids and generally lower metabolite levels of Cr, Cho, and mI (upper trace). This patient was too sick for therapy at the time of diagnosis and died soon after above examination. There was no clear evidence for citrate in the spectra.

Conclusions

A pontine glioma that appeared to have progressed at initial presentation showed no clear evidence for citrate. Other metabolite features of the spectrum acquired from the solid part of the lesion were consistent with pontine glioma.

Case 26: Diffuse Pontine Glioma IV, Metabolic Progression

Clinical Background

7-year-old female with pontine mass.

MRS Method

1.5 T, single-voxel PRESS, TE 35 ms, lesion, baseline and follow-up.

Interpretation/Discussion

At baseline, MRI showed a nonenhancing mass centered in the pons consistent with a pontine glioma. MR spectroscopy showed elevated lactate, significant residual NAA, and a signal consistent with citrate (Fig. 22.26). Both Cr and Cho were close to or below normal levels for brainstem whereas mI was above normal. MRS was consistent with a pontine glioma. This patient subsequently underwent standard radiation therapy. MRS immediately after completion of radiation therapy was not performed. MRS at 5 months showed now more prominent lipids and lactate, reduced NAA and Cr, and Cho elevated and more prominent relative to Cr, whereas mI was slightly lower than at baseline. At that time the patient was clinically stable albeit MRS would be suggestive for progressing disease. Clinical progression was noticed around 6 months after initial diagnosis. MRS at that time was comparable with the previous scan at 5 months. The patient underwent one more study at 8 months where lipids and Cho had increased further. The patient died soon after that scan.

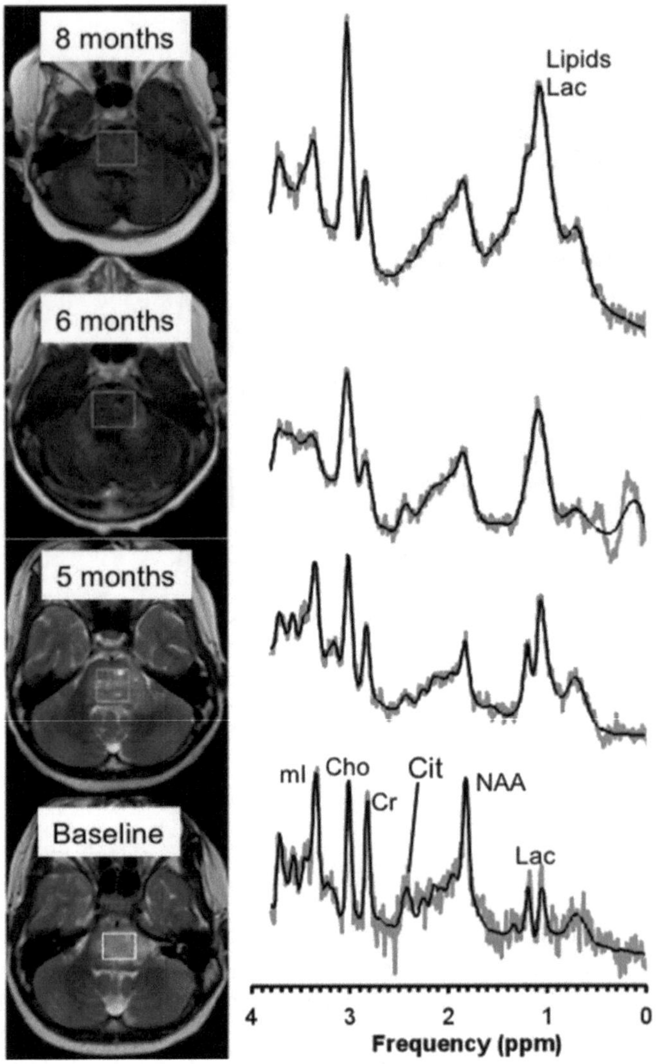

Fig. 22.26 Diffuse Pontine Glioma IV, Metabolic Progression

Conclusions

Metabolic changes consistent with progression, despite radiation and chemotherapy, were observed in this patient prior to clinical progression.

Case 27: Metastatic Pontine Glioma

Clinical Background

10-year-old boy with pontine glioma 9 months after radiation therapy. MRI/MRS was carried out for disease monitoring.

MRS Method

3 T, single-voxel PRESS, TE 35 ms, of brainstem lesion and of suspicious tissue in region of the left frontal ventricle.

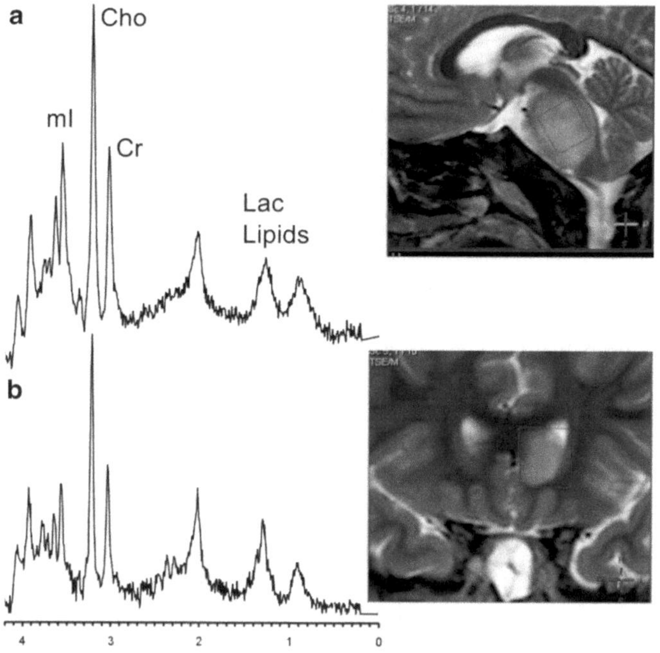

Fig. 22.27 Metastatic Pontine Glioma

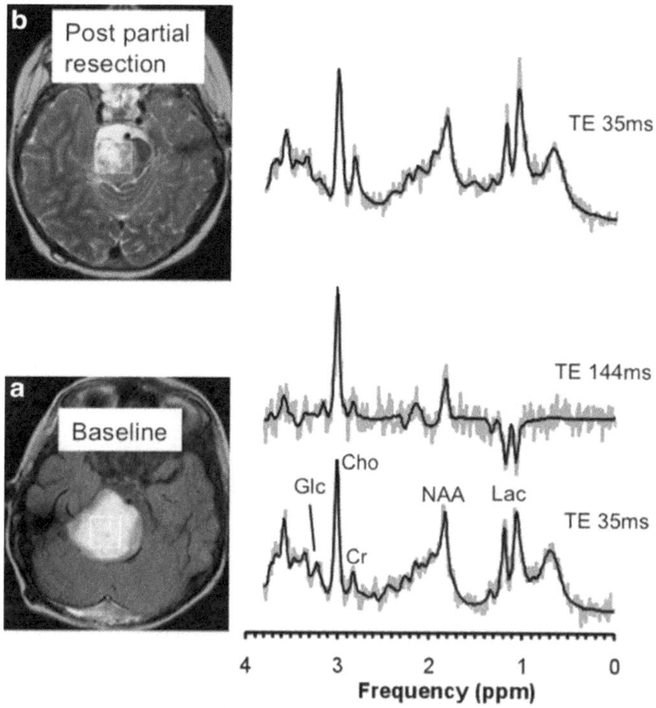

Fig. 22.28 Brainstem Tumor, Exophytic Pilocytic Astrocytoma

Interpretation/Discussion

Albeit being the worst tumor in pediatric neuro-oncology, pontine gliomas do rarely metastasize. In this case, however, a suspicious lesion anatomically not contiguous with the brainstem glioma was noticed. The frontal lesion likely represents a secondary metastatic ependymal seeding of the frontal horn. Spectra, obtained from the brainstem lesion (A) and the metastasis (B), demonstrate similar patterns and confirm disease progression (Fig. 22.27).

Conclusions

MRS of a rare metastatic pontine glioma is shown.

Case 28: Brainstem Tumor, Exophytic Pilocytic Astrocytoma

Clinical Background

7-year-old female with brainstem tumor, initially suspected to be a diffuse intrinsic pontine glioma.

MRS Method

1.5 T, single-voxel PRESS, TE 35 ms and TE 144 ms, lesion at baseline and residual lesion after partial resection.

Interpretation/Discussion

MRI showed an intrinsic eccentrically located mass centered at the right side of the pons. The lesion demonstrated heterogeneous enhancement. MRI was consistent with an exophytic brainstem tumor, which are often pilocytic lesions. The MR spectrum at baseline (A) showed prominent lactate, residual NAA, and significantly reduced Cr. Cho was prominent (Fig. 22.28). However, absolute Cho concentrations were close to normal tissue levels. mI was low. A peak from likely glucose (Glc) was noted. A spectrum acquired with a long echo time of 144 ms showed an inverted lactate signal. The lesion was subsequently partially resected and a pilocytic astrocytoma was confirmed. MRS of the residual tumor was essentially unchanged from the baseline scan and consistent with a pilocytic astrocytoma (B).

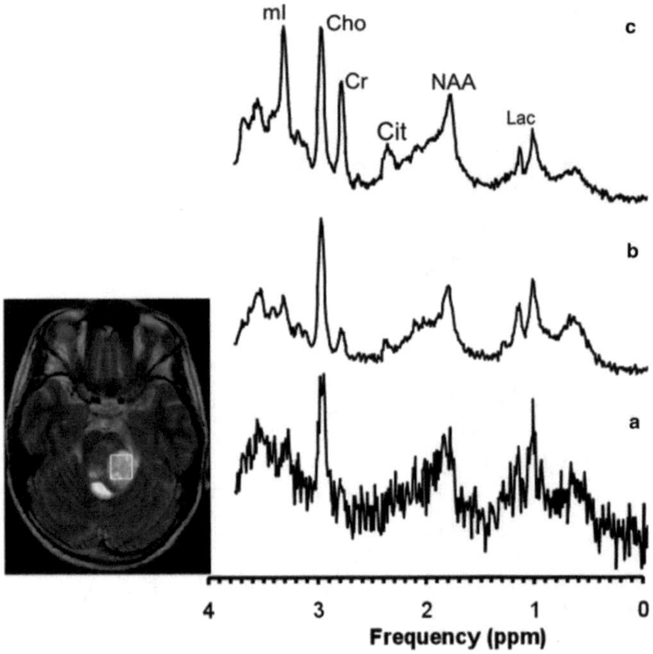

Fig. 22.29 Brainstem Tumor, Atypical Long-Term Survivor

Conclusions

MRS may be useful for characterization of exophytic brainstem tumors and help distinguish them from diffuse intrinsic pontine gliomas or other brainstem tumors.

Case 29: Brainstem Tumor, Atypical Long-Term Survivor

Clinical Background

11-year-old female with brainstem tumor, atypical long term survivor.

MRS Method

3 T, single-voxel PRESS, TE 35 ms, lesion.

Interpretation/Discussion

Several previous MRI studies showed a mass in the belly of the pons with inhomogeneous enhancement following contrast. The mass extended to the midbrain but not into the thalami. The impression from MRI was that the lesion was consistent with a diffuse pontine glioma. A spectrum acquired from a T2-hyperintense part of the lesion (A) showed generally low metabolite concentrations (Fig. 22.29). Lactate was present and Cho was prominent, albeit absolute Cho concentrations were low. Cr was not detectable and mI was very low. This profile is not typical for pontine gliomas but more typical for the pattern observed in pilocytic astrocytoma. For illustration, averaged spectra of infratentorial pilocytic astrocytoma (B) and pontine gliomas (C) are shown. Clinically, this patient did very well and was alive and stable until at least 8 years after the lesion was diagnosed. This patient was treated with radiation therapy and chemotherapy. Radiation therapy has significant adverse long-term effects in children. One may wonder whether advanced imaging could help to identify subtypes of brainstem tumors that require less aggressive therapy to maintain a good quality of life for patients.

Conclusions

An unusual brainstem glioma with atypical long survival shows a spectrum more typical for a pilocytic lesion than for a diffuse pontine glioma. MRS may be useful in differentiating different types of brainstem tumors, which may overlap in conventional MRI findings with diffuse intrinsic pontine glioma.

Case 30: Brainstem Tumor, Stable, Exophytic

Clinical Background

11-year-old male with history of exophytic brainstem tumor dating back 7 years—no biopsy.

MRS Method

3 T, single-voxel PRESS, TE 35 ms, of lesion with small partial volume of surrounding tissue.

Interpretation/Discussion

On MRI, an expansile mass centered on the left-sided superior cerebellar peduncle was seen. The imaging characteristics were stable when compared with earlier studies. MRS showed no clear evidence for elevated lactate (Fig. 22.30). NAA was reduced whereas Cr was slightly above normal. Both Cho and mI were above normal. MRS was not typical for pilocytic astrocytoma. This pattern was felt to be more typical for other low-grade tumors. However, the location and clinical history is nevertheless suggestive for a now indolent pilocytic lesion. It is thus possible that the biochemical profile observed is that of an indolent pilocytic lesion that may have become “gliotic” and thus changed its biochemical profile.

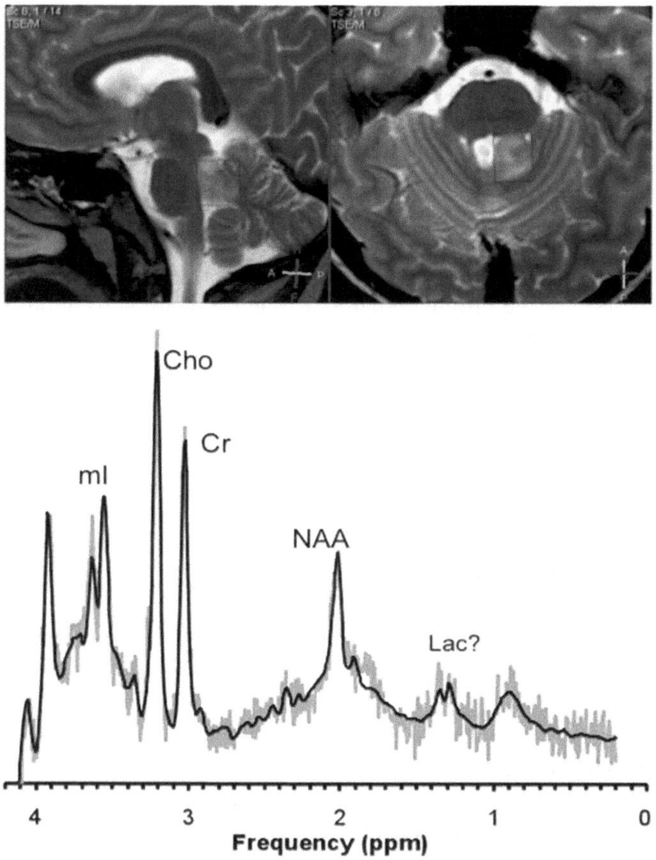

Fig. 22.30 Brainstem Tumor, Stable, Exophytic

Conclusions

MRS of a long-term stable exophytic brainstem tumor showed a profile of a low-grade lesion. Considering the long history of stable appearance of this lesion, one might speculate that this lesion might present an old indolent and gliotic pilocytic lesion.

Case 31: Citrate, Anaplastic Astrocytoma

Clinical Background

Seven-year-old female with brain lesion. MRS was performed for lesion characterization.

MRS Method

1.5 T, single-voxel PRESS, TE 35 ms.

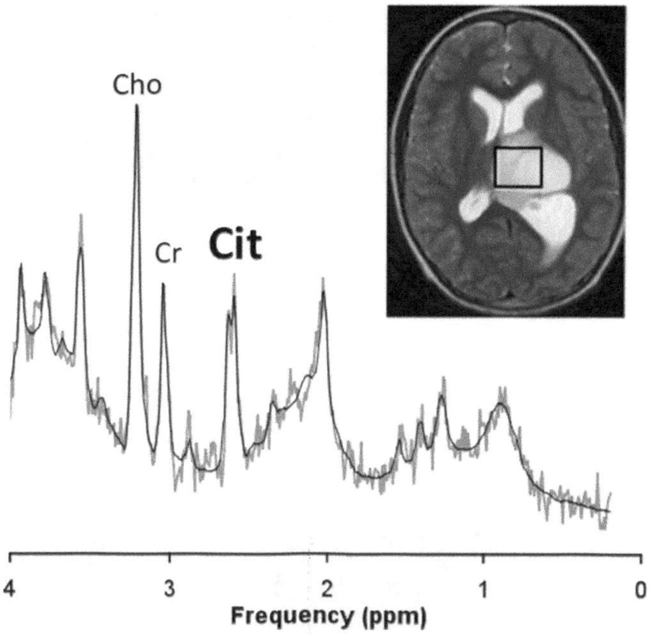

Fig. 22.31 Citrate, Anaplastic Astrocytoma

Interpretation/Discussion

On MRI a left thalamic/left intraventricular solid-cystic hypocellular mass most likely presenting a pilocytic astrocytoma was reported. Perfusion MRI was also performed and indicated a hypoperfused tumor (Fig. 22.31). MRS was not consistent with pilocytic astrocytoma and a regular glial tumor was suggested. Subsequent resection revealed an anaplastic astrocytoma. The unusual peak at ≈2.6 ppm was consistent with citrate, which has previously been observed most consistently in diffuse brainstem gliomas but also in other grade II and grade III gliomas [1]. Despite surgical resection and chemotherapy, disease progression was noted at 5 months after initial diagnosis and the patient died within 1 year after diagnosis.

Conclusions

Citrate may be observed in subgroups of pediatric brain tumors, mostly likely in glial tumors. The role of citrate and its potential value as a predictor for malignant progression is currently being investigated [2].

Case 32A: Citrate, 3 T, Short TE

Clinical Background

Seven-year-old male with brain lesion. MRS was performed for lesion characterization.

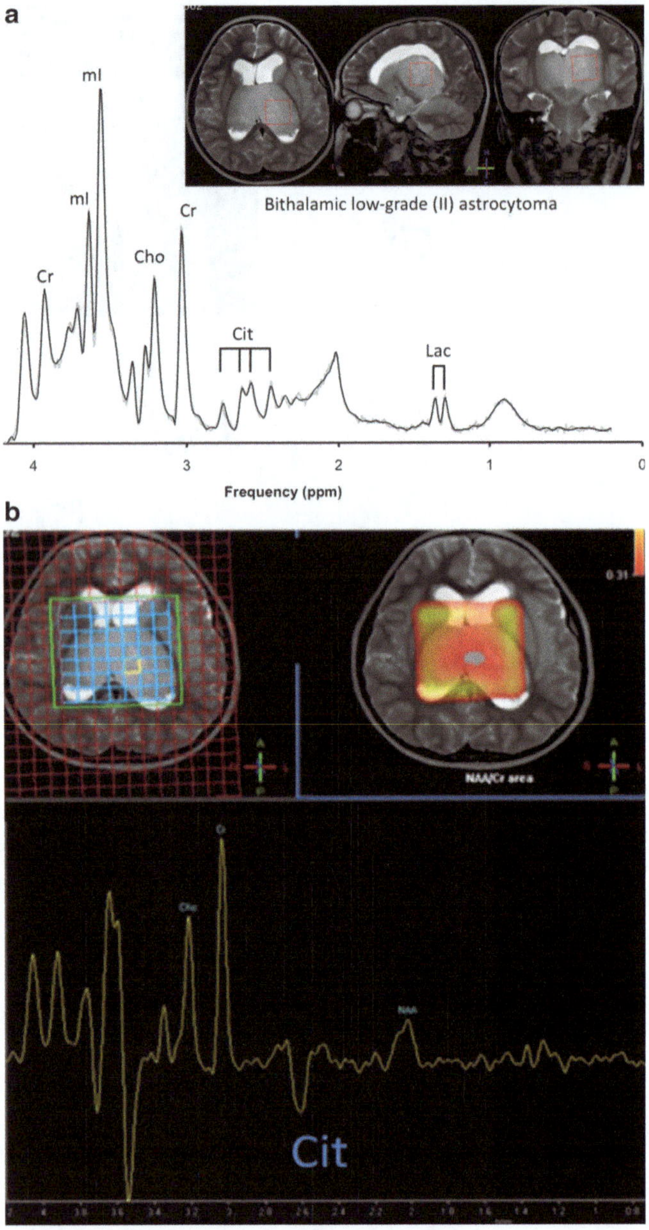

Fig. 22.32 Citrate, 3 T, Short TE (*top*), Citrate, 3 T, Long TE (*bottom*)

MRS Method

3 T, single-voxel PRESS, TE 35 ms, lesion.

Interpretation/Discussion

On MRI a bithalamic/left nonenhancing lesion was detected. Subsequent biopsy revealed a low-grade (WHO II) astrocytoma (Fig. 22.32a). Perfusion MRI was also performed and indicated a hypoperfused tumor. MRS was consistent in a low-grade glioma. Moderate levels of Cho are more typical for lower grade lesions albeit there is a significant overlap. The unusual signal at ≈2.4–2.8 ppm was consistent with citrate. This tumor eventually progressed and the patient died from the disease.

Conclusions

Note that the citrate signal at 1.5 and 3 T are substantially different even when the same acquisition method is used. Citrate may predict poor outcome despite the low grade of the lesion.

Case 32B: Citrate, 3 T, Long TE

Clinical Background

Seven-year-old male with brain lesion. MRS was performed for lesion characterization.

MRS Method

3 T, 2D-CSI, TE 85 ms, lesion and surrounding tissue. A TE of 85 ms was selected as citrate is inverted at this echo time at 3 T.

Interpretation/Discussion

Multivoxel MRS confirms moderate levels of Cho throughout lesion (not shown in detail) (Fig. 22.32b). An inverted peak consistent with citrate was observed.

Conclusions

Note that the citrate signal is inverted at 3 T when an echo time of 85 ms is selected.

Case 33: Choroid Plexus Carcinoma

Clinical Background

14-month-old male with new tumor in right lateral ventricle.

MRS Method

1.5 T, single-voxel PRESS, TE 35 ms, lesion.

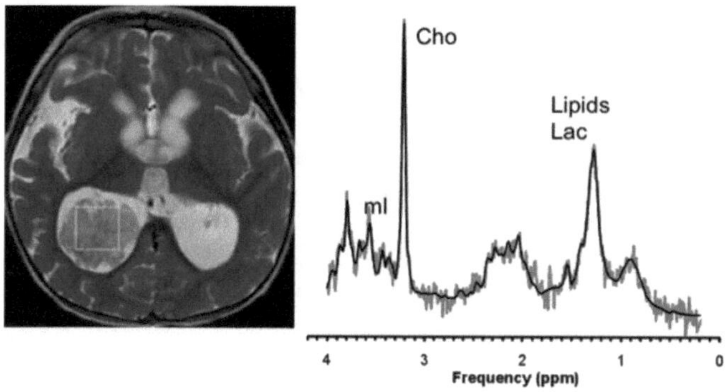

Fig. 22.33 Choroid Plexus Carcinoma

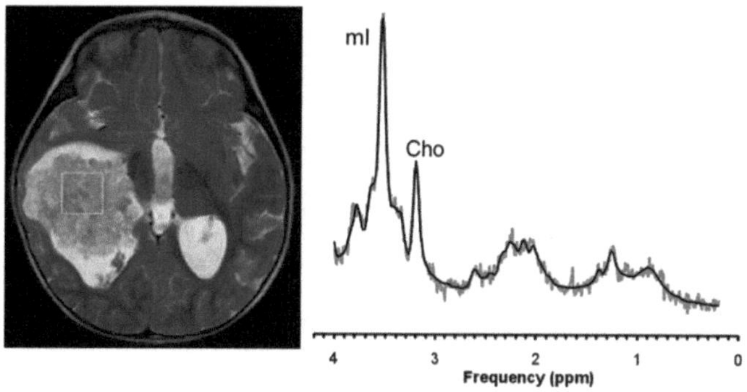

Fig. 22.34 Choroid Plexus Papilloma

Interpretation/Discussion

MRI showed a multilobular avidly enhancing mass in the atria of the right lateral ventricle without invasion of the surrounding brain parenchyma most consistent with a grade I choroid plexus papilloma (Fig. 22.33). MR spectroscopy showed elevated lipids (and possibly lactate), depleted NAA, and depleted Cr. Cho was prominent, whereas mI was below normal. MRS was not consistent with choroid plexus papilloma. Instead, a grade III choroid plexus carcinoma was suggested. This was subsequently confirmed after the lesion was resected.

Conclusions

MRS can readily distinguish between grade I choroid plexus papilloma versus grade III choroid plexus carcinoma, particularly in regards to the relationship between mI and Cho (cf. *Case 34*).

Case 34: Choroid Plexus Papilloma

Clinical Background

22-month-old female with new ventricular tumor.

MRS Method

1.5 T, single-voxel PRESS, TE 35 ms, lesion.

Interpretation/Discussion

MRI showed a large lobulated avidly enhancing mass in the atria of the right lateral ventricle with minimal transependymal edema on the right side (Fig. 22.34). MRI mentioned grade III choroid plexus carcinoma as the most likely tumor type. MR spectroscopy showed only minimal elevated lipids (and possibly lactate), depleted NAA, and depleted Cr. Cho was elevated but much less prominent than mI. MRS was consistent choroid plexus papilloma. This was subsequently confirmed after the lesion was resected.

Conclusions

MRS can readily distinguish between grade I choroid plexus papilloma versus grade III choroid plexus carcinoma particularly in regards to the relationship between mI and Cho.

Case 35: Choroid Plexus Papilloma, 3 T

Clinical Background

2-year-old female with new ventricular tumor.

MRS Method

3 T, single-voxel PRESS, TE 35 ms, lesion.

Interpretation/Discussion

MRI showed an intraventricular lesion consistent with a choroid plexus papilloma (Fig. 22.35). MR spectroscopy showed only minimal elevated lipids (and possibly lactate), depleted NAA, and depleted Cr. Cho was elevated but much less prominent than mI. Note that at 3 T the mI peak is more complex than at 1.5 T.

Conclusions

An example of choroid plexus papilloma spectrum acquired at 3 T is shown with more complex rendered mI signal.

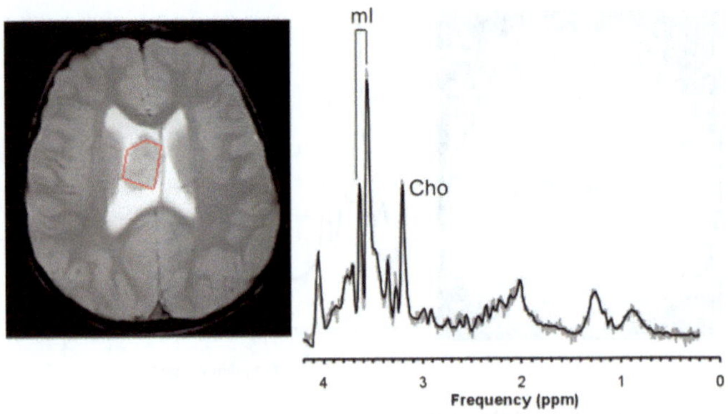

Fig. 22.35 Choroid Plexus Papilloma, 3 T

Case 36: Choroid Plexus Carcinoma, 3 T

Clinical Background

14-month-old male with left parietal/temporal mass.

MRS Method

3 T, single-voxel PRESS, TE 35 ms and 144 ms, of lesion.

Interpretation/Discussion

The MRI showed an avidly enhancing, hemorrhagic mass centered in the atrium of the left lateral ventricle with findings suggestive of invasion of the adjacent brain parenchyma (Fig. 22.36). Primary consideration was that of a choroid plexus neoplastic process. Given the posterior mediastinal mass on the concurrent spine MRI, favored etiology was that of metastatic neuroblastoma. Other potential etiologies based on the appearance include high-grade primary neoplasms of the choroid plexus such as carcinoma, PNET/ATRT, and anaplastic ependymoma. The MRS showed elevated lipids, no evidence for lactate, and NAA and Cr were depleted. Cho was prominent and mI was significantly above normal but less prominent than Cho. MRS was not typical for PNET/ATRT or ependymoma. It was concluded that the MRS was consistent with choroid plexus carcinoma. This was subsequently confirmed after surgical resection of the lesion.

Conclusions

MRS can provide additional information to improve initial diagnoses.

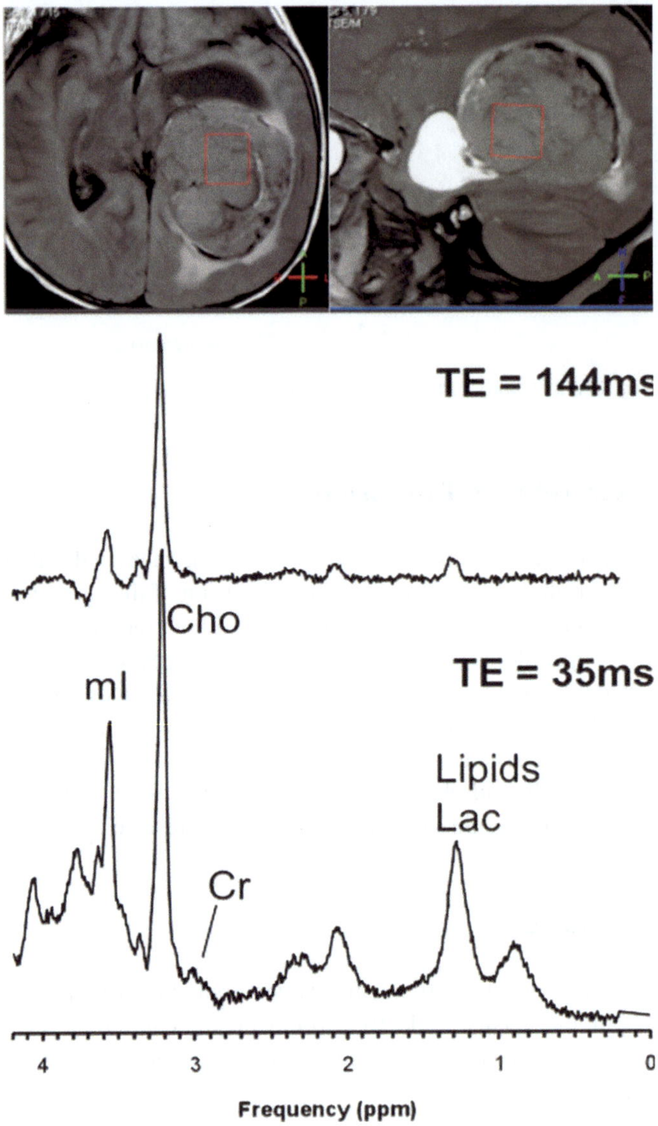

Fig. 22.36 Choroid Plexus Carcinoma, 3 T

Case 37: Atypical Choroid Plexus Papilloma

Clinical Background

10-year-old girl presenting with chronic headaches. A tumor was found on CT in the cerebellar region.

MRS Method

1.5 T, single-voxel PRESS, TE 35 ms, of lesion and surrounding tissue.

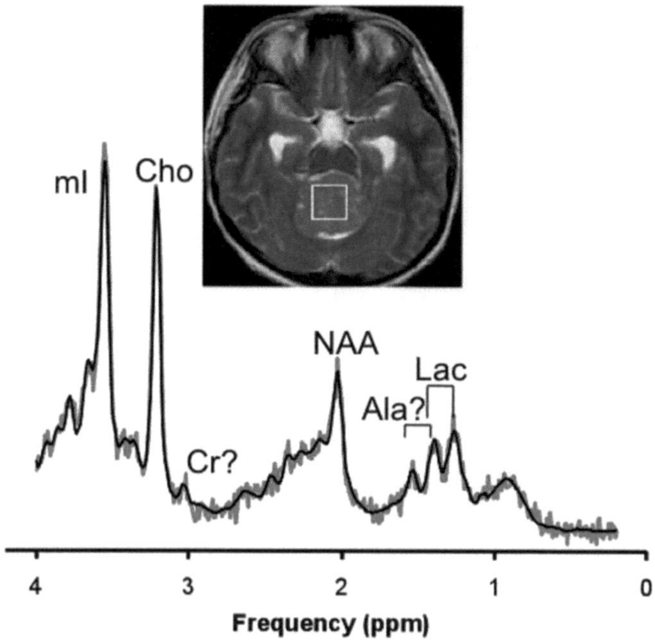

Fig. 22.37 Atypical Choroid Plexus Papilloma

Interpretation/Discussion

The MRI of this enhancing lesion was suggestive for a choroid plexus tumor or an ependymoma. Ependymoma often present with prominent lipids, which were unremarkable in this case (Fig. 22.37). Depleted Cr, as observed in this case, would also be unusual for ependymoma. On the other hand, in choroid plexus papilloma, mI is highly prominent, whereas Cho is the most prominent in choroid plexus carcinoma. Neither was observed and it was thus felt that the above case might fall between grade I papilloma and grade III carcinoma and represent an atypical choroid plexus papilloma (WHO II). This pathological diagnosis was subsequently confirmed after the lesion was resected. Lactate was observed and possibly also alanine (Ala).

Conclusions

Combined MRI/MRS improves initial diagnoses of posterior fossa tumors.

Case 38: Craniopharyngioma, NAA?

Clinical Background

Patient 1: 7-year-old boy with hydrocphalus and suprasellar mass with CT suggestive for craniopharyngioma. Patient 2: 11-year-old male with head ache, vomiting, and fatigue for 8 months. CT suggestive for craniopharyngioma.

MRS Method

1.5 T, single-voxel PRESS, TE 35 ms and 144 ms, of lesion and surrounding tissues.

Interpretation/Discussion

Patient 1: The MRI showed a complex cystic and partially solid enhancing suprasellar mass with areas calcification, suggestive of craniopharyngioma. Short TE MRS showed elevated lipids/macromolecules at 0.9 ppm, prominent lactate, and a prominent peak at around 2.0 ppm (Fig. 22.38). This peak is not consistent with NAA, which has a more complex spectrum. The signal was substantially diminished in a spectrum acquired with a long TE of 144 ms. Patient 2: A comparable spectrum was obtained from another craniopharyngioma confirming the presence of the unusual peak.

Conclusions

Spectra of craniopharyngioma may show an unusual peak at approximately 2.0 ppm. The signal appears to be not consistent with NAA.

Case 39: Disseminated, Rare Atypical Neurocytoma

Clinical Background

5-year-old female with a disseminated atypical neurocytoma.

MRS Method

3 T, single-voxel PRESS, TE 35 ms, of lesion and surrounding tissues.

Interpretation/Discussion

The MRI showed a diffuse leptomeningeal, basilar cistern, and perivascular space tumor (Fig. 22.39). The tumor appeared to have slowly progressed in size of overall tumor volume from previous studies. MRS was performed in three regions of interest: within resection cavity (ROI1), cystic appearing tumor tissue in right parietal tissue (ROI2), and right cerebellar tumor (ROI3). Cho was most prominent in ROI1 but also elevated relative to Cr in ROI2. There was considerable residual NAA in ROI3. However, residual NAA

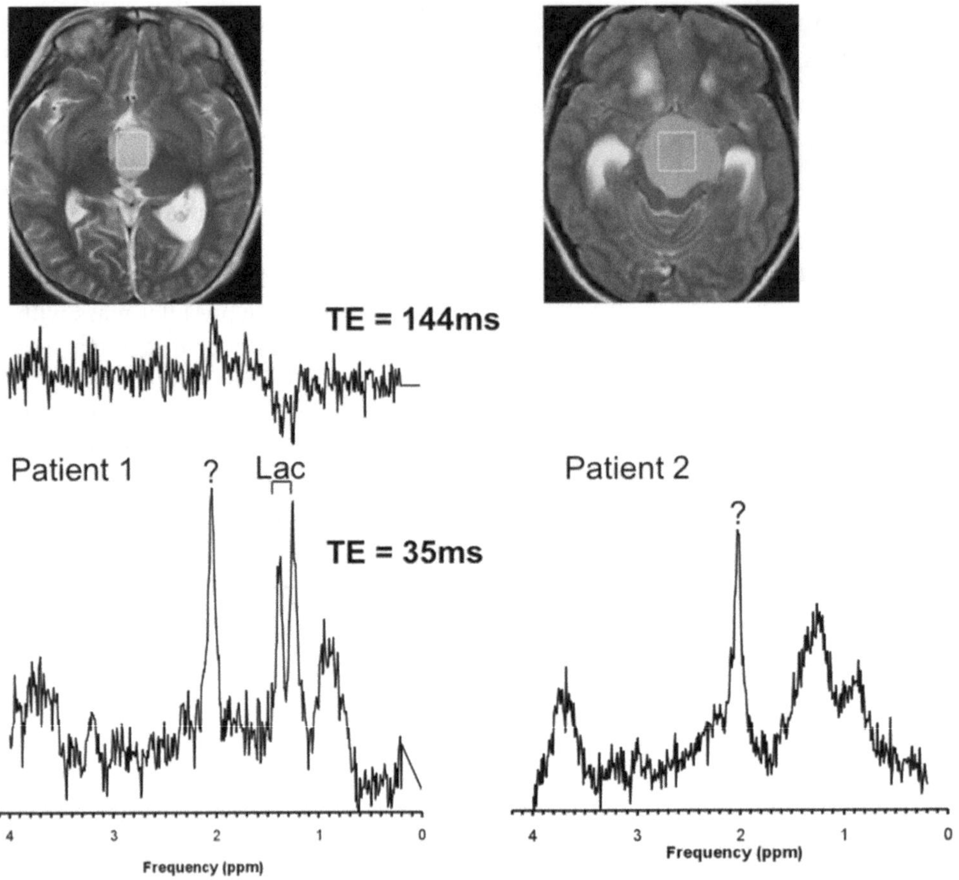

Fig. 22.38 Craniopharyngioma, NAA?

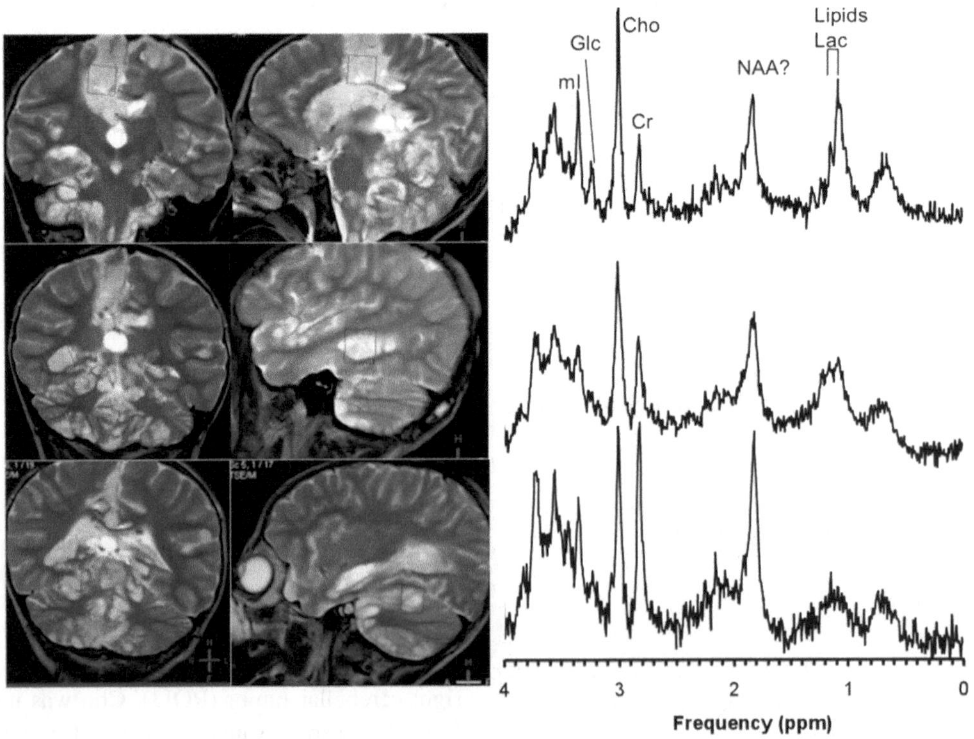

Fig. 22.39 Disseminated, Rare Atypical Neurocytoma

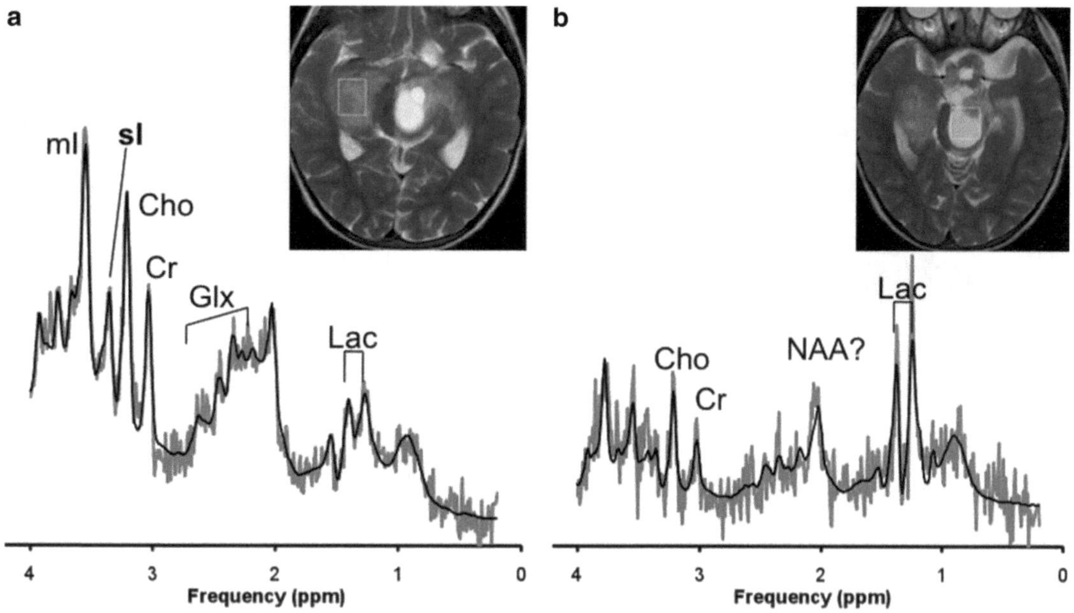

Fig. 22.40 Astrocytoma, High Scyllo-Inositol

was also observed for ROI2 and ROI1, where there is little partial volume of surrounding normal tissue. Lactate was elevated in ROI1, which also showed a comparably prominent Glc peak. Other tumors that may show signal consistent with NAA even when partial volume with surrounding tissue can be ruled out are pilocytic astrocytoma and mixed neuronal-glial tumors.

Conclusions

Spectra of a disseminated neurocytoma showed a peak consistent with NAA despite no partial volume with surrounding normal tissue.

Case 40: Astrocytoma, High Scyllo-Inositol

Clinical Background

4-year-old girl is presenting progressive right-sided weakness. Started as limp, progressed to include arm. Prior CT showed a brain lesion. MRI/MRS was performed for lesion characterization.

MRS Method

1.5 T, single-voxel PRESS, TE 35 ms of solid lesion and cystic lesion.

Interpretation/Discussion

The MRI showed a multicentric mass involving the right hippocampus, chiasm, hypothalamus, left thalamus, and midbrain (Fig. 22.40). Following contrast administration, the multilobulated tumors showed inhomogeneous enhancement. There was a 2 cm in diameter cyst within the midbrain with a 12 mm enhancing nodule along the wall. A glial tumor was suggested. MRS of the solid tumor showed elevated lactate and depleted NAA. Cho was only moderately more prominent than Cr. mI was prominent. Noted was an unusual prominent peak consistent with scyllo-inositol (sI). The tumor was resected and was determined to be a grade II astrocytoma. The tumor eventually progressed and outcome was poor.

Conclusions

An unusual high scyllo-inositol peak was detected in a grade II astrocytoma. The significance of high sI is unclear.

Case 41: Acute Myeloid Leukemia, Myeloid Sarcoma

Clinical Background

23-year-old male with history of acute myeloid leukemia (AML), swelling of right mastoid and mandible, vertigo and headache. CT showed right cerebellar mass.

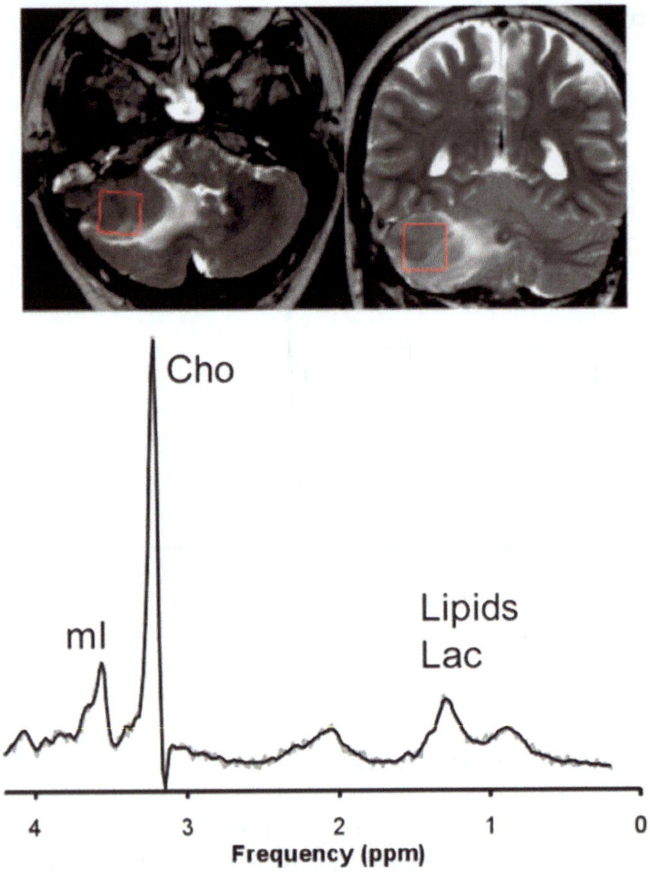

Fig. 22.41 Acute Myeloid Leukemia, Myeloid Sarcoma

MRS Method

1.5 T, single-voxel PRESS, TE 35 ms, of lesion.

Interpretation/Discussion

On MRI, an avidly enhancing extra-axial mass in the right aspect of the posterior fossa involving the right temporal bone, right parotid space, and extending into and occluding the right sigmoid sinus and internal jugular vein was seen (Fig. 22.41). Findings were consistent with a neoplastic process such as a myeloid sarcoma (chloroma, granulocytic sarcoma) correlating with patient's history of AML. MRS confirms impression from MRI of an extra-axial tumor by showing a spectrum with depleted Cr and NAA. Cho was very prominent suggestive for a malignant lesion.

Conclusions

MRS of a myeloid sarcoma shows prominent Cho and depleted Cr.

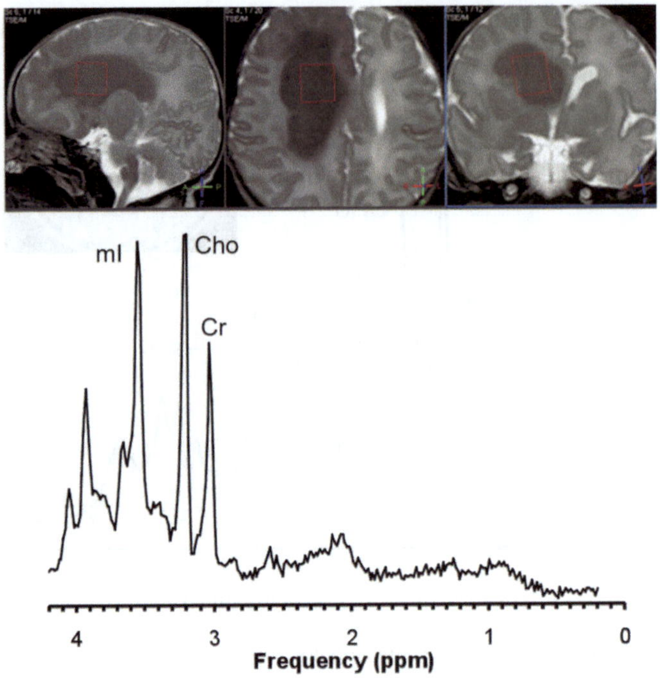

Fig. 22.42 Gemistocytic Astrocytoma: Newborn Tumor

Case 42: Gemistocytic Astrocytoma: Newborn Tumor

Clinical Background

4-day-old female baby (36 weeks gestational age at birth) with intracranial mass versus hemorrhage.

MRS Method

3 T, single-voxel PRESS, TE 35 ms, of lesion and surrounding tissues.

Interpretation/Discussion

The incidence of primary brain tumors in newborns is very low. An example for a rare gemistocytic astrocytoma is shown (Fig. 22.42). There was no evidence for lactate or lipids. NAA is depleted. Cr, Cho, and mI were above normal tissue concentrations for a normal neonatal MRS study in this location. Overall, the MRS is similar to the pattern of regular grade II astrocytoma observed in pediatrics.

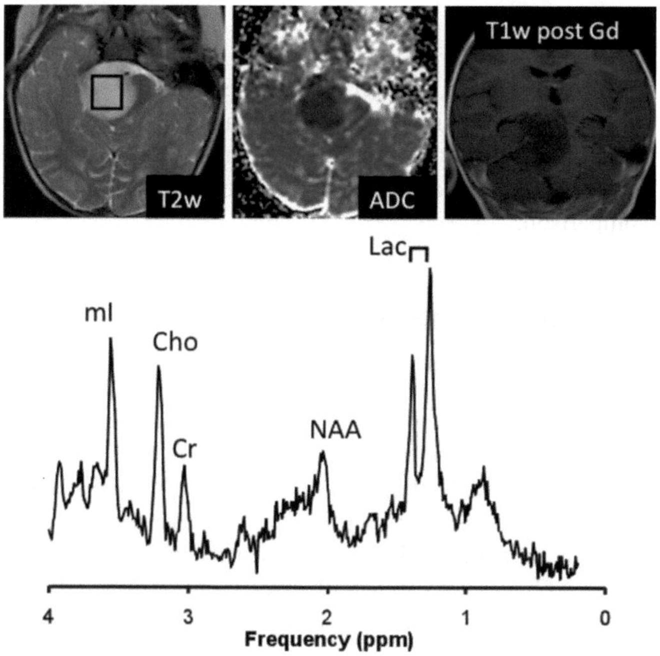

Fig. 22.43 Brainstem PNET, Glioma

Conclusions

A rare case of gemistocytic astrocytoma in a newborn is shown. The pattern is comparable with the profile of regular pediatric diffuse astrocytoma.

Case 43: Brainstem PNET, Glioma

Clinical Background

15-month-old boy with left-sided weakness.

MRS Method

1.5 T, repeated single-voxel PRESS, TE 35 ms, lesion, at presentation

Interpretation/Discussion

On MRI a well-circumscribed nonenhancing lesion, which is bright on T2w images was detected (Fig. 22.43). The diffusion signal is hyperintense with a low ADC value. The lesion was hypointense on T1w images but nevertheless considered to be consistent with large epidermoid tumor. MRS was not consistent with epidermoid, where previous studies have shown mostly lactate. The MR spectrum showed prominent lactate and a small residual signal from NAA. Both Cho and mI were elevated relative to Cr. However, absolute Cho and mI were below normal tissue levels. There is no evidence for Tau. The MRS pattern fits best the pattern of a glial tumor. Due to the absence of Tau, the low concentration of Cho, and relatively prominent mI it was felt that MRS was not consistent with a primitive neuroectodermal tumor (PNET). However, the tumor was biopsied/partially resected and the pathologist classified the tumor as a PNET. The tumor was treated with radiation therapy but with limited response, which is unusual for PNET. The patient died approximately two years after initial diagnosis.

Conclusion

The typical MRS pattern of brainstem PNETs is unknown. However, this individual study indicates that brainstem PNET do not necessarily present with elevated Tau.

Case 44: Meningioma, Alanine, Unusual MRI

Clinical Background

12-year-old previously healthy male with left-sided lower CNS dysfunction. MRS was carried out to improve initial lesion characterization.

MRS Method

3 T, single-voxel PRESS with TE = 35 ms (A) and TE = 144 ms (B), centered in lesion without partial volume of surrounding tissue.

Interpretation/Discussion

On MRI an enhancing extra-axial posterior fossa lesion was seen (Fig. 22.44). A nerve sheath tumor was suggested as the most likely tumor type due to the growth pattern. The MRS showed elevated lipids. A doublet consistent with *alanine* was noted. Cr appeared depleted whereas Cho was the most prominent peak. The long TE spectrum confirmed the presence of *alanine*. MRS was suggestive for meningioma as the most likely tumor type since alanine has frequently been reported in these tumors. The pathology was confirmed by biopsy.

Case 45: Anaplastic Astrocytoma, Disease Monitoring, Metabolic Progression

Clinical Background

Nine-year-old girl with history of recurrent anaplastic astrocytoma post gross total resection. MRS was carried to distinguish between treatment-related changes versus residual/ recurrent disease.

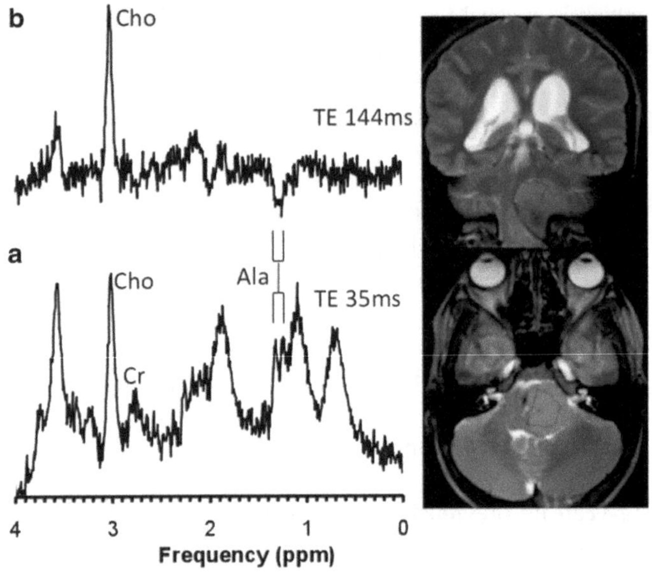

Fig. 22.44 Meningioma, Alanine, Unusual MRI

MRS Method

1.5 T, repeated single-voxel PRESS, TE 35 ms, of enhancing tissue adjacent to site of resection 2 days (A), 1 month (B), 2½ months (C), and 7 months (D) after surgery. Spectra are scaled to present absolute concentrations to allow direct comparison.

Interpretation/Discussion

The MRI at 1 month (B) suggested "*...interval decrease of ... edema, enhancement ... probably due to resolution of post-op changes and ongoing therapy...*". In contrast, MRS demonstrates relatively increased levels of Cho and reduced NAA suggesting recurrent/residual disease already at 1 month after surgery (Fig. 22.45). The subsequent MRI at 2½ months (C) was consistent with disease progression. MRS at that time was interpreted as likely grade IV glioblastoma. The MRI performed at 7 months (D) shows dramatic disease progression.

Conclusions

Increasing levels of Cho (either absolute concentrations or relative to NAA and/or Cr) in serial MRS studies may indicate recurrent disease.

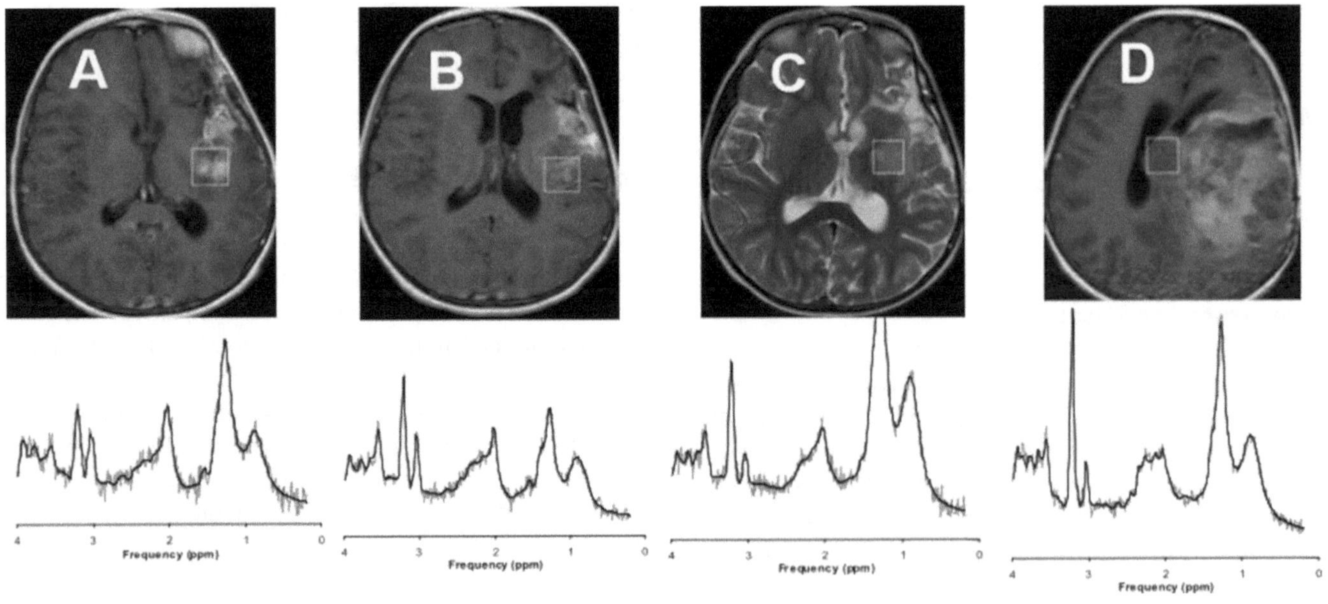

Fig. 22.45 Anaplastic Astrocytoma, Disease Monitoring, Metabolic Progression

Case 46: Serial MRS, Low-Grade Astrocytoma Versus High Grade Astrocytoma

Clinical Background

16-year-old male with a cerebellar/brainstem lesion. History of left temporal rhabdomyosarcoma at seven years of age. MRI/MRS was performed to rule out glioblastoma or anaplastic astrocytoma.

MRS Method

1.5 T and 3 T, single-voxel, TE 35 ms PRESS of the lesion at initial diagnosis and at several follow-up examinations.

Interpretation/Discussion

MRI at diagnosis: T2 hyperintense lesion at left-sided middle cerebellar peduncle, extending into the left pons and medulla and left cerebellar hemisphere, with mass effect and mild heterogeneous enhancement, suggestive of a tumor such as a glioma (Fig. 22.46). Given the patient's history, it was suggested that this tumor might have been a radiation-induced glioma. MRS showed slightly elevated lipids whereas NAA was reduced. Cr was below normal levels. Cho is very prominent and mI is slightly elevated. Considering the very high Cho, MRS was interpreted as being consistent with a malignant tumor such as anaplastic astrocytoma (Grade III) or grade IV glioblastoma. Subsequent to the initial (baseline) MRI/S study, the lesion was biopsied and an astrocytoma grade II (!) was diagnosed. The patient was nevertheless treated

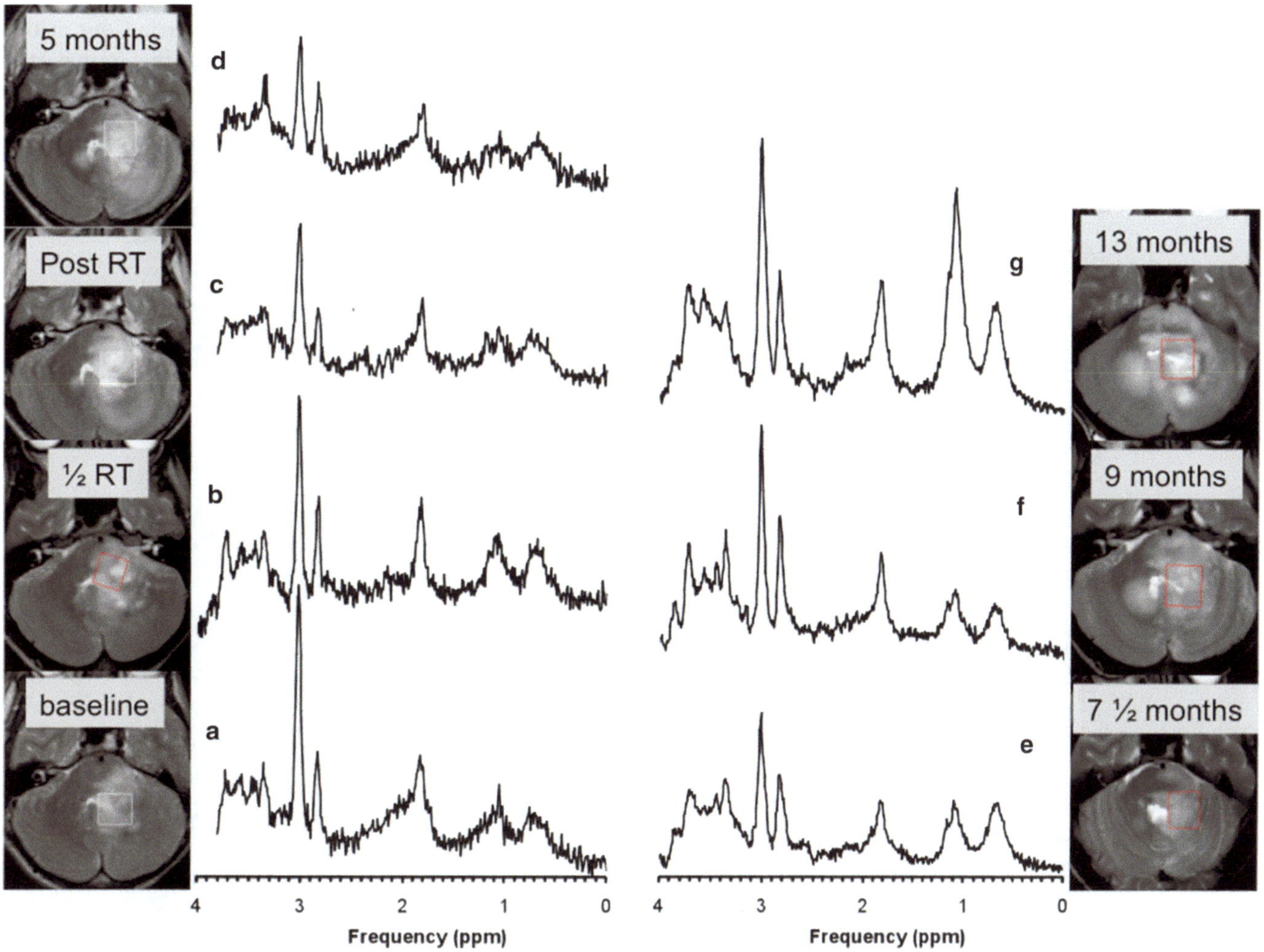

Fig. 22.46 Serial MRS, Low-Grade Astrocytoma Versus High Grade Astrocytoma

aggressively with radiation therapy considering clinical history and the features of the lesion on MRI and MRS. The lesion initially appeared to respond to therapy as Cho concentrations declined during and immediately after therapy. However, lipids remained unremarkable indicating no substantial necrosis after therapy. Cho levels started to increase again at 7 months after diagnosis (3½ months after completion of RT). On subsequent MRI, progression of the disease was noted. The patient succumbed to the disease approximately 18 months after initial diagnosis. It is noteworthy that MRI and MRS are "out of sync" with MRS preceding observations on MRI. For example, between 5 months and 7½ months post-baseline, the MRI appearance of the lesion improved, whereas on MRS, Cho was past its minimum and started to increase again. In addition, lipids increased at that time, both observations consistent with a worsening of the disease.

Conclusions

Prominent Cho may be helpful for identifying patients at high risk for progression and for disease monitoring.

Case 47: Tectal Glioma, Spontaneous Change, Serial MRS

Clinical Background

7-year-old female presenting with headache.

MRS Method

1.5 T and 3 T, single-voxel PRESS, TE 35 ms, of lesion at diagnosis and follow-up for 4½ years.

Interpretation/Discussion

A tectal lesion extending into the left thalamic region was diagnosed. Patient had enlarged ventricles and a third ventriculostomy was performed to address the clinical symptoms. A biopsy was considered not beneficial. Two single-voxel MRS studies were carried out at that time (Fig. 22.47). The MRS of the more thalamic part of

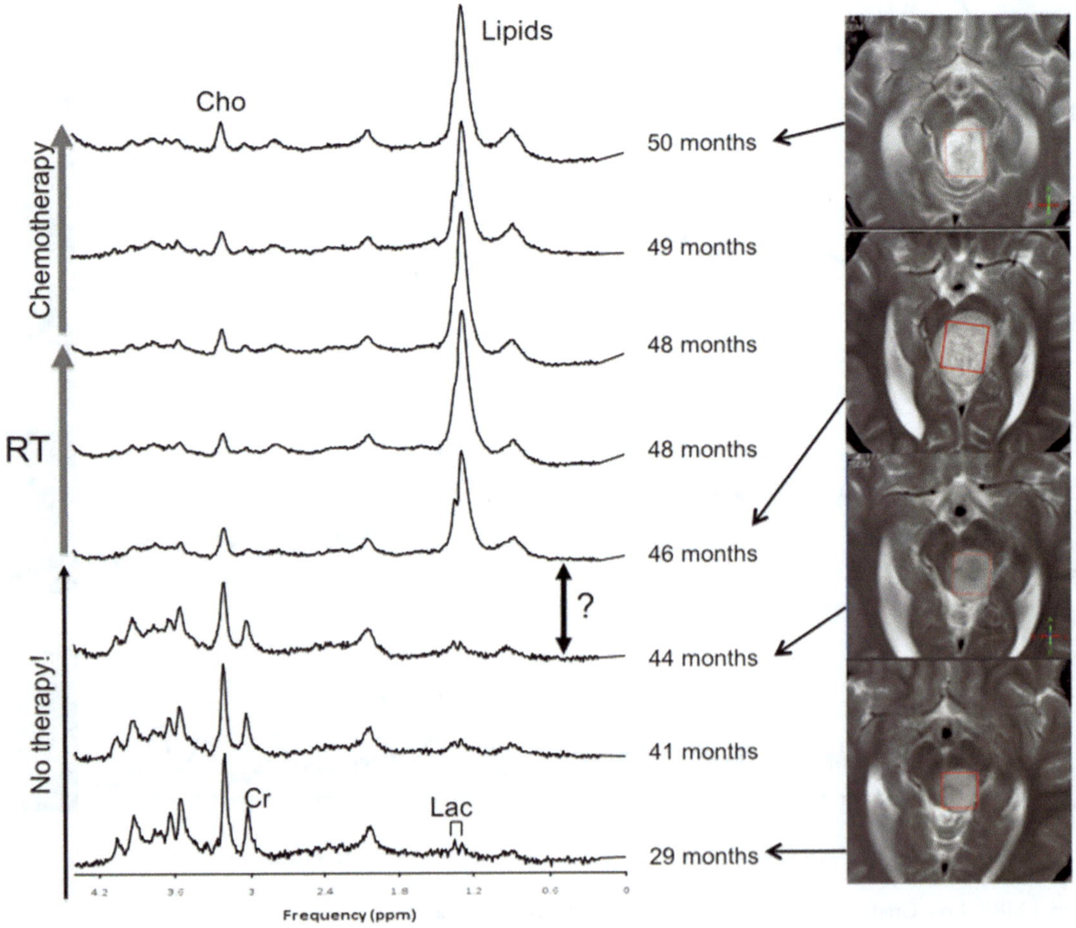

Fig. 22.47 Tectal Glioma, Spontaneous Change, Serial MRS

the lesion was consistent with a low-grade lesion and remained stable as of today (not shown). MRS of the tectal part was more concerning as Cho was more prominent. Close monitoring with MRI and MRS was recommended. Eight studies (all 3 T) are shown in the figure. The lesion remained stable for more than 3 years. Forty-four months after initial diagnosis the patient experienced increased clinical symptoms. On MRI, the tectal lesion increased significantly in size within 2 months. Spectroscopy showed decreased metabolite levels (for example a 55% reduction of Cho) and dramatically increased lipids. Only after these changes were observed, radiation therapy was initiated at 46 months. The lesion reached its maximum size at the end of radiation therapy. Two months after radiation therapy, the size of the lesions was considerably reduced.

Conclusion

This study demonstrates that lesions can undergo spontaneous and dramatic metabolic changes. The cause of the observed anatomical and metabolic changes is unclear.

Case 48: Unusual Disease Course of High-Grade Glioma

Clinical Background

16-year-old female with new intracranial mass on CT. MRI/MRS was carried out for initial lesion characterization for treatment monitoring.

MRS Method

1.5 T, single-voxel PRESS, TE 35 ms, of lesion and surrounding tissues.

Interpretation/Discussion

Baseline: On MRI a large heterogeneous and enhancing mass involving the left-sided frontal and temporal lobes, with additional foci of abnormal enhancement within the posterior right temporal lobe, and with associated mild midline shift from the left to the right was noted (Fig. 22.48). The appearance of this mass was interpreted to be consistent with a multifocal high-grade glioma. As other, less likely, diagnostic considerations based on MRI, supratentorial ependymoma or primitive neuroectodermal tumors were

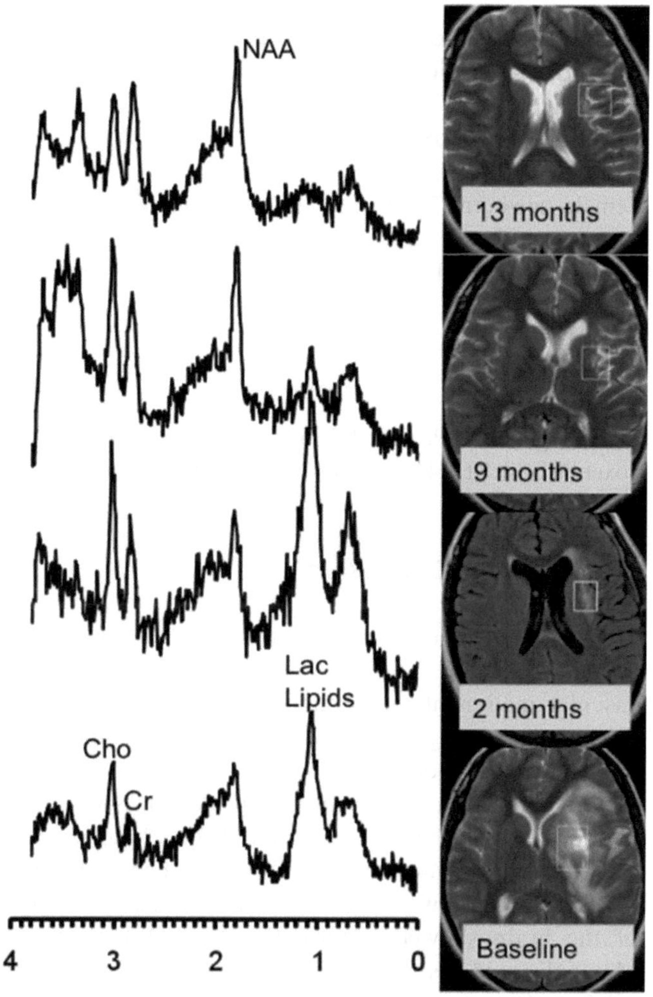

Fig. 22.48 Unusual Disease Course of High-Grade Glioma

suggested. The MRS was not typical for a high-grade glioma. Although, Cho was the most prominent peak, absolute Cho concentration was low. A biopsy and a resection were performed. A grade IV glioblastoma was diagnosed.

Follow-up studies: MRI appearance and MRS improved considerably in follow-up studies. The MRI/S performed 13 months after initial diagnosis was not consistent with tumor. A NAA peak indicates considerable normal tissue at the original site of the lesion. The most recently performed MRI study (without MRS, not shown), more than two years after diagnosis, was also stable.

Conclusions

Posttreatment MRS indicates considerable "normal" tissue at location of original tumor. It is unclear whether the observation of low Cho at baseline correlates with the, as of now, unusually good clinical course.

Case 49: Newborn, Rhabdoid Tumor, Metabolic Acidosis

Clinical Background

Female newborn (34 weeks gestational age at birth) with large facial/scalp mass (suspected hemangioma) and hepatosplenomegaly.

MRS Method

1.5 T, single-voxel PRESS, TE 35 ms of left frontal WM single-voxel PRESS, TE 144 ms of lesion in the right upper neck.

Interpretation/Discussion

MR imaging features of the lesion were atypical for a hemangioma (Fig. 22.49). Instead, concerns for a highly vascular malignant tumor such as hemangiopericytoma, fibrosarcoma, angiosarcoma, or other sarcoma were raised. MRS supports suspicion of a malignant lesion by identification of a prominent Cho peak (B). No discernable peak would have been expected for a hemangioma. This lesion was later confirmed to be a rhabdoid tumor. MRI of the brain was reported to be unremarkable. MRS of the brain showed abnormally elevated lactate (A). Metabolic acidosis was confirmed 2 weeks after the MRI/MRS study.

Conclusions

MRS can help with distinguishing benign from malignant lesions. Abnormally elevated lactate could indicate metabolic acidosis.

Case 50: Glioneuronal Tumor, Pre/Postradiation Therapy

Clinical Background

4-year-old female with brain tumor, evaluation for surgery.

MRS Method

3 T, single-voxel PRESS, TE 35 ms, of lesion at baseline and of lesion and parietal WM at postradiation therapy follow-up.

Interpretation/Discussion

On MRI, an expansile partially exophytic mass involving the pons, medulla, and cervical cord was observed. The MRI was suggestive for an exophytic pilocytic astrocytoma or a diffuse astrocytoma. The MRS (A) showed elevated lipids and lactate and an NAA peak that exceeded the intensity of the Cr peak (Fig. 22.50). Cho was prominent; however, absolute levels of Cho were close to nor-

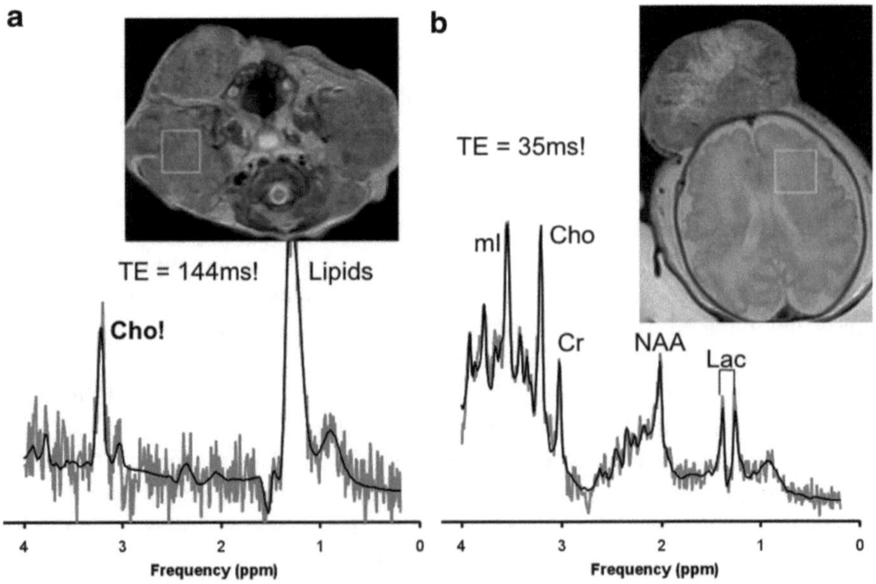

Fig. 22.49 Newborn, Rhabdoid Tumor, Metabolic Acidosis

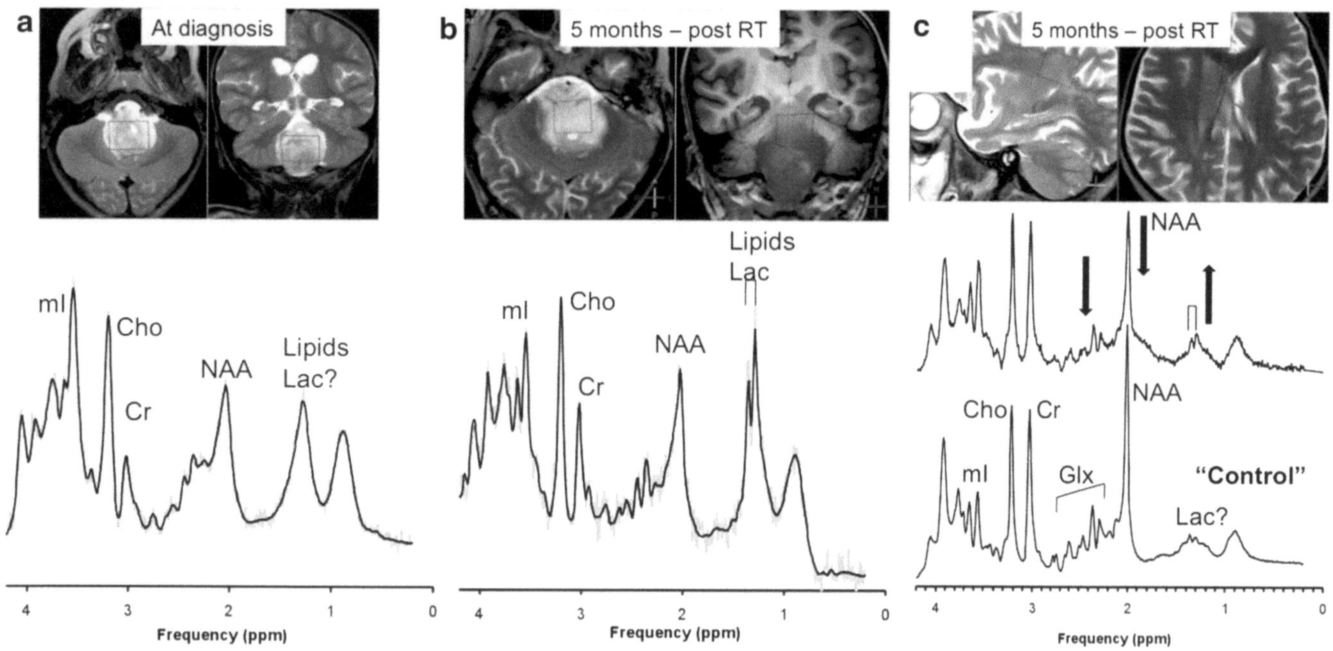

Fig. 22.50 Glioneuronal Tumor, Pre/Postradiation Therapy

mal levels. MI was above normal levels and there was no citrate detectable. Albeit, elevated mI is unusual for pilocytic lesions, MRS pattern was more consistent with a pilocytic astrocytoma but was not typical for regular astrocytoma. In a subsequently performed biopsy, a rare glioneuronal tumor was diagnosed. The lesion was inoperable and was treated with radiation therapy. Post therapy, the lesion had changed little and the MRS spectrum was comparable with the profile obtained at initial presentation (B). A spectrum obtained at that time from right parietal WM (C) showed elevated lactate, significantly reduced NAA, and reduced Glu + Gln (=Glx).

Conclusions

A glioneuronal tumor showed residual signal consistent with NAA—similar to what is being observed in pilocytic astrocytomas. MRS provided evidence for axonal damage/loss likely caused by radiation therapy.

Case 51: PNET, Rapid Disease Progression? Leucine?

Clinical Background

13-year-old female with supratentorial primitive neuroectodermal tumors (PNET) diagnosed 10 months earlier. The tumor was resected and radiation and chemotherapy was performed. MRI/MRS was performed for disease monitoring.

MRS Method

1.5 T and 3 T, single voxel PRESS, TE 35 ms and TE 144 ms, of lesion and surrounding tissues.

Interpretation/Discussion

The MRI study performed 8 months after diagnosis (A) showed a large resection cavity in the right parietal lobe with no evidence of residual or recurrent tumor (Fig. 22.51). Diffuse areas of white matter T2 hyperintensity involving the bilateral cerebral hemispheres were interpreted as most likely treatment related. Similarly, signal abnormalities involving the bilateral basal ganglia were interpreted as treatment related. No areas suspicious for recurrent or residual tumor were reported. MRS at that time was consistent with MRI. Although, NAA of a spectrum acquired of abnormal parietal white matter was clearly reduced, in the absence of evidence for elevated Cho, this was interpreted as treatment related. Albeit diffuse areas of white matter T2 hyperintensity involving the increased over the next 2½ months were noticed, these were nevertheless interpreted as most likely treatment related (B). At that time, MRS showed increased lactate and possibly leucine at 0.9 ppm (see inset in B—inverted peaks in long TE spectrum) but otherwise similar to the previous study and thus interpreted as consistent with treatment-related changes but not recurrent disease. However, 3½ months later, bilateral abnormal parenchymal areas of focal abnormal signal intensity with abnormal enhancement were noted (C). This was interpreted as likely due to progression of patient's primary PNET. The MR spectrum acquired from the parietal lobe showed increased lipids

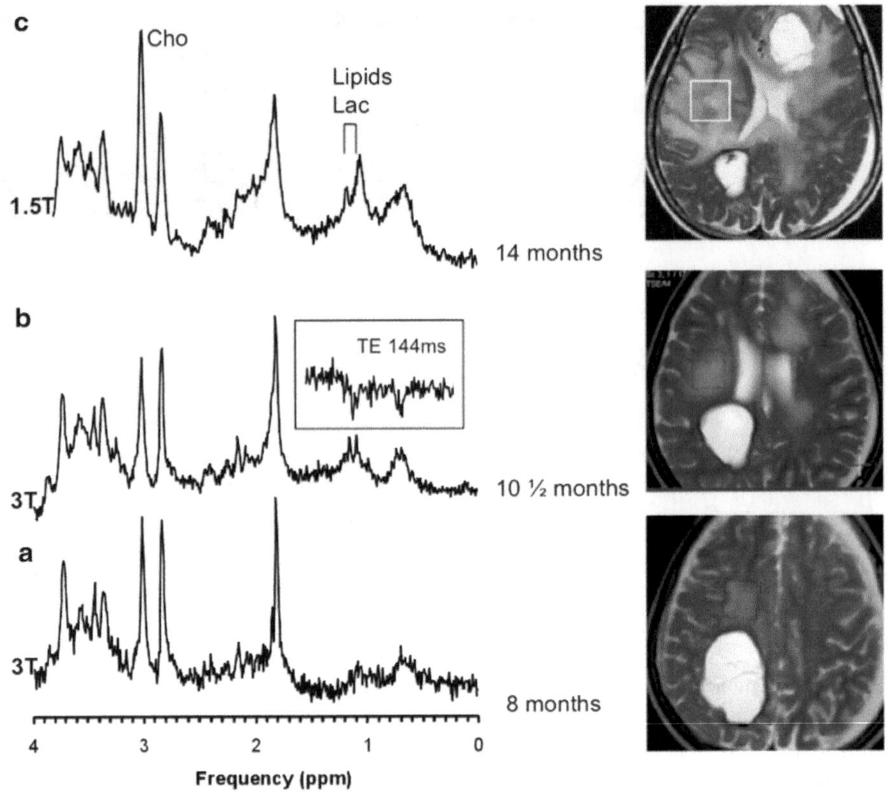

Fig. 22.51 PNET, Rapid Disease Progression? Leucine?

and lactate, reduced NAA, and increased Cho. The MR spectrum was interpreted to be consistent with recurrent disease. The patient died soon after the study at 14 months.

Conclusions

A dramatic change of the spectral appearance (and MRI) was noted. MRS indicates that disease progression accompanied by a striking change of the metabolic profile can occur very rapidly for some tumors. A resonance at 0.9 ppm consistent with leucine was detected in short TE and long TE spectra. Since Leucine has frequently been observed in infections one could speculate that other processes have contributed to rapid change of the MRS profile.

Case 52: Residual Tumor?

Clinical Background

8-year-old girl status post left temporal resection of a pilocytic astrocytoma after experiencing a seizure-like episode. MRI/MRS was performed to evaluate for tumor residual.

MRS Method

1.5 T, single-voxel PRESS, TE 35 ms, of lesion and surrounding tissues.

Interpretation/Discussion

On MRI there was no evidence of significant residual abnormal enhancing tumor. It was cautioned that areas of T2 hyperintensity posterior to of the resection margin may represent areas of vasogenic edema, but also areas of infiltrate nonenhancing tumor (administration of steroids can dimish contrast uptake of tumors) (Fig. 22.52). Close follow-up was recommended. On MRS, lipids and lactate were unremarkable. Absolute NAA was reduced but was well preserved relative to Cr. Cho was slightly above normal and mI within normal range. MRS appeared to be consistent with mostly normal tissue. The slightly relative (when compared with Cr) prominence of Cho was of concern as it may reflect a small partial volume of residual tumor tissue in region of interest. Still, 2 years later (not shown) no evidence for residual tumor was detectable.

Conclusions

MRS can assist MRI with assessment of postoperative edema versus residual tumor.

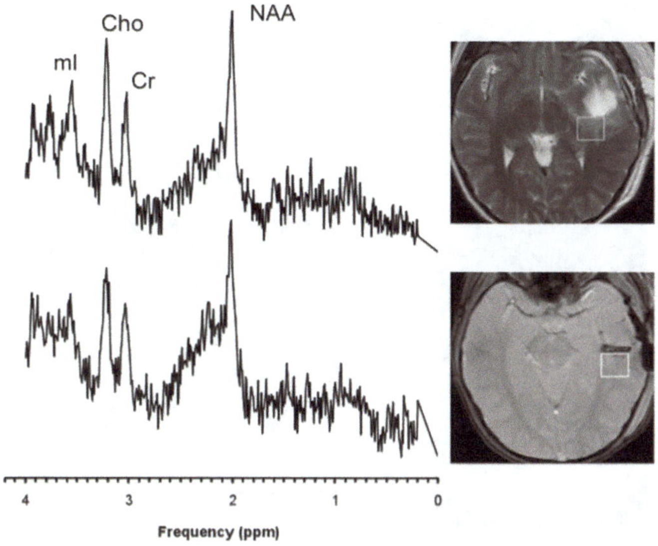

Fig. 22.52 Residual Tumor?

Case 53: Pilocytic Astrocytoma, Recurrent Versus Edema

Clinical Background

8-year-old female with recurrent pilocytic astrocytoma seven years after initial diagnosis. MRI/MRS was performed at diagnosis and several studies were performed to evaluate for the extent of the disease at the time of recurrent disease and thereafter.

MRS Method

1.5 T and 3 T, single-voxel PRESS, TE 35 ms, of lesion and surrounding tissues.

Interpretation/Discussion

MRS at initial presentation (A, lower trace) was consistent with a pilocytic astrocytoma (Fig. 22.53). The tumor was subsequently resected. Due to the location of the lesion complete resection was not achieved and the residual tumor was

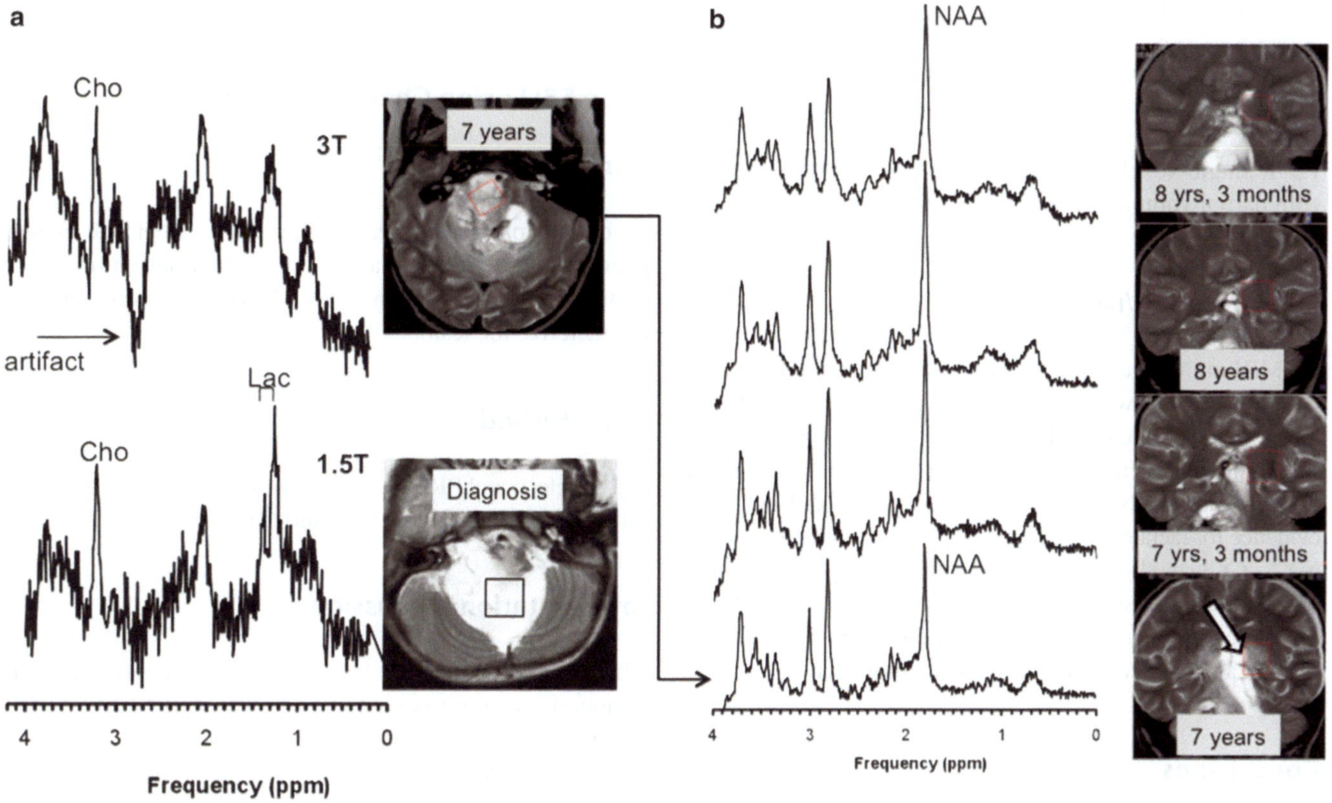

Fig. 22.53 Pilocytic Astrocytoma, Recurrent Versus Edema

monitored by MRI (no MRS studies) over several years. Multiple resections were carried out and the patient was treated with chemotherapies. Seven years after initial diagnosis, MRI was again suggestive for tumor growth. MRS performed at that time was consistent with tumor (A, upper trace). Also noticed, at that time were white matter abnormalities and there were concerns for spreading disease versus edema due to increased size of adjacent lesions. MRS showed reduced NAA (B, lowest trace) but was not consistent tumor and more suggestive for edema. Subsequently, the abnormality on MRI resolved and the MRS pattern returned to a profile close to that of normal white matter (B, upper traces).

Conclusion

MRS helped to distinguish edema from recurrent/disseminated pilocytic astrocytoma.

Case 54: Anaplastic Astrocytoma, Follow-up

Clinical Background

14-year-old female with a history of thalamic anaplastic astrocytoma. Post (incomplete?) resection and radiation therapy eight years ago. MRI/MRS was performed for disease status monitoring.

MRS Method

1.5 T, single-voxel PRESS, TE 35 ms, of suspicious lesions with partial volumes of surrounding tissue.

Interpretation/Discussion

On MRI multiple cysts in the brain parenchyma of both cerebral hemispheres which were unchanged in appearance from the prior examinations. There was increased signal present within the putamen and globus pallidus and within the thalamus on the unenhanced images. MR spectra did not show evidence for lactate (Fig. 22.54). There was significant residual NAA, Cr was slightly reduced, and Cho slightly elevated. MRS pattern of tissue in region of interest was interpreted as not typical for astrocytoma. This patient has remained stable 5 years after above studies have been completed.

Conclusions

MRS is useful to distinguish treatment-related changes from recurrent tumor.

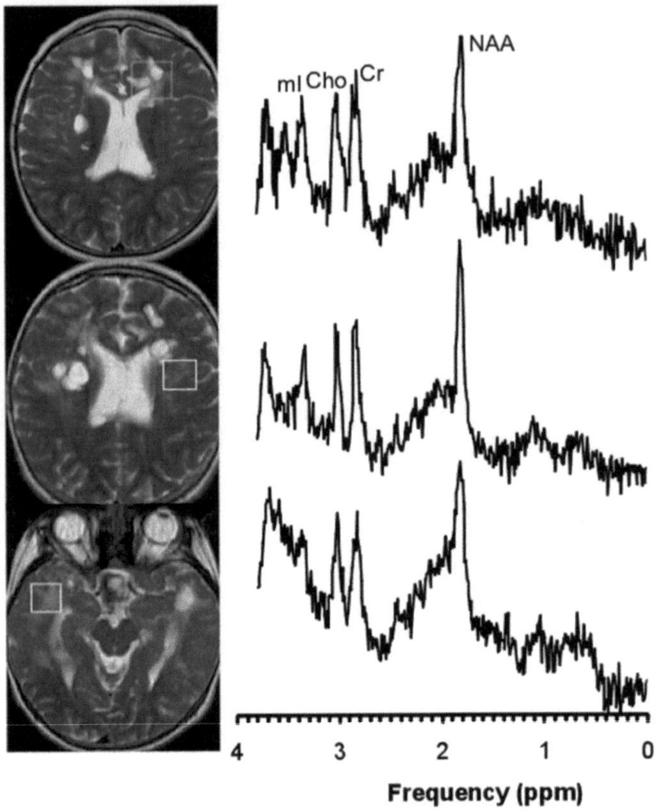

Fig. 22.54 Anaplastic Astrocytoma, Follow-up

Case 55: Lesion Characterization

Clinical Background

5-year-old previously healthy boy after an episode of near drowning. A CT scan was reported abnormal with an incidental finding of a brain lesion. MRI/S was performed to characterize the lesion.

MRS Method

3 T, single-voxel PRESS, TE 35 ms, of lesion in right occipital lobe—partial volume with surrounding tissue.

Interpretation/Discussion

MRI: A T2-hyperintense lesion involving the posterior right temporal and right occipital lobes was noted (Fig. 22.55). The imaging characteristics for the lesion were suggestive of a focus of cortical dysplasia/cortical tuber. MRI was interpreted as less likely to be consistent with a focus of demyelination or an alternative inflammatory or infectious etiology. A low-grade tumor was also considered less likely.

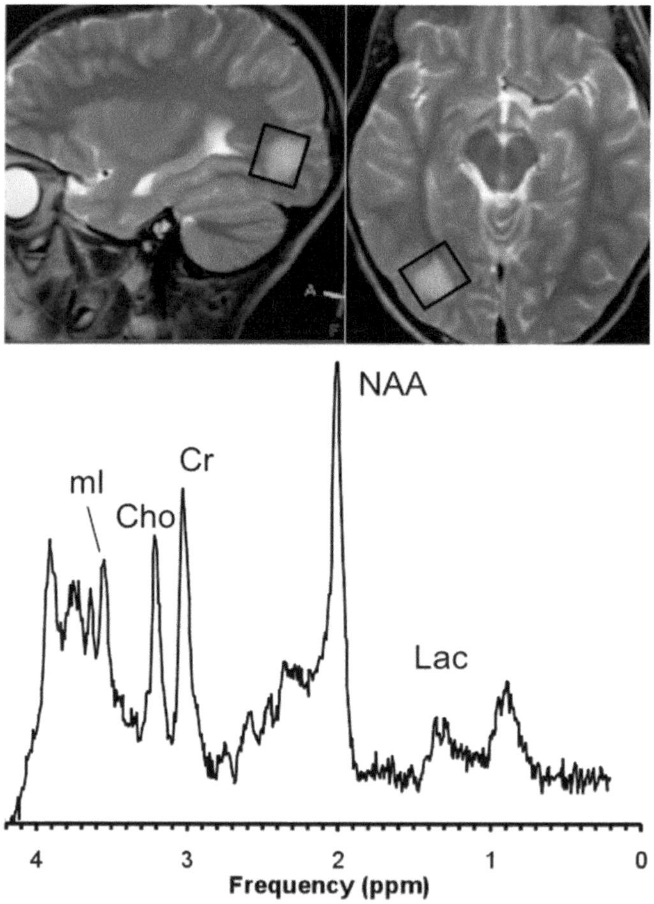

Fig. 22.55 Lesion Characterization

MRS: Lactate was mildly above normal. Other metabolites were close to or below normal levels. Cho was unremarkable when compared with Cr. mI also within normal range. MRS was not typical for glial tumor or other neoplastic process. Low levels of lactate and lipids are not typical for acute inflammatory processes. MRS is not consistent with an infection.

Conclusions

MRS confirms impression from MRI of a benign lesion.

Case 56: Aspergilloma

Clinical Background

10-year-old male with history of acute myeloid leukemia (AML), multifocal osteoma, and pulmonary aspergillosis. Now with 3 days of headache and emesis. CT showed mass in left side of brain.

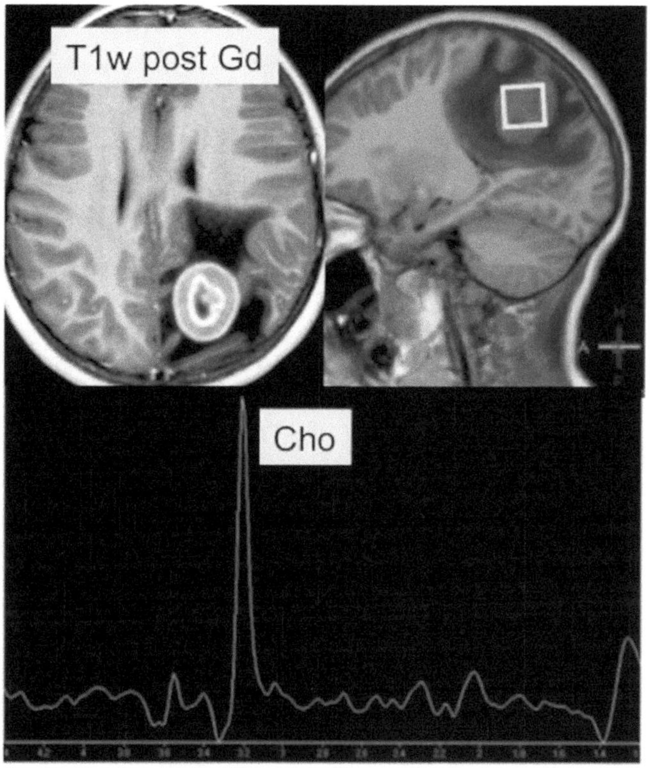

Fig. 22.56 Aspergilloma

MRS Method

1.5 T, single-voxel PRESS, TE 35 ms, of the lesion.

Interpretation/Discussion

Aspergilloma (or mycetoma) is a fungus ball inside tissue. The conventional MRI showed a ring enhancing lesion with significant surrounding vasogenic edema in the left parietal lobe (Fig. 22.56). A highly unusual spectrum was observed with Cho the only readily detectable peak.

Conclusions

Aspergilloma (or mycetoma) have prominent Cho. If MRS is interpreted alone without MRI, the spectrum could be confused with a tumor spectrum.

Case 57: Pontine Lesion, Cerebral Dysgenesis

Clinical Background

10-month-old male with microcephaly, schizencephaly with fluid collections on CT.

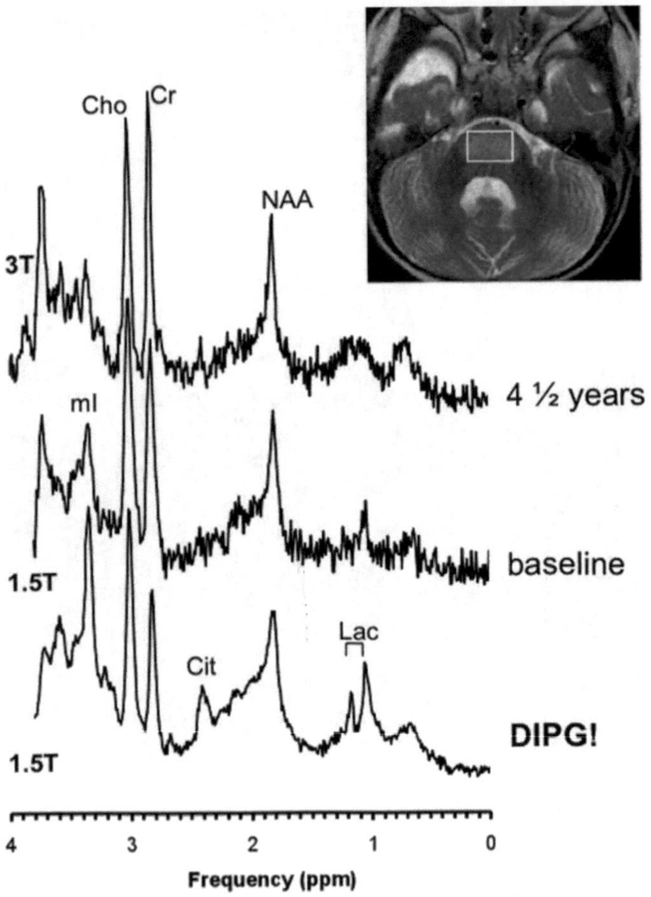

Fig. 22.57 Pontine Lesion, Cerebral Dysgenesis

MRS Method

1.5 T and 3 T, single-voxel PRESS, TE 35 ms, of lesion with small partial volume of surrounding normal appearing tissue.

Interpretation/Discussion

On MRI, a dysplastic frontal lobe cortex and a dysplastic corpus callosum were noticed. An abnormal focus of edema in the center of the pons was also described and the differential included a demyelinating lesion, encephalitis, or possibly a pontine tumor (Fig. 22.57). The MR spectroscopy at initial presentation (baseline) showed elevated Cho and decreased NAA relative to age-matched controls. There was no evidence for lactate or citrate, two metabolites that are frequently detectable in diffuse intrinsic pontine gliomas (lower trace: DIPG—average MRS of 20 patients at diagnosis). mI was also low when compared with a typical spectrum of DIPG. It was felt that MRS was not consistent with a DIPG. The MRS was also not consistent with encephalitis where lipids, lactate, and Gln are elevated and mI is reduced (acute encephalitis, cf. *Cases 60, 61, 68, and 71*). Follow-up 4½ years after diagnosis showed an essentially unchanged spectrum of the same lesion.

Conclusion

MR spectroscopy is helpful for initial characterization of brainstem lesions, which are in the differential for diffuse intrinsic pontine gliomas.

Case 58: Edema, Moderate, Severe

Clinical Background

Patient A: 2-year-old boy with suspicion for brain tumor. MRI/MRS was performed for lesion characterization. Patient B: 3-year-old girl with choroid plexus carcinoma after resection.

MRS Method

Patient A: 3 T, single-voxel PRESS, TE 35 ms, of lesion (pilocytic astrocytoma, not shown) and edema. Patient B: 1.5 T, single-voxel PRESS, TE 35 ms, of edema.

Interpretation/Discussion

Patient A: The lesion obstructed CSF flow and caused periventricular edema. The spectrum of edema (Fig. 22.58a, upper trace) showed generally reduced metabolite concentrations (cf. control, figure A lower trace, spectra are scaled to concentrations) and lactate was elevated. MI appeared to be disproportionally reduced whereas the relative concentrations of NAA, Cr, and Cho appeared to be similar in edema and in the control spectrum.

Patient B: This patient appeared to have had more severe edema. Metabolite concentrations were below normal with the exception of Gln, which was above normal. NAA was reduced consistent with axonal/neuronal damage/loss. Seven years after the MRS study was performed, a follow-up MRI revealed large extra-axial fluid collection along the margin of the right cerebral hemisphere.

Conclusions

There appears to be a wide range of spectral appearances for edema. MRS might potentially be useful to predict recovery from edema versus permanent tissue damage.

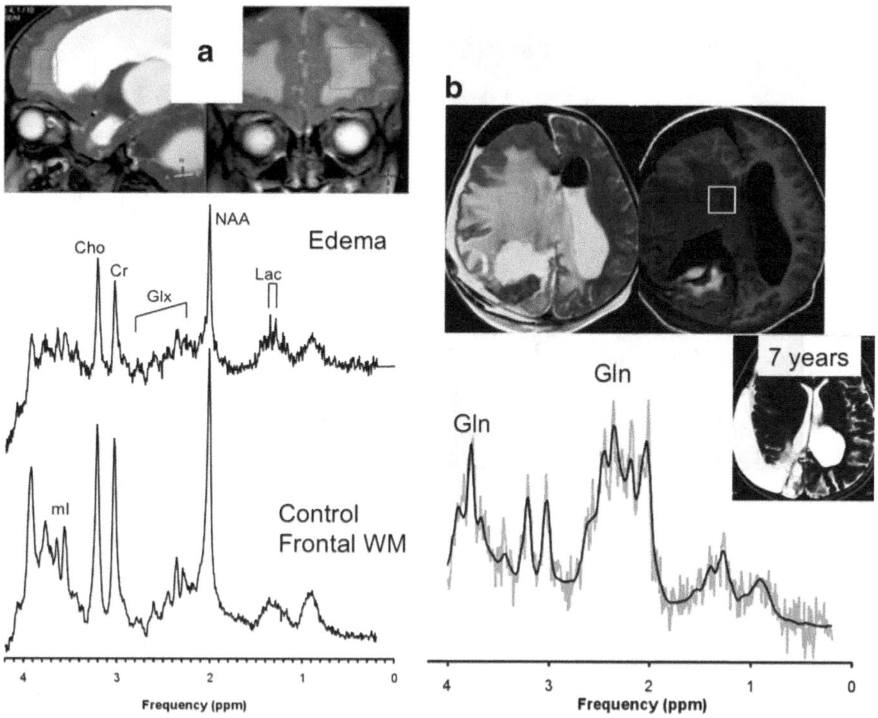

Fig. 22.58 Edema, Moderate, Severe

Case 59: Extreme Edema, Glutamine, NF1, Unusual Tumor

Clinical Background

12-year-old boy with neurofibromatosis 1 and right frontal lobe mass.

MRS Method

1.5 T, SV-PRESS TE 35 ms, lesion and surrounding edema.

Interpretation/Discussion

MRI showed a large enhancing mass involving the anterior right frontal lobe. There was adjacent extensive T2 hyperintensity, which was thought to represent vasogenic edema, infiltrating tumor, or a combination of the two (Fig. 22.59). The lesion demonstrated restricted diffusion consistent with a high-grade lesion. Spectroscopy of the lesion (A) showed prominent lipids and only moderately above normal absolute Cho levels. Spectroscopy of the surrounding edema showed elevated lactate and strikingly elevated Gln. NAA was reduced (approximately 15% of normal) and mI was depleted (0%). The causes for the striking accumulation of Gln are unclear. Increased Gln has been observed in acute hypoxic/ischemic injury and in hepatic encephalopathy believed to be secondary to ammonia accumulation. Gln is an osmolyte and mI might be depleted to counterbalance the Gln accumulation. This spectrum was interpreted as not consistent with tumor infiltration. The pattern of significantly below normal NAA may indicate permanent damage. However, long-term follow-up of this patient was not available to confirm this interpretation.

Conclusions

A case of extreme edema is presented with strikingly high Gln. MRS may be useful in distinguishing vasogenic edema from infiltrative tumor edema.

Case 60: Acute Herpes Encephalitis, 7 Months Old

Clinical Background

7-month-old male with focal seizures, oral herpetic sores.

MRS Method

1.5 T, single-voxel PRESS, TE 35 ms and 144 ms, of suspicious tissue and of contralateral side.

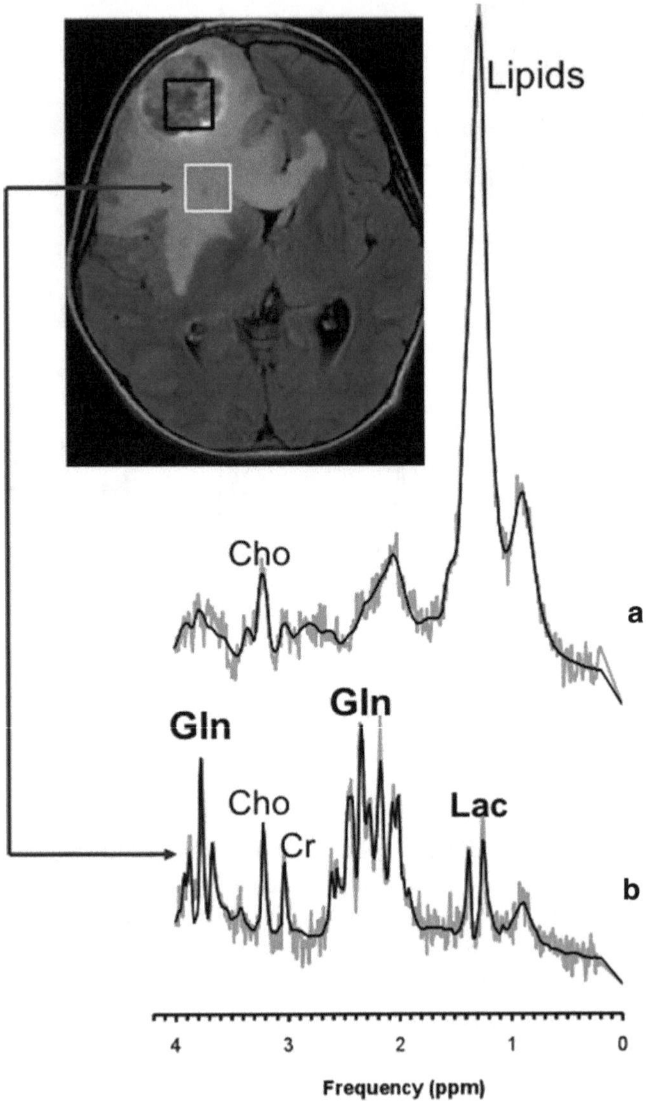

Fig. 22.59 Extreme Edema, Glutamine, NF1, Unusual Tumor

Interpretation/Discussion

The MRI showed multiple areas of abnormal T2 hyperintensity (Fig. 22.60). These showed correlative DWI/ADC restriction suggestive of a cytotoxic process. The distribution was interpreted as compatible with HSV encephalitis, although an ischemic process could have had a similar appearance with the caveat that the distribution would have been unusual. The MRS of abnormal appearing tissue (A) showed elevated lactate, reduced NAA, and elevated (likely) Gln. Cho was normal for age of 7 months whereas mI was below normal. The spectrum acquired from the brain hemisphere from normal appearing tissue was within normal limits.

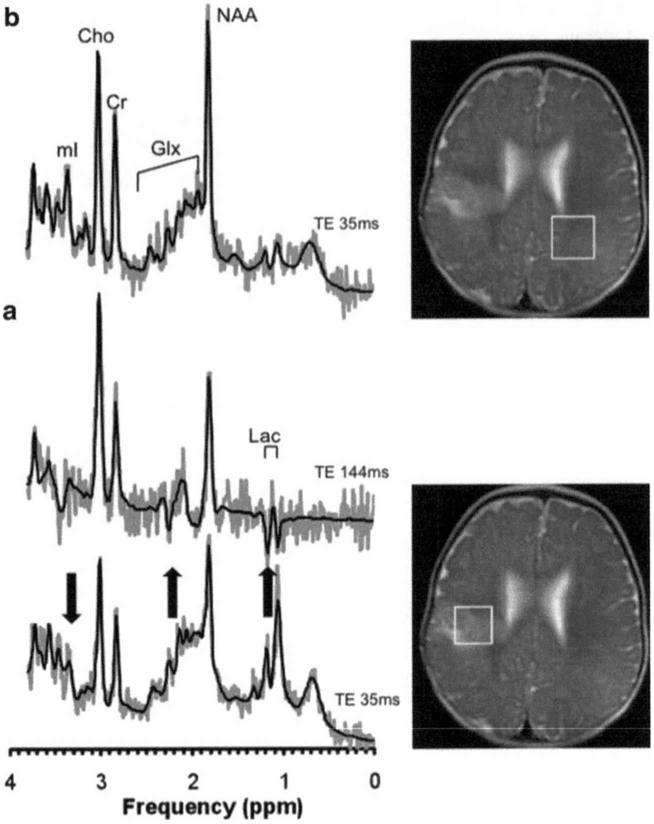

Fig. 22.60 Acute Herpes Encephalitis, 7 Months Old

Conclusions

MRS of a 7 months old with acute herpes encephalitis shows high lactate, elevated Gln, and reduced mI. NAA was also reduced.

Case 61: Acute Encephalitis

Clinical Background

2-year-old female with acute onset of left arm and leg weakness.

MRS Method

1.5 T, single-voxel PRESS, TE 35 ms, of abnormal basal ganglia tissue, two studies 11 days apart.

Interpretation/Discussion

On MRI abnormal signal intensity, involving the bilateral basal ganglia, subcortical white matter, and cortex of the

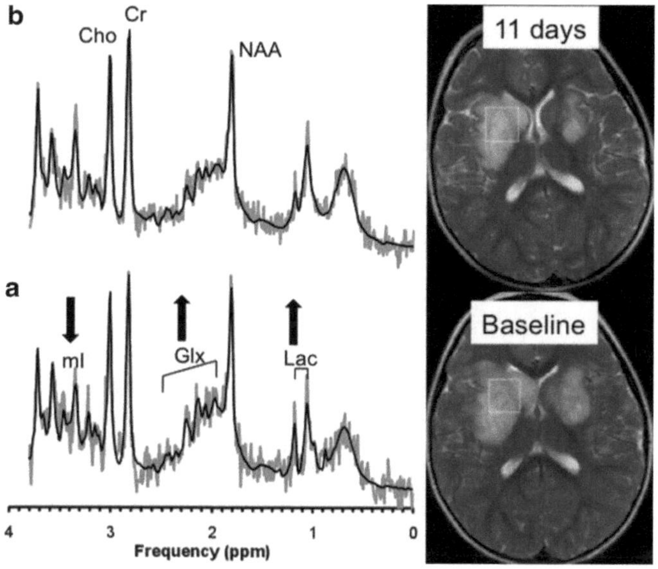

Fig. 22.61 Acute Encephalitis

bilateral frontal and parietal lobes was noted (Fig. 22.61). MRI was consistent with severe encephalitis. The MRS showed elevated lactate, reduced NAA, and elevated (likely) Gln. mI was below normal. Eleven days later, MRS of the same lesion showed decreased lactate, decreased Gln, and further reduced mI. At that time areas of abnormal signal intensity on MRI had decreased.

Conclusions

MRS of a 2-year-old girl with acute viral encephalitis shows high lactate, elevated Gln, and reduced mI. NAA was also reduced. Improved appearance on MRI correlated with reduced levels of Gln.

Case 62: Systematic Lupus Erythromatosis

Clinical Background

16-year-old female with history of systematic lupus erythromatosis (SLE), now with multiple hospitalizations in past 2 months for diffuse pain of unclear etiology, possible increase in depressive symptoms, assess for neuropsychiatric lupus.

MRS Method

1.5 T, single-voxel PRESS, TE 35 ms, parietal WM (WM) and parietal–occipital GM (GM).

Interpretation/Discussion

The MRI was interpreted as normal (Fig. 22.62). MRS of GM also appeared to be within normal range when compared with controls. The somewhat lower Cho in the patient may be due to the slightly lower age of the subjects included in the control group (approximately 10 years versus the 16-year-old patient), considering that Cho continues to decrease relative to Cr through adolescence. In WM, on the other hand, NAA was reduced whereas Cho was increased in the patient.

Conclusions

MRS of systematic lupus erythromatosis (SLE) can be abnormal when MRI is unremarkable. WM appears to be more affected than GM.

Case 63: Citrullinemia I

Clinical Background

Seven-year-old boy with new-onset seizures and tremors, prior diagnosis of citrullinemia.

MRS Method

1.5 T, single-voxel PRESS, TE 35 ms, occipital mostly gray matter-containing tissue.

Interpretation/Discussion

Citrullinemia is an autosomal recessive urea cycle disorder that causes ammonia to accumulate in the blood. The MRI showed moderate diffuse volume loss and hyperintensity on FLAIR images in subcortical and periventricular white matter (Fig. 22.63). MRS of normal appearing occipital gray matter was strikingly abnormal with prominent Gln and depleted mI. NAA was only slightly reduced in this patient.

Conclusion

MRS of citrullinemia is consistent with acute hyperammonia and accumulation of Gln.

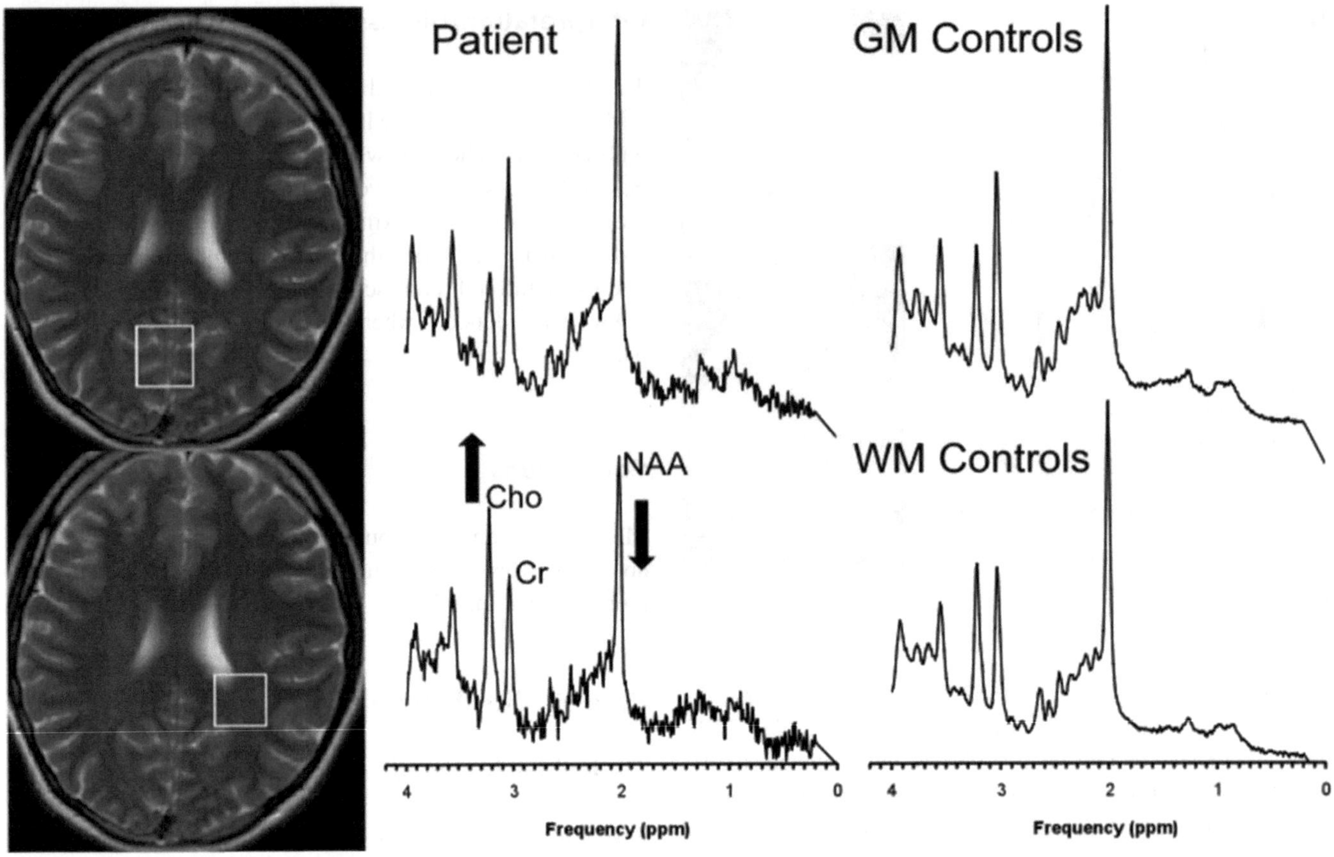

Fig. 22.62 Systematic Lupus Erythromatosis

Case 64: Status Post-Bone Marrow Transplant (BMT), Posterior Reversible Encephalopathy Syndrome (PRES)

Clinical Background

3-year-old girl with history of rhabdoid tumor, status post-BMT, now with acute vision loss, CT concerning for PRES following FK-506 administration for immunosuppression.

MRS Method

3 T, single-voxel PRESS, TE 35 ms, of lesions in white matter and in right occipital/visual cortex.

Interpretation/Discussion

On MRI, evolving parenchymal findings compatible with posterior reversal encephalopathy syndrome (PRES) with some areas that were improved but some areas that had worsened when compared with an earlier MRI of this patient (Fig. 22.64). The MRS showed slightly elevated lactate and lipids. NAA was moderately but significantly reduced, whereas Cr was close to normal. Cho was slightly above normal and mI was reduced. Glc was consistently observed and was significantly above normal levels. Elevated Glc may indicate abnormal Glc energy metabolism.

Conclusions

MRS provided evidence for moderate but significant neuronal/axonal damage/loss in regions examined.

Case 65: Newborn Infarct, Lactate, Propylene Glycol

Clinical Background

22-day-old baby boy with congenital heart defect, after surgical procedure (Blalock Taussig shunt), now with focal left hand seizure. Concerns for stroke.

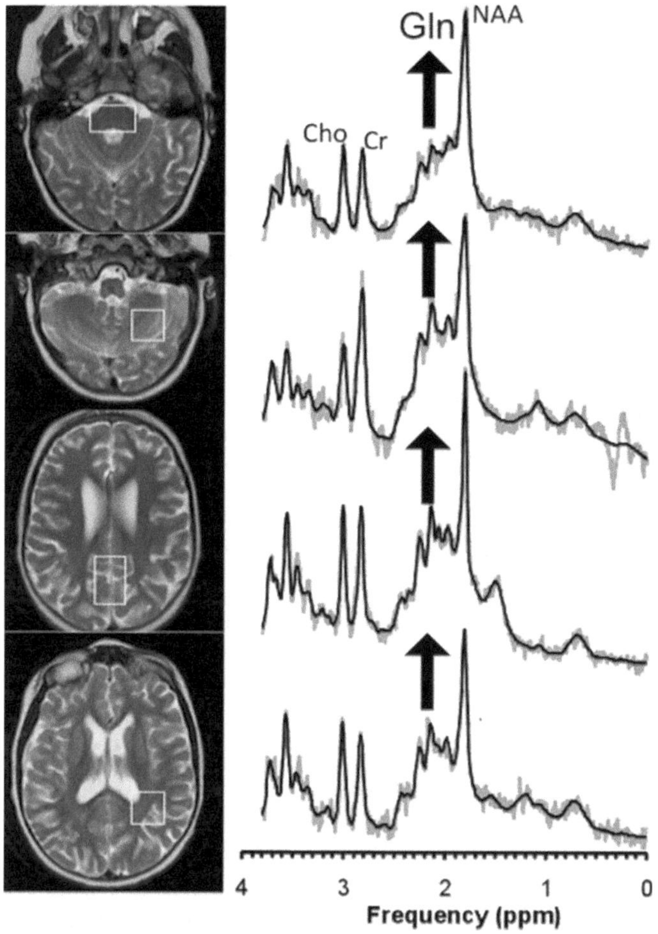

Fig. 22.63 Citrullinemia I

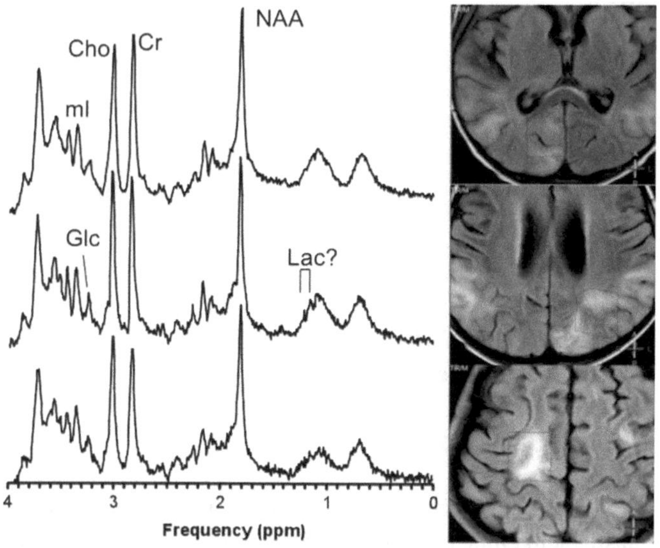

Fig. 22.64 Status Post-Bone Marrow Transplant (BMT), Posterior Reversible Encephalopathy Syndrome (PRES)

MRS Method

3 T, single-voxel PRESS, TE 35 ms, of parieto/occipital GM (GM) and right parietal infarct lobe.

Interpretation/Discussion

On MRI, an acute infarction involving approximately two-thirds of the right MCA distribution, with sparing of the majority of the right temporal lobe was observed (Fig. 22.65). MRS of the infracted area shows overall reduced metabolite concentrations when compared with spared areas (spectra in figure are scaled to concentrations), except lactate, which was elevated. Also, observed was signal consistent with propylene glycol in both spectra. Note that lactate was also detectable in normal appearing parieto/occipital GM. Also note the unusual shoulder of the Cho peak in the stroke spectrum.

Conclusions

Metabolites were generally reduced in a newborn infarct when compared with normal appearing brain tissue. Propylene glycol was likely used as a solvent for drugs administered to this patient and can sometimes be confused for lactate and lipids in the clinical setting.

Case 66: Low ml: Posterior Reversible Encephalopathy Syndrome (PRES)

Clinical Background

12-year-old male with T-cell acute lymphoblastic leukemia (ALL) who is undergoing chemotherapy began to have new seizures and found to have scattered lesion in brain. A previous MRI from a few days before was suggestive for either an infectious or a neoplastic process. MRS was ordered to specify nature of lesion(s).

MRS Method

3 T, single-voxel PRESS, TE 35 ms, of lesions and surrounding tissues.

Interpretation/Discussion

NAA was well preserved relative to Cr (Fig. 22.66). Cho, considering a mixed gray matter/white matter ROI as reference, was unremarkable. mI was markedly reduced.

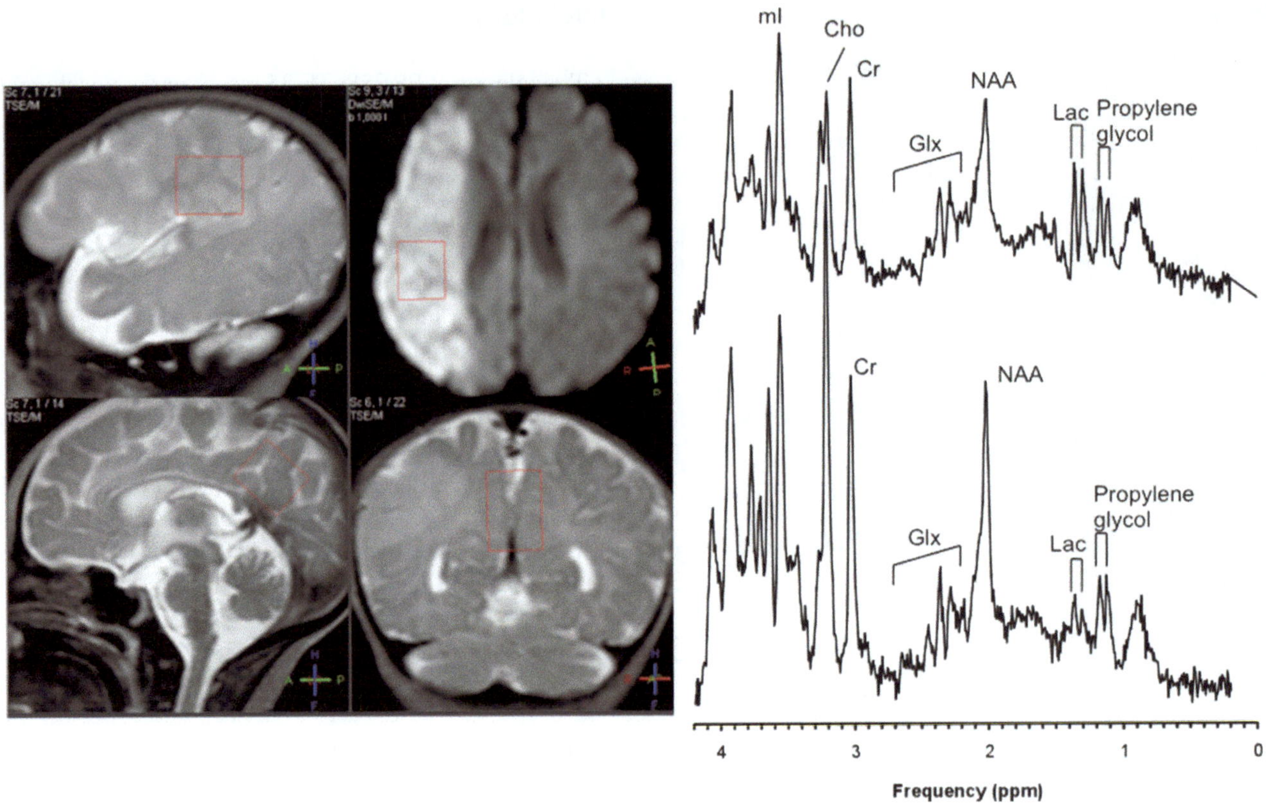

Fig. 22.65 Newborn Infarct, Lactate, Propylene Glycol

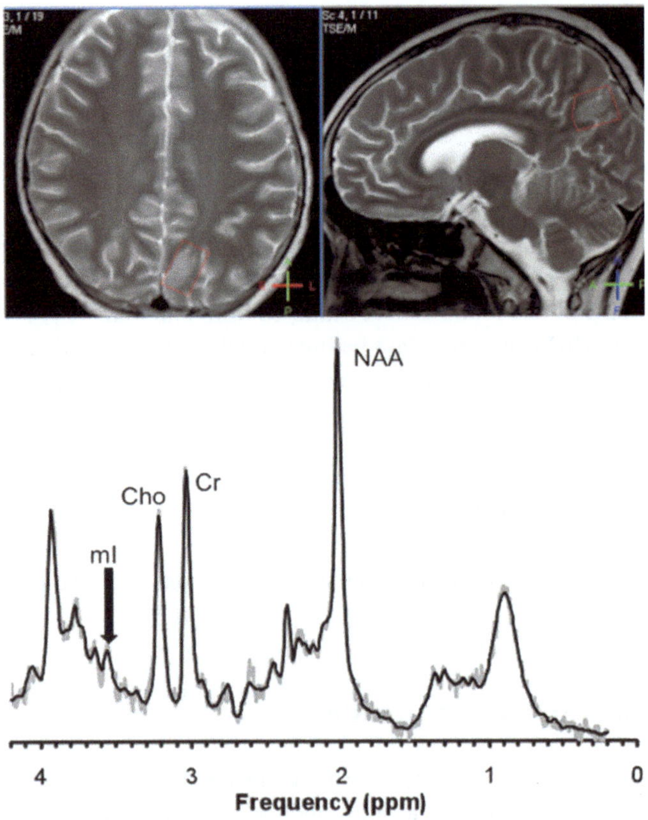

Fig. 22.66 Low mI: Posterior Reversible Encephalopathy Syndrome (PRES)

This pattern was observed also in two other locations (not shown). MRS was not consistent with significant neuronal/axonal loss. MRS was not typical for a neoplastic process or an acute infection. A third MRI study conducted a few days later showed interval near resolution of numerous bilateral white matter lesions compared with prior examinations. This was interpreted as being most suggestive of resolving PRES.

Conclusions

MRI/MRS can be used to characterize lesions better than with MRI alone.

Case 67: Liver Failure, Comatose, High Glutamine

Clinical Background

15-year-old male with new diagnosis of T-cell acute lymphoblastic leukemia (ALL) with new onset of disorientation, headache, with coagulopathy, then liver failure and comatose, possible intracranial hemorrhage.

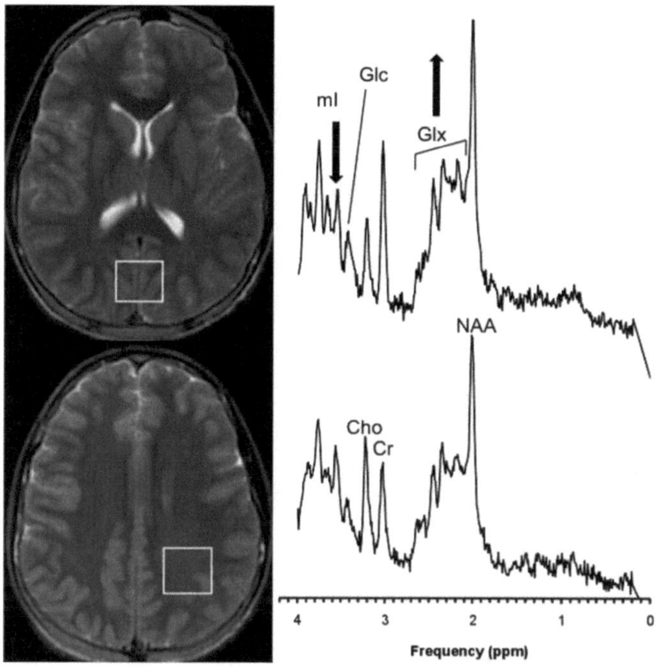

Fig. 22.67 Liver Failure, Comatose, High Glutamine

MRS Method

1.5 T, single-voxel PRESS, TE 35 ms, of the standard occipital GM and parietal WM.

Interpretation/Discussion

The MRI was reported to be unremarkable with the brain parenchyma of normal signal intensity on all sequences and without focal abnormalities (Fig. 22.67). The MRS demonstrated severely elevated levels of (likely) Gln and moderately reduced mI. These findings were reported to be consistent with hepatic encephalopathy. Noticed were also above normal Glc levels.

Conclusions

MRS of hepatic encephalopathy can be strikingly abnormal when MRI is unremarkable.

Case 68: Acute Cerebellar Encephalitis

Clinical Background

7-year-old male with history of headache for 1 week.

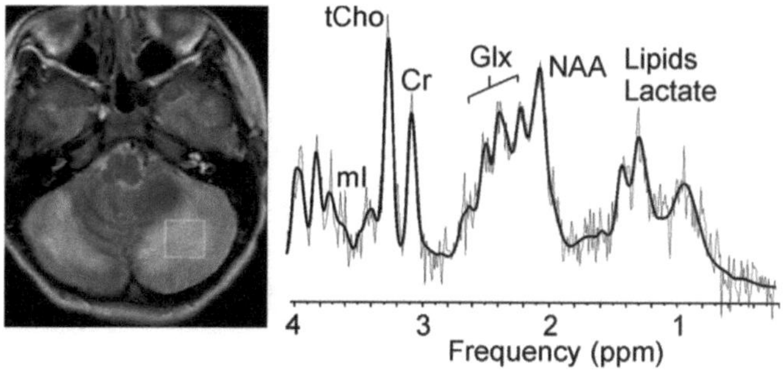

Fig. 22.68 Acute Cerebellar Encephalitis

MRS Method

1.5 T, single-voxel PRESS, TE 35 ms, of cerebellar tissue.

Interpretation/Discussion

On MRI, increased T2 signal was noted within cerebellar hemispheres with sparing of the vermis (Fig. 22.68). MRI was consistent with cerebellar encephalitis and was less suggestive for a low-grade glioma. MRS showed elevated lactate and NAA significantly reduced. Gln was elevated and Cho was slightly prominent relative to Cr, whereas mI was depleted. These findings were interpreted as consistent with encephalitis. The almost depleted NAA would suggest significant long-term tissue damage. Unfortunately, there has been no follow-up of this patient to confirm this hypothesis.

Conclusions

Encephalitis can sometimes be confused with low-grade gliomas on MRI. Note that the spectrum of acute encephalitis is quite different from spectra of low-grade gliomas—particularly with regards to the depletion of the mI peak.

Case 69: Hypertensive Encephalopathy, Posthypertensive Crisis, Acute Lymphoblastic Leukemia

Clinical Background

12-year-old female with acute lymphoblastic leukemia after treatment and bone marrow transplant. Hypertensive crisis, now with new seizures of unknown etiology.

MRS Method

1.5 T, single-voxel PRESS, TE 35 ms, two studies.

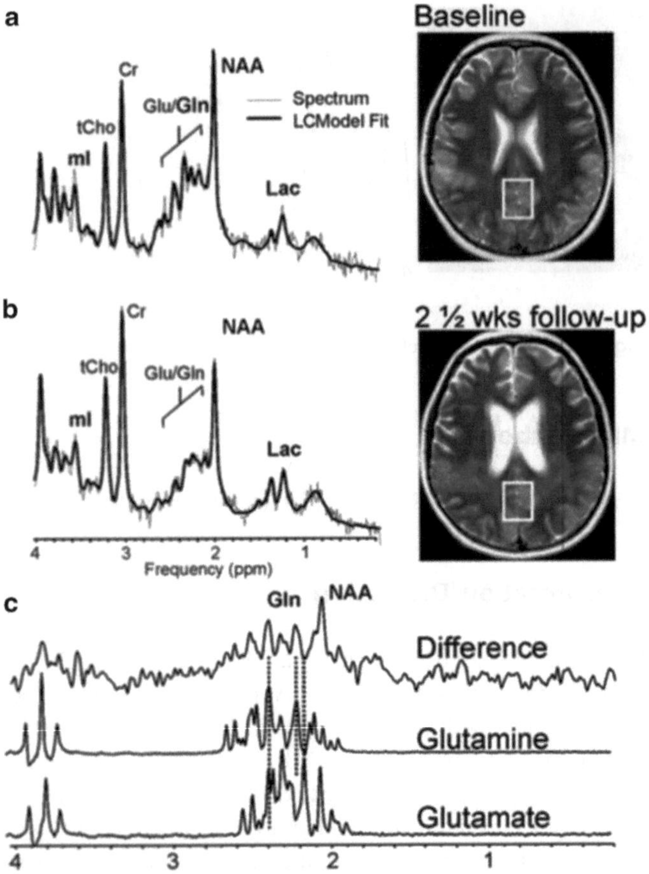

Fig. 22.69 Hypertensive Encephalopathy, Posthypertensive Crisis, Acute Lymphoblastic Leukemia

Interpretation/Discussion

On the first MRI multifocal lesions within the cerebral hemispheres involving cortical and subcortical white matter with some brain stem and presumably pulvinar changes were noted immediately after a hypertensive crisis (Fig. 22.69). 2½ weeks later, a follow-up MRI showed resolving multifocal lesions consistent with the history of hypertensive encephalopathy. The initial MRS (A) study demonstrated elevated lactate and moderately reduced NAA. Gln was also elevated. At follow-up (B), lactate had increased whereas NAA was slightly further reduced. There was no apparent increase of Gln detectable at that time. The difference spectrum between the two MR studies was computed and compared with model solution spectra of Glu and Gln (C). This comparison showed that indeed Gln was initially elevated. Of note, the increased lactate and the further reduced NAA suggest some neuronal loss/damage has occurred in this patient.

Conclusions

MRS of hypertensive encephalopathy can be considerably abnormal. MRS may be useful to assess the extent of tissue damage.

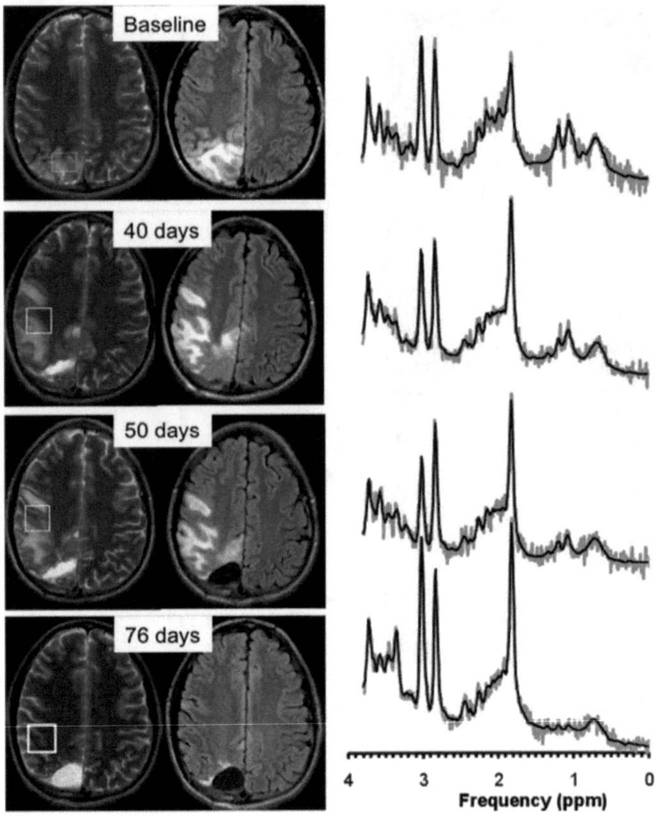

Fig. 22.70 Acute and Subacute Encephalitis, Serial MRS

Case 70: Acute and Subacute Encephalitis, Serial MRS

Clinical Background

16-year-old boy with new onset seizures, suspicion for tumor.

MRS Method

1.5 T, single-voxel PRESS, TE 35 ms, of suspicious tissue, serial MRS.

Interpretation/Discussion

The MRI performed at baseline spectroscopy showed an abnormal right parietal lesion associated with abnormal cortical thickening and edema and leptomeningeal enhancement (Fig. 22.70). The differential from MRI included encephalitis and infiltrating glioma. The MRS showed significantly decreased mI, decreased NAA, slightly elevated Cho, and slightly reduced Cr relative to normal gray matter values. Lactate, lipids, and Gln (or Gln + Glu) were elevated. MRS was interpreted as not consistent with glioma. Due to the clinical impression, favoring tumor a biopsy was obtained which was interpreted as consistent with a low-grade glioma. The patient subsequently underwent surgery. After surgery, increased abnormalities on MRI were noticed with MRS again showing a spectrum not suggestive for a low-grade tumor. At that time tissue samples were reviewed again and it was concluded that the original interpretation might have been wrong. The patient was subsequently treated for encephalitis. Two more MRI/S studies were performed. In the final study, 76 days after baseline, abnormalities on MRI had improved. On MRS, lactate and lipids were not detectable and mI had returned to close to normal levels.

Conclusions

MRS may be useful for distinguishing encephalitis from neoplastic processes particularly with regards to the depletion of mI.

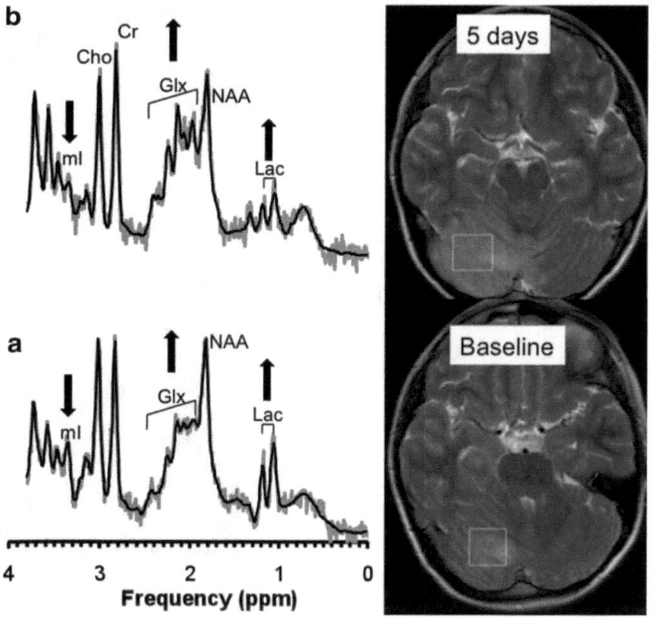

Fig. 22.71 Acute Cerebellar Encephalitis, 10 Years Old, Serial MRS

Case 71: Acute Cerebellar Encephalitis, 10 Years Old, Serial MRS

Clinical Background

10-year-old female with abnormal appearing pons on previous CT, vomiting, MRI/MRS for lesion characterization.

MRS Method

1.5 T, single-voxel PRESS, TE 35 ms, of suspicious tissue, follow-up 5 days later.

Interpretation/Discussion

A mass effect and T2 signal abnormality was noted in the right cerebellar hemisphere. Apart from the mass effect from the cerebellum, the pons itself was unremarkable (Fig. 22.71). Abnormal contrast enhancement was identified in the adjacent meninges more suggestive of meningoencephalitis (cerebellitis) albeit it was felt that a diffuse glioma remained in the differential. The MRS at baseline (A) showed elevated lactate, reduced NAA, and elevated (likely) Gln. mI was below normal. Five days later, MRS of the same lesion showed decreased lactate but increased Gln and further reduced mI.

Conclusions

Acute viral encephalitis can sometimes be confused with low-grade gliomas on MRI. MRS can reaffirm the impression from MRI.

Case 72: Multicentric Gliomatosis Versus Encephalitis

Clinical Background

9-year-old female with suspicion of posterior fossa lesion.

MRS Method

1.5 T, single-voxel PRESS, TE 35 ms, of suspicious cerebellar tissue and of abnormal tissue in right basal ganglia/thalamus.

Interpretation/Discussion

The MRI showed multifocal edema in the right cerebellum, brainstem, thalami, right basal ganglia, and selected areas of the cortex (Fig. 22.72). The differential included multicentric gliomatosis and encephalitis. MRS of the cerebellar abnormality showed high lactate, depleted NAA, prominent

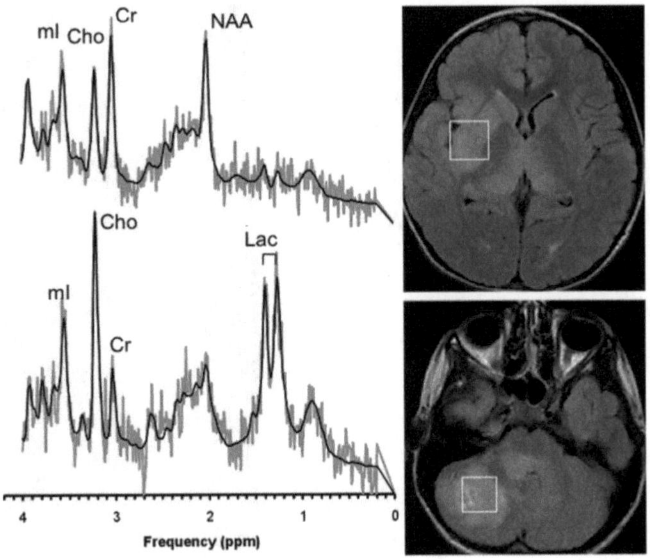

Fig. 22.72 Multicentric Gliomatosis Versus Encephalitis

Cho, and mI above normal. The prominent Cho and high mI is not typical for acute encephalitis. The MRS of the abnormality in the basal ganglia showed reduced NAA, unremarkable Cho, and elevated mI. Again, this pattern is not typical for encephalitis. MRS was interpreted to be consistent with a multifocal tumor. MRS of the cerebellar lesion was more suggestive for a higher grade tumor whereas in the basal ganglia MRS was more compatible with a low-grade lesion. Subsequent biopsy confirmed an anaplastic astrocytoma in the cerebellum. Other parts of the brain were not biopsied.

Conclusions

MRS may be useful to distinguish multifocal tumors from acute viral encephalitis.

Case 73: Gliomatosis Cerebri Versus Encephalitis

Clinical Background

14-year-old female with suspected encephalitis presenting with new onset seizure and right cerebral hemisphere lesion seen on a previous MRI from an outside hospital.

MRS Method

1.5 T, single-voxel PRESS, TE 35 ms, of suspicious tissue at several occasions.

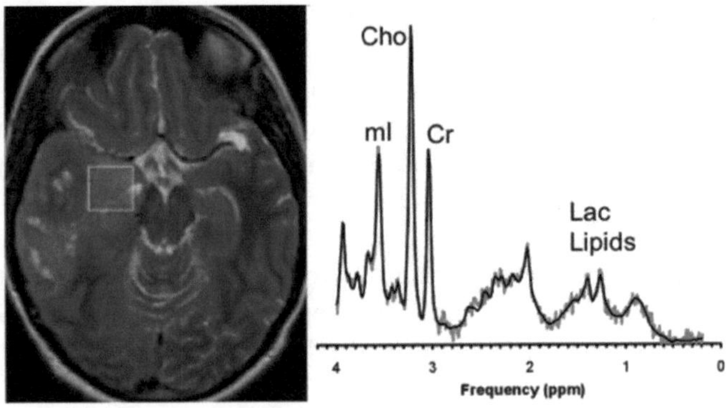

Fig. 22.73 Gliomatosis Cerebri Versus Encephalitis

Interpretation/Discussion

MRI showed abnormal edema seen in the right temporal lobe, including the medial temporal lobe and hippocampus, with extension into the right insular cortex and right basal ganglia (Fig. 22.73). These findings were interpreted as being consistent encephalitis with herpes encephalitis as the main differential. MRS, on the other hand, showed a spectrum with elevated lipids and lactate, low or depleted NAA, prominent Cho, and elevated mI. This pattern was interpreted as being not consistent with acute encephalitis. Subsequent biopsy and clinical course confirmed an anaplastic astrocytoma and gliomatosis cerebri.

Conclusions

MRS may be useful to distinguish brain tumors from acute viral encephalitis.

Case 74: Canavan Disease

Clinical Background

4-month-old male infant with truncal hypotonia and spastic extremities.

MRS Method

1.5 T, SV-PRESS TE 35 ms, parietal WM.

Interpretation/Discussion

On MRI diffuse T2 white and deep gray matter signal abnormality were observed (Fig. 22.74). The MR spectrum demonstrated elevated NAA (and mI), consistent with Canavan

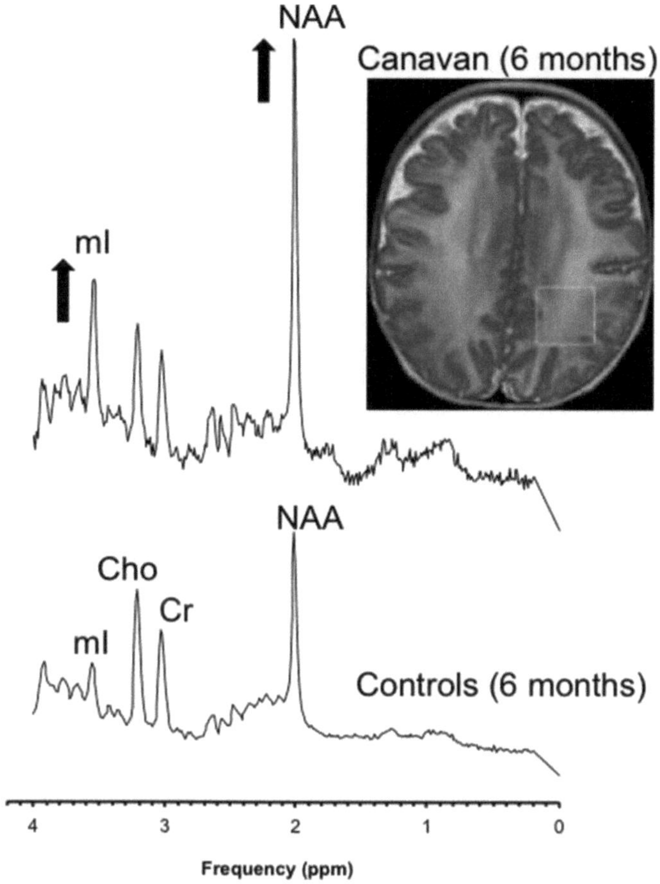

Fig. 22.74 Canavan Disease

disease. In Canavan disease the enzyme that breaks down NAA (aspartoacylase) in the brain is deficient. Thus, NAA accumulates to abnormally high concentrations.

Conclusions

Canavan disease is readily diagnosed by MRS by strikingly elevated NAA.

Case 75: Leukodystrophy (Unknown Etiology), Hypomyelination?

Clinical Background

6-year-old girl with familial history of leukodystrophy.

MRS Method

1.5 T, SV-PRESS TE 35 ms, parietal abnormal appearing WM.

Interpretation/Discussion

On MRI abnormal signal in all of the cerebral white matter with some sparing of the corpus callosum and subcortical fibers was noted and white matter volume was reduced (Fig. 22.75). Findings were interpreted with consistent hypomyelination and leukodystrophy of unknown type with involvement of most of the white matter of both cerebral hemispheres. The MR spectrum showed no evidence for elevated lactate or lipids. NAA was well within normal levels for age. Cho was at or slightly below normal levels whereas mI was close to or slightly above normal levels. A follow-up study 1 year later showed no significant changes on MRI and MRS.

Conclusions

MRS of child with abnormal WM interpreted as hypomyelination and leukodystrophy showed close to normal pattern with well-preserved NAA and moderately below normal Cho.

Case 76: Leukodystrophy (ALD), Symptomatic

Clinical Background

14-year-old male with symptomatic frontal adrenoleukodystrophy (ALD).

MRS Method

1.5 T, SV-PRESS TE 35 ms, frontal and parietal white matter pre- and 9 months post-bone marrow transplant (BMT).

Interpretation/Discussion

On MRI the findings were consistent with leukodystrophy, suggestive for an unusual variant of adrenal leukodystrophy with white matter signal abnormalities in the anterior rather than in the posterior part of the brain (Fig. 22.76a). The follow-up exam after BMT (B) showed again extensive bifrontal leukoencephalopathy with new changes representing volume loss. MRS of normal appearing parietal white matter was within normal limits for age. Both pre- and post-BMT of frontal white matter showed depleted NAA. Pre-BMT, lipids, and lactate were elevated and Cho was more prominent relative to the post-BMT study. mI, on the other hand, was more prominent in the post-BMT study. The pre-BMT study is more consistent with acute damage/tissue stress (lactate and lipids), whereas the post-MRS is more consistent with chronic abnormalities. Depleted NAA is consistent with the widespread destruction/damage to axons already prior to BMT.

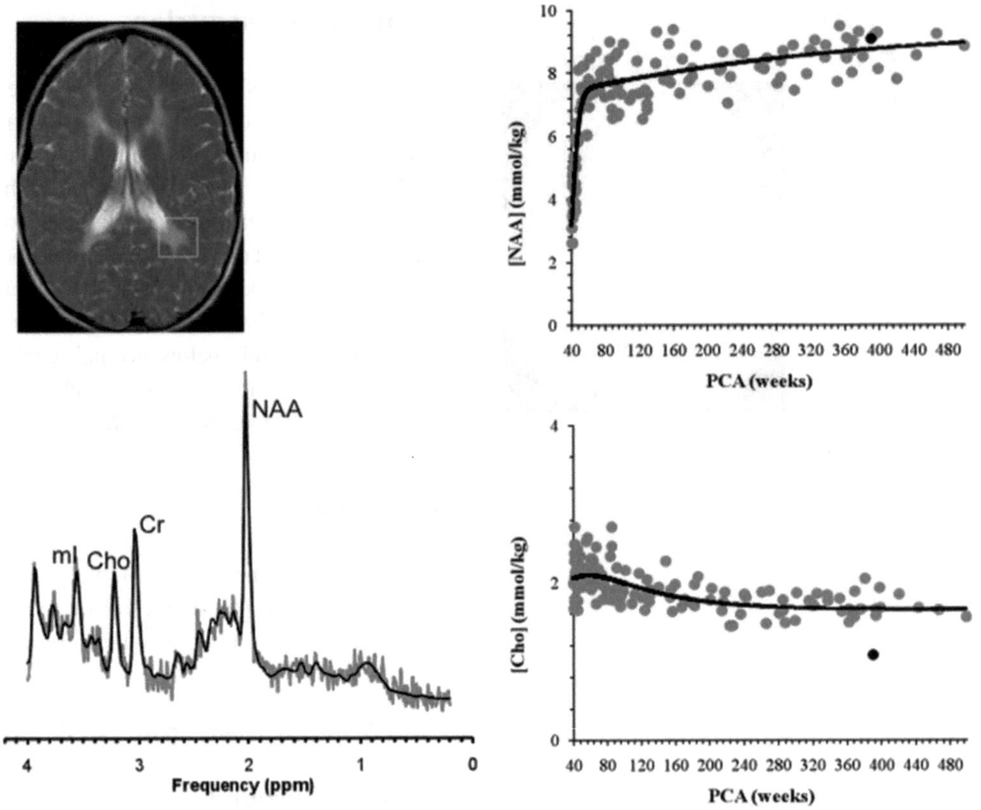

Fig. 22.75 Leukodystrophy (Unknown Etiology), Hypomyelination?

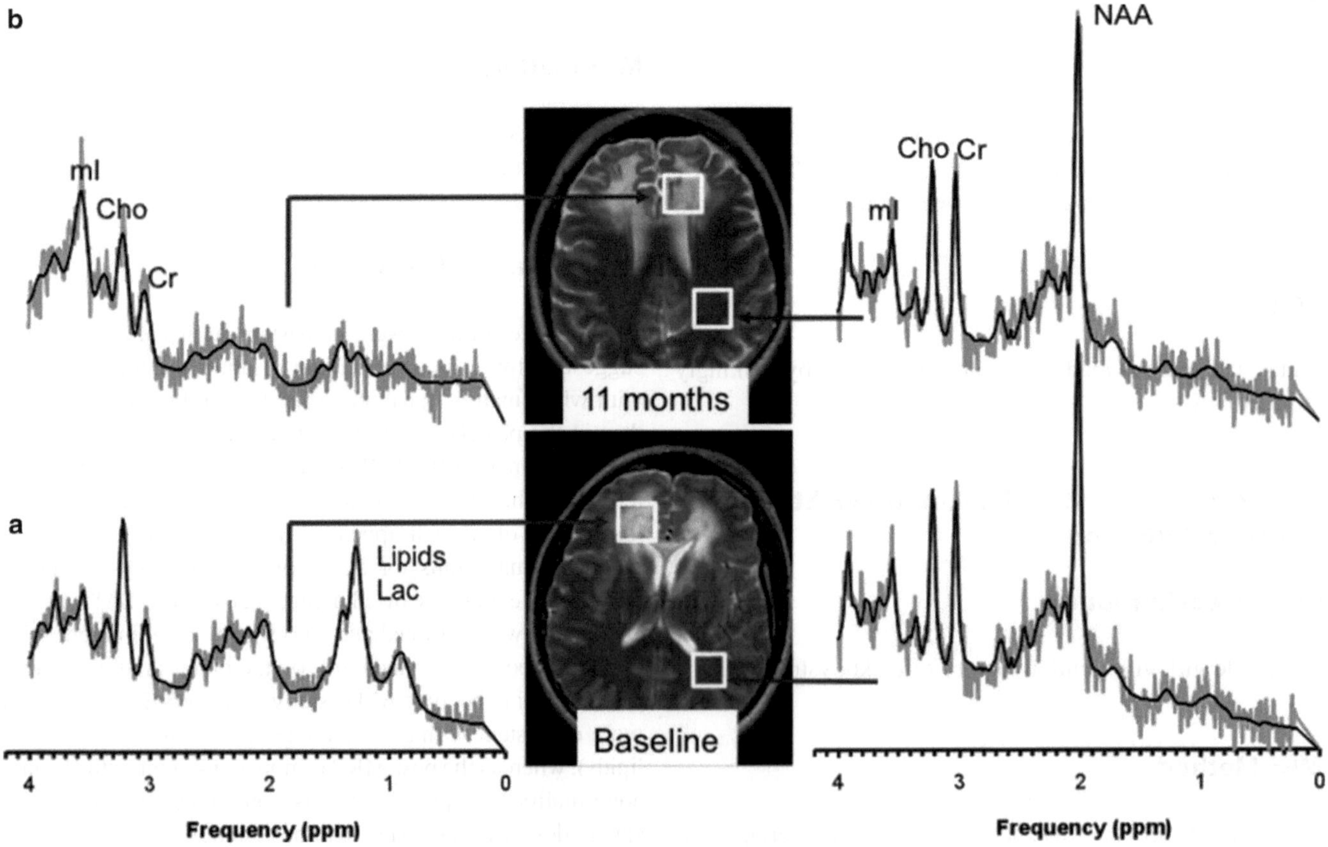

Fig. 22.76 Leukodystrophy (ALD), Symptomatic

Conclusions

MRS can be used to assess the extent of white matter damage in leukodystrophies.

Case 77: Leukodystrophy (ALD)

Clinical Background

5-year-old male with symptomatic adrenoleukodystrophy (ALD).

MRS Method

1.5 T, SV-PRESS TE 35 ms, abnormal white matter, pre/post-bone marrow transplant.

Interpretation/Discussion

Baseline (Fig. 22.77a): On MRI abnormal confluent T2/FLAIR hyperintensity in the periatrial white matter with extension into the splenium of the corpus callosum consistent with adrenoleukodystrophy were observed. The MR spectrum showed increased lipids and lactate. NAA was significantly reduced. Cho and mI were elevated. *2 months (B, post-BMT)*: Abnormalities were consistent with the earlier pre-BMT scan. In addition, there has been interval development of edema in the bilateral posterior parietal and occipital regions. This was interpreted as being consistent with FK-506 toxicity. FK-506 has been administered to reduce likelihood of BMT rejection. Lipid levels were lower than pre-BMT. However, lactate was now more prominent. Cho and Cr appeared to be unchanged whereas mI was lower than in the pre-BMT MRS. It is unclear whether the increase in lactate is due to FK-506 toxicity. *3 years (C):* MRI demonstrated continued abnormalities as described in earlier studies. However, abnormal white matter lesions appear to have consolidated and were less prominent in size. MRS was remarkably different when compared with the previous studies. There was no evidence for elevated lipids or lactate. NAA, albeit not normal, was more readily detectable. Cho was unremarkable and mI was elevated. Another MRS observation worth mentioning is the apparent similarity of MRS in this case of leukodystrophy with tumor MRS. Lactate, reduced NAA, prominent Cho, and elevated mI (especially study B) are frequently observed in tumors, particularly in astrocytoma.

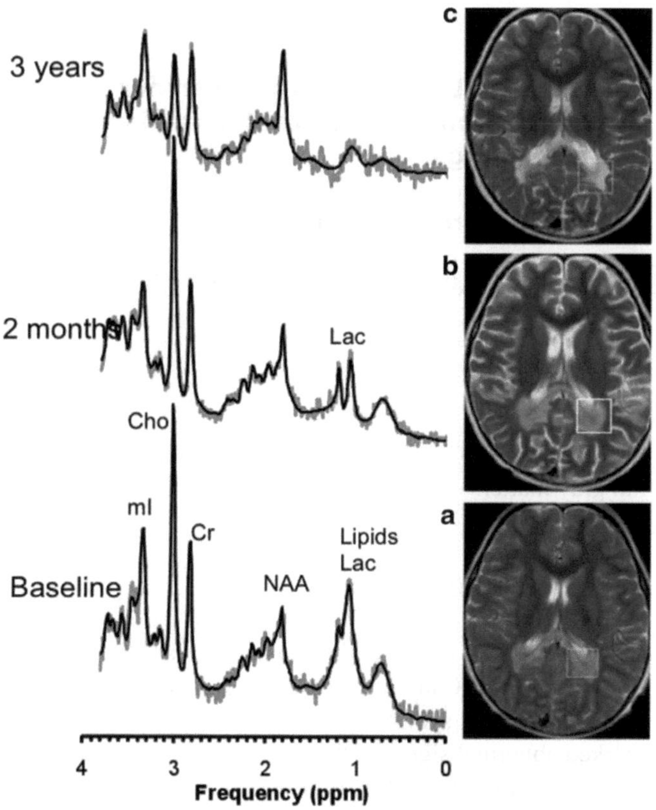

Fig. 22.77 Leukodystrophy (ALD)

Conclusions

MRS of abnormal parietal white matter improved significantly in a case of ALD, despite only minor changes on MRI. There appears to be an overlap in the spectra appearances of leukodystrophies and tumors such as astrocytomas.

Case 78: Leukoencephalopathy

Clinical Background

4-year-old male with leukoencephalopathy of unknown etiology, intractable epilepsy.

MRS Method

1.5 T, SV-PRESS TE 35 ms, five studies over a period of 14 months, abnormal parietal and frontal white matter.

Interpretation/Discussion

Baseline MRI showed extensive white matter and gray matter abnormalities (Fig. 22.78). Over time a decreased involvement of subcortical white matter and cerebellum as well as the deep gray nuclei and thalami was observed. There was

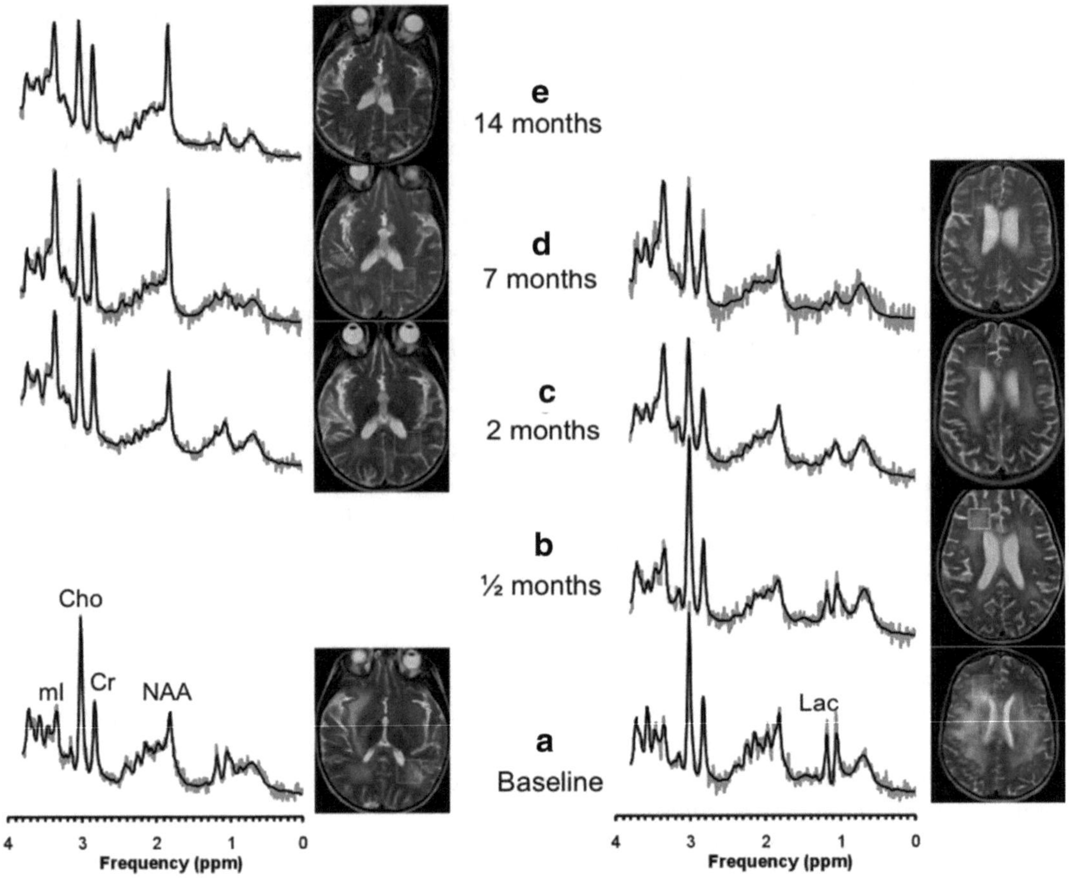

Fig. 22.78 Leukoencephalopathy

no significant interval change in the overall volume of the cerebral hemispheres. Spectroscopy, at baseline showed for both white matter locations elevated lactate, severely decreased NAA, and possibly elevated Gln (likely) or Glu (less likely). Cho was prominent whereas mI was below normal. In subsequent MR spectra lactate levels declined, NAA remained unchanged in frontal white matter whereas it increased in parietal white matter, albeit to levels significantly below normal. Cho levels decreased and mI increased over time. Overall, the pattern of MRS changed from a more acute appearing profile (elevated lactate, Gln) to a more chronic appearing profile. An additional MRI (no MRS) study carried out 2 years later (38 months after initial presentation) showed stable MRI abnormalities. For this patient, no final diagnosis has been made. The patient continues to suffer from weakness, intractable epilepsy, and seizures.

Conclusions

Serial MRS over 14 months demonstrates progressive changes from "acutely" abnormal appearing profile of frontal and parietal WM to a more "chronic" abnormal profile in a patient with abnormal white matter of unknown etiology.

Cases 79–82: Leukodystrophy, van der Knaap or "Vanishing White Matter Disease" in Four Siblings

Clinical Background (*sibling 1*)

5-year-old male being evaluated for possible Canavan disease.

MRS Method

1.5 T, SV-PRESS TE 35 ms, parietal white matter and occipital gray matter.

Interpretation/Discussion

This was the first of the siblings to undergo an MR examination (Fig. 22.79). Canavan disease was discussed as a possible cause for clinical symptoms at that time. On MRI there was marked abnormal signal of the white matter throughout both cerebral hemispheres. No focal absence of tissue is noted. Findings were interpreted as consistent with leukodystrophy.

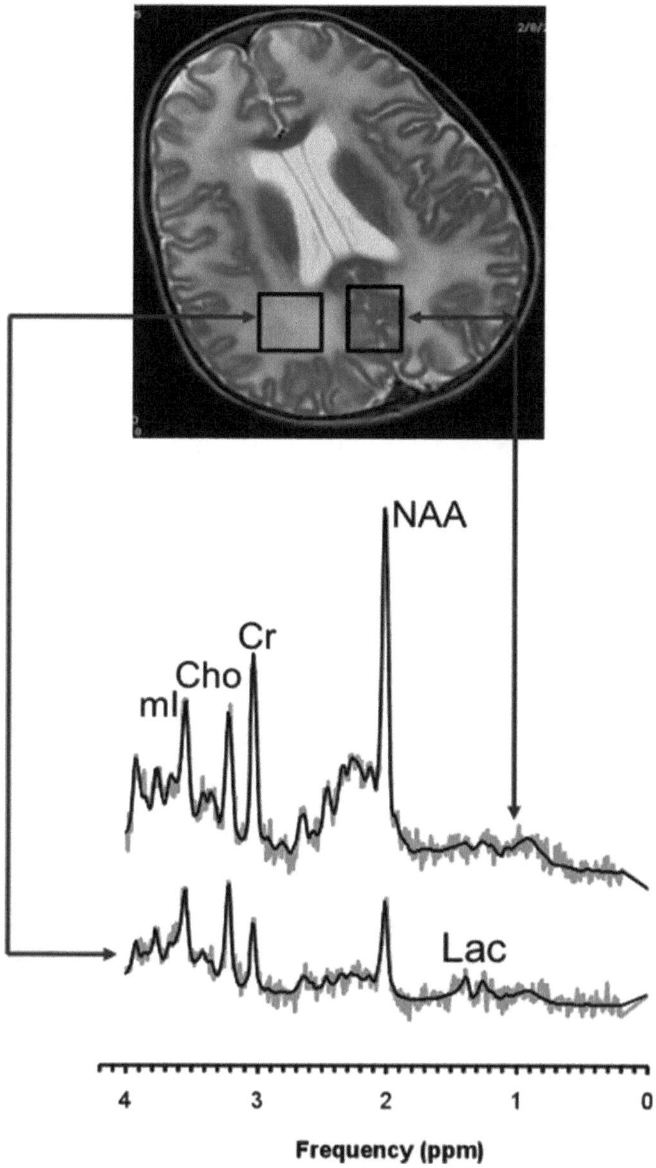

Fig. 22.79 Leukodystrophy, van der Knaap or "Vanishing White Matter Disease" in Four Siblings

MR spectroscopy did not demonstrate elevated NAA and Canavan disease was ruled out. Indeed, MRS showed generally reduced metabolites in white matter (spectra are scaled to absolute concentrations to allow direct comparison). These features, together with the MRI presentation, were suggestive for van der Knaap leukodystrophy. MRS of gray matter showed only minor abnormalities, possibly due to partial volume of white matter.

Conclusions

MRS of Van der Knaap leukodystrophy or "Vanishing White Matter Disease" showed severely abnormal MRS of white

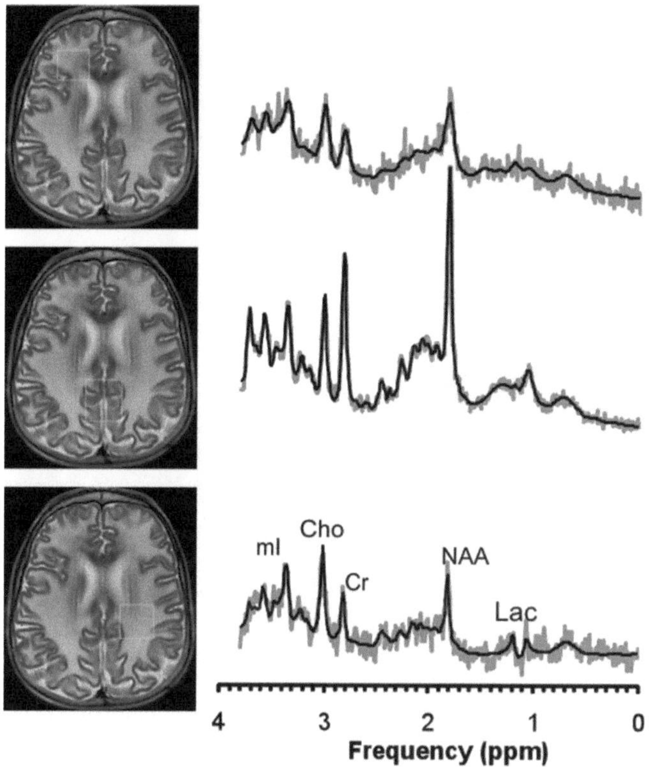

Fig. 22.80 Leukodystrophy, van der Knaap or "Vanishing White Matter Disease" in Four Siblings

matter with all metabolites significantly reduced. MRS of gray matter was close to normal.

Clinical Background (*sibling 2*)

2-year-old female being evaluated for possible Canavan disease.

MRS Method

1.5 T, SV-PRESS TE 35 ms, parietal/frontal white matter and occipital gray matter.

Interpretation/Discussion

This sibling was examined at the same time as her older brother with Canavan disease discussed as a possible cause for clinical symptoms. MRI and MRS were comparable with what has been observed in her older sibling (Fig. 22.80).

Conclusions

MRS of Van der Knaap leukodystrophy or "Vanishing White Matter Disease" showed severely abnormal MRS of white

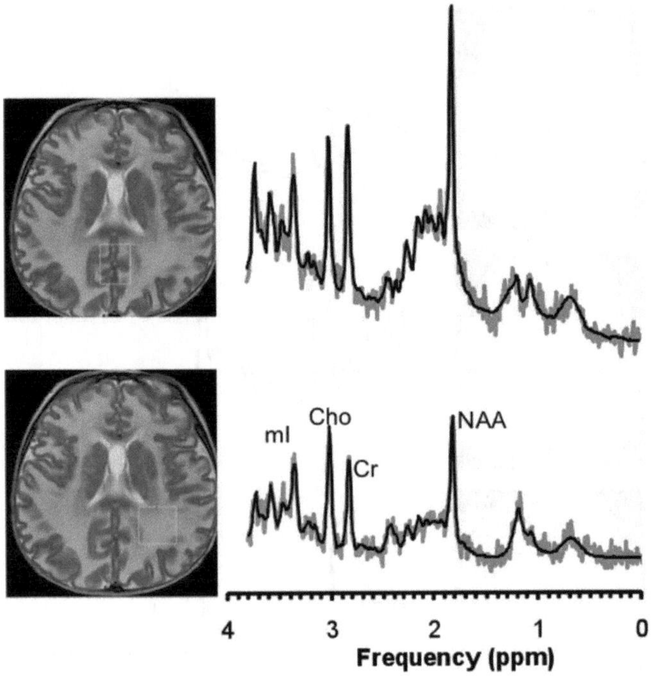

Fig. 22.81 Leukodystrophy, van der Knaap or "Vanishing White Matter Disease" in Four Siblings

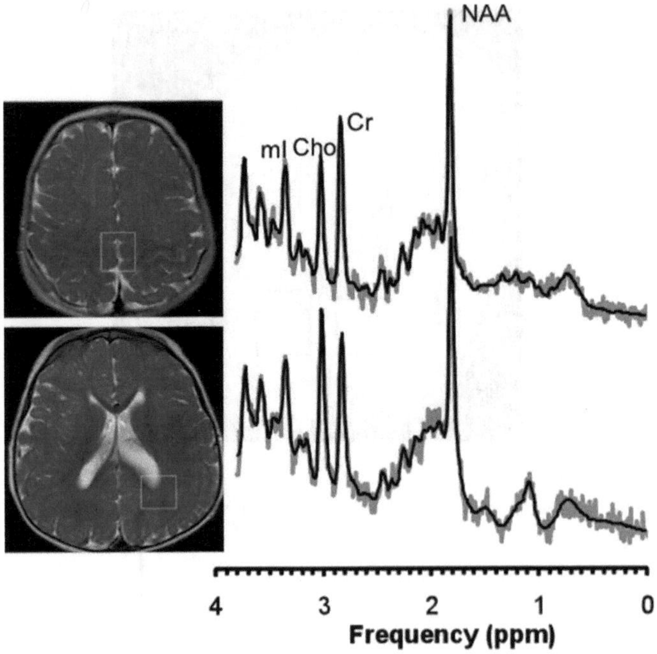

Fig. 22.82 Leukodystrophy, van der Knaap or "Vanishing White Matter Disease" in Four Siblings

matter with all metabolites significantly reduced. MRS of gray matter was close to normal.

Clinical Background (*sibling 3*)

9-month-old boy with two siblings with known leukodystrophy.

MRS Method

1.5 T, SV-PRESS TE 35 ms, parietal white matter and occipital gray matter.

Interpretation/Discussion

MRI and MRS were comparable with what has been observed in the two older siblings (Fig. 22.81).

Conclusions

MRS of Van der Knaap leukodystrophy or "Vanishing White Matter Disease" showed severely abnormal MRS of white matter with all metabolites significantly reduced. MRS of gray matter was close to normal.

Clinical Background (*sibling 4*)

12-month-old male with three siblings with known leukodystrophy, developmental delay.

MRS Method

1.5 T, SV-PRESS TE 35 ms, parietal white matter and occipital gray matter.

Interpretation/Discussion

MRI and MRS were interpreted as within normal range for age (Fig. 22.82). There is no follow-up examination available for this child.

Conclusions

Normal MRS in a child with three siblings that has previously been diagnosed with of Van der Knaap leukodystrophy or "Vanishing White Matter Disease."

Case 83: Unusual 0.9 ppm: High Glucose

Clinical Background

4-month-old female with congenital heart disease (Truncus Arteriosus) status post repair, congenital cystic adenomatoid malformation (CCAM) with right lower lobe (RLL) lung resection, ventilator dependent, and seizure disorder. MRI and MRS were performed to assess the extent of tissue damage.

MRS Method

3 T, single-voxel PRESS, TE 35 ms, of the left occipital white matter—partial volume with ventricle and the left thalamus.

Interpretation/Discussion

On MRI, diffuse signal abnormality of the bilateral cerebral hemispheres with associated volume loss was noted (Fig. 22.83). This was interpreted as likely representing the sequela of acute, subacute, and chronic areas of infarction. MRS demonstrated significantly elevated lactate, whereas NAA was depleted. In both spectra acquired, Glc was prominent. The depleted NAA is suggestive for substantial neuronal/axonal loss in the remaining tissue and poor outcome. The prominent Glc may indicate reduced glycolysis in apoptotic and necrotic tissue. The resonance at 0.9 ppm, generally believed to represent methyl ($-CH_3$) end-groups of lipids and macromolecules, was prominent. For lipids, in the absence of equally prominent signal from CH_2-groups (at 1.2 ppm), this would indicate the accumulation of small and short-chain lipids in this case. More regular lipid molecules have several CH_2-groups for each molecule-terminating $-CH_3$ group. Thus, generally the 1.2 ppm is more prominent than the peak at 0.9 ppm.

Conclusions

An unusually prominent signal at 0.9 ppm was observed. The origin of the signal is unclear. Prominent Glc may indicate impaired glycolysis.

Case 84: Unusual "Local" Global Hypoxia

Clinical Background

2-year-old female status post drowning for unknown amount of time.

MRS Method

3 T, single-voxel PRESS, TE 35 ms, of the occipital abnormal appearing GM, right frontal WM, and standard parietal WM.

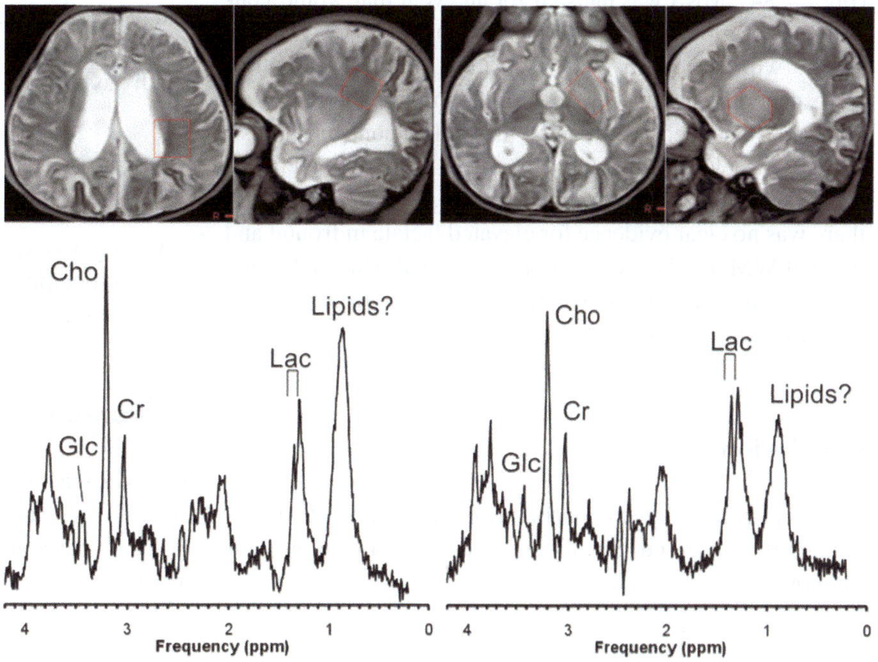

Fig. 22.83 Unusual 0.9 ppm: High Glucose

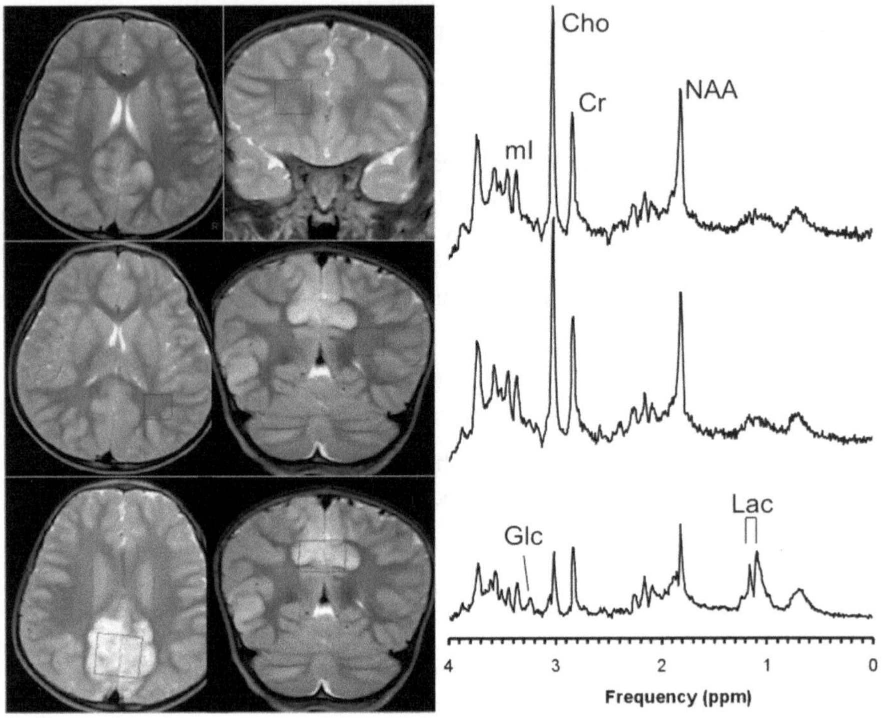

Fig. 22.84 Unusual "Local" Global Hypoxia

Interpretation/Discussion

On MRI extensive swelling, T2 prolongation, and restricted diffusion involving the paramedian parietal lobes, paramedian posterior frontal lobes, bilateral occipital lobes, right posterior temporal lobe, and right cerebellar hemisphere compatible with acute to subacute infarctions was observed (Fig. 22.84). MRS was unusual for an event that would generally cause global damages. The gray matter MRS was consistent with severe hypoxic/ischemic injury. Metabolites were generally reduced with NAA approximately 30% of normal levels (spectra are scaled to absolute concentrations). Lactate was elevated and Gln was above normal. In addition, it was noted that Glc was above normal. On the other hand, there was no clear evidence for elevated lactate in frontal and parietal WM and NAA was close to normal. Unusual, however, was the Cho signal, which was above normal levels in both white matter locations.

Conclusions

Unusual "global" hypoxic/ischemic injury with white matter apparently preserved. Significance of the high Cho levels is unknown.

Case 85: Acute Seizures

Clinical Background

15-year-old female with hemolytic uremic syndrome, acute renal failure, had seizures 5 h before MR examination. Thereafter, the patient had no coherent verbalizations and had decreased strength in the right arm. MRI/MRS was performed to rule out stroke and posterior reversible encephalopathy syndrome (PRES).

MRS Method

3 T, single-voxel PRESS, TE 35 ms, of left parietal WM, parietal–occipital GM, right visual/occipital cortex, and basal ganglia.

Interpretation/Discussion

The MRS acquired from left parietal WM appeared to be close to normal (cf. Fig. 22.85a, upper and lower traces). MRS of parietal–occipital GM showed reduced NAA and increased Cho (cf. B, upper and lower traces). Noted was

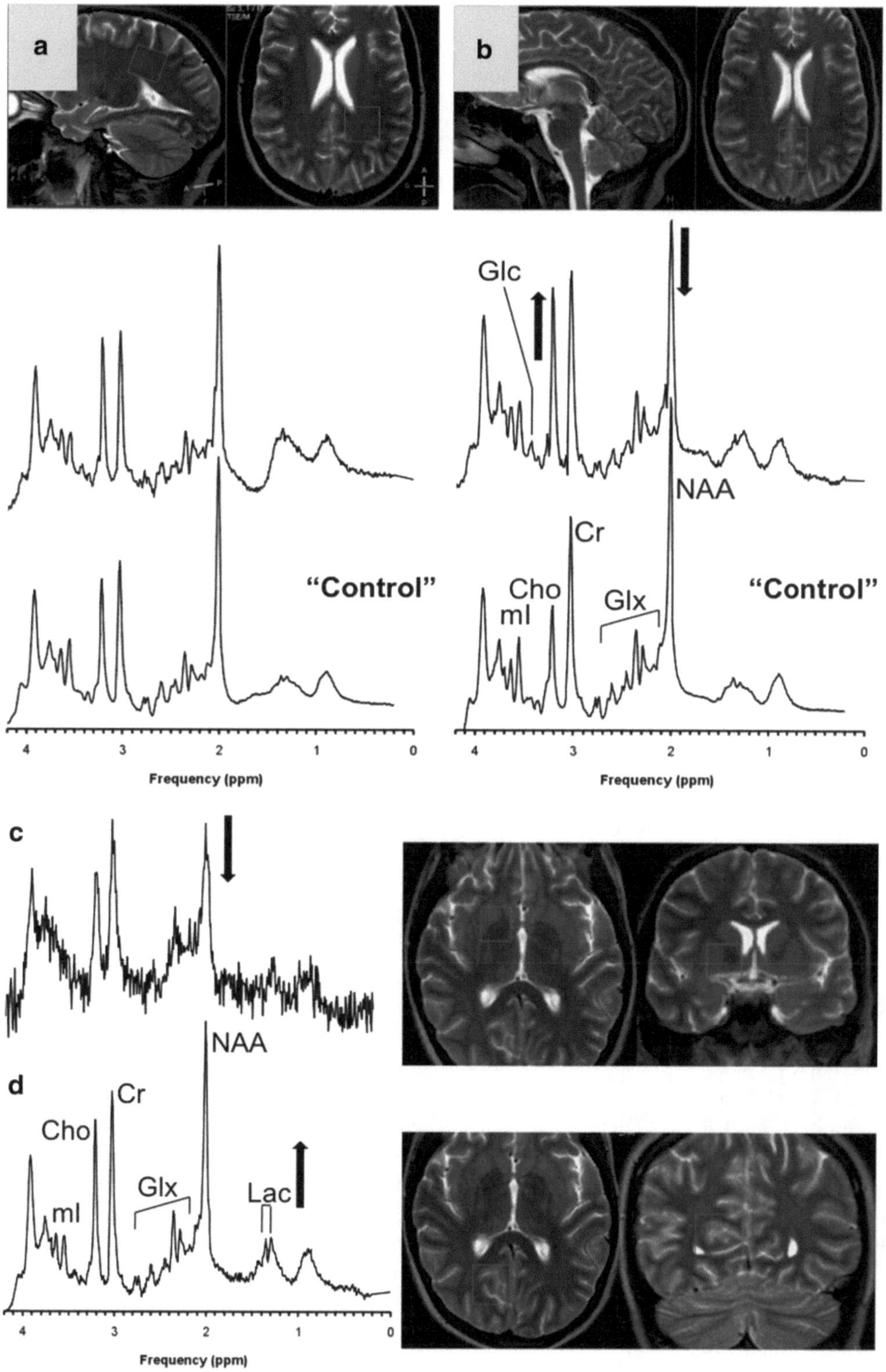

Fig. 22.85 Acute Seizures

also a Glc peak slightly more prominent than generally observed. NAA appeared to be reduced in the spectrum obtained from the basal ganglia (C), whereas there was evidence for elevated lactate in the right visual/occipital cortex spectrum (D). Lactate could indicate a more acute metabolic imbalance whereas the low NAA in the basal ganglia could raise concerns for more permanent/chronic abnormalities. The MRI was reported to be normal. Follow-up MRI one year later was also reported to be unremarkable (no MRS performed).

Conclusions

MRS showed significant abnormalities in a patient with acute seizures.

Case 86: Newborn Trauma (Negative), Follow-up

Clinical Background

2-month-old male, CT scan chronic extra-axial hemorrhage, concern for nonaccidental trauma (NAT).

MRS Method

1.5 T, SV-PRESS TE 35 ms, parietal WM, occipital/parietal GM, baseline and 6-months follow-up.

Interpretation/Discussion

Initial study (at 2 months): The MRI showed cerebral extra-axial fluid collections and acute/subacute subdural hemorrhage (Fig. 22.86). There was no evidence for acute infarction (diffusion negative). The MRS of parietal WM was interpreted as unremarkable with no evidence of elevated lactate and other metabolites within normal range for age. *Follow-up (at 8 months):* MRI showed a small residual left subdural hematoma with well-defined membranes reduced in size. Also, extracerebral fluid collections were resolved and the MRI was otherwise normal. The MR spectrum obtained from a comparable position showed markedly increased NAA consistent with normal developmental changes. Other metabolites were also within normal range for age.

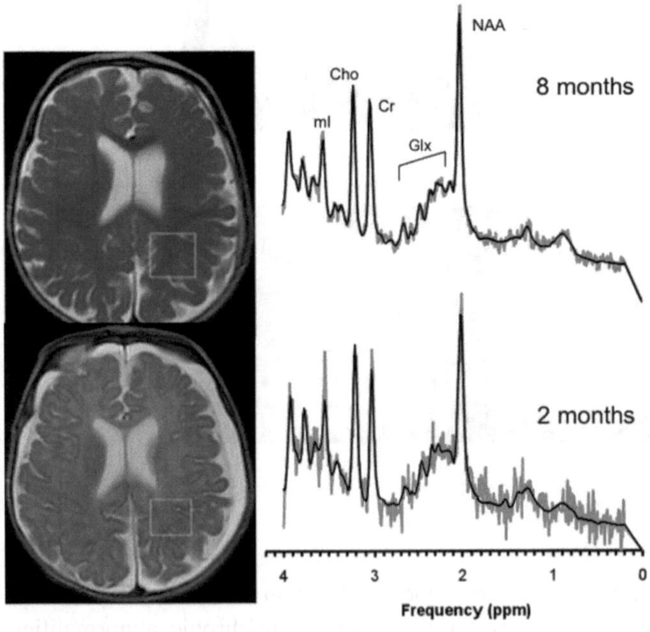

Fig. 22.86 Newborn Trauma (Negative), Follow-up

Conclusions

No evidence from MRS for traumatic brain injury. Metabolic changes between initial and follow-up MRS consistent with normal biochemical maturation.

Case 87: Intractable Seizures

Clinical Background

6-month-old male with seizures of unknown etiology.

MRS Method

1.5 T, SV-PRESS TE 35 ms, parietal WM, occipital/parietal GM, re-examined at 11 months.

Interpretation/Discussion

Initial MRI at 6 months (Fig. 22.87a) was interpreted as normal. At that time, MRS was interpreted as borderline normal with, for example, NAA concentrations approximately 86% of what has been established for normal at this age at Children's Hospital Los Angeles. Other metabolites were also close to normal for age. At 11 months (B), the brain parenchyma was of normal signal intensity on all sequences without focal abnormality. Myelination was appropriate for the patient's age. However, a slight increase in the size of the lateral ventricles and sulci suggesting mild diffuse volume loss was noted on MRI. Spectroscopy was clearly abnormal with NAA reaching only 65% of normal (C). On the other hand, Cr did not change significantly (D). The same pattern was observed for occipital/parietal gray matter (not shown). These changes are consistent with progressive neuronal/axonal damage/loss. Four years after theses studies were conducted the patient exhibits global developmental delays and continues to have seizures.

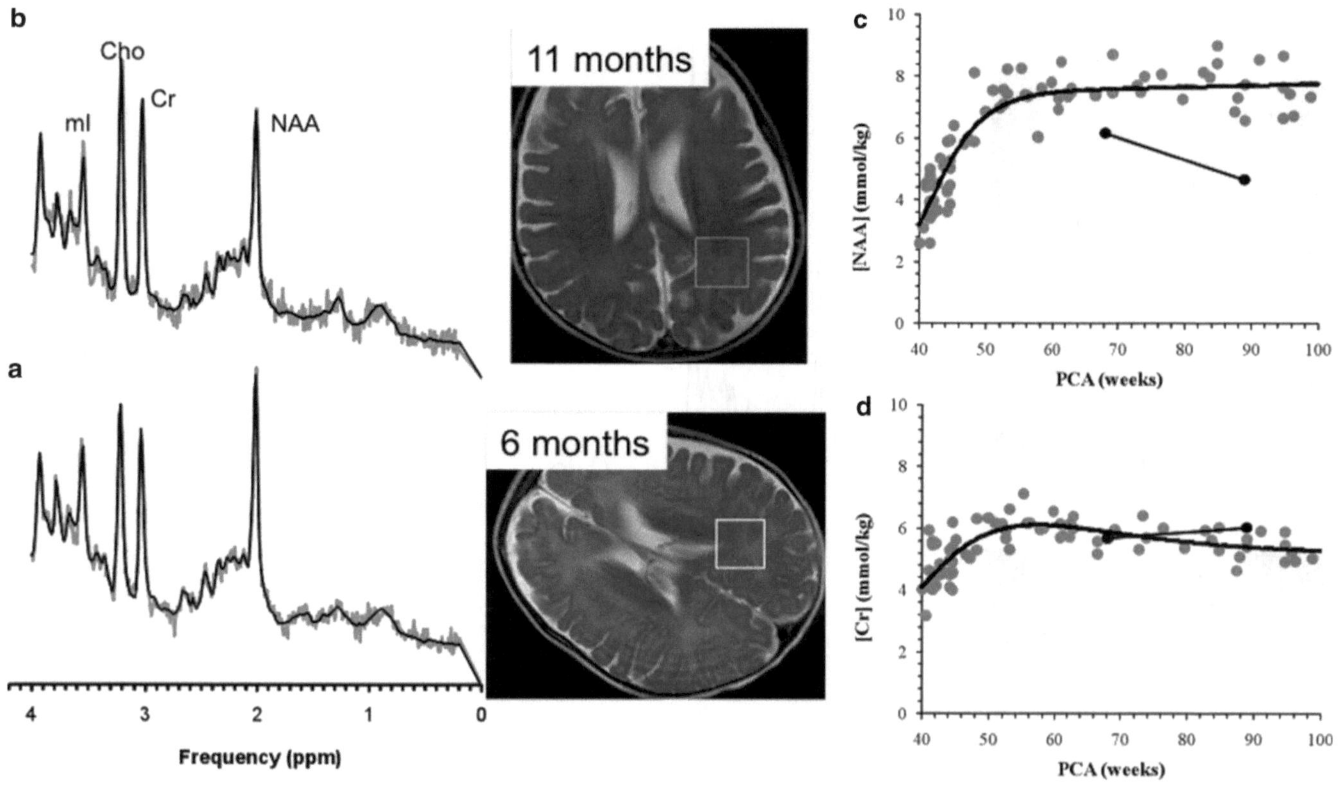

Fig. 22.87 Intractable Seizures

Conclusions

MR spectroscopy identified progressive neuronal/axonal damage/loss in a patient with intractable seizures of unknown etiology.

Case 88: Newborn Hypotonia, "Normal" Age-Dependent Changes

Clinical Background

7-day-old boy with hypotonia and seizures.

MRS Method

1.5 T, SV-PRESS TE 35 ms, parietal WM, occipital/parietal GM, re-examined at 9½ months.

Interpretation/Discussion

The initial MRI demonstrated multiple foci of parenchymal necrosis in the white matter of the left frontal and parietal lobes (black arrow, Fig. 22.88). The gray matter was unremarkable. At the 9½ months follow-up WM necrosis was still present but had improved, although associated with white matter volume loss. Gray matter was again unremarkable and appropriate for age. The MR spectrum showed a significant increase of NAA, slightly increased Cr, and reduced mI consistent with the expected age-dependent changes.

Conclusions

Serial MRS in a patient with hypotonia and seizures and focal white matter necrosis showed normal age-dependent changes in parietal/occipital gray matter.

Case 89: Nonaccidental Trauma, Severe Hypoxic/Ischemic Injury Pattern, Progression

Clinical Background

2-month-old boy, admitted with suspicion for nonaccidental trauma 3 days before the initial study.

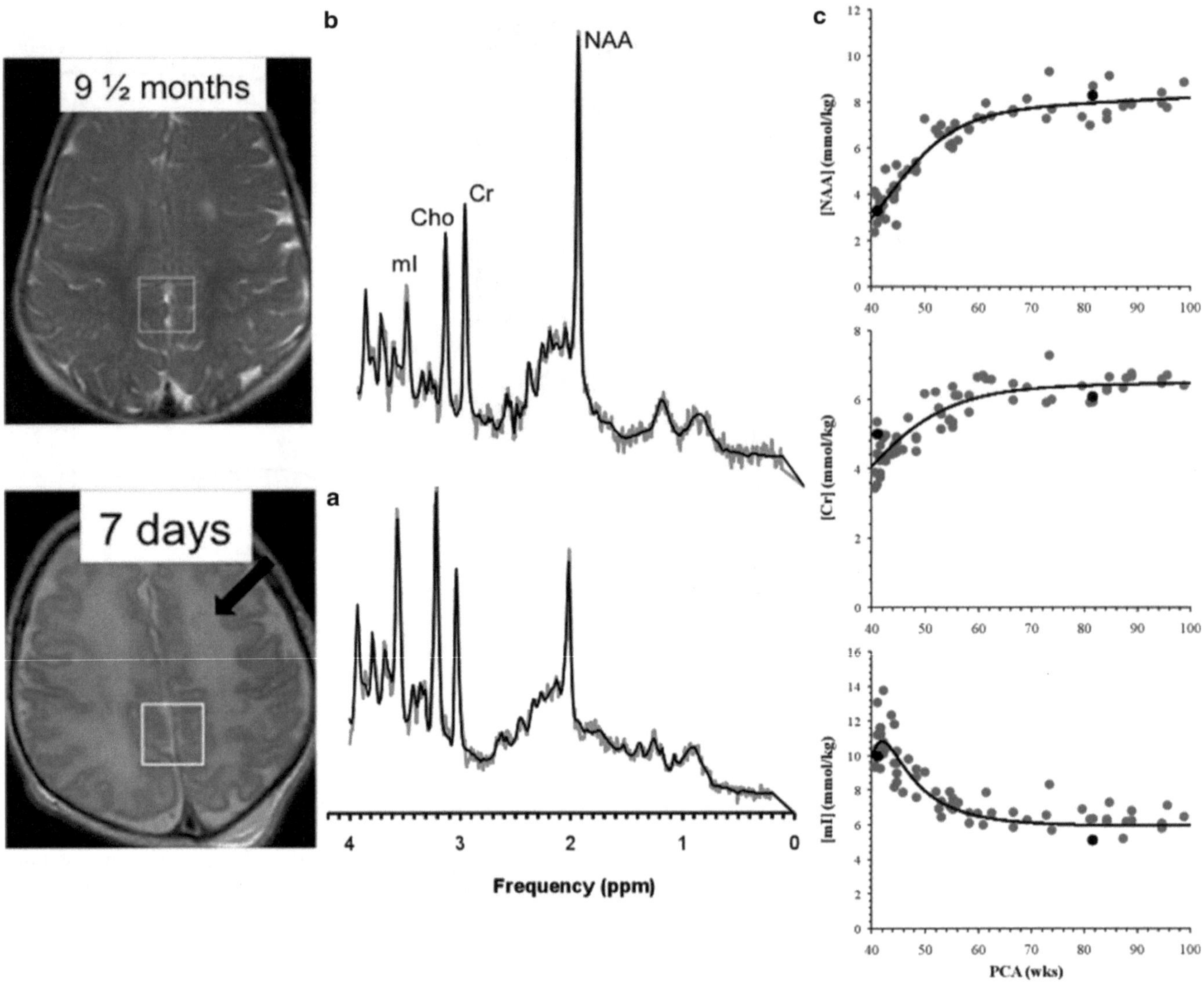

Fig. 22.88 Newborn Hypotonia, "Normal" Age-Dependent Changes

MRS Method

1.5 T, SV-PRESS TE 35 ms, occipital/parietal GM, baseline and one-month follow-up.

Interpretation/Discussion

Initial study: On MRI there was evidence of diffuse cerebral edema with diffusion pattern of abnormality suggestive of a bilateral border zone (low perfusion) acute infarct, with acute subdural hemorrhage in the posterior fossa (Fig. 22.89). Spectroscopy demonstrated elevated lactate and lipids, reduced NAA, and increased (likely) Gln. MRS was consistent with severe, acute hypoxic/ischemic injury. *One-month follow-up*: MRI showed evidence of diffuse cerebral multicystic volume loss secondary to the previously seen diffuse cerebral edema with diffusion pattern suggestive of a bilateral border zone (low perfusion) acute infarcts. Spectroscopy showed now lipids to be more prominent than lactate. NAA was not detectable and Gln, which was increased previously, was now depleted.

Conclusions

An example for progression of severe hypoxic/ischemic injury at 1-month postinsult in a 2-month-old baby is shown.

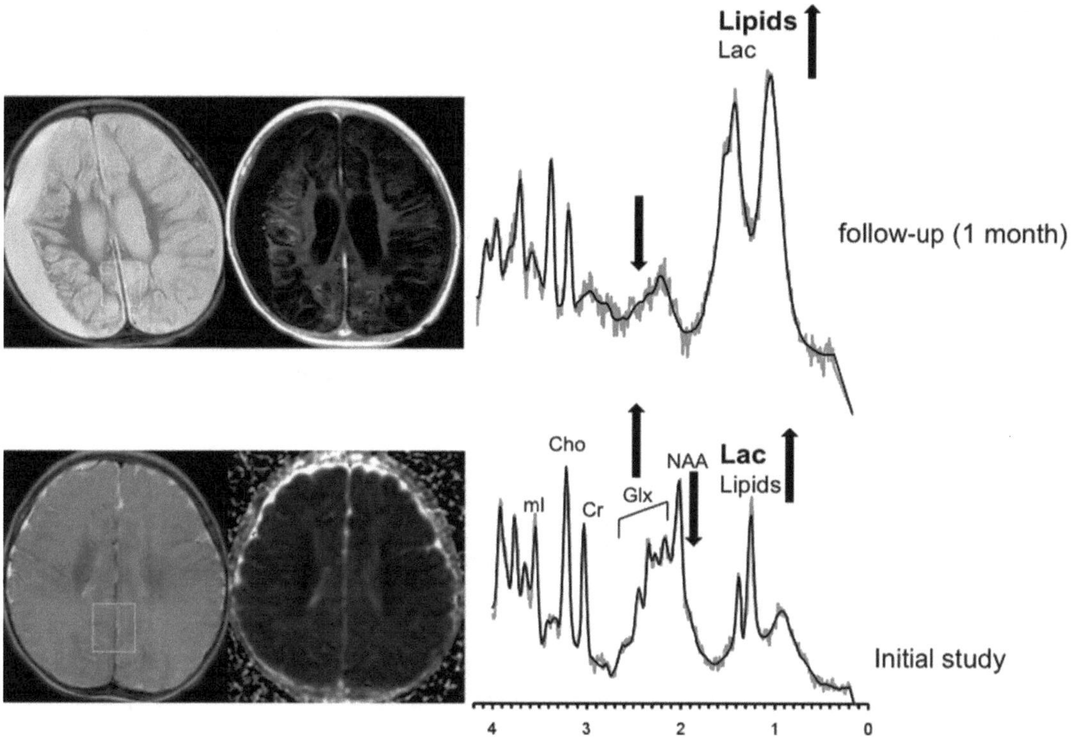

Fig. 22.89 Nonaccidental Trauma, Severe Hypoxic/Ischemic Injury Pattern, Progression

Case 90: Hypoxic/Ischemic Injury, Newborn, Citrate

Clinical Background

11-day-old male with perinatal depression, asphyxia now seizures, born at 34 weeks gestational age.

MRS Method

1.5 T, single-voxel PRESS, TE 35 ms, parietal and frontal white matter, parieto/occipital gray matter.

Interpretation/Discussion

The MRI showed multiple areas of signal abnormality and restricted diffusion involving the basal ganglia, thalami, internal capsule, and corona radiata bilaterally most likely related to areas of hyperperfusion injury given the provided history of birth asphyxia (Fig. 22.90). An underlying metabolic abnormality cannot be excluded. MRS was significantly abnormal. It showed increased lactate and lipids in all regions examined suggesting acute or subacute injury. NAA was possibly slightly reduced for age. Cr, Cho, and mI appear to be close to normal for age. Noted was a signal consistent with citrate in all three spectra. The significance of citrate is unclear. In normal brain, citrate is involved in energy metabolism and is the first intermediate in the TCA cycle.

Conclusions

A slightly unusual pattern in a newborn with ischemic/hypoxic was observed. The presence of citrate may raise the possibility of an underlying inborn error with abnormal energy metabolism.

Case 91: Charge Syndrome

Clinical Background

14-day-old infant (38 weeks gestational age at birth) with CHARGE association, hearing loss.

MRS Method

1.5 T, SV-PRESS TE 35 ms, parietal WM, occipital/parietal GM, re-examined at 2½ months.

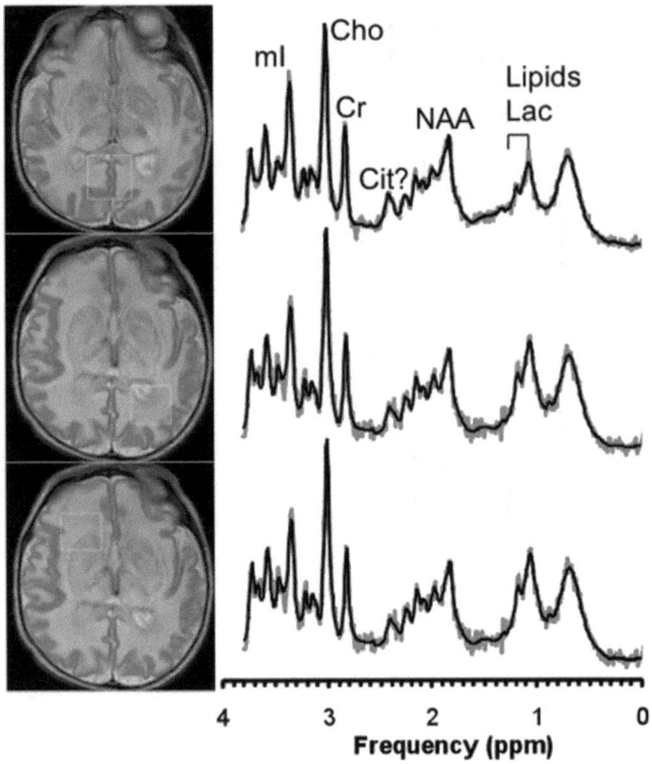

Fig. 22.90 Hypoxic/Ischemic Injury, Newborn, Citrate

Interpretation/Discussion

First study (Fig. 22.91a): Structural abnormalities such as absent olfactory tracks and bulbs were noted on MR images (not shown). The brain parenchyma demonstrated bands of migrating cells in the white matter of both cerebral hemispheres of unknown significance, but can be seen in case of congenital heart disease and other congenital syndromic cases. These may represent makers of immature white matter maturation. Myelination was appropriate for the patient's age and the ventricles were normal in size and configuration. MR spectroscopy showed a biochemical profile close to normal for age. The exception was mI, which appeared to be slightly above normal levels. Second study (B): The MRI interpretation did not change with structural abnormalities noted as above but with brain parenchyma and myelination appropriate for age. MR spectroscopy was also consistent with the initial study showing only mI to be slightly above normal levels (C).

Conclusions

Increased mI, possibly incidental, was observed in Charge syndrome in two studies of the same patient. Other metabolites were within the normal range.

Case 92: Scyllo-Inositol, Prominent

Clinical Background

18 month old with hypotonia and respiratory failure, MRI/S was performed to rule out ischemic event and to explain decreased respiratory function.

MRS Method

1.5 T, SV-PRESS TE 35 ms, parietal WM, occipital/parietal GM.

Interpretation/Discussion

On MRI there was no evidence of acute infarction. However, bilateral striatal (basal ganglia) T2 hyperintensity was noticed (Fig. 22.92). The differential included chronic hypoxic–ischemic injury. Other differential considerations were toxic injury and metabolic disease. The spectra did not show evidence for elevated lactate and/or reduced NAA. Cho was prominent relative to Cr. In both white matter and gray matter, scyllo-inositol (sI) was prominent. Scyllo-inositol is often too small for reliable detection. In this case, it was readily detectable and estimated to be 500–700% above normal levels.

Conclusions

A case with prominent scyllo-inositol is shown. The cause and significance of prominent sI is unclear. Cho was also elevated in this patient.

Case 93: Focal White Matter Necrosis, Periventricular Leukomalacia (PVL)

Clinical Background

6-week-old male with seizures, born at 31 weeks gestational age.

MRS Method

1.5 T, single-voxel PRESS, TE 35 ms, parietal and frontal white matter, parieto/occipital gray matter.

Interpretation/Discussion

The MRI showed ventricles that were normal in size and configuration (Fig. 22.93). However, there were multiple

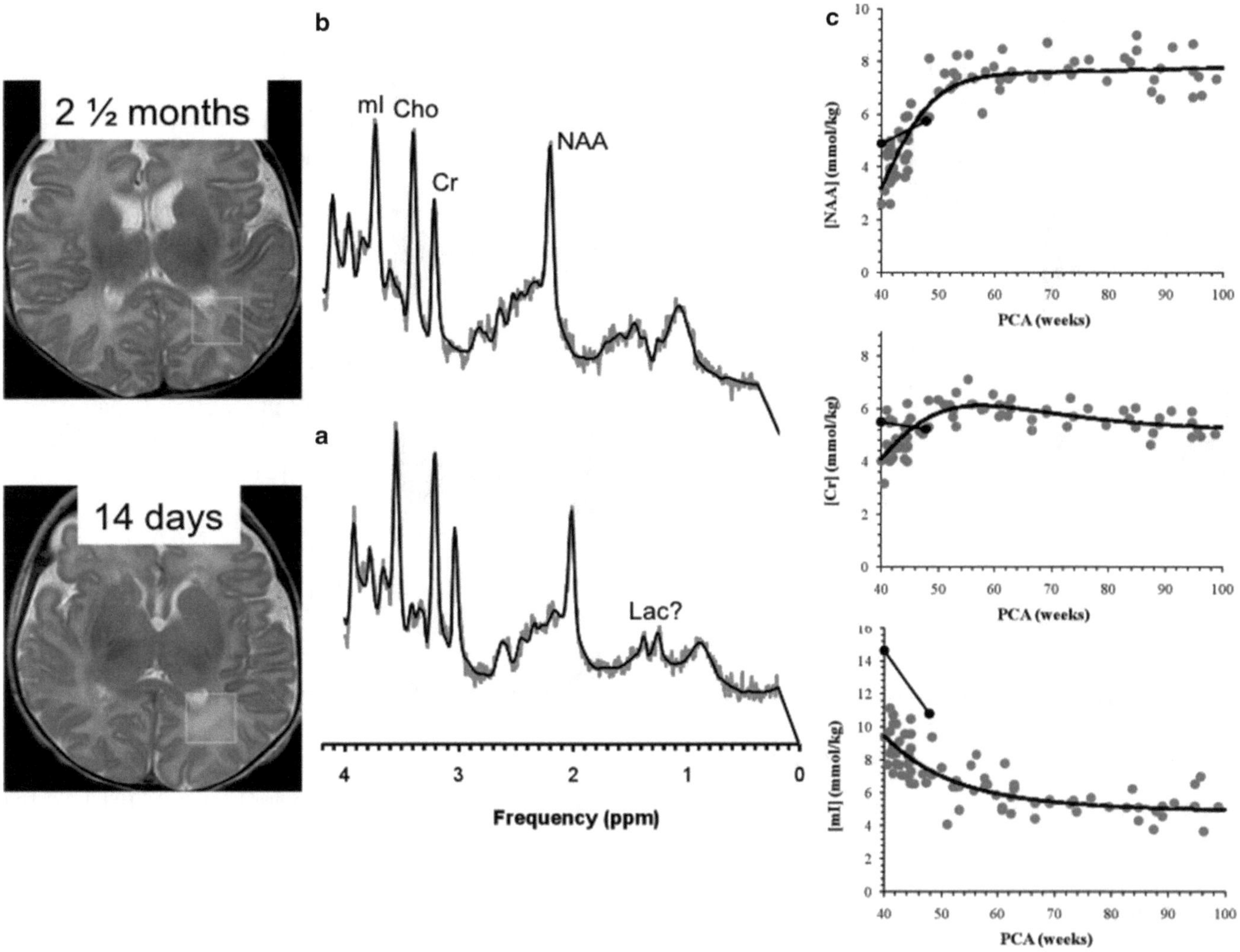

Fig. 22.91 Charge Syndrome

Fig. 22.92 Scyllo-Inositol, Prominent

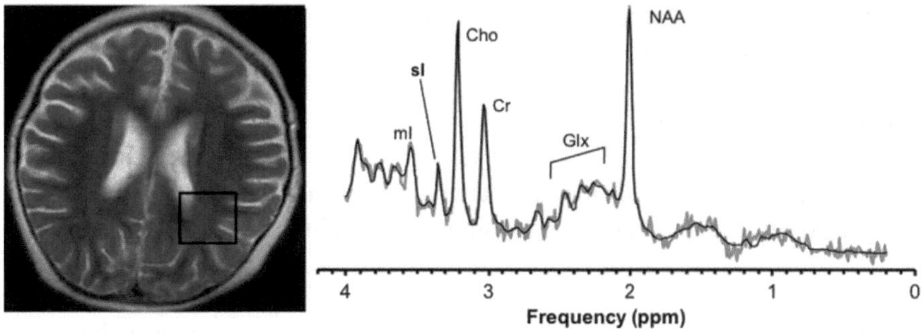

1–2 mm focal areas of coagulation necrosis in the white matter of both cerebral hemispheres which was detected on 3D spoiled gradient-echo imaging (not shown). Myelination was deemed appropriate for the patient's age. No malformations were identified. The MRS appeared to be mostly unremarkable for age. Only in parietal white matter, lactate appeared to be slightly abnormal. As all studies in very small babies, the interpretation of the spectra is complicated by the lack of appropriate control data.

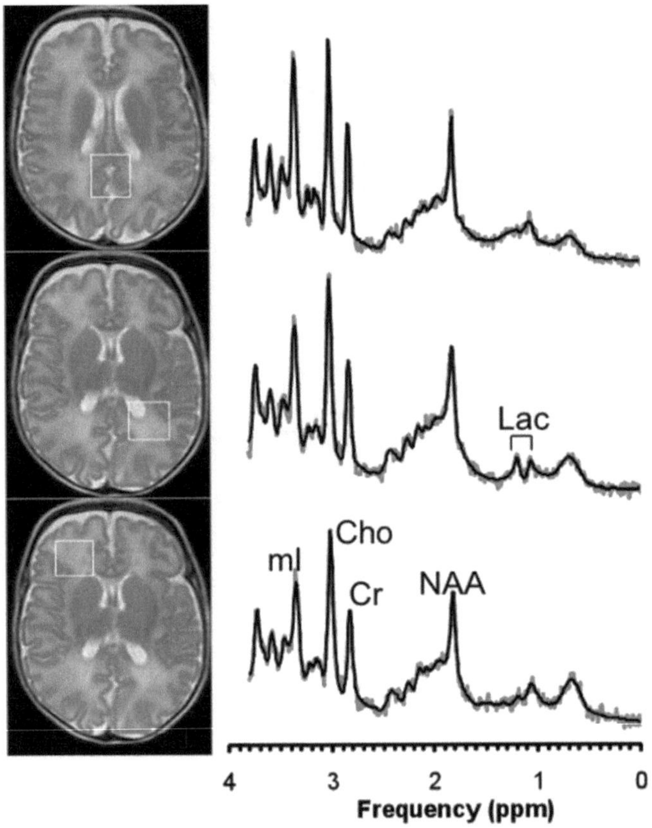

Fig. 22.93 Focal White Matter Necrosis, Periventricular Leukomalacia (PVL)

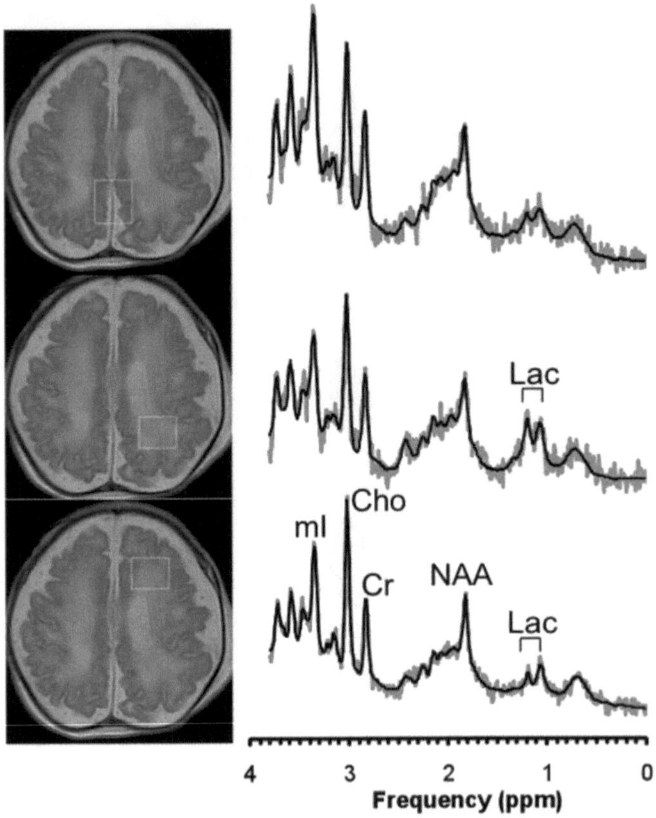

Fig. 22.94 Diffuse Excessive High Signal Intensity (DEHSI) I, Newborn

Conclusions

A patient with focal white matter necrosis presents with slightly abnormal lactate in parietal white matter.

Case 94: Diffuse Excessive High Signal Intensity (DEHSI) I, Newborn

Clinical Background

2-week-old male with congenital heart defect, born at 34 weeks gestational age, examined for brain abnormalities.

MRS Method

1.5 T, single-voxel PRESS, TE 35 ms, parietal and frontal white matter, parieto/occipital gray matter.

Interpretation/Discussion

The MRI showed features consistent with severe Diffuse Excessive High Signal Intensity (DEHSI), an abnormality putatively thought to represent diffuse WM gliosis within the spectrum of perinatal white matter injury (Fig. 22.94). In addition, the ventricles were enlarged and there was above normal extra-axial fluid accumulation. The MRS showed in both white matter locations evidence for slightly elevated lactate. Other metabolites appear to be within normal range. However, the interpretation of the spectra is complicated by the lack of appropriate control data.

Conclusions

A patient with severe DEHSI shows readily detectable lactate. A more detailed interpretation of data from very young babies is complicated by the unavailability of appropriate control data.

Case 95: Diffuse Excessive High Signal Intensity (DEHSI) II, Newborn

Clinical Background

Newborn male with abnormal perfusion examined to rule out infarction, born at 33 weeks gestational age.

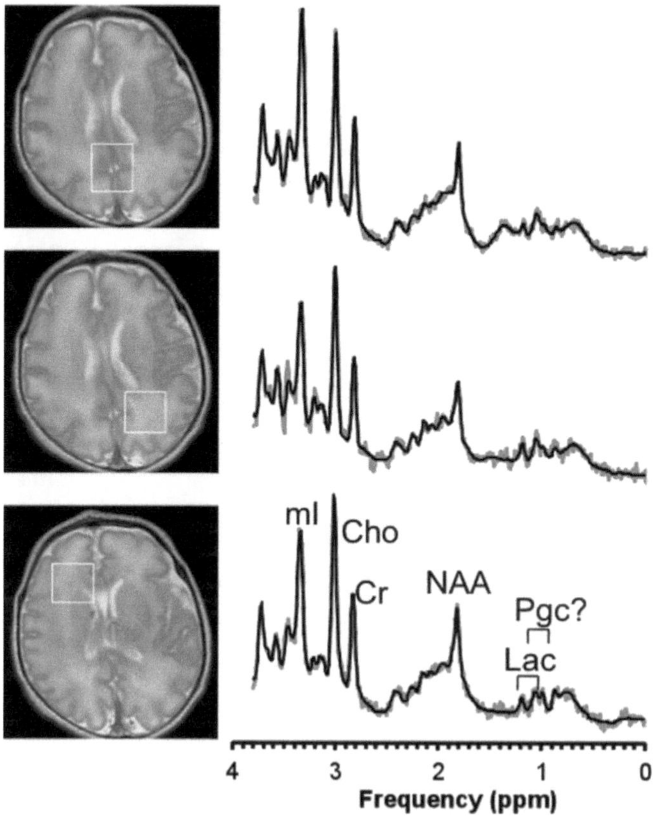

Fig. 22.95 Diffuse Excessive High Signal Intensity (DEHSI) II, Newborn

MRS Method

1.5 T, single-voxel PRESS, TE 35 ms, parietal and frontal white matter, parieto/occipital gray matter.

Interpretation/Discussion

The MRI showed features consistent with severe Diffuse Excessive High Signal Intensity (DEHSI), an abnormality putatively thought to represent diffuse WM gliosis (Fig. 22.95). The MRS showed in both white matter locations evidence for slightly elevated lactate. It is also possible that there were small amounts of propylene glycol, which has often been used as a solvent for medication administered to patients. Other metabolites appear to be within normal range. However, the interpretation of the spectra is complicated by the lack of appropriate control data.

Conclusions

A patient with severe DEHSI shows lactate. A more detailed interpretation of data from very young babies is complicated by the unavailability of appropriate control data.

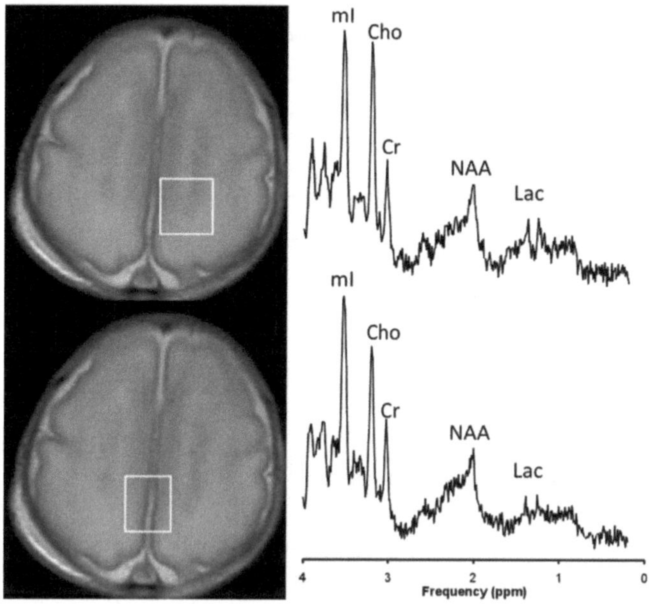

Fig. 22.96 Extreme Prematurity, Normal MRI, Lactate

Case 96: Extreme Prematurity, Normal MRI, Lactate

Clinical Background

Premature baby with respiratory distress. Gestational age at birth was 25 weeks. The patient was studied 1 week after birth.

MRS Method

1.5 T, single-voxel PRESS, TE 35 ms, two locations in undifferentiated brain tissue

Interpretation/Discussion

MRI was reported to be within normal limits and clinical follow-up of more than 4 years after the study was unremarkable for this patient (Fig. 22.96). Lactate is present in both spectra. NAA is very low, whereas mI is the most prominent peak.

Conclusions

Lactate detected at very early brain development (prematurity) does not necessarily indicate brain injury. Similarly, very low NAA and elevated mI levels are normal at this age.

Case 97: Newborn, Propylene Glycol, *Not* Lactate

Clinical Background

Two-month-old male with hemorrhage and suspected head trauma. MRS was performed to rule out axonal/neuronal injury.

MRS Method

1.5 T, single-voxel PRESS, TE=35 ms, occipital gray matter.

Interpretation/Discussion

On MRI, the brain parenchyma appeared normal on all sequences and the ventricles were of normal size (Fig. 22.97). An acute subdural hemorrhage along the falx and tentorium was noted. A prominent signal from propylene glycol (Pgc), also known as propan-1,2-diol, was detected in the MR spectrum. Pgc presents with a doublet that can be confused with the lactate doublet. The concentration of Pgc in brain tissue was ≈20 mmol/kg. Additionally, NAA was reduced in this patient indicating significant brain damage. A later CT scan revealed shrunken gyri and ventriculomegaly suggesting parenchymal volume loss in both hemispheres.

Conclusions

To ensure proper identification of lactate and/or propylene glycol the chemical shift of the downfield doublet needs to be checked carefully. Note that the Pgc doublet is centered at ≈1.2 ppm whereas the double from lactate is centered at ≈1.3 ppm. Propylene glycol is often used as a solvent for drugs (antiseizure drugs) and its accumulation in brain tissue of small babies has been reported by several groups (1). It is unknown whether Pgc by itself can cause brain damage.

Case 98: Cockayne Syndrome

Clinical Background

3-month-old female with dysmorphic features.

MRS Method

1.5 T, single-voxel PRESS, TE 35 ms, of parietal WM, occipital GM.

Interpretation/Discussion

The initial MRI study showed enlarged lateral ventricles and a cystic lesion at right posterior ventricle (Fig. 22.98). Extensive diffuse predominantly white matter signal abnormality was noted. The spectrum showed significantly elevated lactate. NAA was slightly reduced, Cr and Cho were close to normal, and mI was elevated. Glc appeared to be slightly prominent. A repeat MRI (no MRS performed) 3 months later showed significant volume loss. At that time the patient suffered from uncontrollable hyperglycemia. Cockayne syndrome is currently discussed as the underlying disease of this patient.

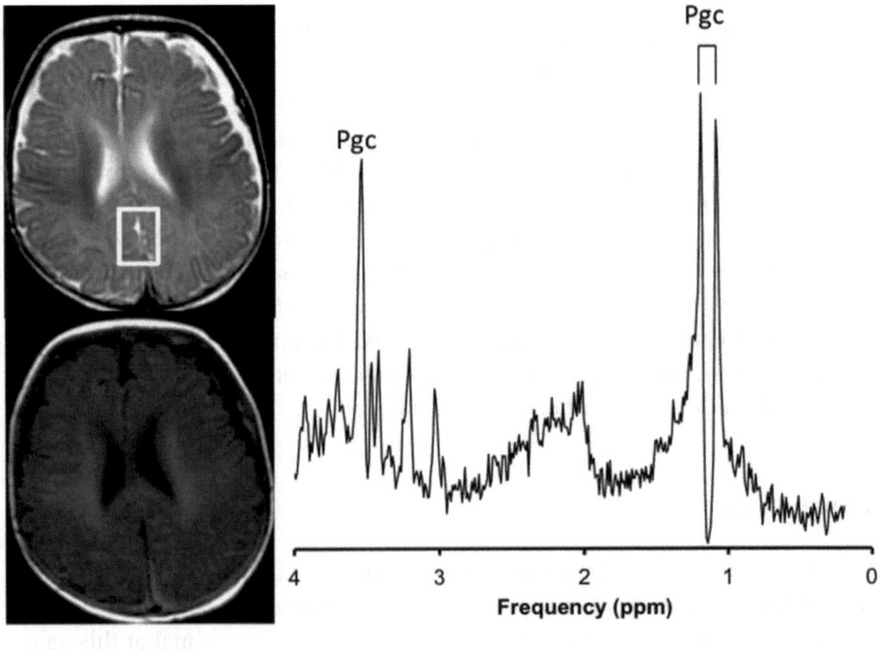

Fig. 22.97 Newborn, Propylene Glycol, *Not* Lactate

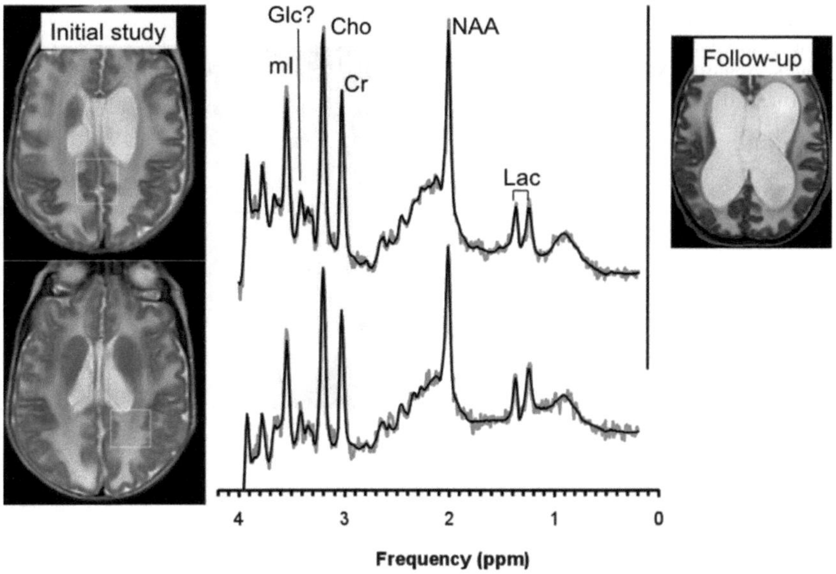

Fig. 22.98 Cockayne Syndrome

Conclusions

A spectrum of a patient tentatively diagnosed with Cockayne syndrome showed elevated lactate.

Case 99: Leigh's Disease

Clinical Background

17-month-old male with developmental delay.

MRS Method

1.5 T, single-voxel PRESS, TE 35 ms, basal ganglia, occipital GM.

Interpretation/Discussion

The MRI showed abnormal edema in the midbrain and basal ganglia, which is suggestive of Leigh's disease (Fig. 22.99). There was high diffusion signal seen within the lesion suggesting an acute etiology. MRS of basal ganglia showed prominent lactate. MRS of gray matter was close to normal with only a small amount of lactate detectable.

Conclusions

A patient with suspected Leigh's disease had prominent lactate in a spectrum obtained from abnormal basal ganglia. Gray matter MRS was close to normal.

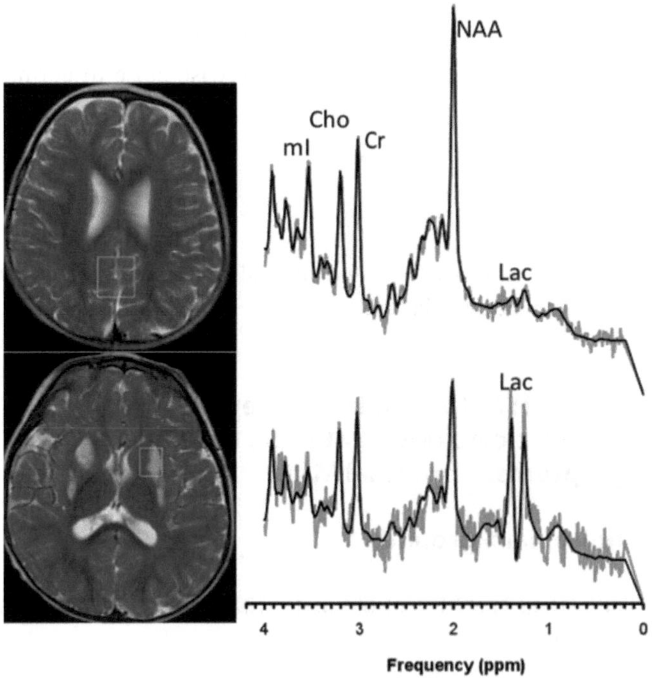

Fig. 22.99 Leigh's Disease

Case 100: Mitochondrial Encephalomyopathy with Lactic Acidosis (MELAS), Normal MRI

Clinical Background

12-year-old male with MELAS syndrome.

MRS Method

1.5 T, single-voxel PRESS, TE 35 ms, occipital GM.

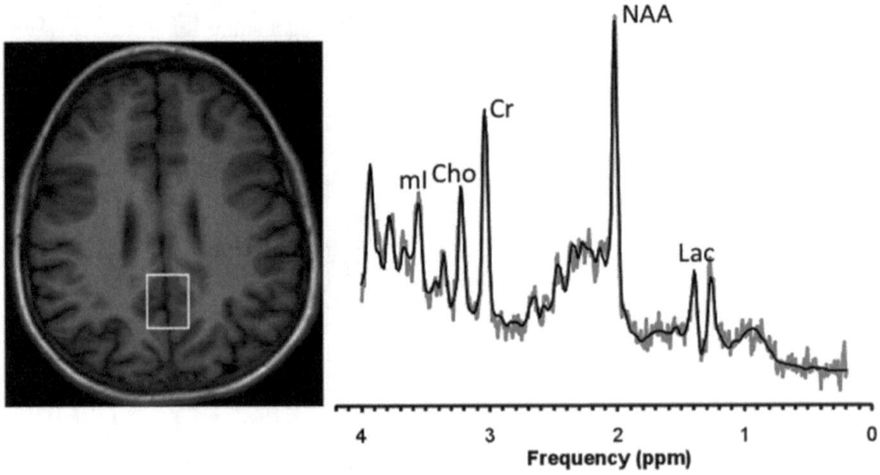

Fig. 22.100 Mitochondrial Encephalomyopathy with Lactic Acidosis (MELAS), Normal MRI

Interpretation/Discussion

The MRI was interpreted as normal. MRS of gray matter showed elevated lactate but was otherwise close to normal (Fig. 22.100).

Conclusions

A patient with MELAS and normal MRI showed readily detectable elevated lactate.

Case 101: Mitochondrial Encephalomyopathy with Lactic Acidosis (MELAS), New Acute Symptoms, Abnormal MRI

Clinical Background

The patient is a 14-year-old male with a history of MELAS syndrome.

MRS Method

1.5 T, single-voxel PRESS, TE 35 ms, occipital GM, lesion.

Interpretation/Discussion

The MRI showed multiple acute and subacute infarcts (Fig. 22.101). MRS of gray matter showed elevated lactate and reduced NAA. MRS of abnormal periventricular white matter showed more significantly elevated lactate and significantly reduced NAA. Reduced NAA is consistent with neuronal/axonal damage/loss.

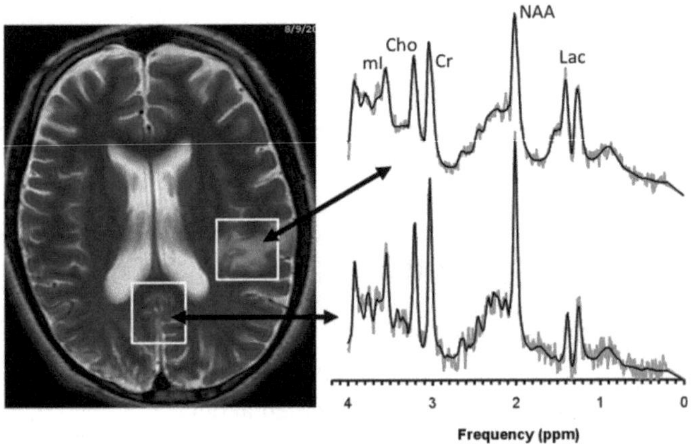

Fig. 22.101 Mitochondrial Encephalomyopathy with Lactic Acidosis (MELAS), New Acute Symptoms, Abnormal MRI

Conclusions

A patient with MELAS and abnormal MRI showed readily detectable elevated lactate and reduced NAA.

Case 102: Reproducibility of MRS, State-of-the-Art

Clinical Background

Healthy adult control.

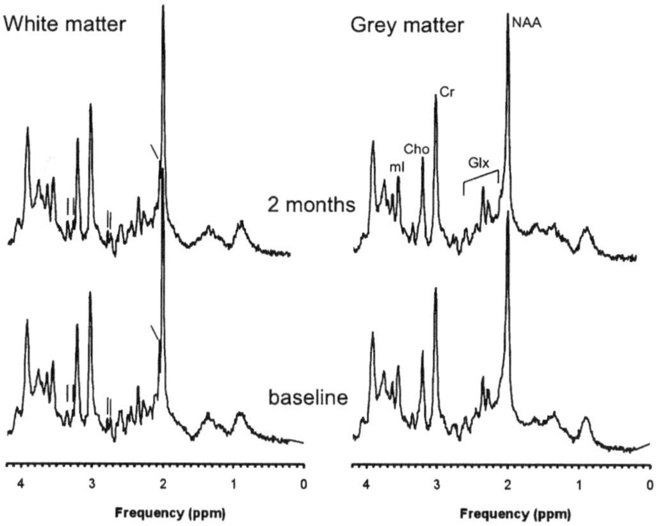

Fig. 22.102 Reproducibility of MRS, State-of-the-Art

MRS Method

3 T, SV-PRESS TE 35 ms, occipital/parietal GM, two studies 2 months apart.

Interpretation/Discussion

MRS has often been perceived as being an unreliable methodology (Fig. 22.102). However, significant advances in hardware have improved the reliability of MRS considerably. In the above study, the volunteer was examined twice—2 months apart. The ROIs were carefully placed in standard parietal white matter and parietal/occipital gray matter. Both white matter and gray matter spectra obtained at the session were highly comparable. This not only includes the major peaks of the proton spectrum such as NAA, Cr, Cho, or mI but also smaller details of the spectra (e.g., see "ticks" in white matter spectra).

Conclusions

With an appropriate effort, proton MRS on modern scanners is highly reproducible.

Case 103: Stability, State-of-the-Art

Clinical Background

Healthy adult control.

MRS Method

3 T, SV-PRESS TE 35 ms, parietal WM and occipital/parietal GM, repeated MRS studies after oral administration of a Glc solution (oral Glc tolerance test (OGT)).

Interpretation/Discussion

This study was undertaken to demonstrate the excellent stability provided by modern MR scanners and thus sensitivity to detect small changes in individual subjects. A healthy adult control (over-night fasting) was examined after the administration of oral Glc. Spectra were acquired from two locations repeatedly (Fig. 22.103). Highly consistent data were obtained with variations of the major peaks (NAA, Cr, Cho, and mI) of less than 10% over the duration of this study (A). The only metabolite with significant not-random changes was Glc, which, as expected, increased in both GM (B) and WM (not shown).

Conclusions

Modern scanners provide excellent stability for proton MRS.

Case 104: Cerebrospinal Fluid (CSF)

Clinical Background

3-day-old boy with congenital hydrocephalus.

MRS Method

1.5 T, single-voxel PRESS, TE 35 ms, three locations with increasing partial volume of CSF.

Interpretation/Discussion

Metabolites are mostly intracellular and thus little signal is observed in spectra containing substantial amounts of CSF (Fig. 22.104). CSF itself, however, does not necessarily degrade the quality of the MRS. The linewidths of peaks in the spectra were excellent. Considering the partial volume of CSF is important when absolute quantitation is attempted. In this example, metabolite concentrations would be underestimated without applying a correction for the small amount of tissue enclosed in the ROI.

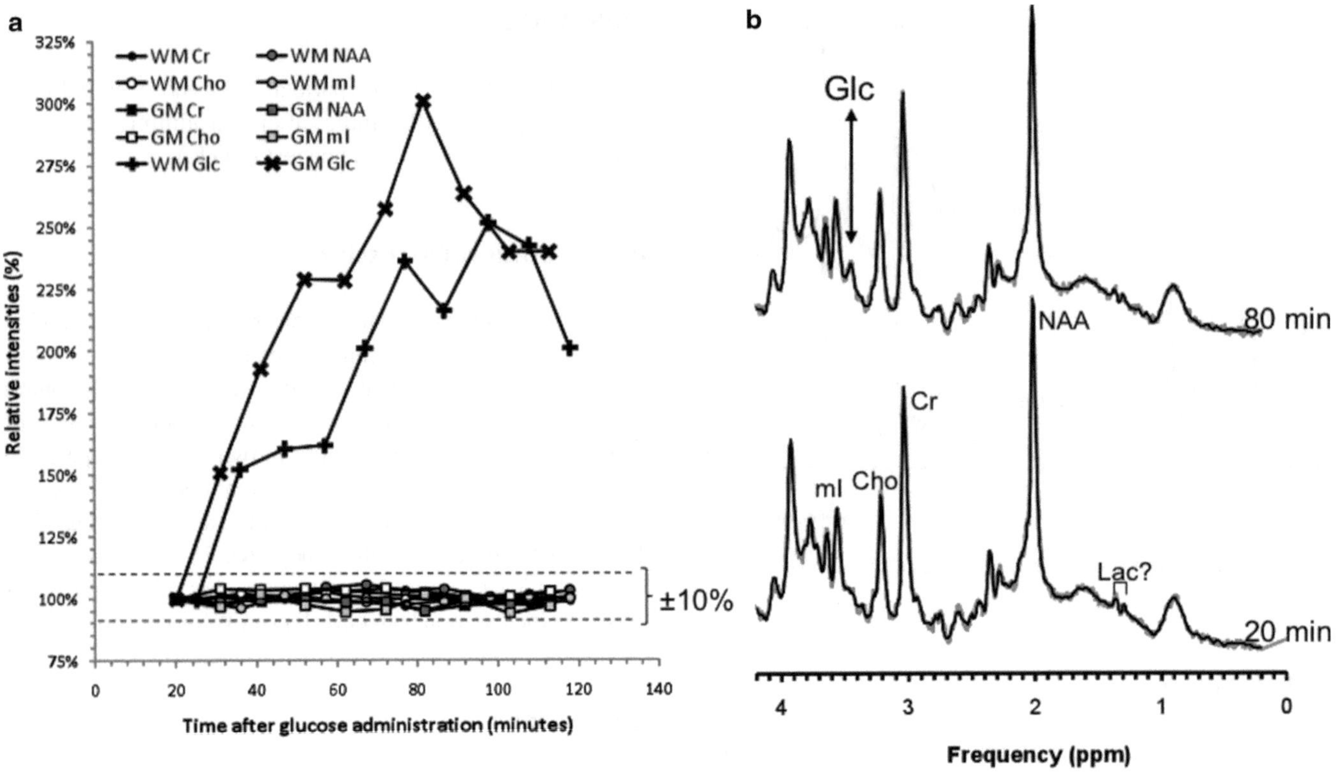

Fig. 22.103 Stability, State-of-the-Art

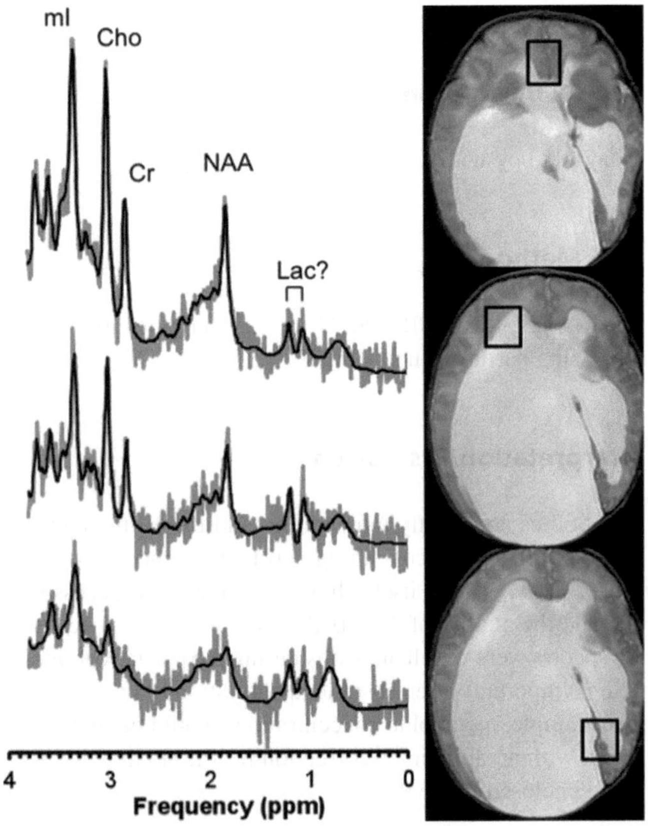

Fig. 22.104 Cerebrospinal Fluid (CSF)

Conclusions

CSF does not degrade spectral linewidth. Spectra from ROIs with large partial volume of CSF may be compromised by low SNR. For absolute quantitation, a correction for the amount of CSF enclosed in the ROI is required.

Case 105: Voxel Size and Signal to Noise

Clinical Background

Three infants with various indications for MRI/S.

MRS Method

1.5 T, single-voxel PRESS, TE 35 ms, 128 averages.

Interpretation/Discussion

These cases illustrate the importance for a realistic assessment of the impact of the voxel size on the signal-to-noise ratio (SNR). Shown are the original measured spectra (gray lines) with superimposed fits (black lines) (Fig. 22.105). The SNR

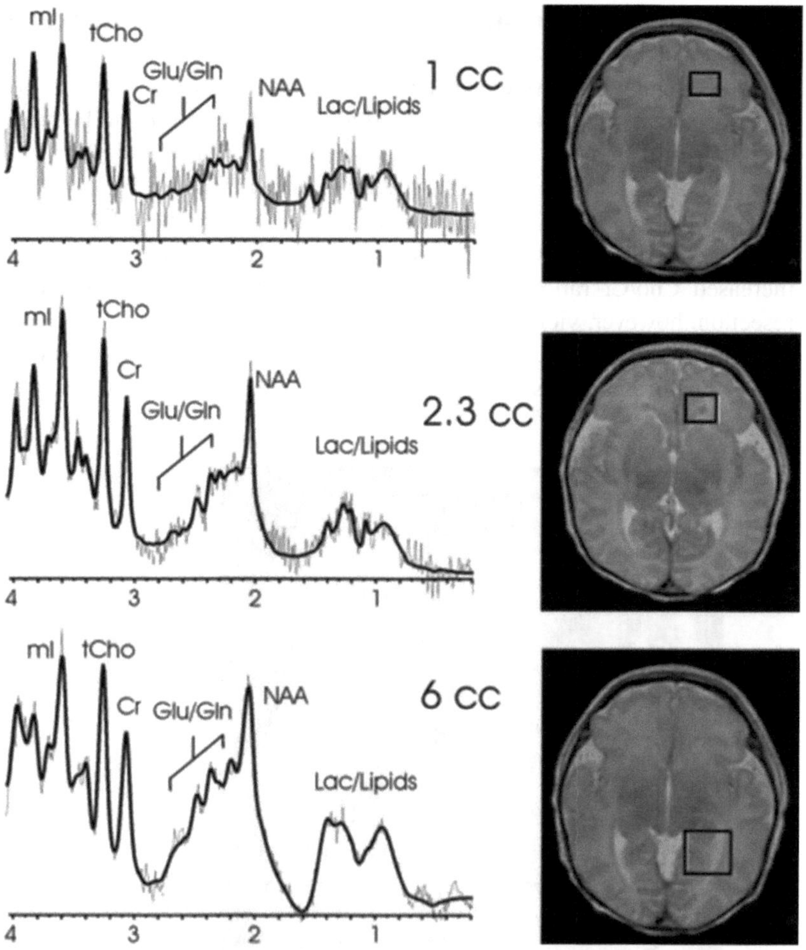

Fig. 22.105 Voxel Size and Signal to Noise

increases (decreases) linearly with the volume of the region of interest. Fitting the low SNR spectrum (top trace), a spectrum with readily recognizable features such as peaks from NAA, Cr, Cho, and mI is produced. However, fitting procedures generally "assume" that there are resonances at predefined positions. So it is not a surprise that a readily recognizable pattern is generated by the fit. For the interpretation, the random noise needs to be considered before arriving at any conclusions. That means, for this case, very little can be concluded from the spectrum shown on the top. With all parameters identical, except the volume of the voxel, the bottom spectrum has a sixfold higher SNR and can be interpreted with much more confidence. For the upper spectrum to have the same SNR without increasing the voxel size, the acquisition time would need to be increased by a factor of 36 (SNR increases with the square root of the acquisition time). A compromise between an acquisition with a voxel too small for sufficient SNR and an example of somewhat large and not very specific box in a small child is shown in the middle.

Conclusions

The random noise of a spectrum needs to be considered when interpreting a study.

Case 106: Low Signal to Noise

Clinical Background

14-year-old boy with history of pineal germinoma, postradiation therapy.

MRS Method

1.5 T, single-voxel PRESS, TE 35 ms, lesion, 2D CSI, TE 144 ms, lesion and surrounding tissue.

Interpretation/Discussion

On MRI a small focus of enhancement in the region of the superior tectal plate was detected. Single-voxel and 2D chemical shift imaging (CSI) was attempted (Fig. 22.106). The single-voxel MRS of the lesion was not interpreted due to low signal to noise. On CSI, in the spectrum covering the suspicious lesion, Cho was the most prominent peak and an increased Cho/Cr ratio was reported. Subsequent surgical resection, however, yielded only scar tissue. The patient has been followed and is currently, 6 years later, free of any residual/recurrent disease.

Conclusions

Spectra of low quality, in this case low signal to noise, need to be interpreted carefully.

Case 107: Quality Compromised, Poor SHIM

Clinical Background

18-year-old male after resection of a posterior fossa pilocytic astrocytoma being evaluated for residual disease.

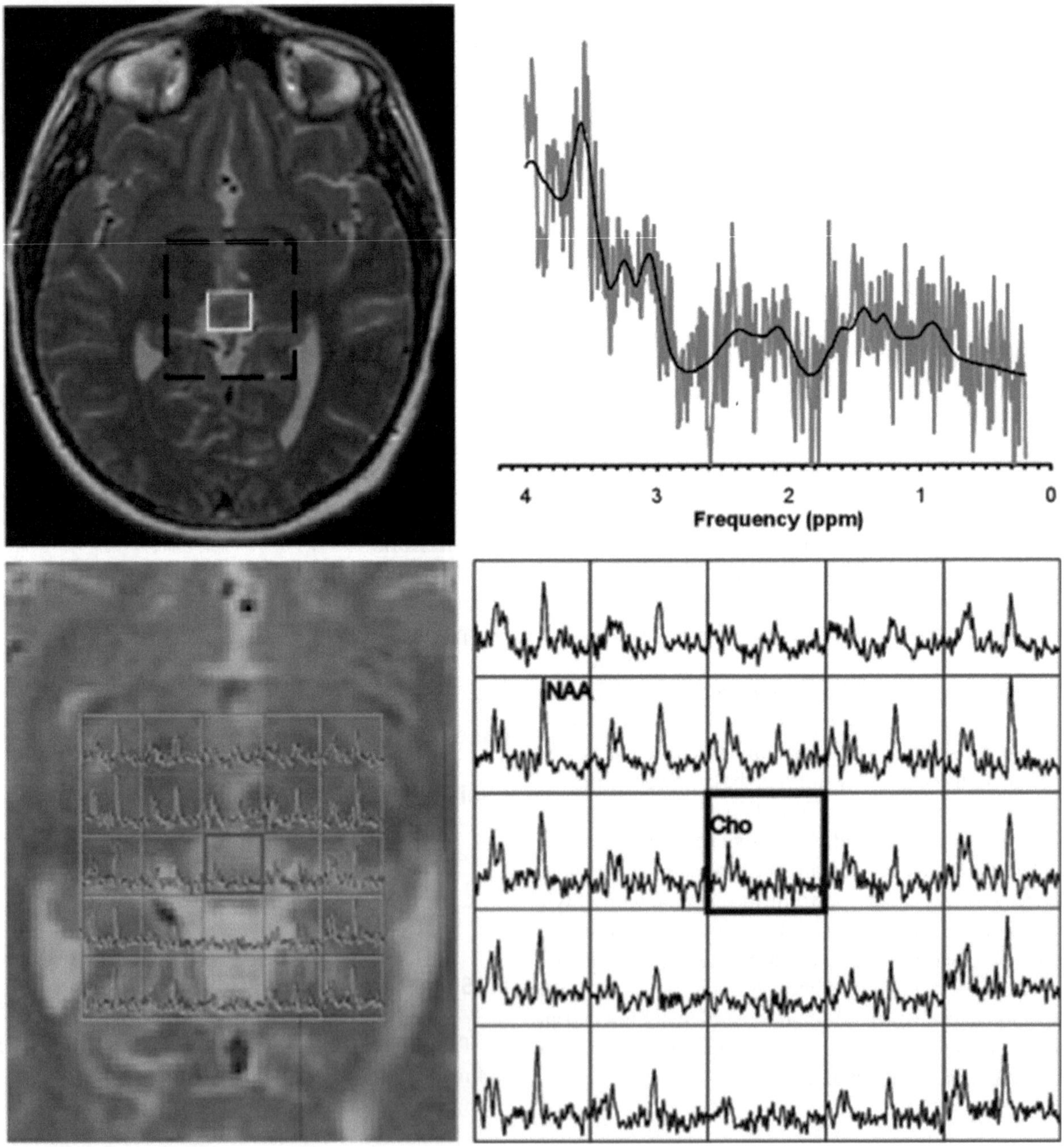

Fig. 22.106 Low Signal to Noise

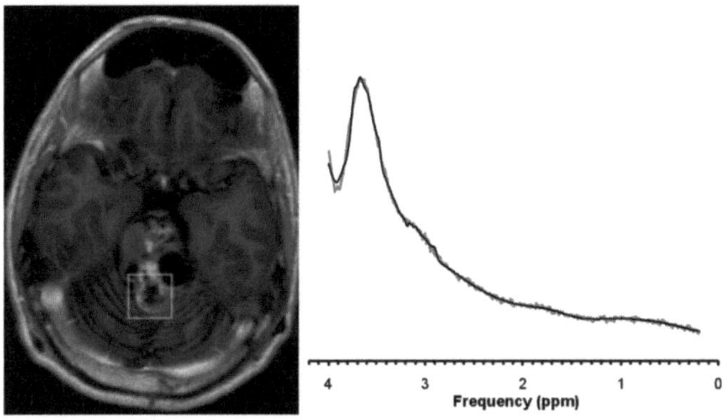

Fig. 22.107 Quality Compromised, Poor SHIM

MRS Method

1.5 T, single-voxel PRESS, TE 35 ms, of partially enhancing/suspicious tissue.

Interpretation/Discussion

The MRI was interpreted to be consistent with residual tumor. The MRS showed a spectrum with no metabolites discernable (Fig. 22.107). Inspection of the quality parameters showed that the linewidth (18 Hz) was more than 10 standard deviations above the linewidth routinely achieved. MRS was thus not reported. Blood in the surgical cavity may have caused poor magnetic field homogeneity in the region of interest.

Conclusions

The quality of MRS may be severely compromised by poor magnetic field homogeneity. In severe cases, MRS should not be reported. If there are concerns for bleeds it might be useful to have T2*weighted GRE or SWI imaging available when planning voxel placement for neoplasms.

Case 108: Quality Compromised, Braces, Poor SHIM

Clinical Background

17-year-old female with cerebellar lesion believed to be low grade.

MRS Method

1.5 T, single-voxel PRESS, TE 35 ms, of lesion with partial volume of surrounding tissue. The patient was wearing braces. 3 T, single-voxel PRESS, TE 35 ms, repeat study without braces.

Interpretation/Discussion

On MRI, a nonenhancing cerebellar lesion consistent with a low-grade lesion was observed. Image distortions due to the braces were noticed (Fig. 22.108). The MRS (A) showed a low-quality spectrum with a linewidth four standard deviations above the linewidth routinely achieved. There was no evidence for NAA. There appears to be a Cho peak more prominent than Cr and mI is possibly detectable. Nevertheless, MRS was reported as "*cannot be interpreted*". In a later study (B) a spectrum was obtained that is more typical for a low-grade lesion (but not pilocytic astrocytoma). The patient has been stable with no evidence of lesion growth since initial diagnosis.

Conclusions

Braces may have a significant impact on the quality of MRS. MRS may not be interpretable. Programmable shunts may also cause similar artifacts.

Case 109: Artifact, Voxel Placement, Prominent Lipids

Clinical Background

3-week-old female admitted for concern of central hypoventilation, for evaluation of brain structures.

MRS Method

3 T, single-voxel PRESS, TE 35 ms.

Interpretation/Discussion

The MR spectrum showed a massive lipid peak (Fig. 22.109). However, other MR spectra obtained from this patient had unremarkable lipids (not shown). When reviewing the position of the ROI it was noticed that it has not been carefully placed and that it partially overlapped lipid-containing tissue next to the eye.

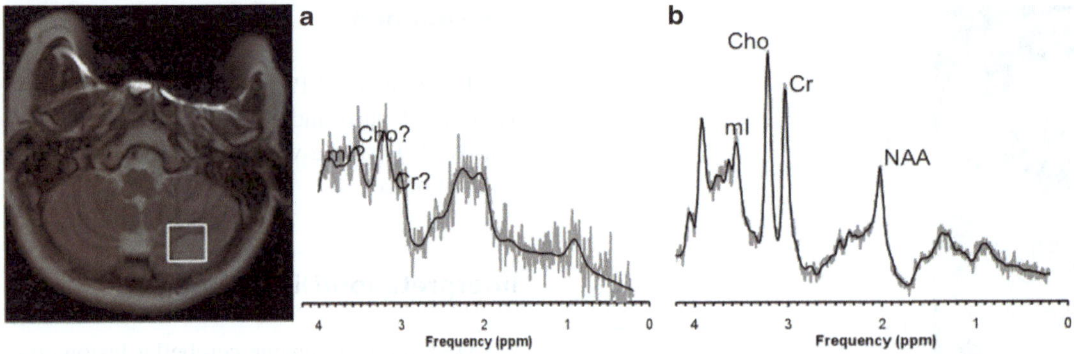

Fig. 22.108 Quality Compromised, Braces, Poor SHIM

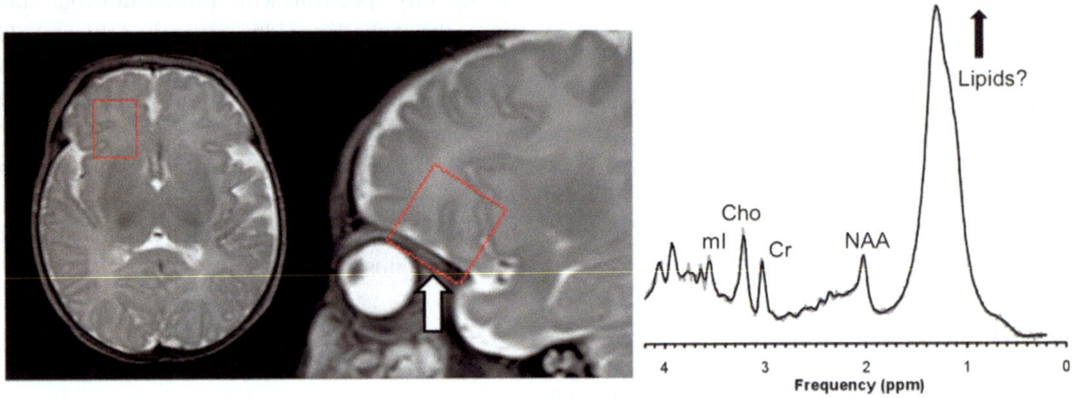

Fig. 22.109 Artifact, Voxel Placement, Prominent Lipids

Conclusions

An important part of the interpretation of MRS is the careful review of the position of the ROI. In this case, the prominent lipids are explained by the "sloppy" positioning of the ROI.

Case 110: Shifted Head Position Relative to Localizer MRI

Clinical Background

16-year-old female with pilocytic astrocytoma.

MRS Method

1.5 T, single-voxel PRESS, TE 35 ms, lesion.

Interpretation/Discussion

The MR spectrum of an vividly enhancing lesion (suspected pilocytic astrocytoma) showed a spectrum close to normal with NAA being the most prominent peak and Cho

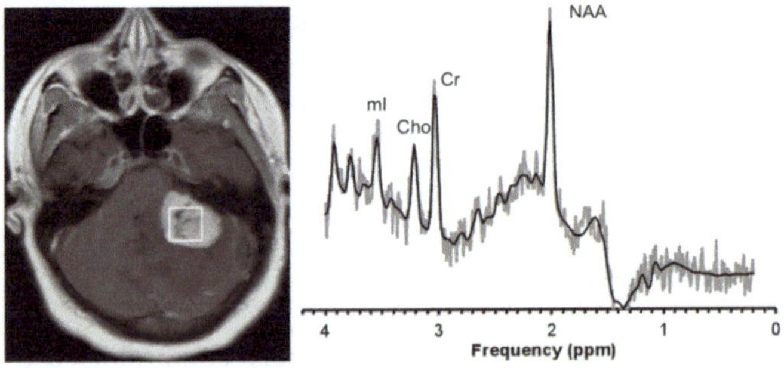

Fig. 22.110 Shifted Head Position Relative to Localizer MRI

unremarkable relative to Cr (Fig. 22.110). MR images before and after MRS were compared and it was noticed that the patient shifted the head significantly. The scan was repeated and a spectrum consistent with a pilocytic astrocytoma was obtained (not shown).

Conclusions

In case the MR spectrum of a lesion is obviously not compatible with metabolic pattern generally observed in lesions (e.g., low NAA), MR images before and after the MRS study should be compared to rule out significant shifts of the head. For this to be possible, the MRS should not be the very last sequence of an MR examination. If there is concern for the length of an examination, the number signal averages can be changed (decrease) to help acquire the spectra faster (at the risk of having less SNR).

Case 111: Frequency Jump, Patient Moving?

Clinical Background

7-year-old boy with posterior fossa tumor.

MRS Method

1.5 T, SV-MRS PRESS, TE 35 ms, lesion.

Interpretation/Discussion

The first spectrum acquired (Fig. 22.111a) showed lipids and depleted NAA. Instead of Cr peak, a broad shoulder next to Cho peak was noticed. The Cho peak itself was split in what looked like two peaks. The same was observed for mI. An artifact or a technical problem was suspected and the scan was repeated (B). The repeat scan showed "clean" peaks for Cr, Cho, and mI. The exact cause that resulted in the artifact in spectrum A is unclear. However, it is apparent that at approximately half way through data acquisition, a distinct "jump" of the frequency must have occurred. A more gradual shifting of the frequency can be ruled out, as this would have resulted in a spectrum with broad lines instead of two distinct peaks for Cho and mI, respectively. A slow/steady shifting of the position of the head as cause for the frequency jump appears thus unlikely. It is possible is that the head moved at some stage from one distinct position to another one.

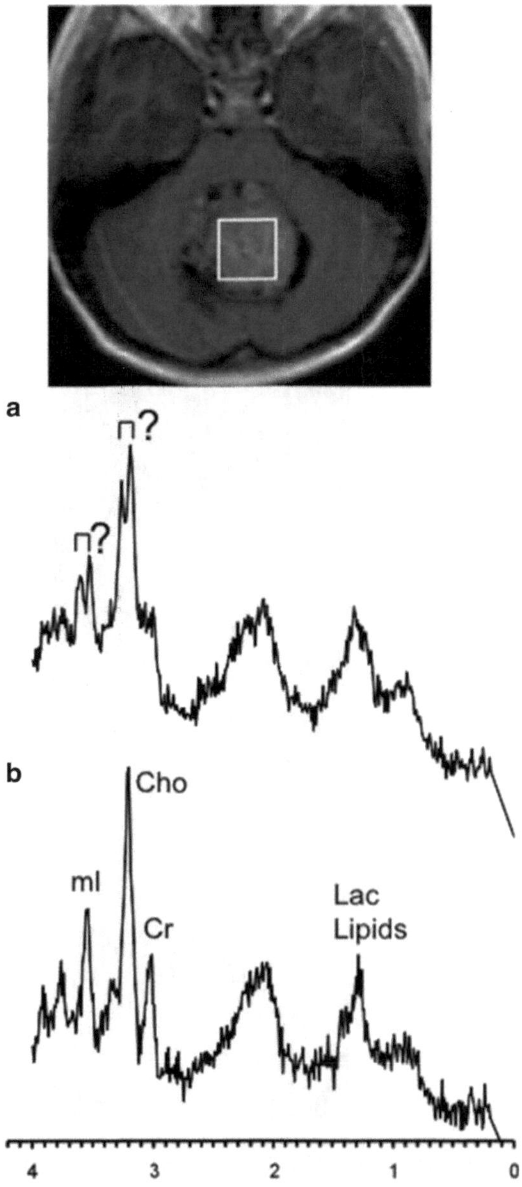

Fig. 22.111 Frequency Jump, Patient Moving?

Conclusions

Unexpected "splitting" of peaks was observed. A repeat MRS without "splitting" of lines indicated that this was likely due to the patient moving the head between two distinct positions.

Case 112: Hemorrhage, MRS Degradation by Blood Products

Clinical Background

Patient 1: Frontal lobe hemorrhage, diagnosed 1 year earlier.

Patient 2: Acute parenchymal hemorrhage in the superior vermis of the cerebellum.

Patient 3: Ependymoma, 4 months postresection.

MRS Method

1.5 T (patients 1 + 3), 3 T (patient 2), single-voxel PRESS, TE 35 ms, lesion.

Interpretation/Discussion

All spectra were of low quality with broad lines (Fig. 22.112). No metabolites were detectable in any of the spectra. Note that for patient three, a good quality spectrum (inset) was acquired from a ROI adjacent to the hemorrhagic part of the lesion. That spectrum showed elevated Cho consistent with residual/recurrent disease, which was subsequently confirmed.

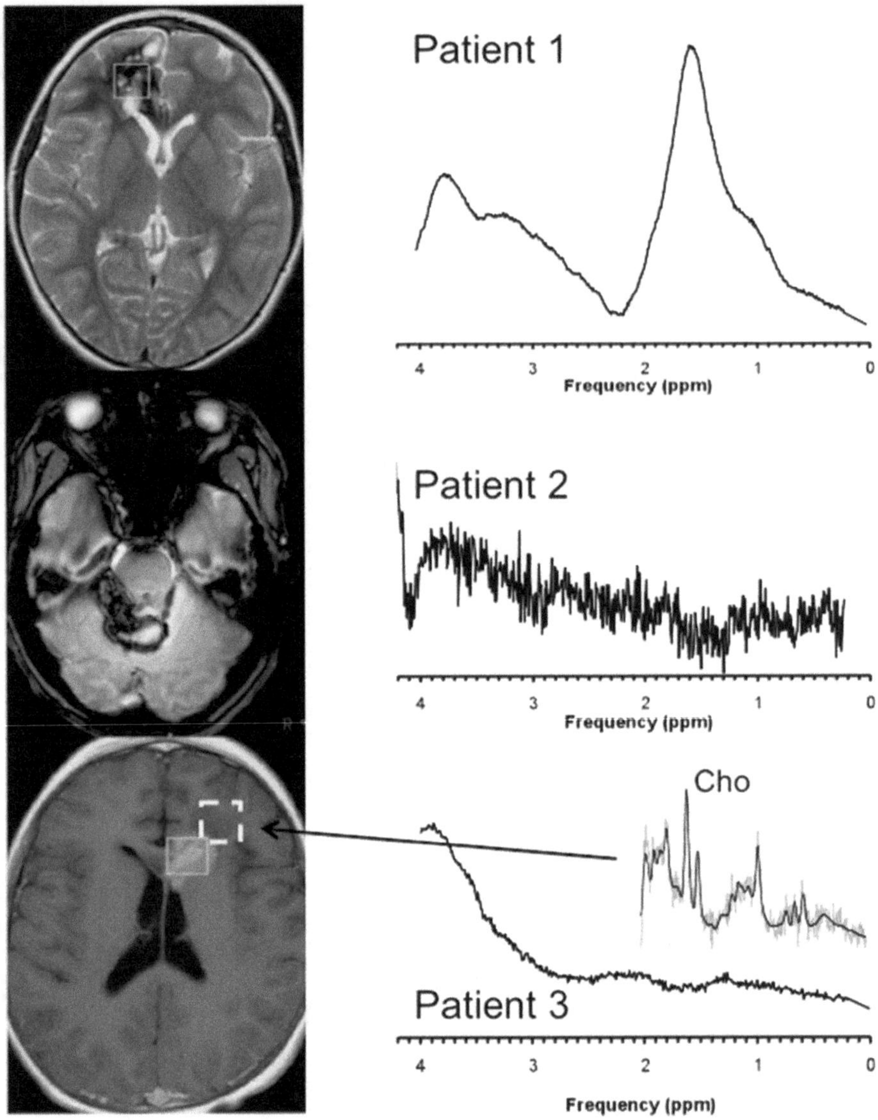

Fig. 22.112 Hemorrhage, MRS Degradation by Blood Products

Conclusions

Quality of MRS is severely compromised by the presence of blood products. It should be noted that cavernoma lesions can also cause this type of spectra. Cavernoma are sometimes in the differential diagnosis of brain tumors.

Case 113: Calcification

Clinical Background

7-year-old boy postresection of an anaplastic oligoastrocytoma with residual disease 3 years after surgery.

MRS Method

1.5 T, single-voxel PRESS, TE 35 ms, lesion.

Interpretation/Discussion

MRI/CT showed a large calcified mass, which involved the tectal plate and the left thalamus consistent with residual tumor (Fig. 22.113). The MR spectrum was acquired from an ROI that included calcified parts of the lesion. Despite the calcification, a spectrum with sufficient quality for interpretation was obtained. Although, the linewidth of the spectrum was worse than generally observed, peaks of Cho, Cr, and mI

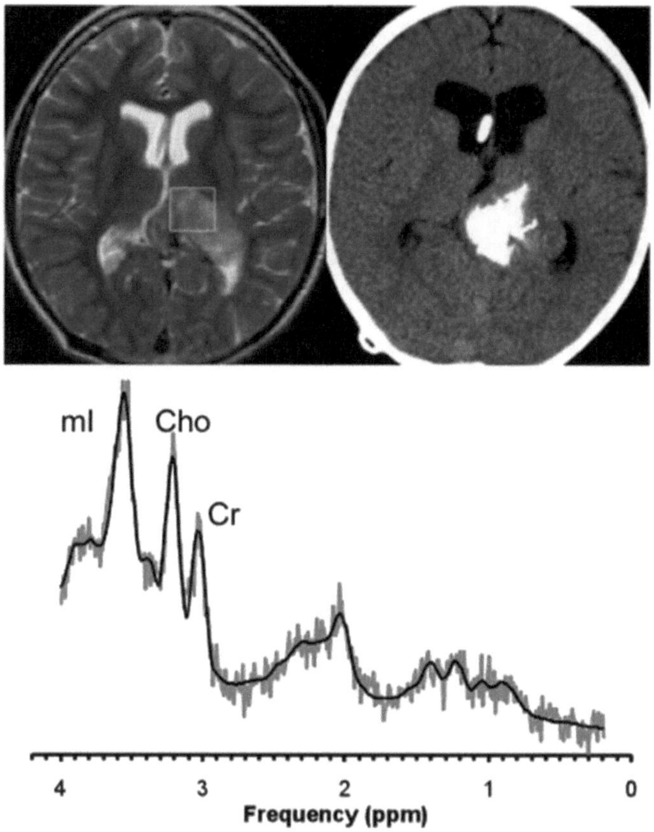

Fig. 22.113 Calcification

were well separated. Generally, the quality of MR depends on the extent of calcification. In extreme cases, the spectrum may not be interpretable.

Conclusions

Calcification apparent on CT does not necessarily rule out MRS based on technical grounds.

Case 114: Medulloblastoma (Classic), High Lipids, Atypical, Scaling: Advantage of Absolute Quantitation

Clinical Background

12-year-old male with new posterior fossa tumor.

MRS Method

1.5 T, SV-PRESS TE 35 ms.

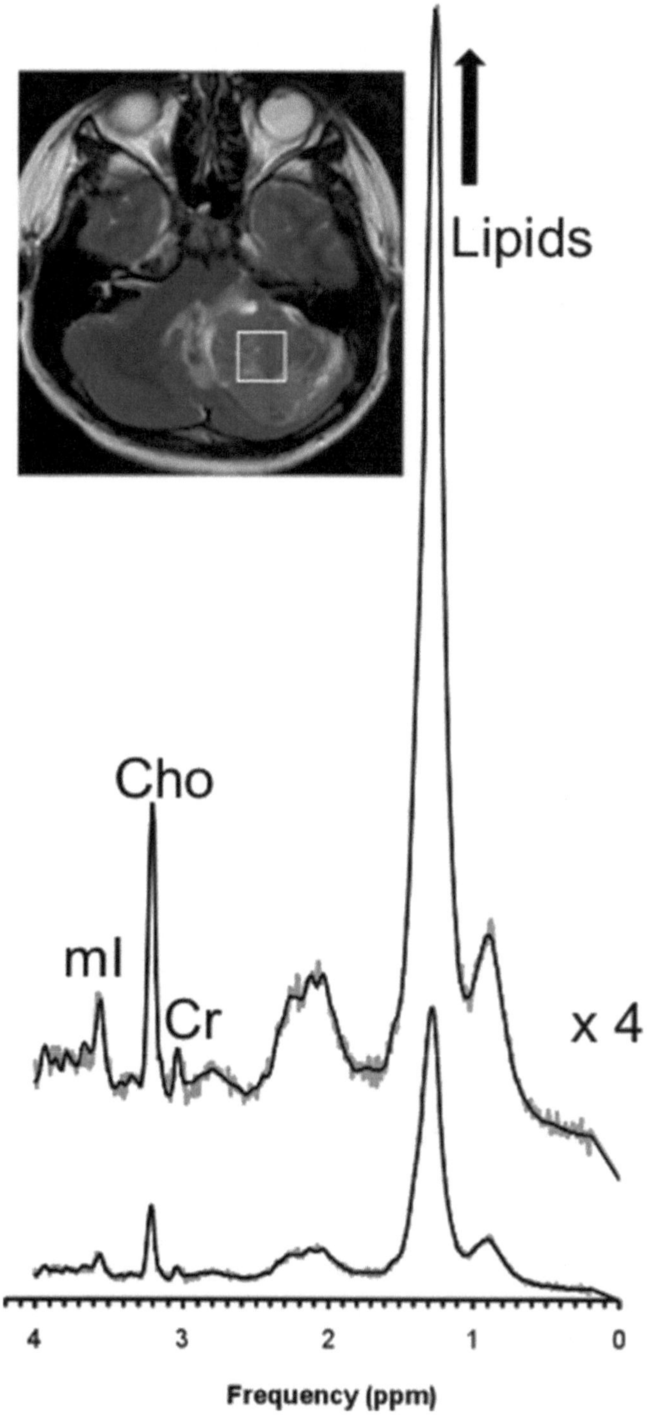

Fig. 22.114 Medulloblastoma (Classic), High Lipids, Atypical, Scaling: Advantage of Absolute Quantitation

Interpretation/Discussion

A left cerebellar tumor consistent with medulloblastoma was seen on MRI (Fig. 22.114). The tumor was resected and initially classified as desmoplastic medulloblastoma based on frozen sections. The diagnosis was changed after a more thorough review of tissue samples to classic medulloblastoma. MRS showed an unusually prominent lipid signal—more than 10 standard deviations higher than the mean lipid signal observed in other medulloblastomas. Spectra are often arbitrarily scaled to the most prominent peak and this spectrum. In this case, the Cho peak appeared to be of low intensity, when compared with the lipid signal (lower trace). The same spectrum with rescaled by a factor of four is shown in the upper trace. Indeed, absolute quantitation revealed that Cho was prominent and consistent with an aggressive tumor. Tau was not readily detectable, Cr was very low, and mI was unremarkable.

Conclusions

Spectra with unusual prominent signal from lipids need to be interpreted carefully as manufacturer provided software often scales the spectra to the peaks with the highest intensity. Absolute quantitation removes this ambiguity.

Case 115: Out-of-Voxel Lipid Artifact

Clinical Background

13-year-old girl with brain tumor postradiation therapy.

MRS Method

3 T, single-voxel PRESS, TE 35 ms, parietal WM.

Interpretation/Discussion

The spectrum showed metabolites were close to normal. However, unusual and prominent lipid signal was observed (Fig. 22.115). This signal is most likely contamination by lipids outside the region of interest due to a combination of effects. First, this patient may have moved the head slightly between the MRI used for the placement of the voxel and the MRS study. This is documented by comparing MR images from the same absolute position before and after the acquisition of the MR spectrum. Second, the chemical shift artifact causes the ROI to be slightly different for each chemical depending on their resonance frequencies. In this case, the ROI for lipids was shifted closer to the skull. Third, RF pulses are not perfect and will excite tissue outside the ROI. This can be a problem if the signal from the tissue outside the ROI is very strong, as can be the case with lipids. In the example above, the lipid signal is "out-of-phase," which is a strong indicator that the signal originates from tissue outside the ROI.

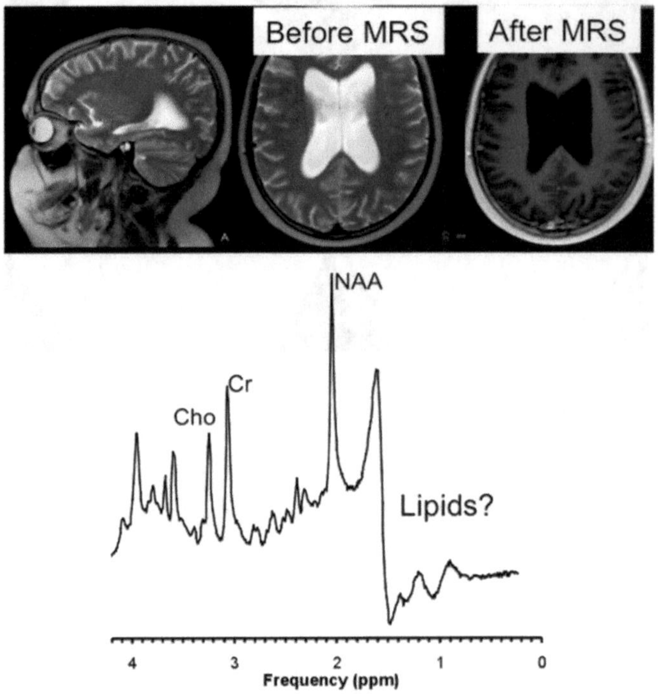

Fig. 22.115 Out-of-Voxel Lipid Artifact

Conclusions

Lipid contamination can occur even when ROIs do not include tissues with a high lipid content due to the imperfections of slice selective RF pulses, patient movement, and chemical shift artifact. "Out-of-phase" appearance is a strong indicator for the signal not originating from within the ROI. Saturation bands can sometimes be placed on bone structures that are adjacent to regions for MRS voxel placement, in order to help reduce lipid contamination.

References

1. Moreno-Torres A, Martinez-Perez I, Baquero M, Campistol J, Capdevila A, Arus C, et al. Tau detection by proton magnetic resonance spectroscopy in medulloblastoma: contribution to noninvasive differential diagnosis with cerebellar astrocytomas. Neurosurgery. 2004;55:824–9.
2. Kovanlikaya A, Panigrahy A, Krieger MD, Gonzalez-Gomez I, Ghugre N, McComb JG, et al. Untreated pediatric primitive neuroectodermal tumor in vivo: quantitation of Tau with MR spectroscopy. Radiology. 2005;236(3):1020–5.
3. Delikatny EJ, Chawla S, Leung DJ, Poptani H. MR-visible lipids and the tumor microenvironment. NMR Biomed. 2011;24(6):592–611.

4. Seymour ZA, Panigrahy A, Finlay JL, Nelson Jr MD, Bluml S. Citrate in pediatric CNS tumors? AJNR Am J Neuroradiol. 2008;29(5):1006–11.
5. Blüml S, Panigrahy A, Laskov M, Dhall G, Krieger MD, Nelson MD, et al. Elevated citrate in pediatric astrocytomas with malignant progression. Neuro Oncol. 2011;13:1107–17.
6. Cady EB, Lorek A, Penrice J, Reynolds EO, Iles RA, Burns SP, et al. Detection of propan-1,2-diol in neonatal brain by in vivo proton magnetic resonance spectroscopy. Magn Reson Med. 1994; 32(6):764–7.

Index

S. Blüml and A. Panigrahy (eds.), *MR Spectroscopy of Pediatric Brain Disorders*,
DOI 10.1007/978-1-4419-5864-8, © Springer Science+Business Media, LLC 2013

G

H

MIX
Papier aus verantwortungsvollen Quellen
Paper from responsible sources
FSC® C105338
FSC
www.fsc.org

If you have any concerns about our products,
you can contact us on
ProductSafety@springernature.com

In case Publisher is established outside the EU,
the EU authorized representative is:
Springer Nature Customer Service Center GmbH
Europaplatz 3, 69115 Heidelberg, Germany

Printed by Libri Plureos GmbH
in Hamburg, Germany